Medical Genetics

Medical Genetics

Editor: Ellie Peyton

AMERICAN
MEDICAL PUBLISHERS
www.americanmedicalpublishers.com

AMERICAN
MEDICAL PUBLISHERS
www.americanmedicalpublishers.com

Cataloging-in-Publication Data

Medical genetics / edited by Ellie Peyton.
p. cm.
Includes bibliographical references and index.
ISBN 978-1-63927-256-3
1. Medical genetics. 2. Human genetics. 3. Medical sciences. 4. Genetic disorders. I. Peyton, Ellie.
RB155 .M43 2022
616.042--dc23

American Medical Publishers,
41 Flatbush Avenue,
1st Floor, New York,
NY 11217, USA

ISBN 978-1-63927-256-3 (Hardback)

Contents

Preface

The branch of medicine, which involves the diagnosis and management of hereditary disorders is known as medical genetics. It encompasses the areas of personalized medicine, gene therapy and predictive medicine. Birth defects, mental retardation, cancer genetics, prenatal diagnosis, autism, etc. also fall within the scope of medical genetics. Some of the sub-specialties within this field are cytogenetics, clinical genetics, molecular genetics, mitochondrial genetics, etc. Basic metabolic studies, chromosome studies and molecular studies are used as diagnostic evaluation tools to determine inborn errors of metabolism, chromosomal disorders and single gene disorders. Symptoms of genetic disorders can be managed with medication and diet. Research in this field is actively seeking new medications and gene therapies for treating genetic disorders. This book elucidates new techniques and applications of medical genetics in a multidisciplinary manner. It provides significant information of this discipline to help develop a good understanding of medical genetics and related fields. This book aims to serve as a resource guide for students and experts alike and contribute to the growth of the field.

This book is a result of research of several months to collate the most relevant data in the field.

When I was approached with the idea of this book and the proposal to edit it, I was overwhelmed. It gave me an opportunity to reach out to all those who share a common interest with me in this field. I had 3 main parameters for editing this text:

1. Accuracy - The data and information provided in this book should be up-to-date and valuable to the readers.

2. Structure - The data must be presented in a structured format for easy understanding and better grasping of the readers.

3. Universal Approach - This book not only targets students but also experts and innovators in the field, thus my aim was to present topics which are of use to all.

Thus, it took me a couple of months to finish the editing of this book.

I would like to make a special mention of my publisher who considered me worthy of this opportunity and also supported me throughout the editing process. I would also like to thank the editing team at the back-end who extended their help whenever required.

Editor

1

Mitochondrial and nuclear genomics and the emergence of personalized medicine

Ryan L Parr* and Luis H Martin

Abstract

Developing early detection biosensors for disease has been the long-held goal of the Human Genome Project, but with little success. Conversely, the biological properties of the mitochondrion coupled with the relative simplicity of the mitochondrial genome give this organelle extraordinary functionality as a biosensor and places the field of mitochondrial genomics in a position of strategic advantage to launch significant advances in personalized medicine. Numerous factors make the mitochondrion organelle uniquely suited to be an early detection biosensor with applications in oncology as well as many other aspects of human health and disease. Early detection of disease translates into more effective, less expensive treatments for disease and overall better prognoses for those at greater risk for developing diseases.

Keywords: Mitochondrial genomics, Mitogenome, Genomic deletions, Cancerization field, Biosensor, Heteroplasmy

Introduction

Nascentes Morimur—from the moment we are born, we begin to die. This Latin phrase succinctly expresses the motivations behind personalized medicine and genomic research. The goal is to detect the earliest indications of disease process initiation within the human body and prevent disease advancement through early treatment. Ideally, this leads to extended human life spans coupled with enhanced quality of life. While the genetic root of many diseases has been known for decades, the '-omics' revolution starting with the Human Genome Project (HGP) was the flashpoint that began the personalized medicine movement.

Direct medical advances resulting from the HGP have been minimal compared to the expectations of its champions. Most currently available gene-specific treatments for cancers, novel therapies for inherited disorders, companion diagnostic genetic markers for drug responsiveness, and gene-based risk assessments for specific diseases are founded on research that predates the HGP. Very little HGP research has made the transition into practical use in the clinical setting [1].

The greatest hindrance has been the sheer expansiveness of the human genome. Consisting of nearly 6 billion base pairs (bp), finding specific and actionable connections with diseases requires filtering through enormous data sets. Scientists are still developing tools to decipher this information, and applications in the clinical setting are not yet a reality, despite the cost of sequencing an entire genome now at about $1,000.

However, there is a branch of genomic research, specifically mitochondrial genomics (mtgenomics), that is poised to begin entering clinical practice, and in some instances, it already has. Though much emphasis was initially placed on the HGP as a paradigm shift in modern medicine, this declaration would more accurately be made of mtgenomics for a number of reasons that will be outlined in this article.

Simply stating that a new technology or field of knowledge represents a paradigm shift in medicine does not justify its adoption into mainstream medical practice. Utility must be shown on a number of levels. This paper outlines why the mitochondrion organelle is a suitable biosensor for detecting the early onset of disease; how its use could decrease the cost of health care or lessen the impact of disease; and how a mitochondrion biosensor can be utilized to detect a range of disorders, for which oncology will be presented as an example throughout this article.

* Correspondence: r.parr@mitomicsinc.com
Mitomics Inc, Thunder Bay, Ontario P7A 7T1, Canada

Mitochondrial genomics: a paradigm shift in medicine

The field of mtgenomics, from its inception in 1909 with the discovery of extranuclear inheritance to the completed sequencing of the human mitochondrial genome (mtgenome) in 1981, has been firmly established as a primary arena for the development of genomic biosensors for early cancer detection. Although mtgenomics has been overshadowed in the last two decades by the extraordinary amount of funding and effort directed toward the HGP, it is a more practical backdrop for the discovery and implementation of diagnostic and early detection tools for numerous types of cancers. Historically, cancers such as ovarian, prostate, and colorectal cancer have been very difficult to detect before a devastating prognosis is the result. Utilizing the entire genome of the mitochondrion as a biosensor to detect the onset of these and other diseases is a highly significant medical advancement that could save lives and also makes sound economic sense.

The prospect of discovering countless treatments and possibly even cures for diseases that have a genetic or heritable origin has always surrounded the HGP. Early on genomics was hailed as the beginning of a medical revolution where personalized medicine or health care and treatments tailored to individual genomic profiles would become the norm. However, the enormity and complexity of the human genome, comprised of over 6 billion base pairs, have made this task of developing new medical therapies more complex than originally anticipated by many. What was initially acclaimed as a paradigm shift in modern medicine has become a long process and has necessitated additional programs such as the sequencing of disease specific genomes and characterization of the proteasome as well. Currently, risk assessments based on nuclear genomic data can do little more than provide motivation to encourage diet and lifestyle changes, and since this can be suitably addressed through public wellness campaigns, it becomes hard to justify the expense of offering complete routine genomic evaluations in medicine.

Paradigm shifts are not sudden rearrangements of the world order. They are in fact a series of concepts, theories, and discoveries that gradually build upon one another until enough knowledge accumulates for a larger picture to emerge. The function of all the constituent parts must be understood before an understanding of the overall form can be achieved. When this process of dissection has been completed, in theory, a map should exist that delineates links between each of those parts and their function. How fast these paradigm shifts can occur is directly related to the complexity of the object of study. In stark contrast to the nuclear genome, the human mtgenome is composed of 16,568 base pairs and 37 genes, which by comparison is strikingly simple. If one were to anticipate a paradigm shift towards personalized medicine, particularly where tools for detecting the onset of diseases such as cancer are concerned, a logical place to look would be within the field of mtgenomics. Mathematically, the odds favor a mtgenomic solution. This is suggested by the compactness of the mtgenome and exemplified by mtDNA mutations found in association with numerous diseases, including cancer. A detailed review of these oncologic associations has been presented by Parr et al. in 2007 [2].

mtGenomics is also favored by time since paradigm shifts are not sudden events, but rather the culmination of a series of discoveries and innovations. In 1981, the entire mtgenome was already sequenced, but it would not be until 2006, a full quarter of a century later, when the complete human genome would be sequenced. The field of mtgenomics has had more time to mature, giving scientists substantial opportunities to understand the intricacies of this knowledge base. The benefit of lead time combined with the relative simplicity of the mtgenome and specific biological properties of the mitochondria gives mtgenomics a significant advantage over the larger field of genomics when prospecting for biosensors, especially since mitochondrion organelles can be utilized collectively as a biosensor. From this standpoint, mtgenomics may become an organizational model for the larger body of data that is the HGP.

Table 1 [3-8] provides a brief overview of the most significant events in the development of mtgenomics, and for comparison, it includes some of the more recent milestones in the field of genomics.

Mitochondrial genomics and biosensor prospecting

Utilizing mtgenomics as a clinical tool to detect the onset of disease is part of a larger shift towards prevention in medicine. Western medical systems have traditionally focused on treating disease once symptoms have become overt and often acute. This is not a function of intent but a result of the primary diagnostic tools at hand. Instruments like the microscope and stethoscope were the only means of detecting disease available to physicians prior to about 1895 when X-rays came into use. X-ray technology made it possible to see into the body without creating a surgical opening; however, its utility was limited primarily to visualizing bones and the outline of dense masses. Until the mid 1950s with the founding of companies like the Thermo Electron Corporation and the subsequent increased access to mass spectrometric instruments, even physiologists primarily conducted nutritional studies by direct physical observation and measurement. However, from this point on, various types of instrumentation began to develop that

Table 1 Milestones in mitochondrial genomics

Year	Milestone
1909	Correns and Baur independently identify the first cases of extranuclear inheritance
1934	Goldschmidt suggests that causes for color differences in gypsy moths may reside in the mitochondria
1940	Winge and Laustsen observe 'inbreeding degeneration' in diploid yeast which they suggest is due to mitochondrial heredity
1944	Slaughter presents the idea of field cancerization in oral cancer
1949	Ephrussi uses genetic analysis to show that respiration-deficient baker's yeast is due to mutations in the cytoplasm, not the nucleus. Soon after, Slonimski and Ephrussi show the deficiency is due to mitochondrial dysfunction
1953	Slaughter formalizes the concept of field cancerization as preconditioning of tissues for the onset of an 'as-yet-unknown carcinogenic agent' which later turns out to be mitochondrial mutation
1963	Nass and Nass use an electron microscope to show that chick embryo mitochondria contain DNA
1964	Schatz et al. shows biochemically that baker's yeast mitochondria contains DNA
Late 1970s	Groundwork for the field of mitochondrial genomics is firmly established
1981	Anderson et al. publishes the sequence and organization of the human mitochondrial genome as 16,569 base pairs long
1990[a]	The US Department of Energy and the National Institute of Health present a 5-year plan to Congress for the Human Genome Project
1999[a]	Chromosome 22 becomes the first human chromosome to be completely sequenced
2000[a]	Working draft of the human genome is completed
2004[a]	Human gene count estimated at 20,000 to 25,000
2006[a]	Human genome completely sequenced in high resolution and is about 3 billion base pairs long

[a]Recent milestones in genomics.

made numerous types of remote imaging and biochemical analysis possible. This is the era in which mtgenomics came of age. Coinciding with the advent of technology that made it possible to peer into the workings of the human body from many different perspectives, mtgenomics became part of the movement towards developing preventive medicine as opposed to being absorbed into acute care medicine.

There are a number of factors that make mitochondrion organelles well suited for use as a biosensor:

1. Mitochondria contain multiple copies of their own genome, and each cell contains multiple mitochondria, resulting in a 10- to 100-fold copy advantage over nuclear DNA. This means that smaller samples can yield reliable results, and body fluids with low cellularity can be readily evaluated for their mtgenomic content.
2. Mitochondria have their own unique genome which is transmitted clonally through the mother and should remain the same from generation to generation.
3. Mitochondria do not contain histones and are more prone to somatic or spontaneous DNA mutations. The rate of somatic mutation in mtDNA is 10- to 17-fold that of the mutation rate within nuclear DNA. Hence, molecular changes associated with malignant transformations may be detectable much earlier in mtDNA than nuclear DNA.
4. Genomic deletions within mitochondria begin to happen long before traditional histology can identify disease. Biochemical signatures can identify genomic deletions associated with a disease and predict its onset much earlier than a pathologist can observe a problem, thus creating a greater window of time for treatment possibilities.
5. The cancerization field associated with mitochondrial deletions provides a distinct molecular signature that mtgenomic assessment can detect. Though conventional histology of a biopsy sample might not display evidence of malignancy, if the tissue comes from an area that is within the cancerization field, disease onset will be detectable via this signature. Coupling conventional biopsy methodology with mtgenomic assessment to detect this cancerization field provides vital clinical information.
6. The small size of the mtgenome (16,568 bp) places it at a cost advantage compared to the nuclear genome (6,000,000,000 bp) when it comes to analyses. Its compact nature also makes it possible to analyze the entire mtgenome rapidly to identify specific molecular markers with great accuracy.
7. Somatic mutations which affect ATP synthesis by inhibiting OXPHOS also increase the production of reactive oxygen species (ROS) and promote tumor cell proliferation. Detecting these mutations can serve to identify the onset of cancer [9].
8. The mtgenome often displays heteroplasmy, a subset of altered/deleted genomes within the mitochondria. Human tumor tissues that have undergone somatic mutations often display heteroplasmy. Differential rates of heteroplasmy in mitochondria are associated with specific types of tumors and can be used to identify different types of cancer [9].
9. Mutations in the mtgenome have been identified in a wide variety of cancers [2]. Individual as well as combinations of mtgenome deletions can accurately detect cancerization field effects [10].
10. Mitochondria mediate multiple metabolic pathways and are sensitive to physiological changes.

Within a cell, the mitochondrial and nuclear genomes function symbiotically, and their resulting interactions make it possible to detect dysfunction within the cell. Though mitochondria execute various metabolic functions outside of the nucleus of a cell, including synthesizing 95% of cellular metabolic fuel, 1,200 nuclear genes drive and participate in mitochondrial function. While there are 37 genes coded by the mitochondrial genome, 24 of these genes are dedicated to processing 13 genes within the mtgenome that produce protein subunits essential to electron transport. These 13 genes work in concert with 93 nuclear proteins. Some mutations in mitochondrial genes alter the biochemical behavior of the overall mitochondrial/nuclear protein complexes, increasing pools of ROS, which in turn enable tumor growth and may bestow proliferative advantages to the cell [11]. Despite its miniscule size and the small number of genes that comprise the mtgenome, somatic alterations that occur in this molecule directly contribute to tumorigenesis.

There is a deep body of literature describing mitochondrial-nuclear interactions [e.g. 12-14]. The somatic mutations that alter these interactions occur very early in the process of disease onset, even before histopathological changes to cells and tissues are evident to the pathologist. mtGenomic technology makes it possible to exploit these molecular signatures as a biosensor for early indications of disease—detection that would not otherwise be possible for many disorders in the current clinical setting [15]. For example, the sampling error of prostate biopsy is reduced to a 3.4-kb mtgenome deletion which is present in prostate tumor as well as the surrounding normal-appearing tissue [16,17].

There are already mtgenomic tests available for the detection of disease onset, such as Prostate Core Mitomic Test™ (PCMT) offered by Mitomics™ (Thunder Bay, Ontario, Canada). This test, as will other mtgenomic tests, utilizes the cancerization field effect and mtDNA deletions to anticipate the onset and/or presence of hidden or occult cancer. Ideally, this test and others like it act to identify changes in tissue biopsies or other types of biological samples that are indicative of the onset of tumorigenesis. Mitochondrion biosensor tests such as these provide the largest time frame possible to ward off the onset of disease or prevent it altogether (Figure 1).

mtGenomic and complete genomic evaluations will eventually become available with standard medical evaluations and annual physicals. This will provide physicians with comparative longitudinal genomic records and enable the earliest possible routine identification of somatic mutations and the initiation of disease processes. It will also ensure that patients have access to the latest preventative therapies developed in concordance with the field of genomics. Having access to longitudinal genomic records and targeted therapies ascertains the best prognosis for patients. Targeted therapies attack specific types of tissues and are often more tolerable systemically than older chemotherapies which were designed to be aggressive for treating diseases such as cancer identified in acute stages of development.

Lessening personal and economic costs of disease

Though mtgenomics removes technological barriers for developing early detection biosensor platforms, there are also other considerations to be made. Specifically, developing tools for detecting diseases necessitates the need for early response treatments. This is one of the primary reasons why some of the first mtgenomic tests being developed are for various types of cancer. A number of cancers are difficult to detect using standard medical investigative practices because their symptoms do not become obvious until they reach a very late stage and have become difficult to treat. However, numerous chemopreventive treatments can be used at the earliest stages of these diseases to either suppress or prevent the initiation of carcinogenesis. These treatments are suitable for those deemed at greater risk for developing particular cancers but do not yet have any indications of disease onset, and for those who have begun to display signs of disease, these treatments may halt the progression of precancerous lesions into cancer [18,19].

The National Cancer Institute (NCI) began conducting research on chemopreventive compounds in the early 1980s. To date, about 400 compounds are being actively studied as chemopreventive agents, and more than 40 compounds are being evaluated in a clinical trial setting. Of those agents being studied in a clinical setting, five classes of agents have shown promise, and the NCI considers these classes of compounds to be priority substances for study [20]. Table 2 [20,21] briefly summarizes these priority compounds.

Toxicity studies can also make use of mtgenomic research. A crucial aspect of evaluating new chemical entities (NCE) for their chemopreventive properties is ensuring that while the compounds disrupt the advance of the disease process, they do not also result in contraindications that are more damaging than the disease itself. A major problem with many new compounds is perturbation of mitochondrial function, resulting in toxic cellular effects. Integrating mitochondrial function studies during the early stages of NCE evaluation provides the opportunity to identify toxic effects from these compounds before they reach later stage development or even human trials. This can save extraordinary amounts of research dollars and time [23].

Additionally, mtgenomic research conducted along with NCE evaluation can stratify the study population into two groups—those that respond to the compound and those that do not. This could keep many drugs from being unnecessarily ejected from the NCE pipeline while

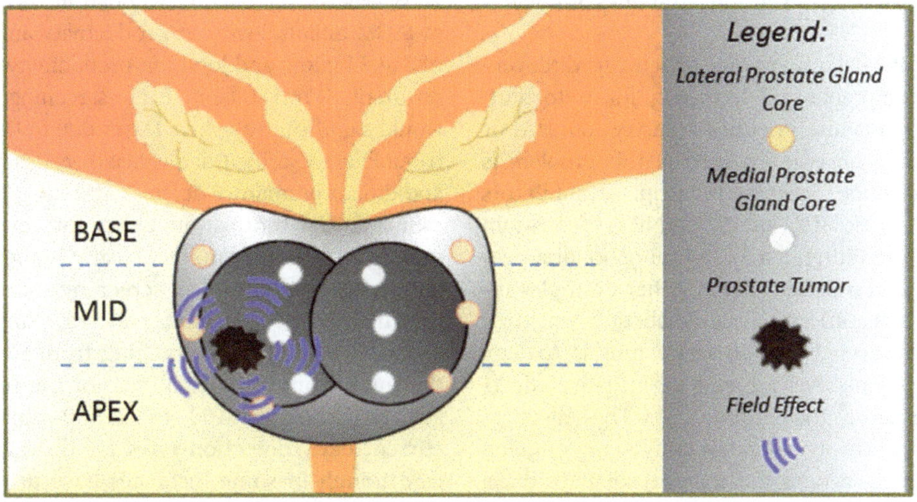

Figure 1 The cancerization field effect and prostate cancer. Real-time PCR can be used to identify underlying molecular alterations in normal-appearing tissues, thereby detecting the presence of malignant cells via a cancerization field effect. Though prostate needle biopsy cores may fail to collect a tumor sample, the chemical signature of the tumor cancerization field may be detected in these same samples, optimizing the biopsy procedure and the outcome for the patient [16,17].

also resulting in cleaner, more accurate clinical trial results by removing non-responders from the study population. This strategy has been used in breast cancer; 5–10% of women are homozygous for low-activity CYP2D6 alleles, and these women cannot properly metabolize Tamoxifen. For women with this genotype, Raloxifene is the chemopreventive therapy of choice. CYP2D6 protein has been indentified and is metabolically active in liver cell mitochondria and functional in drug metabolism. Variants of CYP2D6 alter the efficiency of mitochondrial targeting, suggesting individual responses to drug therapy based on the CYP2D6 protein and mitochondrial interactions [24]. Kelloff et al. [23] summarizes this strategy in the following statement: 'Molecular Targets that are relevant to risk assessment and patient selection, drug development and outcome evaluation will streamline chemoprevention research. In turn, these molecular targets will lead to effective, safe

Table 2 Priority cancer chemopreventive agents

Class of agent	Chemical/brand name	Preventive targets
Selective estrogen receptor modulators and other hormonal agents	Tamoxifen	Breast
	Arzoxifene	Breast
	Acolbifene	Breast
	Raxoxifene/Evista®	Breast
	Finasteride	Prostate
Nonsteroidal anti-inflammatory drugs	Celecoxib/Celebrex®	Colon, breast, prostate, bladder
	Sulindac/Clinoril®	Esophagus, skin
	Aspirin	
Minerals and micronutrients	Calcium compounds	Colon
Glucocorticoids	Budesonide	Lung
Retinoids	All-trans-retinoic acid tretinoin/Retin-A®	Cervix, esophagus, larynx, lung,
	9-cis-Retinoic acid alitretinoin/Panretin®	Nasopharynx, oral cavity, ovary
	13-cis-Retinoic acid isotreninoin/Accutane®	
	4-Hydroxyretinamide, (4-HPR) fenretinide	

Adapted from [21,22].

and personalized cancer prevention strategies for widespread clinical use.'

Moreover, it is of vital importance that drug discovery regimes include comprehensive screening for mitochondrial toxicity to avoid failure in either industry standard or regulatory programs. A classic example of this problem is illustrated by nucleoside reverse transcriptase inhibitors (NRTIs) used to treat HIV infection. NRTIs constrain mtDNA replication resulting in a loss of mitochondria over time, causing liver and muscle toxicity. Other examples include a statin (cerivastatin) and an antidiabetic agent (troglitazone) that have been found to cause muscle toxicity and hepatotoxicity, respectively, due to the negative effects these drugs have on mitochondria [25]. The effect of pharmacological agents on mitochondria is an ongoing concern [26] especially where the majority of individuals benefit while others experience severe contraindications when taking such medications.

mtGenomics has the potential to make meaningful contributions to the area of pharmacogenomics since patients receive obvious benefits from this approach, but making these options available begins with ensuring that the process of disease onset is clearly understood. Michael B. Sporn, former Chief of the Laboratory of Chemoprevention at the NCI and the scientist who coined the term and developed the concept of chemoprevention in the early 1970s, points out that 'There is still tremendous resistance to the idea of telling people they have early changes in their cells that could someday lead to invasive cancer. The emphasis should be on suppressing carcinogenesis, the development of cancer, before it becomes evident as invasive or metastatic cancer. We need a whole educational mission to get people to think about cancer before they go to the doctor, for example, with a lump in their breast [27].' For many cancers, the molecular preamble leading to the discovery of a physically observable malignant lesion generally occurs over a 20- to 30-year period. This is a huge window of opportunity for detecting the onset of these diseases. Early detection enables minimally invasive and generally well-tolerated therapies for treatment of these diseases. This means that the impact on quality of life for the patient is minimized to the greatest extent possible.

The economic benefits are also clearly visible. The retail cost for a 30-day supply of Tamoxifen is about \$60, and a 5-year supply would cost about \$3,700; a 30-day supply of Raloxifene is about \$97 with a 5-year supply cost of about \$5,800 [28]. Given that in 2006, the first year of treatment for breast cancer in the US cost an average of \$30,000 per patient [29,30], utilizing options that prevent the need for any kind of treatment beyond chemoprevention strategies, and monitoring represents a savings to the health care system of more than 80% in the first 12 months alone.

More broadly, figures from the American Cancer Society [19] indicate that the total economic impact of cancer in 2008 was \$228.1 billion. Included in this were direct costs of \$93.2 billion, losses in productivity amounting to a cost of \$18.8 billion, and losses in productivity due to premature death of \$116.1 billion. Early screening to detect cancer would significantly reduce losses due to lost productivity attributable to sudden acute health crises for these patients and due to premature death.

Substantial motivation exists for investing in the research and development of early screening methodologies. Multi-billion-dollar screening markets exist for the top five most prevalent cancers (lung, colon, breast, prostate, and ovarian), ranging from \$24 to \$401 billion dependent upon the final cost of the tests, which typically range from \$100 to \$3,500 dollars. Incidentally, current early detection rates for these five types of cancer, though in some instances have improved over what they were even 20 years ago, are still unacceptably low.

Mitochondrial genomics and human health

While a significant portion of biosensor research has focused on oncology, mtgenomics is applicable to human health in general. Because mitochondria are responsible for converting energy stores into a useable form for our cells, any disorder that affects mitochondrial function could be evaluated using mtgenomics. Mitochondrial function disorders can be caused by mutations or deletions occurring either in the mtgenome or in the nuclear genome (occurring in genes that code for proteins that contribute to mitochondrial function). Mutations in nuclear genes can be inherited from either parent, while heritable mutations in the mtgenome will be transmitted maternally. Heritable mtgenomic mutations can be identified by the presence of heteroplasmy; however, the degree to which these disorders will affect mitochondrial function is generally dependent on the degree of heteroplasmy. If enough copies of unaffected mtDNA are present within a cell, these copies of mtDNA will compensate for the dysfunction of the heteroplasmic copies of mtDNA. Unless individuals with relatively minimal levels of heteroplasmy undergo some sort of trauma or extreme physiological stress that makes it impossible for the unaffected mtDNA to compensate for the heteroplasmic DNA, overt indications of these disorders may never occur. Assessing the degree of heteroplasmy may help these individuals take preventative measures to ensure they minimize the possibility of experiencing such physiological effects.

mtGenomic function may also be affected suddenly by physiological traumas such as hemorrhage or a cardiac event that induces hypoxia and forces mitochondrial function to occur temporarily in an oxygen-reduced environment. These events may induce mitochondrial damage similar to age-related declines in mitochondrial function that, as free-radical theory-of-aging proponents hypothesize, is due to increased and prolonged exposure to ROS [31]. Other diseases and conditions that increase exposure to ROS and affect circulatory process, such as diabetes mellitus, type II diabetes, and obesity, may also contribute to cumulative disruptions in mitochondrial function. Because the effects of many of these types of disorders accumulate over time, associated somatic mtDNA mutations will also likely accumulate over time. Depending on the degree of severity of these conditions, mitochondrial dysfunction and mtgenomic evidence of dysfunction can occur at any age and ultimately drives the aging process.

Many noncancerous clinical disorders have been associated with mitochondrial dysfunction. Disorders involving the brain and the heart, organs which are high consumers of energy and would suffer from a downturn in mitochondrial production of energy, are notably present in this list. Disorders falling into the neurological category include migraine, strokes, epilepsy, dementia, myopathy, peripheral neuropathy, speech disturbances, and sensorineural deafness. Cardiac disorders include heart failure, heart block, and cardiomyopathy. Gastrointestinal conditions include constipation and irritable bowel syndrome. Respiratory conditions associated with mitochondrial dysfunction include respiratory failure, nocturnal hyperventilation, recurrent aspiration, and pneumonia. Endocrine disorders include diabetes, thyroid disease, parathyroid disease, and ovarian failure. Ophthalmological disorders include optic atrophy, cataracts, and ophthalmoplegia [32]. While this listing is not comprehensive, it shows that the effects of mitochondrial dysfunction are far reaching. While prevalence varies in different populations, research suggests that mtDNA disease is surprisingly high. For example, in a working-age population (>16 and <60/65 years for female/male patients, respectively) in the north east of England, 9.2 in 100,000 people were found to have manifest mtDNA disease [33].

Presently, mtgenomics is better situated than nuclear genomics for the evaluation of mtDNA disorders due to the smaller size of the mtgenome and number of constituent genes. However, evaluating mtDNA disorders is an area of research where mtgenomics and nuclear genomics could be applied in conjunction since a considerable number of mitochondrial disorders are associated with nuclear genetic inheritance. To exemplify this, the Mitochondria Phenome Knowledgebase cites 174 genes that are associated with 502 different phenotypic features spanning the following categories: oncologic, musculoskeletal, gastrointestinal, respiratory, neurologic, ophthalmologic, genitourinary, cardiovascular, hematologic, dermatologic, metabolic, endocrinologic, immunologic, psychiatric, and numerous miscellaneous categories [34].

While second-generation technologies have been useful for mtgenomic and nuclear genomic discovery and determining the genetic basis of disease, the rapid action and low cost of genomic sequencing that will become available with third-generation genomic instrumentation will make it possible to move those discoveries more generally into the clinical setting and widespread medical use [35].

It should not be overlooked that mtgenomics requires careful experimental considerations. Population and group variations in mtgenome sequences may alter or preclude the absence or presence of a specific SNP or deletion(s), leading to incorrect data interpretations for certain populations. Mitochondrial sequencing data must be compared to germ plasma on an individual patient basis if point mutations are to be used as a diagnostic reference. Using published mitochondrial genome standards is inappropriate as these references are not representative of either the individual or the specific disease under study. Moreover, mitochondrial pseudogenes are embedded in the nucleus and often obscure results or lead to inaccurate data interpretation since pseudogene contamination is often mistaken for nucleotide heteroplasmy particularly in sequencing data [36]. This is a noteworthy concern given the sensitivity of next-generation sequencing technology as opposed to dideoxy chemistry, and extreme care must be taken to preclude co-amplification of nuclear and mitochondrial pseudogenes. Finally, caution is warranted when comparing malignant lesions and normal tissue from the same organ and individual. The field effect is often operative in the normal tissue and may have many mutations in common with the tumor site. Use of normal tissue as a comparative control may preclude reliable results [10].

Summary and conclusions

Both simplicity of structure and historical timing have placed mtgenomics ahead of the HGP as a technology leader for the development of early detection biosensors for many diseases. Numerous mtgenomic-based tests are currently in development, and some have already entered the marketplace, signaling a transformation in medicine towards prevention as the preferred strategy for treating disease. Early detection biosensors have premiered in oncology, as many types of cancer can be associated with mtDNA deletions. Oncology-based chemopreventive strategies have been in development since the 1970s and are now available to be paired with early detection strategies. Following closely is the development of biosensors for other mitochondrial disorders. Since these disorders are more frequently hereditary than are many cancers, examining them from the perspective of both mtgenomics and nuclear genomics will provide insight into illness and also serve to develop strategies for dealing with the extraordinary amounts of data generated from the HGP.

Developing mtgenomic-based technologies presents significant economic benefits for health care management and the development of new drugs. Pairing mtDNA studies with clinical trials stratifies study populations into responders and non-responders, making the development and usage of these drugs as efficient and effective as possible. Coupling this with the pending release of cheaper and faster third-generation sequencing technologies creates an opportunity to make mtgenomic-based early detection biosensors widely available in the near future. This stands to revolutionize the conventional medical experience we are all familiar with into a personalized experience specifically tailored to the well-being of every individual.

Competing interests

RP and LM are employed by Mitomics, and RP holds shares in the company.

Acknowledgement

Organization, writing, and formatting of the manuscript were completed by Rebecca Friend-Heath using the information and research provided by Ryan L. Parr and Luis H. Martin.

Authors' contributions

RP and LM participated in the design and coordination of this manuscript. Both authors read and approved the final manuscript.

References

1. Varmus H: **Ten years on - the human genome and medicine.** *N Eng J Med* 2010, **362:**21.
2. Parr RL, Jakupciak JP, Birch-Machin MA, Dakubo GD: **The mitochondrial genome: a biosensor for early cancer detection?** *Expert Opin Med Diagn* 2007, **1**(2):169–182.
3. Hagemann R: **The foundation of extranuclear inheritance: plastid and mitochondrial genetics.** *Mol Genet Genomics* 2010, **283:**199–209.
4. Slaughter D, Southwick H, Smejkal W: **Field cancerization in oral stratified squamous epithelium: clinical implications of multicentric origin.** *Cancer* 1953, **6:**963–968.
5. Nass MMK, Nass S: **Intramitochondrial fibers with DNA characteristics.** *J Cell Biol* 1963, **19**(3):593–611.
6. Schatz G, Halsbrunner E, Tuppy H: **Deoxyribonucleic acid associated with yeast mitochondria.** *Biochem Biophys Res Commun* 1964, **15**(2):127–132.
7. Anderson S, Bankier AT, Barrell BG, de Bruijn MH, Coulson AR, Drouin J, Eperon IC, Nierlich DP, Roe BA, Sanger F, Schreier PH, Smith AJ, Staden R, Young IG: **Sequence and organization of the human mitochondrial genome.** *Nature* 1981, **290**(5806):457–465.
8. DoE: **Human Genome Project Information.**, . http://www.ornl.gov/sci/techresources/Human_Genome/project/timeline.shtml.
9. Brandon M, Baldi P, Wallace DC: **Mitochondrial mutations in cancer.** *Oncogene* 2006, **25**(34):4647–4662.
10. Dakubo GD, Jakupciak JP, Birch-Machin MA, Parr RL: **Clinical implications and utility of field cancerization.** *Cancer Cell International* 2007, **7:**2.
11. Greaves LC, Reeve AK, Taylor RW, Turnbull DM: **Mitochondrial DNA and disease.** *J Pathol* 2012, **226**(2):274–286.
12. Hock MB, Kralli A: **Transcriptional control of mitochondrial biogenesis and function.** *Annu Rev Physiol* 2009, **71:**177–203.
13. Cannino G, Di Liegro CM, Rinaldi AM: **Nuclear-mitochondrial interaction.** *Mitochondrion* 2007, **7:**359–366.
14. Ryan MT, Hoogenraad NJ: **Mitochondrial-nuclear communications.** *Annu Rev Biochem* 2007, **76:**701–722.
15. Ohta S: **Contribution of somatic mutations in the mitochondrial genome to the development of cancer and tolerance against anticancer drugs.** *Oncogene* 2006, **25**(34):4768–4776.
16. Maki J, Robinson K, Reguly B, Alexander J, Wittock R, Aguirre A, Diamandis EP, Escott N, Skehan A, Prowse O, Thayer RE, Froberg MK, Wilson MJ, Maragh S, Jakupciak JP, Wagner PD, Srivastava S, Dakubo GD, Parr RL: **Mitochondrial genome deletion aids in the identification of false- and true-negative prostate needle core biopsy specimens.** *Am J Clin Pathol* 2008, **129**(1):57–66.
17. Robinson K, Creed J, Reguly B, Powell C, Wittock R, Klein D, Maggrah A, Klotz L, Parr RL, Dakubo GD: **Accurate prediction of repeat prostate biopsy outcomes by a mitochondrial DNA deletion assay.** *Prostate Cancer Prostatic Dis* 2010, **13**(2):126–131.
18. William WN Jr, Heymach JV, Kim ES, Lippman SM: **Molecular targets for cancer chemoprevention.** *Nat Rev Drug Discov* 2009, **8**(3):213–225.
19. American Cancer Society: *Cancer Facts & Figures.* Atlanta: American Cancer Society; 2009.
20. Cancer Information Network: **Chemoprevention.**, . http://www.cancerlinksusa.com/chemo/chemoprevention.asp.
21. National Cancer Institute: *Chemopreventive Agents.* Bethesda: NCI - Division of Cancer Prevention; 2011.
22. Cancer Information Network: **Chemoprevention.** 2011, http://prevention.cancer.gov/programs-resources/resources/agents.
23. Kelloff G, O'Shaughnessy J, Gordon G, Hawk E, Sigman C: **Counterpoint: because some surrogate end point biomarkers measure the neoplastic process they will have high utility in the development of cancer chemopreventive agents against sporadic cancers.** *Cancer Epidemiol Biomarkers Prev* 2003, **12**(7):593–596.
24. Sangar MC, Hindupur KA, Martin MV, Guengerich FP, Avadhani NG: **Identification of genetic variants of human cytochrome P450 2D6 with impaired mitochondrial targeting.** *Mol Genet Metab* 2010, **99**(1):90–97.
25. Dykens JA, Marroquin LD, Will Y: **Strategies to reduce late-stage drug attrition due to mitochondrial toxicity.** *Expert Rev Mol Diagn* 2007, **7**(2):161–175.
26. Pereira CV, Moreira AC, Pereira SP, Machado NG, Carvalho FS, Sardão VA, Oliveira PJ: **Investigating drug-induced mitochondrial toxicity: a biosensor to increase drug safety?** *Curr Drug Saf* 2009, **4**(1):34–54.
27. American Association for Cancer Research, Michael B: **Sporn, M.D., to receive inaugural cancer prevention award.** http://scienceblog.com/community/older/2002/G/2002019.html.
28. Fabian C: **Tamoxifen or taloxifene in postmenopausal women for prevention of breast cancer: a tale of two choices - counterpoint.** *Cancer Epidemiol Biomarkers Prev* 2007, **16**(11):2210–2212.
29. National Cancer Institute: *Surveillance Epidemiology and End Results: SEER Stat Fact Sheets: Breast.* Bethesda: National Cancer Institute; 2010.
30. National Center for Health Statistics: *Health, United States, 2009 - With Special Feature on Medical Technology.* Hyattsville: Centers for Disease Control and Prevention; 2009.
31. Raju R, Jian B, Hubbard W, Chaudry I: **The mitoscriptome in aging and disease.** *Aging and Disease* 2011, **2**(2):174–180.
32. Chial H, Craig J: **mtDNA and mitochondrial diseases.** *Nature Education* 2008, **1.**
33. Schaefer AM, McFarland R, Blakely EL, He L, Whittaker RG, Taylor RW, Chinnery PF, Turnbull DM: **Prevalence of mitochondrial DNA disease in adults.** *Ann Neurol* 2008, **63**(1):35–39.
34. Mitophenome [database on the Internet]: **Mitochondria Phenome Knowledgebase.** http://www.mitophenome.org/phenotypes/list.
35. Glaser V: **Third-generation sequencing debuts: single-molecule detection solutions push the techniques to new levels.** *Genetic Engineering & Biotechnology News* 2010, **30**(6).
36. Parr RLM J, Reguly B, Dakubo GD, Aguirre A, Wittock R, Robinson K, Jakupciak JP, Thayer RE: **The pseudo-mitochondrial genome influences mistakes in heteroplasmy interpretation.** *BMC Genomics* 2006, **7:**185.

2

Prediction of complex human diseases from pathway-focused candidate markers by joint estimation of marker effects: case of chronic fatigue syndrome

Madhuchhanda Bhattacharjee[1*], Mangalathu S. Rajeevan[2] and Mikko J. Sillanpää[3]

Abstract

Background: The current practice of using only a few strongly associated genetic markers in regression models results in generally low power in prediction or accounting for heritability of complex human traits.

Purpose: We illustrate here a Bayesian joint estimation of single nucleotide polymorphism (SNP) effects principle to improve prediction of phenotype status from pathway-focused sets of SNPs. Chronic fatigue syndrome (CFS), a complex disease of unknown etiology with no laboratory methods for diagnosis, was chosen to demonstrate the power of this Bayesian method. For CFS, such a genetic predictive model in combination with clinical evidence might lead to an earlier diagnosis than one based solely on clinical findings.

Methods: One of our goals is to model disease status using Bayesian statistics which perform variable selection and parameter estimation simultaneously and which can induce the sparseness and smoothness of the SNP effects. Smoothness of the SNP effects is obtained by explicit modeling of the covariance structure of the SNP effects.

Results: The Bayesian model achieved perfect goodness of fit when tested within the sampled data. Tenfold cross-validation resulted in 80 % accuracy, one of the best so far for CFS in comparison to previous prediction models. Model reduction aspects were investigated in a computationally feasible manner. Additionally, genetic variation estimates provided by the model identified specific genetic markers for their biological role in the disease pathophysiology.

Conclusions: This proof-of-principle study provides a powerful approach combining Bayesian methods, SNPs representing multiple pathways and rigorous case ascertainment for accurate genetic risk prediction modeling of complex diseases like CFS and other chronic diseases.

Keywords: Chronic fatigue syndrome, Phenotype prediction, Cross-validation, SNP, Bayesian analysis

Introduction

Human genetic studies generally focus on identifying genes associated with diseases and subsequently using the significant genetic information for phenotypic predictions. Statistical methods vary with each of these goals, with methods for gene identification becoming increasingly effective with genome-wide association studies (GWAS). However, modeling principles for phenotypic predictions of complex human diseases remain largely unexplored even in this era of GWAS [1, 2]. Phenotypic predictions in human data sets have been modeled using regression models with a few single nucleotide polymorphisms (SNPs) having strong association identified by GWAS, but this practice of using only a few genetic markers has been disappointing due to its low predictive power [3]. A similar problem known as "the problem of missing heritability" is encountered when only highly associated markers are used to estimate heritability of complex traits [4, 5]. However, as demonstrated recently with human height and complex diseases, the missing heritability problem

* Correspondence: mbsm@uohyd.ernet.in
[1]School of Mathematics and Statistics, University of Hyderabad, Hyderabad 500046, India
Full list of author information is available at the end of the article

can be alleviated when linear regression models include information from all markers in the GWAS [6–8]. Such models can be seen as finite locus approximations for polygenic models, being representative for linkage disequilibrium (LD) structure in population, and they should therefore provide useful predictions even in the presence of a large number of rare variants.

Bayesian variable selection [9, 10] and the frequentist regularization methods [11, 12] have gained attention to perform parameter estimation and variable selection simultaneously in phenotype-marker association analysis. These methods generally perform well in selecting trait-associated loci or loci in LD to estimate genomic breeding values in animals and plants [13, 14]. Lee et al. [15] considered that methods for predictions of phenotypes and genomic breeding values may employ similar tasks and can be successfully substituted for one another. Generally, it is known that the marker density (the length of the genome), population LD, and number of individuals in the learning sample will all have a strong influence on the prediction accuracy [1]. Moreover, simplicity of the genetic architecture and heritability of the trait are also the key factors for the prediction success. Animal and plant breeding literature includes numerous simulation studies on how these factors influence prediction accuracy, see, e.g., references in [1]. Generally, from studies of different prediction methods applied to plant and animal data sets, one can conclude that variable selection approaches seem to work most efficiently for oligogenic traits with sparse genetic architectures in the presence of moderate LD among markers. On the other hand, approaches based on mixed models and marker-estimated covariance structures [1, 16] seem to work well for polygenic traits or oligogenic traits in the presence of strong LD among markers (which will make oligogenic data sets to have large numbers of trait-associated markers like polygenic traits). Certain modern classification methods [17] and Bayesian subset selection methods [18, 19] have been applied to predict chronic disease or to find important subsets of SNPs contributing to chronic diseases with small data sets. In general, combining multiple sources of information may lead to more accurate phenotype prediction [12, 20, 21]. This approach has been confirmed with simulations but its benefit with real data is still questionable, especially with complex phenotypes [19]. We consider here information from a carefully selected set of pathway-focused SNPs and applied Bayesian methods in the context of association mapping to model phenotype status. In association studies with SNPs, it is difficult to distinguish the most associated SNPs in regions of high LD. In such situations, it may be informative to inspect for stable association signals after first smoothing the signals in regions of high LD [22]. On this basis, we hypothesize that more stable and accurate phenotypic prediction may be achieved after smoothing pathway-focused SNP effects in regions of high LD. Our goals here are to provide genomic prediction of an individual's disease status as a sum of SNP effects, which depend on individual's genotype pattern at SNPs. This is done by means of model-averaged estimation of genetic effects used to weight individual SNPs. For this, we use Bayesian methods in genetic association studies and model-averaged estimate of genetic effects that we call as weighted genetic variation (WGV) [23]. Our Bayesian methods can perform variable selection and parameter estimation simultaneously and can induce the sparseness and smoothness of the estimated SNP effects [19, 23]. Smoothness of the SNP effects is obtained by the explicit modeling of the covariance structure of the SNP effects. We evaluated our Bayesian modeling principle and methods for modeling of chronic fatigue syndrome (CFS), as an example of a complex disease where its diagnosis remains elusive with the need for improved analytical approaches for gene identification and accurate phenotypic prediction [24].

Methods

Subjects and illness classification

This study adhered to human experimental guidelines of US Department of Health and Human Services and the Helsinki Declaration. The Centers for Disease Control Human Subjects committee approved the study protocol, and all subjects gave written informed consent. Subject recruitment, clinical evaluation, laboratory tests, and their classification were described previously [25]. Briefly, 227 subjects were recruited from Wichita, KS, USA, as part of a 2-day in-hospital evaluation of unexplained fatigue. These subjects were identified from a surveillance cohort of 7162 fatigued and non-fatigued subjects who were originally screened from 56,146 adult residents, 18 to 69 years of age. During the 2-day hospital stay, symptoms and exclusionary medical and psychiatric conditions were reevaluated for all 227 subjects. Following the 2-day hospital study, all subjects were classified based on all aspects specified in 1994 CFS case definition [26] and Medical Outcomes Short-Form, Multidimensional Fatigue Inventory and Symptom Inventory cutoff scores to include measures on the functional impairment, fatigue, and accompanying symptom complex that characterize CFS. Following this classification, 124 subjects were excluded because of medical or psychiatric exclusionary conditions or insufficient criteria to classify as CFS. Of the 103 remaining subjects, 101 subjects with genotype data were classified as CFS (43 subjects) and non-fatigued (NF; 58 subjects) healthy controls. The demographic characteristics along with the type of disease onset (gradual vs. sudden) of subjects in this study are given in Table 1.

Table 1 Demographic and other characteristics of the subjects selected for analysis

Factor	Categories	NF subjects ($n = 58$)	CFS subjects ($n = 43$)
Age (years)	MQMQM[a]	31.0/44.3/51.5/ 56.0/69.0	27.0/46.5/51.0/ 57.5/69.0
Sex (n)	Female/male	46/12	36/7
Race (n)	White/Black/others	54/2/2	40/1/2
BMI	MQMQM	16.0/25.3/29.0/ 32.0/40.0	23.0/26.0/29.0/ 32.5/40.0
Onset[b]	Gradual/sudden	14/1	36/6

[a]MQMQM represents the minimum, first quartile, median, third quartile, and maximum, respectively
[b]Onset represents gradual vs. sudden onset of illness. This information is available for all but one CFS subject. For NF subjects, onset information is relevant to only 15 individuals with past report of chronic fatigue

SNP selection, genotyping, and annotation

Because of the reported associations of CFS with perturbations in hypothalamic-pituitary-adrenal (HPA) axis and immune functions, we selected a total of 39 candidate genes implicated with the central nervous system (CNS) (30 genes) or immune and inflammation functions (nine genes) to determine the accuracy CFS prediction based on combinations of SNPs (Additional file 1: Table S1). There were a total of 167 SNPs in all candidate genes (137 SNPs in genes implicated with CNS and 30 SNPs in genes implicated with immune and inflammation). There were a total of 23 SNPs in X-chromosomes, and these were in two genes of serotonergic neurotransmission (*HTR2C* and *MAOA*). SNPs were selected from the SNP database (dbSNP) of National Center for Biotechnology Information database, Applied Biosystem's SNPBrowser™ or from the literature. All SNP markers had a minor allele frequency ≥10 % with the exception of *HTR2A* rs6314 (6.2 %), a non-synonymous SNP. DNA extraction and genotyping were done as described earlier [27]. Most SNPs (158 out of 167) were genotyped using validated TaqMan genotyping assay kits (Applied Biosystems, CA, USA) and the 7900 Sequence detection system (Applied Biosystems). Eight SNPs were genotyped by pyrosequencing. Genotyping for one polymorphism in *SLC6A4* designated 5-HTTLPR was conducted using gel-based assays [28]. SNP annotation was done using SPOT algorithm as implemented in the web-based tool accessible at https://spot.cgsmd.isi.edu/submit.php [29]. It may be noted that SNP selection was done in the design stage of this study before genotyping while in some other studies, statistical prescreening procedures such as sure independent screening were applied after genotyping to reduce the dimensionality [30, 31].

Model

We applied Bayesian logistic association models [18, 19] using subset of SNPs to predict disease status (y_i) of the individual i. Our hierarchical model structure underlying our predictive model is almost identical to that presented earlier by us [23] for LD mapping.

The logistic association model for SNP data (of individual i) can be written as:

$$\text{Logit}(p_i) = \alpha + \sum_{l \in M_A} \left(\beta_{l,1}(2-m_{i,l}) + \beta_{l,2}m_{i,l}\right) I_l + \sum_{l \in M_S} \frac{1}{2}\left(\beta_{l,1}(2-m_{i,l}) + \beta_{l,2}m_{i,l}\right) I_l.$$

Here, the logistic link function, $\text{Logit}(p_i) = \ln\left[\frac{p_i}{1-p_i}\right] = \ln\left[\frac{P(y_i=1|m)}{1-P(y_i=1|m)}\right]$, α is an intercept, ($\beta_{l,1}$ and $\beta_{l,2}$) are genetic effects of SNP l. I_l's are the indicator variables taking care of variable selection to select subset of SNPs to the model (see below for more details). The SNPs have been reorganized into two groups according to whether they are on sex chromosomes (i.e., $l \in M_S$) or autosomal chromosomes (i.e., $l \in M_A$). The genotype value $m_{i,l}$ of individual i at SNP l is represented numerically by 0 for homozygote AA, 1 for heterozygote AB, and 2 for homozygote BB. Our model for the genetic effects assumes an additive model, where an effect of the heterozygote ($\beta_{l,1} + \beta_{l,2}$) is in the middle of the effects of two homozygotes ($\beta_{l,1} + \beta_{l,1}$ and $\beta_{l,2} + \beta_{l,2}$). It is over-parameterized to improve the mixing and convergence properties of the Markov chain Monte Carlo (MCMC) sampling algorithm to yield better parameter estimates. The usual practice would be to set the first genetic effect to zero and have one parameter only for the other genetic effect. The absolute difference of the two effects here reflects the effect size of the SNP. Note that the factor of one half is introduced for the SNPs on the sex chromosome due to female X-chromosome mosaicism and the adjustment by half can be used for male only after assuming all SNPs on their X-chromosome are homozygous (cf. [32]).

We assume a priori that there is only a small subset of important SNPs that are useful to predict disease status. In these predictive models, subset selection of important SNP effects to the predictive model is based on the use of indicator variables (I_l, $l = 1,\ldots, M$), all of which either equals one (inclusion) or zero (exclusion) depending on the importance of particular SNP (see, e.g., [9]). Here, M is a number of SNPs. However, in reality for closely situated SNPs, it is difficult to distinguish the effects of individual SNPs due to LD. Thus, LD pattern among SNPs in the linked region is explicitly modeled as dependency prior for variable selection indicators in our model as described below and reported earlier in [23].

Model for missing SNP data

Missing SNP data are handled in a similar manner as any other model parameter. Thus, prior distributions are assigned to all missing SNP data. We assume a priori that the missing SNP genotypes occur at random and independently within and across SNPs (in the sense that the probability that the genotype is missing is not dependent on the true genotype pattern at the locus or at any of its neighboring loci). The prior distribution $p(m_{i,l})$ of a missing genotype $m_{i,l}$ under the Hardy-Weinberg equilibrium is a binomial distribution, where both alleles have equal occurrence probabilities within the locus (i.e., $p(m_{i,l})$ = 0.25, 0.5, and 0.25 for three genotypes AA, AB, and BB, respectively). Additionally, an independence over loci (linkage equilibrium) is assumed for missing SNP genotypes as $p(m) = \prod_{i=1}^{N} p(m_{i,1}, \ldots, m_{i,M}) = \prod_{i=1}^{N}\prod_{l=1}^{M} p(m_{i,l})$. During MCMC sampling, our phenotypic model (likelihood) gives information on which genotype value is most likely in the light of the data. Thus, we let the data to speak in our missing data model. For meta-analysis purposes, where SNP genotypes at some data sets may be missing for all the individuals, one may want to consider to predict the SNP genotypes with reasonable accuracy using genotype imputation methods (utilizing LD correlation structure between neighboring SNPs) based on HapMap and 1000 genomes project reference panels [33, 34].

Priors for α, β, I

Prior specification is intrinsically subjective, and specifying prior that will satisfy everyone and/or every aspect might be unachievable. We adopt the method where priors reflect our intuitive knowledge but are also useful in avoiding some potential pitfalls and help reduce the computational burden. The parameter α relates to the intercept term of the regression which in this case with the Logit function would be close to zero (with 43 CFS cases and 58 NF controls). In the case of regression modeling a quantitative phenotype, the variance of the intercept parameter can be related to the scale of the phenotype. Here, we have binary phenotype; thus, without further information on the variability, we assume a standard normal distribution for the intercept parameter α.

The parameters β and I together determine which SNPs potentially have effect on the phenotype and the extent of this effect.

Following [23], we denote the vector of (genetic or physical) distances between the SNPs with $d = (d_2, \ldots, d_M)$. We also use a smoothing parameter λ for neighboring SNPs which allows us to model dependence of two adjacent SNPs. Our prior probability for each SNP to be involved in the model is $P(I_l = 1|s) = s = \frac{1}{M}$, which corresponds to assuming only a single marker to be important predictor in the model (see [23] for details). However, SNPs exhibiting strong LD in a single genomic region would change these probabilities, and we model this by a Markov model where the extent of LD is decaying according to the distance information [23]. This is, $P(I_1, \ldots, I_N|s, \lambda, d) = P(I_1|s)\prod_{l=2}^{M} P(I_l|I_{l-1}, s, \lambda, d_l)$. Given the state of inclusion indicators at locus $(l-1)$, the transition matrix for the inclusion indicators for locus l is given by

$$\begin{pmatrix} e^{-\lambda d_l} + (1-e^{-\lambda d_l})(1-s) & (1-e^{-\lambda d_l})s \\ (1-e^{-\lambda d_l})(1-s) & e^{-\lambda d_l} + (1-e^{-\lambda d_l})s \end{pmatrix}.$$

Genetic effects ($\beta_{l,1}$ and $\beta_{l,2}$) of each locus are assigned marginally a priori using a scale-mixture representation of Student's t distribution (e.g., [35]). This means that genetic effects at each locus are first assumed to be normally distributed with common variance σ_l^2 which again is assumed to be a priori inverse gamma distributed. In this model, a vector of locus-specific genetic variance components $\sigma^2 = (\sigma_1^2, \ldots, \sigma_M^2)$, over the M loci, controls the corresponding genetic effect parameters under a normal model. We further make the following conditional independence assumption that given σ^2 and s, the locus indicators I and genetic effects β are independent. Thus, prior distribution $P(\beta_{l,k}|\sigma_l^2)$ for genetic effects $\beta_{l,k}(k = 1,2)$ was assumed to be normal $N(0, \sigma_l^2)$ with locus-specific variance component σ_l^2.

Priors for hyper-parameters σ_l^2, λ

The prior for genetic variance $P(\sigma_l^2)$ at locus l was given an inverse *gamma* (1, 1), and consequently, $P(\sigma^2) = \Pi_{l=1}^{M} P(\sigma_l^2)$. The smoothing parameter λ is given a wide prior of *gamma* (1, 0.01) which has both the mean and standard deviation as 100. This parameter helps to eliminate spurious associations but strengthens the real association signals. However, since we utilize a common smoothing parameter over multiple locations of the genome, it lacks intuitive explanation compared to situation where it is used for a single densely mapped genomic region. There, this parameter can be thought to roughly represent the time since the relevant mutation affecting the phenotype (see [23]).

Complete model

The relevant joint density to derive the posterior of the parameters of interest is then obtained using the following expression which is based on the above and utilizes appropriate conditional independence assumptions:

$$\begin{aligned} p(y, I, \alpha, \beta, \sigma^2, \lambda, m|s, d) &= p(y|m, I, \alpha, \beta) \\ &\times p(I|\lambda, s, d)p(\lambda) \\ &\times p(\alpha)p(\beta|\sigma^2)p(\sigma^2) \\ &\times p(m) \end{aligned}$$

Weighted genetic variation and heuristic model reduction

The weighted genetic variation ($WGV_l = |\beta_{l,1} - \beta_{l,2}|I_l$) at locus l, ($l = 1,..., M$), is computed as a product of absolute difference of the genetic effects $|\beta_{l,1} - \beta_{l,2}|$ and the inclusion indicator (I_l).

A heuristic model reduction method was used to speed up the estimation by determining the number of SNP predictors that can be reduced without loss of predictive ability. Using the percentiles of WGV (Additional file 1: Table S2) as cutoff/threshold, a selected set of SNPs was retained in the model with two critical components derived from the overall model as follows. For the indicators, the joint posterior distribution of the indicators from the full model was used where the outcome of the spike-n-slab technique over the MCMC simulation for full model was stored and reused for model reduction purposes. For the remaining SNPs (with WGV lower than the threshold value), the individual-level genotype information were not used, and thus, these SNPs would effectively cease to act as covariates in the model (see Additional file 1 for detailed information on WGV and heuristic model reduction).

K-fold cross-validation

Cross-validation methods [36] give a better assessment of model predictive performance for new data, i.e., phenotypic predictions of individuals whose phenotypes and genotypes have not been involved in the learning sample. The hold-out or split-sample method, in which the data is split into training and testing sets, is the simplest kind of cross-validation. While this method assesses model performance on real prediction situation with new data, it is subjective to the choice of the partition of the data into training and testing sets. *K*-fold cross-validation is one way to improve over the split-sample method. The data set is divided into K (approximately) equal subsets, and the hold-out method is repeated K times, by which every data point gets to be in a test set exactly once and gets to be in a training set $K - 1$ times. We have used $K = 10$ which is also one of the most popular choices of K [37].

One major disadvantage of *K*-fold cross-validation is that the time taken would also be typically K times that required for estimation based on whole data. Using data on all 167 SNPs, a tenfold cross-validation would require approximately 150 min per MCMC iteration. We retained information from all SNPs since CFS phenotype is complex and there could be loss of predictive ability with reduced number of SNPs. Therefore, instead of reducing the number of SNPs in the model to reduce the time, we made a few modifications to the full model ("Model" section) as noted in the supplementary file.

Model implementation

The models were implemented in WinBUGS software [38], a special software to carry out MCMC simulation from posterior of complex models. The simulations were started with random initial values and were run for several thousands of iterations. Convergence of MCMC chains was monitored by visual inspection of MCMC trace plots with respect to several different model parameters and also by assuring that low values of the MCMC error have been reached for all critical model parameters. Software codes are available in the supplementary file and at http://www.rni.helsinki.fi/~mjs/.

Comparison with competing prediction methods

To compare our method, certain predictions were made for the same data set with generalized linear model versions of LASSO and ridge regression [11, 12] using R-package "penalized" [39]. LASSO model assumes independence among predictors while ridge regression can handle collinearity among them. We also compared our Bayesian model assuming independence between predictors (i.e., prior independence among indicator variables). This can provide information on the importance of the dependence structure to the model. LASSO and ridge regression analyses were performed using the same overparameterized model as in the Bayesian analysis which had own coefficient for each allele. Before LASSO and ridge regression analyses, we imputed missing data (once) using the Bayesian missing data model. However, this resulted in rank-deficient data matrix in which we eliminated 15 markers to make matrix acceptable for the R-package. To find the best tuning parameter value in LASSO (and ridge regression), we tried 55 (and 94) different values in range [0.1, 1000] (and [0.01, 25000]), respectively. In the Bayesian analysis, the priors and other settings were kept the same as earlier.

Results

CFS in-data prediction using full model

In-data prediction basically uses the training data itself to model the phenotype outcome. The data described earlier in the "Subjects and illness classification" and "SNP selection, genotyping, and annotation" sections and the model developed by us (presented in the "Model" section) were used to evaluate the goodness of fit of the model to predict CFS for 101 subjects (with 43 CFS and 58 NF individuals) using all the SNP data. This in-data prediction model, among other things, provided estimates of WGV of the SNPs, which are combined measures of their selection probability in the model and degree of effect on the phenotype (Additional file 1: Table S2). This is computed as a random variable based on the product of the indicator and absolute difference of the genetic effects for a locus, i.e.

$WGV_l = |\beta_{l,1} - \beta_{l,2}|I_l$ for the l-th locus, $l = 1,..., M$. The MCMC sampling from the posterior also enables us to estimate the WGVs. SNPs rs2288831 (*IL12B*), rs2071376

(*IL1A*), rs2069718 (*IFNG*), rs846906 (*HSD11B1*), rs1923884 (*HTR2A*), rs1799836 (*MAOA*), and rs1396862 (*CRHR1*) were among the top 10 SNPs with the highest genetic effect on the phenotype as measured by WGV (Table 2). For this particular CFS data using all 167 SNPs, this full model showed 100 % goodness of fit, probably due to over-fitting in a small data set. This necessitates extensive cross-validation of the model with unseen test data.

Impact of CFS prediction using variable number of SNPs

We examined if the number of SNP predictors can be reduced without loss of predictive ability by implementing a heuristic model reduction. Using percentiles from the estimated WGV, an increasing number of SNPs were included in the model with appropriate parameters, while the effect of the rest was adjusted as described above. As expected, with the increased number of SNPs, there was a corresponding increase in the model prediction accuracy (see Fig. 1 and Table 3). Although prediction accuracy reached near perfection (accuracy 97 %) with nearly all SNPs (159 out of 167), accuracy remained still close to perfection (accuracy 95 %) using a combination of close to 100 SNPs (35th percentile of WGV). Accuracy remained high (90 %) even with the top 70 SNPs in WGV. Accuracy decreased with fewer SNPs in the model, although we also obtained 79 % accuracy with combinations of 26 SNPs ranked top in WGV.

The above utilized the cutoff probability of 0.5 to declare a case as CFS or otherwise. However, this threshold could also be varied. Figure 2 presents the predictive performance as measured by accuracy of prediction while varying the threshold probability and number of (unadjusted) SNPs in the model. As stated earlier, SNPs were considered in the increasing order of their WGV for inclusion/exclusion in the model. Thus, least effective SNPs are removed from the model at first. This illustrates that model accuracy is not highly susceptible to the choice of cutoff and is capable of staying at high level in an interval around the chosen 0.5 used for this analysis.

Tenfold cross-validation of CFS prediction

The cross-validation results on prediction are summarized using the standard sensitivity, specificity, false detection rate (FDR), and overall accuracy (Table 4). Computation time per iteration is approximately 50 min. As can be seen, the overall accuracy is still high (79 %) for the tenfold cross-validation. The overall sensitivity and specificity of the tenfold cross-validation were 74.4 and 82.8 %, respectively. Accuracy for individual sets varied between 70 and 100 %. At an individual level, the prediction probabilities were compared for the *K*-fold model and in-data model, and the results are presented as Fig. 3. We observe that those predicted with high probability/accuracy when the data is seen can still be recovered when the respective data is withheld. However, as this accuracy comes down, probability of correct prediction also comes down when the corresponding data is unseen. It should also be noted that the grouping of subjects based on overall cross-validation probability (>0.5) still predicts 14-fold higher risk for a subject to be classified as CFS (OR = 13.963; 95 % confidence interval 5.313–36.69; p value = 6.64×10^{-9}).

For comparison, the same cross-validation analysis was done for LASSO, ridge regression, and Bayesian model without dependence (Table 5). The Bayesian approach (with and without dependence) clearly outperformed LASSO and ridge regression in accuracy and in sensitivity, but specificity was slightly better in penalized regression approaches. Including between SNP dependence to the Bayesian model improved sensitivity from 65.1 to 74.4. Otherwise, accuracy and specificity remained almost at the same levels for the two Bayes models.

There were a total of 21 false predictions out of 101 predictions in this study. We investigated the source of

Table 2 Top 10 genetic markers associated with CFS based on weighted genetic variation (WGV) estimated by the Bayesian model

SNP ID	Proxy SNP	Gene symbol[a]	SNP annotation[a]	WGV	SE of WGV[b]
rs2288831	rs3212227	*IL12B*	Intron (UTR-3)	3.95	0.0299
rs2071376		*IL1A*	intron	3.6	0.0296
rs2069718		*IFNG*	intron	3.34	0.0272
rs846906		*HSD11B1*	intron	3.29	0.0337
rs1923884		*HTR2A*	intron	3.16	0.0324
rs1799836		*MAOB*	Intron	2.56	0.0394
rs363236	rs3814230	*SLC18A2 (PDZD8)*	UTR-3 (synonymous codon)	2.31	0.0272
rs1396862	rs1218523	*CRHR1 (IMP5)*	Intron (missense codon)	2.31	0.0334
rs891512	rs743507	*NOS3*	Intron	2.18	0.0287
rs1124492	rs46220755	*DRD2*	Intron	2.02	0.0312

[a]Gene symbol and SNP annotation in parenthesis correspond to proxy SNPs, if different from the genotyped SNPs for the model
[b]SE of WGV standard error of weighted genetic variation

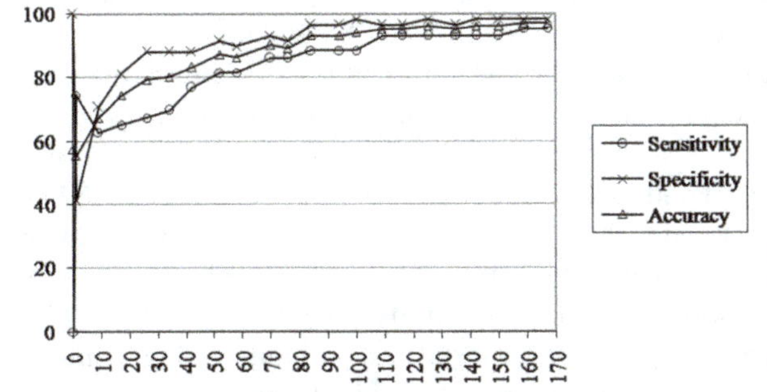

Fig. 1 Impact of varying the number of SNPs on prediction performance, as measured by sensitivity, specificity, and accuracy

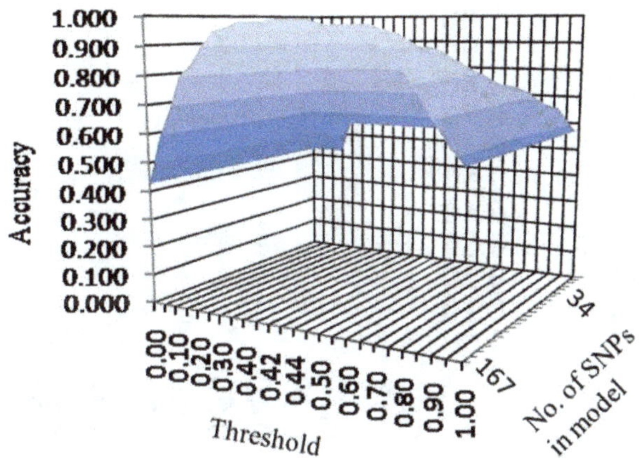

Fig. 2 Impact of varying the threshold and the number of SNPs on prediction performance as assessed by the in-data prediction accuracy

these false predictions in terms of the sudden vs. gradual onset of chronic fatigue as reported by the subjects in the study. It appears that tenfold cross-validation is accurate for all individuals (six out of six) with sudden onset of CFS and one CFS subject with no onset information. All the erroneous predictions for CFS cases occurred only for those CFS cases with gradual onset (11 out of 36 CFS subjects with gradual onset). Among NF controls, 15 subjects reported previously being fatigued (14 gradual and 1 sudden onset) but did not meet the criteria for CFS, and three of these NF controls were predicted incorrectly. The remaining seven false predictions belonged to the 43 NF subjects who reported that they were never chronically fatigued before. These erroneous predictions potentially reflect heterogeneity in both cases and control subjects in the study.

Table 3 Increase in accuracy with increasing number of SNPs in the predictive model with individual-level allelic information

Percentile[a]	Cutoff for weighted genetic variation	No. of SNPs	Sensitivity	Specificity	Accuracy
100	3.95	1	74.42	41.38	0.55
95	2.13	9	62.79	70.69	0.67
90	1.30	17	65.12	81.03	0.74
85	1.07	26	67.44	87.93	0.79
80	0.96	34	69.77	87.93	0.80
75	0.82	42	76.74	87.93	0.83
70	0.79	52	81.40	91.38	0.87
65	0.74	58	81.40	89.66	0.86
60	0.70	70	86.05	93.10	0.90
55	0.68	76	86.05	91.38	0.89
50	0.63	84	88.37	96.55	0.93
45	0.58	94	88.37	96.55	0.93
40	0.54	100	88.37	98.28	0.94
35	0.51	109	93.02	96.55	0.95
30	0.48	116	93.02	96.55	0.95
25	0.45	125	93.02	98.28	0.96
20	0.42	135	93.02	96.55	0.95
15	0.41	142	93.02	98.28	0.96
10	0.36	150	93.02	98.28	0.96
5	0.32	159	95.35	98.28	0.97
0	0.00	167	100	100	1.00

[a]Percentiles are those for the estimated weighted genetic variation (WGV) under the full model

Discussion

This is a proof-of-principle study that presents a powerful genetic approach that can simultaneously rank SNPs based on their genetic effect and for prediction of complex phenotype based on a Bayesian logistic mixture modeling principle combined with biologically meaningful pathway-focused genetic markers and rigorous case ascertainment. We used CFS SNP data as an example to apply our analytical approach and to compare our model

Table 4 CFS prediction from in-data and tenfold cross-validations

Model and prediction type	Accuracy	Sensitivity	Specificity	FDR
In-data-unconstrained model	100.0	100.0	100.0	0.0
In-data-constrained model	100.0	100.0	100.0	0.0
K-fold-constrained model	79.2	74.4	82.8	23.8
K-fold-set1	72.7	60.0	83.3	25.0
K-fold-set2	70.0	75.0	66.7	40.0
K-fold-set3	80.0	75.0	83.3	25.0
K-fold-set4	100.0	100.0	100.0	0.0
K-fold-set5	70.0	50.0	83.3	33.3
K-fold-set6	70.0	50.0	83.3	33.3
K-fold-set7	70.0	75.0	66.7	40.0
K-fold-set8	70.0	75.0	66.7	40.0
K-fold-set9	100.0	100.0	100.0	0.0
K-fold-set10	90.0	80.0	100.0	0.0

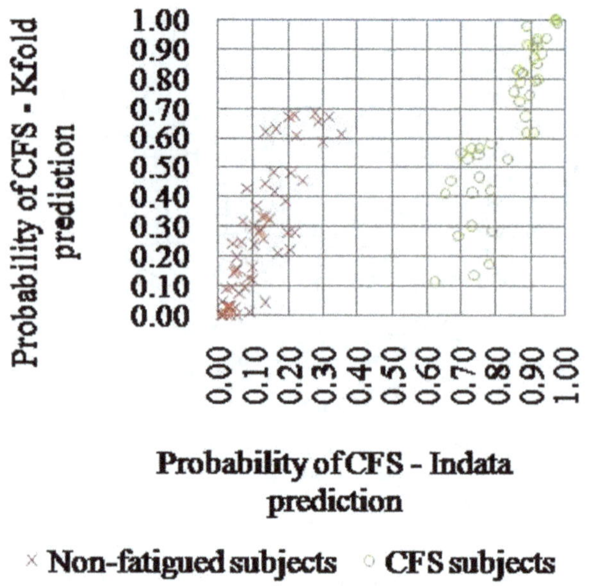

Fig. 3 Probability of CFS at individual level as estimated by the *K*-fold cross-validation model and in-data prediction model

performance with LASSO and ridge regression as well as with results in the literature using other approaches. Our Bayesian prediction model is suitable for any data set that has genotype calls and subjects ascertained into binary phenotype, regardless of whether the illness is specialized or not.

Our modeling approach yielded 80 % accuracy after tenfold cross-validation with CFS data. This prediction accuracy is one of the best so far for this complex disease compared to other prediction models using the same data set. In comparison to other analytical methods, several modeling principles we used may have contributed to this high prediction accuracy. For example, we incorporated covariance due to LD between SNPs so that SNP effects of the predictive model depended on each other and dependence vanishes according to exponential decay with the genetic or physical distance [40]. Originally, closely after the single locus model of Conti and Witte [40], we presented our multi-locus model for genetic association mapping in small chromosomal segments [23]. After that, Malo et al. [41] and Tsai et al. [42] have expressed their own approaches to model covariance between SNP effects in genetic association analyses. Very recently, Fridley and Jenkins [43] also introduced an approach, which is closely related to our earlier model [23] for genetic association studies, see also [35, 44, 45] for the other alternatives.

Table 5 CFS prediction from tenfold cross-validation for competing methods

Model	Accuracy	Sensitivity	Specificity
Bayes with dependence	79.2	74.4	82.8
Bayes with independence	77.2	65.1	86.2
LASSO	59.4	20.9	87.9
Ridge regression	60.4	18.6	91.4

A second methodological enhancement in our model is that it incorporates both sparse selection of trait-associated SNPs and smoothing of estimated SNP effects, and that this enhancement potentially provided competitive and accurate phenotype predictions in comparison to previous methods for CFS prediction. There are two previous reports [17, 46] on testing combinations of SNPs for prediction of CFS using the same subjects but a smaller set of (42 SNPs out of 167) SNPs used in this study. Because of the smaller set of SNPs, Goertzel et al. [46] used an enumerative approach with cross-validation by permutation and reported 76.3 % accuracy in predicting CFS. Huang et al. [17] compared three sets of classification methods (naïve Bayes model, support vector machine, and C4.5 decision tree algorithm) with 42 SNPs and found the naïve Bayes model with the wrapper-based feature selection to give the best overall sensitivity (64 %) and specificity (52 %). This comparison of our model having dependence structure with Huang et al. that does not have dependence structure [17] shows that dependence model like ours provides clear predictive advantage. Our study implies that models with dependence structure should be utilized more in methods addressing the prediction problem. While there are methods that take into account of dependence between SNPs for association mapping [46, 47], to the best of our knowledge, our Bayesian model is the only one that probabilistically models dependence between SNPs for prediction of binary phenotype. Moreover, since there are explicit differences in the models for association mapping and phenotypic prediction, methods developed for association mapping [46, 47] are not necessarily suitable or preferable for phenotypic prediction and vice versa.

Our heuristic model reduction method provided insight into the strength of Bayesian multi-locus association involving 100's of SNPs in comparison to current regression models using a few genetic variants. In this analysis, prediction accuracy reached near perfection (accuracy 97 %) with nearly all SNPs (159 out of 167) and accuracy remained still close to perfection (accuracy 95 %) using a combination of close to 100 SNPs (35th percentile of WGV). Accuracy remained high (90 %) even with the top 70 SNPs in WGV but it decreased with fewer SNPs in the model, although we also obtained 79 % accuracy with 27 SNPs. These results clearly show that the higher the genetic information in the SNP profile, the greater will be the accuracy in prediction of complex diseases. Since the current computational approaches limit multi-locus analysis to only a few genetic variants, each with weak associations, current attempts to predict the individual genetic risk of complex disease traits have not been highly accurate, and their value/relevance was also questioned [48]. However, our results suggest that one can actually achieve reasonable predictive accuracy by using Bayesian predictions based on multi-locus association models involving 100's of SNPs in a small set of genes. Prediction can be further improved with greater accuracy, sensitivity, and specificity, if the model includes genetic variation in hundreds of genes representing expanded set of multiple pathways implicated in immune, inflammation [49], and CNS functions [50]. With additional improvements in genetic variation data, modeling, and sample size, one can also conceive the potential of our approach to generate genetic signatures to delineate heterogeneity/subtypes in complex disease.

Other statistical considerations that favored high accuracy include model selection and estimation (including phenotype predictions) being done simultaneously. By this, we obtained estimates for posterior probability (uncertainty) of disease status and the degree of belief estimate for predicted disease phenotypes. These predictions, which are based on the Bayesian model averaging approach providing robust predictions [51], are however not based on a single best model but rather several different models where prediction of each model is weighted according to the corresponding posterior model probability. Model reduction aspects were investigated in a computationally feasible manner for an otherwise analytically intractable problem. We also showed accurate predictions from partial genotype data. That is, while the learning set contains information on complete set of SNPs, accuracy does not immediately drop if phenotype predictions are made for individuals which have genotypes measured from only a partial set of SNPs. We used indicator variables in the predictive models because they will make it possible to shrink coefficients at some unimportant positions exactly to zero. The same numerical property is difficult to obtain by tuning the value of the shrinkage parameter (which controls amount of shrinkage) in regularization models like the Bayesian LASSO [13], which do not contain indicators in the model. In those models, which have a single shrinkage parameter only, there is always trade-off between obtaining enough shrinkage for unimportant contributors and still maintaining good estimation ability for important positions (without having too much shrinkage).

It was reported recently that in order to achieve accurate prediction of human disease for unrelated individuals, it would take approximately a sample size of 350,000 [52]. This is because accuracy is dependent on the average relatedness between individuals in the population (i.e., effective population size structuring the LD) and genetic architecture of the trait. It was further noted that it can be accurate on small samples only for diseases that are determined by a limited number of genes which is unlikely to be true for a complex disease. It is thus possible that population ascertainment process that involved rigorous clinical evaluation of both cases and control subjects in this study might be an important factor, along with the strength of modeling and SNP selection, for prediction accuracy in this particular case. We are also aware of the rule of thumb that the number of independent predictors should not be greater than the one tenth of the number of samples in the smaller of the two outcome categories in logistic regression modeling. This limitation may be overcome by using the conventional two-stage procedure wherein significant markers are first evaluated from independent analysis, and then, the short-listed markers tested for prediction accuracy. Our analytical approach is to move away from this rule of thumb. Indeed, one of the main focuses of our study is that our Bayesian model estimates good prediction accuracy based on multi-locus/simultaneous association of all SNPs using small data set. This approach in predicting human disease phenotype using the Bayesian multi-locus association model is supported by closely related prediction models in plant breeding research. For example, using 80 markers and 126 soybean lines, Hu et al. demonstrated an increase from 33 to 78 % in explaining the phenotypic variance when markers were collectively accounted for epistatic effects [53]. The findings of Heffner et al. based on a wheat breeding program using a small set of samples [54] and markers also agree with our findings from human studies that jointly estimating all marker effects is able to capture more of the genetic variance than the two-stage conventional approach of first selecting significant markers from independent analysis and then estimating their effects.

Besides, phenotypic prediction using 100's of SNPs, our Bayesian model provided the genetic effect estimated as WGV for each of the SNPs incorporated in the model and thus allowing to rank individual SNPs for exploring their functional role in the pathophysiology of the disease. For example, in our in-data prediction analysis, the top 110 SNPs with over 90 % accuracy were spread on 32 of 39 genes (25 CNS and 7 immune function candidate genes). It is interesting to note that SNPs from 7 out of 9 immune function genes were represented in this group that showed greater prediction, and SNPs in three of them (*IL12B* rs2288831, *IL1A* rs2071376, and *IFNG* rs2069718) showed the highest association with CFS in terms of WGV values. All three SNPs showed replicated or moderate association with other diseases as well. SNP rs2288831 is in complete LD with rs3212227 located in the 3′-untranslated region (3′UTR) of *IL12B* (Table 2), and this proxy SNP was reported to be associated with psoriasis in a large-scale association study, confirming the results of a previous study [55]. rs2071376 located in intron 6 of *IL1A* showed significant association in patients with keratoconus [56]. SNP rs2069718, located in the intron of *IFNG,* was associated with susceptibility to systemic lupus erythematosus in a recessive genetic model [57]. Among the CNS-related genes, the highest measures of genetic effects on CFS prediction were provided by SNPs in *HSD11B1* (rs846906), *HTR2A* (rs1923884), MAOB (rs1799836), *CRHR1* (rs1396862), *SLC18A2* (rs363236), *NOS3* (rs891512), and *DRD2* (rs1124492). Except rs1396862 and rs363236, these SNPs in CNS-related genes were located in introns with no potential function through transcription factor binding or splicing regulation or no proxy SNPs with functional significance. SNP rs891512, although located in intron of *NOS3,* showed protective effect against suicidal behavior [58]. While rs363236 is located in the 3′UTR of *SLC18A2* and is in complete LD with a marker (rs3814230) resulting in synonymous codon change in PDZD8, no functional role or association with disease could be identified with this marker. SNP rs1396862, on the other hand, is in complete LD with rs12185233 that results in a missense codon (R460P) change in *intramembrane protease 5 (IMP5*), a gene associated with Parkinson's disease [59]. Another SNP in *CRHR1* (rs173365) with WGV of 0.58 also showed high LD with another missense codon change (rs242944, H302R) in *IMP5,* suggesting further support of association of this gene region with CFS. Genes with >5 SNPs that contributed to >90 % accuracy included *ACE, DRD2, HTR2A, HTR2C, HTR4, IL1A, MAOA, NR3C1,* and *TPH2.* Thus, at least 16 unique genes (*ACE, CRHR1, DRD2, HSD11B1, HTR2A, HTR2C, HTR4, IL12B, IL1A, IFNG, MAOA, MAOB, NOS3, NR3C1, SLC18A2,* and *TPH2)* appear to be major contributors to CFS prediction by greater genetic effects either through individual or multiple (>5) SNPs. Among these 16 genes, only two (*TPH2* and *NR3C1*) were common with the smaller set of 10 genes in the previous reports [17, 46] illustrating that higher predictive accuracy by multi-locus association is determined by variants with greater genetic effects. Sequence variations in some of these genes were reported to be associated with CFS (*NR3C1*: Rajeevan et al. [60] and *HTR2A*: Smith et al. [27]) or associated with some of the CFS subtypes identified by latent class analyses (*MAOA, MAOB, TPH2,* and *NR3C1*: Smith et al. [61]) or association with allostatic load, a construct that describes cumulative physiological effects of adaptation in response to stress (*ACE*: Smith et al. [62]). Besides estimating prediction accuracy of complex phenotype using multi-locus association, these findings on the association of individual markers/genes with CFS support the hypothesized general applicability of Bayesian model-based WGV estimates to identify specific genetic variations that may play biological roles in the pathophysiology of various diseases.

We concentrated more on the modeling principle rather than implementing the tool for routine phenotype prediction in this study. Thus, we used a general purpose software tool, WinBUGS, for MCMC estimation, which is often slower than tailor-made programs. Moreover, for routine phenotype prediction, maximum a posteriori estimation may be more practical than MCMC estimation (cf. [35, 63]). As is well known, population structure and cryptic relatedness are confounding factors in genetic association studies [64]. We have not corrected for these factors in our models since subjects were collected from a homogeneous population (Caucasians >93 % in both CFS and NF subjects) with no close relatives or complex links between individuals. However, even though such confounding factors may exist in the CFS data, the multi-locus association models have been found to be surprisingly robust to these confounders [31, 65]. Non-genetic risk factors can be included into the model as environmental covariates even if we have not done so here, and their inclusion may improve the accuracy even further. Presently, there is limited clinical/diagnostic utility for this genetic prediction model, since its reproducible performance remains to be evaluated in multiple populations. Further, in order to be clinically useful, it may be advantageous to evaluate prediction models by decision analytic techniques to determine whether models would change medical decisions. This Bayesian model provides an approach to improve phenotypic prediction by exploiting all available genetic information in 100's of loci jointly, an approach that can be extended to the emerging computational field of whole-genome markers-enabled prediction of genetic predisposition in humans.

In conclusion, our results demonstrate, as a proof of principle, the power of using a combination of a Bayesian logistic mixture modeling principle, pathway-focused SNPs, and rigorous subject ascertainment for highly accurate prediction of complex phenotypes. WGV estimates provided by the model can also be useful to identify individual genetic markers/genes with potential biological functions. Future studies are warranted to expand this approach using multiple biological pathways and multiple populations [66] to derive a reproducible genetic profile with greater predictive power than non-genetic risk factors to identify chronic diseases like CFS and its subtypes that have no laboratory-based diagnosis or intermediate markers.

Additional file

Additional file 1: Supplementary information. Figure S1. Scatter plot showing the SNP level differences in the genetic effects estimated under the unconstrained and constrained (with the coefficient of class with higher frequency fixed at zero). **Figure S2.** Box plots of standard deviations over the 167 non-zero genetic effects, where standard deviations were calculated as follows: For each SNP and each (non-zero) genetic effect, the standard deviation over tenfolds was computed from the prior and also from the posterior distribution (under the constrained model used for tenfold cross-validation). **Table S1.** List of genes (along with functions) and SNPs tested for CFS prediction by the Bayesian logistic mixture model. Genes primarily belong to the central nervous system (CNS) including hypothalamic-pituitary-adrenal (HPA) pathway or immune function systems. **Table S2.** Weighted genetic variation in decreasing order for SNPs under full model.

Competing interests
All authors declare that they have no competing interests.

Authors' contributions
MB, MSR, and MJS conceived of the idea. MB and MJS developed the method. MB implemented the method and performed the analyses. MSR made the pathway-based gene and SNP selection and generated the genotype data as part of the genetic association study of CFS. MB, MSR, and MJS interpreted the results and drafted and edited the manuscript. All authors read and approved the final manuscript.

Acknowledgements
The authors appreciate the critical review of the manuscript and suggestions from the referees and Elizabeth Unger, Brian Gurbaxani, and Virginia Falkenberg of Chronic Viral Disease Branch, CDC, Atlanta, GA, USA.

Funding
This work was supported by a research grant (Decision No. 127076) from the Academy of Finland and the University of Helsinki's research funds.

Author details
[1]School of Mathematics and Statistics, University of Hyderabad, Hyderabad 500046, India. [2]Division of High-Consequence Pathogens & Pathology, Centers for Disease Control and Prevention, Atlanta 30333, USA. [3]Departments of Mathematical Sciences, Biocenter Oulu, University of Oulu, Oulu FIN-90014, Finland.

References

1. de los Campos G, Gianola D, Allison DB. Predicting genetic predisposition in humans: the promise of whole-genome markers. Nat Rev Genet. 2010;11:880–6.
2. Jostins L, Barrett JC. Genetic risk prediction in complex disease. Hum Mol Genet. 2011;20:R182–8.
3. Jakobsdottir J, Gorin MB, Conley YP, Ferrell RE, Weeks DE. Interpretation of genetic association studies: markers with replicated highly significant odds ratios may be poor classifiers. PLoS Genet. 2009;5:e1000337.
4. Maher BS. The case of missing heritability. Nature. 2008;456:18–21.
5. Manolio TA, Collins FS, Cox NJ, Goldstein DB, Hindorff LA, Hunter DJ, et al. Finding the missing heritability of complex diseases. Nature. 2009;461:747–53.
6. Lee SH, Wray NR, Goddard ME, Visscher PM. Estimating missing heritability for disease from genome-wide association studies. Am J Hum Genet. 2011;88:294–305.
7. Yang J, Benyamin B, McEvoy BP, Gordon S, Henders AK, Nyholt DR, et al. Common SNPs explain a large proportion of the heritability for human height. Nat Genet. 2010;42:565–9.
8. Yang J, Lee SH, Goddard ME, Visscher PM. GCTA: a tool for genome-wide complex trait analysis. Am J Hum Genet. 2011;88:76–82.
9. O'Hara RB, Sillanpää MJ. A review of Bayesian variable selection methods: what, how and which. Bayesian Anal. 2009;4:85–118.
10. Zhou X, Carbonetto P, Stephens M. Polygenic modeling with Bayesian sparse linear mixed models. PLoS Genet. 2013;9:e1003264.
11. Li Z, Sillanpää MJ. Overview of LASSO-related penalized regression methods for quantitative trait mapping and genomic selection. Theor Appl Genet. 2012;125:419–35.
12. Wu TT, Chen YF, Hastie T, Sobel E, Lange K. Genome-wide association analysis by lasso penalized logistic regression. Bioinformatics. 2009;25:714–21.
13. de los Campos G, Naya H, Gianola D, Crossa J, Legarra A, Manfredi E, et al. Predicting quantitative traits with regression models for dense molecular markers and pedigree. Genetics. 2009;182:375–85.
14. de los Campos G, Hickey JM, Pong-Wong R, Daetwyler HD, Calus MP. Whole-genome regression and prediction methods applied to plant and animal breeding. Genetics. 2013;193:327–45.
15. Lee SH, van der Werf JH, Hayes BJ, Goddard ME, Visscher PM. Predicting unobserved phenotypes for complex traits from whole-genome SNP data. PLoS Genet. 2008;4:e1000231.
16. de los Campos G, Vazquez AI, Fernando R, Klimentidis YC, Sorensen D. Prediction of complex human traits using the genomic best linear unbiased predictor. PLoS Genet. 2013;9:e1003608.
17. Huang LC, Hsu SY, Lin E. A comparison of classification methods for predicting chronic fatigue syndrome based on genetic data. J Transl Med. 2009;7:81.
18. Bhattacharjee M, Sillanpää MJ. Bayesian joint disease-marker-expression analysis applied to clinical characteristics of chronic fatigue syndrome. In: McConnell P, Lin S, Cuticchia AJ, editors. Methods of microarray data analysis VI. (CAMDA). CAMDA 2009, 15–34.
19. Bhattacharjee M, Botting CH, Sillanpää MJ. Bayesian biomarker identification based on marker-expression proteomics data. Genomics. 2008;92:384–92.
20. Bhattacharjee M, Sillanpää MJ. A Bayesian mixed regression based prediction of quantitative traits from molecular marker and gene expression data. PLoS One. 2011;6:e26959.
21. West M, Ginsburg GS, Huang AT, Nevins JR. Embracing the complexity of genomic data for personalized medicine. Genome Res. 2006;16:559–66.
22. Kabán A. On Bayesian classification with Laplace priors. Patt Rec Lett. 2007;28:1271–82.
23. Sillanpää MJ, Bhattacharjee M. Bayesian association-based fine mapping in small chromosomal segments. Genetics. 2005;169:427–39.
24. Vernon SD, Reeves WC. The challenge of integrating disparate high-content data: epidemiological, clinical and laboratory data collected during an in-hospital study of chronic fatigue syndrome. Pharmacogenomics. 2006;7:345–54.
25. Reeves WC, Wagner D, Nisenbaum R, Jones JF, Gurbaxani B, Solomon L, et al. Chronic fatigue syndrome—a clinically empirical approach to its definition and study. BMC Med. 2005;3:19.
26. Fukuda K, Straus SE, Hickie I, Sharpe MC, Dobbins JG, Komaroff A. The chronic fatigue syndrome: a comprehensive approach to its definition and study. International Chronic Fatigue Syndrome Study Group. Ann Intern Med. 1994;121:953–9.
27. Smith AK, Dimulescu I, Falkenberg VR, Narasimhan S, Heim C, Vernon SD, et al. Genetic evaluation of the serotonergic system in chronic fatigue syndrome. Psychoneuroendocrinology. 2008;33:188–97.
28. Narita M, Nishigami N, Narita N, Yamaguti K, Okado N, Watanabe Y, et al. Association between serotonin transporter gene polymorphism and chronic fatigue syndrome. Biochem Biophys Res Commun. 2003;311:264–6.
29. Saccone SF, Bolze R, Thomas P, Quan J, Mehta G, Deelman E, et al. SPOT: a web-based tool for using biological databases to prioritize SNPs after a genome-wide association study. Nucleic Acids Res. 2010;38:W201–9.
30. Fan J, Song R. Sure independence screening in generalized linear models with NP-dimensionality. Ann Stat. 2010;38:3567–604.
31. Kärkkäinen HP, Sillanpää MJ. Robustness of Bayesian multilocus association models to cryptic relatedness. Ann Hum Genet. 2012;76:510–23.
32. Sasieni PD. From genotypes to genes: doubling the sample size. Biometrics. 1997;53:1253–61.
33. Gao X, Haritunians T, Marjoram P, McKean-Cowdin R, Torres M, Taylor KD, et al. Genotype imputation for Latinos using the HapMap and 1000 genomes project reference panels. Front Genet. 2012;3:117.
34. Servin B, Stephens M. Imputation-based analysis of association studies: candidate regions and quantitative traits. PLoS Genet. 2007;3:e114.
35. Mutshinda CM, Sillanpää MJ. Swift block-updating EM and pseudo-EM procedures for Bayesian shrinkage analysis of quantitative trait loci. Theor Appl Genet. 2012;125:1575–87.
36. Stone M. Cross-validatory choice and assessment of statistical predictions. J Roy Stat Soc B. 1974;36:111–47.
37. Hastie T, Tibshirani R, Friedman J. The elements of statistical learning: data mining, inference, and prediction. 2nd ed. Springer; 2009.
38. Spiegelhalter DJ, Thomas A, Best NG. WinBUGS Version 1.2 User Manual. Cambridge: MRC Biostatistics Unit; 1999.
39. Goeman JJ. L-1 penalized estimation in the Cox proportional hazards model. Biometrical J. 2010;52:70–84.
40. Conti DV, Witte JS. Hierarchical modeling of linkage disequilibrium: genetic structure and spatial relations. Am J Hum Genet. 2003;72:351–63.

41. Malo N, Libiger O, Schork NJ. Accommodating linkage disequilibrium in genetic-association analyses via ridge regression. Am J Hum Genet. 2008;82:375–85.
42. Tsai MY, Hsiao CK, Wen SH. A Bayesian spatial multimarker genetic random-effect model for fine-scale mapping. Ann Hum Genet. 2008;72:658–69.
43. Fridley BL, Jenkins GD. Localizing putative markers in genetic association studies by incorporating linkage disequilibrium into Bayesian hierarchical models. Hum Hered. 2010;70:63–73.
44. Yang W, Tempelman RJ. A Bayesian antedependence model for whole genome prediction. Genetics. 2012;190:1491–501.
45. Yi H, Breheny P, Imam N, Liu Y, Hoeschele I. Penalized multimarker vs. single-marker regression methods for genome-wide association studies of quantitative traits. Genetics. 2015;199:205–22.
46. Goertzel BN, Pennachin C, de Souza CL, Gurbaxani B, Maloney EM, Jones JF. Combinations of single nucleotide polymorphisms in neuroendocrine effector and receptor genes predict chronic fatigue syndrome. Pharmacogenomics. 2006;7:475–83.
47. Zuber V, Duarte Silva AP, Strimmer K. A novel algorithm for simultaneous SNP selection in high-dimensional genome-wide association studies. BMC Bioinf. 2012;13:284.
48. Janssens AC, van Duijn CM. Genome-based prediction of common diseases: advances and prospects. Hum Mol Genet. 2008;17:R166–73.
49. Loza MJ, McCall CE, Li L, Isaacs WB, Xu J, Chang BL. Assembly of inflammation-related genes for pathway-focused genetic analysis. PLoS One. 2007;2:e1035.
50. Hattori E, Liu C, Zhu H, Gershon ES. Genetic tests of biologic systems in affective disorders. Mol Psychiatry. 2005;10:719–40.
51. Sillanpää MJ, Corander J. Model choice in gene mapping: what and why. Trends Genet. 2002;18:301–7.
52. Meuwissen TH. Accuracy of breeding values of 'unrelated' individuals predicted by dense SNP genotyping. Genet Sel Evol. 2009;41:35.
53. Hu Z, Li Y, Song X, Han Y, Cai X, Xu S, et al. Genomic value prediction for quantitative traits under the epistatic model. BMC Genet. 2011;12:15.
54. Heffner EL, Jannink J-L, Sorrells ME. Genome selection accuracy using multifamily prediction models in a wheat breeding program. Plant Genome. 2011;4:65–75.
55. Cargill M, Schrodi SJ, Chang M, Garcia VE, Brandon R, Callis KP, et al. A large-scale genetic association study confirms IL12B and leads to the identification of IL23R as psoriasis-risk genes. Am J Hum Genet. 2007;80:273–90.
56. Kim SH, Mok JW, Kim HS, Joo CK. Association of −31T > C and −511 C > T polymorphisms in the interleukin 1 beta (IL1B) promoter in Korean keratoconus patients. Mol Vis. 2008;14:2109–16.
57. Kim K, Cho SK, Sestak A, Namjou B, Kang C, Bae SC. Interferon-gamma gene polymorphisms associated with susceptibility to systemic lupus erythematosus. Ann Rheum Dis. 2010;69:1247–50.
58. Rujescu D, Giegling I, Mandelli L, Schneider B, Hartmann AM, Schnabel A, et al. NOS-I and -III gene variants are differentially associated with facets of suicidal behavior and aggression-related traits. Am J Med Genet B Neuropsychiatr Genet. 2008;147B:42–8.
59. Edwards TL, Scott WK, Almonte C, Burt A, Powell EH, Beecham GW, et al. Genome-wide association study confirms SNPs in SNCA and the MAPT region as common risk factors for Parkinson disease. Ann Hum Genet. 2010;74:97–109.
60. Rajeevan MS, Smith AK, Dimulescu I, Unger ER, Vernon SD, Heim C, et al. Glucocorticoid receptor polymorphisms and haplotypes associated with chronic fatigue syndrome. Genes Brain Behav. 2007;6:167–76.
61. Smith AK, White PD, Aslakson E, Vollmer-Conna U, Rajeevan MS. Polymorphisms in genes regulating the HPA axis associated with empirically delineated classes of unexplained chronic fatigue. Pharmacogenomics. 2006;7:387–94.
62. Smith AK, Maloney EM, Falkenberg VR, Dimulescu I, Rajeevan MS. An angiotensin-1 converting enzyme polymorphism is associated with allostatic load mediated by C-reactive protein, interleukin-6 and cortisol. Psychoneuroendocrinology. 2009;34:597–606.
63. Li Z, Sillanpää MJ. Estimation of quantitative trait locus effects with epistasis by variational Bayes algorithms. Genetics. 2012;190:231–49.
64. Sillanpää MJ. Overview of techniques to account for confounding due to population stratification and cryptic relatedness in genomic data association analyses. Heredity. 2010;106:511–9.
65. Pikkuhookana P, Sillanpää MJ. Correcting for relatedness in Bayesian models for genomic data association analysis. Heredity. 2009;103:223–37.
66. Sillanpää MJ, Bhattacharjee M. Association mapping of complex trait loci with context-dependent effects and unknown context variable. Genetics. 2006;174:1597–611.

3

Success stories in genomic medicine from resource-limited countries

Konstantinos Mitropoulos[1†], Hayat Al Jaibeji[2,3†], Diego A. Forero[4], Paul Laissue[5], Ambroise Wonkam[6], Catalina Lopez-Correa[7], Zahurin Mohamed[8], Wasun Chantratita[9], Ming Ta Michael Lee[10,11], Adrian Llerena[12], Angela Brand[2], Bassam R. Ali[3*] and George P. Patrinos[13*]

Abstract

In recent years, the translation of genomic discoveries into mainstream medical practice and public health has gained momentum, facilitated by the advent of new technologies. However, there are often major discrepancies in the pace of implementation of genomic medicine between developed and developing/resource-limited countries. The main reason does not only lie in the limitation of resources but also in the slow pace of adoption of the new findings and the poor understanding of the potential that this new discipline offers to rationalize medical diagnosis and treatment. Here, we present and critically discuss examples from the successful implementation of genomic medicine in resource-limited countries, focusing on pharmacogenomics, genome informatics, and public health genomics, emphasizing in the latter case genomic education, stakeholder analysis, and economics in pharmacogenomics. These examples can be considered as model cases and be readily replicated for the wide implementation of pharmacogenomics and genomic medicine in other resource-limited environments.

Keywords: Genomic medicine, Pharmacogenomics, Economic evaluation in pharmacogenomics, Genome informatics, Public health genomics, Genetics education, Africa, Latin America, Southeast Asia

Introduction

Advances in genomics and related technologies have revolutionized the practice of medicine by means of better diagnosing and/or prognosing human inherited disorders and cancer and rationalizing drug use [1]. Translation of genomic findings into health care and health systems has been catalyzed by the advent of genome-wide studies, in which next-generation sequencing for either targeted, whole-exome, and/or whole-genome sequence analyses stands as the most powerful approach [2]. These approaches are gradually being adopted by diagnostic laboratories and hospitals in the USA and Western Europe, with several tangible results in the context of the implementation of genomic medicine. In addition, there are several guidelines both from the US Food and Drug Administration (FDA; http://www.fda.gov) and the European Medicines Agency (EMA; http://www.ema.europa.eu) regarding the use of genome-based therapies.

However, the pace of implementation of genomic medicine practices outlined above is not always equally met in developing and resource-limited countries, where significant barriers exist, often related to lack of tangible resources as well as technology and knowledge transfer. Furthermore, biomedical scientists and health care professionals in these countries frequently fail to fully appreciate the potential that this new approach offers to improve medical diagnosis and treatment. As such and taking into consideration that approximately 85 % of the world's population lives in developing/resource-limited countries, making genomic medicine accessible in these countries represents a major opportunity and challenge. There have been recently some significant examples from the successful implementation of genomic medicine in resource-limited settings in Europe and Asia, which could stand as examples for replication in similar environments, towards a broader implementation of genomic medicine and pharmacogenomics.

* Correspondence: bassam.ali@uaeu.ac.ae; gpatrinos@upatras.gr
†Equal contributors
[3]Department of Pathology, College of Medicine and Health Sciences, United Arab Emirates University, Al-Ain, United Arab Emirates
[13]Department of Pharmacy, University of Patras School of Health Sciences, Patras, Greece
Full list of author information is available at the end of the article

Translating genomics into health care of resource-limited countries

Successful translation of genomics into genomic medicine relies on several related disciplines, such as population genomics, pharmacogenomics, or informatics and the approach/task of public health genomics, which are frequently intersected. Below, we describe some examples from successful implementation of genomic medicine related to these disciplines and approaches.

Development of a European-wide pharmacogenomics map: the Euro-PGx project

The implementation rate of pharmacogenomics in the various health systems in Europe is very heterogeneous. This is not only due to the variable degree of harmonization of the national guidelines within Europe, particularly related to health care and education, but also most importantly due to differences in resource availability, making implementation of pharmacogenomics in resource-limited European countries an even more challenging task [3]. Also, there is very little knowledge regarding the pharmacogenomic biomarker allele frequencies in various European countries, to shortlist the different actionable pharmacogenomic biomarkers that would be useful in clinical settings of different countries, on which to base drug dose recommendations. The Euro-PGx project (http://www.goldenhelix.org/index.php/research/pharmacogenomics-in-europe) aims to determine the varying pharmacogenomic biomarkers allele frequencies in a large number of mostly developing European countries in an effort to produce drug dose recommendations for different countries. Preliminary findings from a large-scale genotyping effort using the DMET+ microarray (Affymetrix, Santa Clara, CA, USA), including 1936 pharmacogenomic biomarkers in 231 pharmacogenes, suggest that the allele frequencies of several pharmacogenomic biomarkers vary significantly among different European countries, despite the fact that the vast majority of the European populations have a very strong Caucasian genetic component. In particular, as far as anticoagulation treatment is concerned, significant differences were found in allele frequencies of the *CYP2C9*3* allele in the Serbian population, while there are differences in the average warfarin dosing in the different European countries investigated (Mizzi et al., in preparation). These varying frequencies in the pharmacogenomic biomarkers in different European populations will be made accessible to the scientific community through the FINDbase database (http://www.findbase.org) using the microattribution approach [4]. Also, in an effort to increase pharmacogenomics education and awareness among health care professionals, the Euro-PGx project coordinates the organization of pharmacogenomics educational activities in various European countries, namely the Golden Helix Pharmacogenomics Days (http://pharmacogenomicsdays.goldenhelix.org). Until June 2015, 15 different events have been organized in ten European, mostly developing, countries, with the expectation to expand these activities in other developing nations around the world.

Pharmacogenomics in clinical settings

Perhaps one of the most characteristic and noteworthy examples of success story in pharmacogenomics is the discovery of the association of the HLA-B*1502 allele with the devastating carbamazepine-induced Stevens-Johnson Syndrome/Toxic Epidermal Necrolysis (SJS/TEN) [5] and of the HLA-B*5801 allele with allopurinol-induced severe cutaneous adverse reactions [6] in Southeast Asia and particularly in Taiwan. Subsequently, a large clinical study conducted in Taiwan confirmed the benefit of HLA-B*1502 testing to prevent carbamazepine-induced SJS-TEN by using HLA-B*1502 screening to prospectively identify subjects at genetic risk for the condition [7]. This led the Taiwanese government to cover and reimburse the costs for HLA-B*1502 genetic testing since 2010.

From the numerous pharmacogenomics studies conducted to date, a large number of genomic biomarkers have been shown to be correlated with variable drug efficacy and/or toxicity. However, only a small fraction of these drugs have been approved by regulatory agencies to bear pharmacogenomic information in their labels. To facilitate exploitation of this valuable information from clinicians, who often lack the necessary genomics education, it is of utmost importance to make this knowledge readily available in a format that can be easily digested by clinicians. To fulfill this requirement, DruGeVar database (http://drugevar.genomicmedicinealliance.org) [8] was developed, representing an online knowledge portal for clinical pharmacogenomics which triangulates drugs with genes and pharmacogenomic biomarkers. This online resource includes those pharmacogenomic biomarkers that have been approved by regulatory agencies and allows, through a user-friendly data querying and visualization interface, formulation of queries that would guide clinicians to order the correct genetic test prior to prescribe a drug to a patient and by this, providing an individual theranostic service.

In addition, in order to record patients' pharmacogenomic biomarkers, a pharmacogenomic card has been proposed in Southeast Asia and the Ramathibodi Hospital in Thailand has launched a "pharmacogenomics" wallet card, aiming to summarize patients' HLA gene variant information predicting risk of developing SJS/TEN from specific drugs, a devastating and often fatal cutaneous adverse reaction [9]. Such pharmacogenomics card would be readily expandable to more drug/pharmacogenomic biomarkers to serve patients' needs, depending on the medication that they receive.

In Latin America, the Iberian American Network of Pharmacogenetics and Pharmacogenomics (RIBEF, created in 2006) aims to promote collaborative pharmacogenomics research in Iberoamerica. RIBEF currently consists of 43 research groups and more than 200 researchers with the main goals and principles to promote scientific studies among its members and clinical implementation of pharmacogenomics to improve drug efficacy and security with the ultimate goal of helping the health-care needs of neglected populations. As such, the aims of the Network are to develop human resources training, to produce research and to disseminate information in universities and hospitals, and to promote clinical implementation of pharmacogenomics. Up to date, RIBEF teaching programs and human resources training activities include over 400 events all over Latin America. Also, another goal of the RIBEF network is to develop research projects, among which are population pharmacogenomics studies of Iberoamerican populations. For that purpose, the CEIBA Consortium (Consorcio Europeo e Iberoamericano de Farmacogenética de Poblaciones) was established among the RIBEF members (Ibero-Spain and Portugal and Latino American Network of Pharmacogenomics) to study population pharmacogenomics of these populations. The MESTIFAR project aimed at determining variability of polymorphisms in genes involved in response to drugs in populations of different ethnic origin [Native Americans (Amerindian) and Mestizos (the result of post-Columbian admixture)]. In total, more than 6000 healthy volunteers have been evaluated, constituting one of the largest populations pharmacogenomics study conducted today. Besides population pharmacogenomics, the network has other ongoing projects that are related to clinical pharmacogenomics in neurology, psychiatry, cardiovascular and infectious diseases, etc., with up to a total of 31 scientific articles being published so far.

In Africa, there is a disproportionate burden of disease with the triple challenge caused by HIV/AIDS, tuberculosis, and malaria against a backdrop of an increasing burden of non-communicable diseases [10]. Genomic analyses have found that several genetic variants can provide increased resistance or susceptibility to HIV infections [11]. Moreover, more than 80 % of therapeutic drugs used in the management of these diseases/conditions are metabolized by cytochrome P450 (CYP) enzymes that exhibit genetic polymorphisms. Recent studies have provided evidence of a huge variability in the pattern of genetic variations in the CYP genes among African populations that was translated into differences in drug response [12].

Lastly, in the Middle East, pharmacogenomics research started in 1996 in the United Arab Emirates (UAE), initially involving erythrocyte glucose-6-phosphate dehydrogenase deficiency (G-6-PD) related with drug-induced hemolytic anemia [13] and later arylamine N-acetyltransferase (NAT2) [14]. Also, the *CYP2D6* pharmacogenomic marker allele frequencies were investigated in the Emirati population, including reporting of four novel *CYP2D6* variants [15], while a warfarin pharmacogenomics study is currently under way for the Emirati population [16] (AlJaibeji and coworkers; unpublished). These studies sparked an interest from Dubai Hospital to integrate pharmacogenomics information for chemotherapeutic agents, while the UAE Health Authority policy of reporting adverse drug reaction in the UAE requires expert pharmacogenomics recommendation within the first 24 h related to each adverse drug reactions reported [17].

Mapping of stakeholders in genomic medicine

A plethora of key players and stakeholders compose the genomic medicine puzzle, whose level of genomics awareness and views varies significantly. Systematic mapping of the views and opinions of the various stakeholders on genomic medicine would positively impact on better understanding the corresponding policy environment and the role of the relevant key stakeholders in the field, on identifying the main opportunities and obstacles for evidence-informed policy-making and timely implementation in pharmacogenomics and genomic medicine, and on prioritizing the various stakeholders' needs, in an effort to better plan the undertaking of various measures in genome-based health care, i.e., from the perspective of public health genomics.

Recently, Mitropoulou and coworkers undertook such initiative to assess the level of support or opposition to pharmacogenomics and genomic medicine in Greece [18]. This survey indicated that the majority of the key stakeholders, namely academic institutions and research organizations, the bioethics council, private genetic laboratories, citizens, pharmaceutical and biotechnology companies, genetics and genomics professional associations, private health insurance, industry, pharmacists, and physicians (both geneticists and other specialties), are highly supportive of pharmacogenomics and genomic medicine in Greece. On the contrary, the Ministry of Health and the social health insurance funds oppose to the implementation of genomic medicine, while the Greek National Medicines Organization displays a neutral stance, possibly since the cost-effectiveness and cost-benefit of a pharmacogenomics approach is not yet fully proven, proper legislation to oversee the operation of private genetic testing laboratories is not yet in place, or simply because they fear that reimbursement of genetic testing could increase rather than decrease the overall health-care expenditure. These latter stakeholders have high intervention power against the implementation of pharmacogenomics and genomic medicine into mainstream clinical practice. Subsequently, several opportunities and obstacles in the pharmacogenomics and genomic medicine policy-making in Greece are derived from this analysis, based on the current position and intervention potential of the key stakeholders. Similar analysis is currently on its way in Middle Eastern countries to determine the current position and views of the corresponding stakeholders in these countries.

Also, insufficient genomics education and lack of genomics awareness among health-care professionals and the general public are two perspectives of the same issue, which hinders the smooth incorporation of genomic medicine into clinical practice [19]. On the one hand, the vast majority of health-care professionals state that they feel insufficiently trained in genomics to be able to engage with the delivery of genome-based services [18], while on the other hand, patients and the broader public tend to have low genomic literacy, which impairs their capacity to successfully integrate genome-based information into their personal decision-making, which is a challenge for public health genomics and here especially for the field of health literacy [20]. On top of this, genomics education is not uniformly provided in various academic institutions worldwide, with the USA and Western European countries to lead the way and the Southeastern European countries lagging behind. A recent survey in 175 departments from 98 universities from 11 Southeastern European countries indicated that for a significant number of universities, the topic of pharmacogenetics/pharmacogenomics is not included at all in their undergraduate and postgraduate curricula in health sciences [21]. Also, studies surveyed Greek and Italian physicians indicated that only a small fraction of those feel competent enough either to propose a genetic test for their patients and/or to interpret the results from such a test [21, 22]. These findings are in sharp contrast with the current reality of pharmacogenomics education in northern European countries, where pharmacogenomics are more uniformly and extensively taught and highlight the need for a more in-depth genomics education, either with the incorporation of pharmacogenomics and genomic medicine in their undergraduate or graduate training, or in the form of continuous medical education seminars. These studies might provide the basis to harmonize pharmacogenomics education in southeast European countries with those of northwest European countries, such that it would directly impact on a smoother and timely integration of pharmacogenomics into mainstream medical practice.

As in other resource-limited regions, in Latin America there are very few postgraduate programs focusing on genomics [23]. Finally, in Africa, the high cost of genomic services and low private investment is compounded by a relatively low level of medical professionals with understanding of genomics [24]. In addition, a recent attempt in sub-Saharan Africa to triangulate the views of multiple stakeholders related to sickle-cell disease (SCD), namely doctors, parents with SCD-affected children, and adult SCD patients towards prenatal diagnosis of SCD, showed several discrepancies. The majority accepted the principle of prenatal genetic diagnosis for SCD (78.7, 89.8, and 89.2 %, respectively); however, parents (62.5 %) were more in favor of termination of SCD-affected pregnancy, than doctors and adults patients (36.1 and 40.9 % acceptance, respectively). These differential attitudes signal potential value-based conflicts on the horizon and can usefully inform the future policy actions in the African continent, as OMICS biotechnologies are increasingly employed in global health [25]. Specially, there are encouraging evidence of participation of African-based scientists in studying the genomics of monogenic diseases [26–29] and multifactorial conditions [30]. These data are concretely assisting the effective practice of genomic medicine, that is well established in South Africa [31], in some Northern African countries [32, 33], and recently initiated in Central Africa [34]. In addition, regional initiatives such as the launch of the Southern Africa Human Genome Project by the South African government [35] have been boosted by international funding agencies and academic institutions, through major programs such as the Malaria Genomic Epidemiology Network (MalariaGEN) (http://www.malariagen.net/), the Human Heredity and Health in Africa (H3Africa) program [36], and the African Genome Variation Project [37]. The fortunate association of international consortia efforts will enhance the regional and local initiatives to build the capacity in research skills and overcome the barriers for the use of genomics to address the disease burden of Africans.

Current populations in Latin America are characterized by high and heterogeneous levels of admixture, arising from the history of these regions and corresponding to different patterns of mating between individuals of Native American, European, and African descent [38]. As an interesting international example, the National Institute of Genomic Medicine was built in Mexico with public funds [39], with several publications in the fields of population genomics and medical genomics [40, 41]. Other Latin American countries, such as Brazil and Colombia, have had success in the implementation of genetic and genomic approaches for the study of several human diseases with high epidemiological impact in those resource-limited countries [42–45], while an equally important element that is helping to implement genomics in these countries is the availability of commercial tests, by service providers abroad.

Next-generation sequencing and genomic medicine

The next-generation sequencing (NGS) technology, which was introduced 8 years ago, marked the beginning of a new era concerning the analysis of human genome sequences [46–49]. Before the advent of NGS, Sanger sequencing was widely used for screening variants potentially causing monogenic and complex diseases which were located in coding and regulatory genomic regions. However, studies involving numerous genes or large genomic regions were particularly challenging due to intrinsic technical limitations (e.g., read length encompassing up to 700 base-pairs (bp) per reaction). On the contrary, the NGS approach allows simultaneously analyzing millions of bp in only hours, thereby facilitating large-scale exploration of the human genome [1]. The first NGS studies and many projects nowadays have been focused on researching novel recessive disease-related sequence variants, particularly those caused by homozygous mutations. Such variants are relatively easy to identify because most are novel and/or are exclusively present in several members of the same family. This allows easy screening of candidate variants in public SNP databases and filtering them between affected and non-affected individuals from the same family. Successful screening attempts have also been described for monogenic dominant Mendelian disorders. However, this approach implies more drawbacks because heterozygous mutations (logically) occur more frequently, thereby involving complex filtering to select potentially deleterious mutations. NGS has not been widely used for some complex pathologies in which several variants might contribute towards the phenotype, because data analysis highlights remarkable complexity, especially for simultaneous interactive network exploration.

Three main approaches are normally used at present. They mainly depend on the length of the genome region being analyzed: whole-genome sequencing (WGS), whole-exome sequencing (WES), and custom target sequencing microarrays (TSM) [1]. WGS is mainly used for research purposes while WES and TSM are used for both research and diagnosis. Most academic and private technological platforms for the above are located in high-income countries. This might be due to the high cost of NGS technology, such as new-generation sequencers and bioinformatics platforms. However, resource-limited countries have performed interesting studies by using NGS outsourcing services. For instance, using such NGS services in Colombia has led to identifying novel genes and mutations causing monogenic diseases [43, 44, 50]. Furthermore, innovative diagnostic approaches have been proposed for pathologies having overlapping phenotypes and which are caused by various genes [43, 44]. The available data regarding the genomes of particular mammalian species has enabled large-scale comparative genomics approaches leading to dissecting loci related to evolution mechanisms and potentially contributing towards human diseases [51]. Moreover, complex pathologies such as female infertility have also been explored via NGS (Fonseca et al. in press).

Economic evaluation in pharmacogenomics

Considering the fact that genome-based drug treatment can contribute towards the reduction of national healthcare expenditures, mostly by reducing hospitalization due to the various adverse drug reactions, this need is more than ever urgent, particularly in resource-limited countries, which in many cases have vast fiscal deficits [52].

Although the field of economic evaluation in genomic medicine, pharmacogenomics, and public health genomics is currently in its infancy, the majority of the economic evaluation studies indicate that genotype-guided therapy can be cost-effective and of high cost-benefit in several countries. Particularly related to resource-limited countries, initial economic evaluation studies in the Thai population indicated that HLA-B*15:02-guided carbamazepine treatment is cost-effective in Thailand compared to conventional treatment and can reduce the carbamazepine-induced severe adverse drug reactions [53, 54]. As a result, the Thai government is now providing HLA-B*15:02 testing as a standard of care, while the same findings were reported for the Singaporean population, when cost-effectiveness of HLA-B*1502 genotyping in adult patients with newly diagnosed epilepsy was assessed [55].

Similarly, a recent study to evaluate cost-effectiveness of warfarin treatment in Croatian elderly ischemic stroke patients with atrial fibrillation indicated that 97.07 over 89.12 % of patients belonging to the

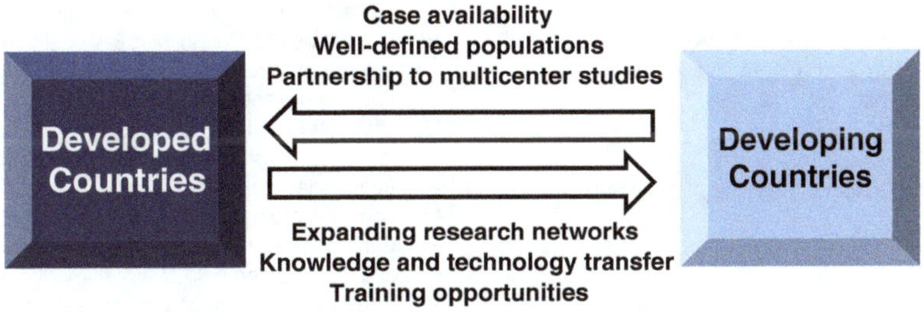

Fig. 1 Encouraging collaboration between developed and developing/resource-limited countries in the field of genomic medicine. While developing countries will benefit from training opportunities, knowledge transfer, and expanding research networks, developed countries are also likely to benefit through comparative work and multicenter projects involving cases with rare diseases or unique clinical features from well-defined populations

pharmacogenomics-based and the control group, respectively, did not present major complications, while the incremental cost-effectiveness ratio of the pharmacogenomics-based versus the control groups was estimated at €31,225/quality-adjusted life year (QALY), indicating that pharmacogenomics-guided warfarin treatment may represent a cost-effective therapy option for the management of elderly patients with atrial fibrillation who developed ischemic stroke in Croatia [56].

Conclusions and future perspectives

Implementation of genomic medicine in resource-limited environments will be only made possible though stronger collaboration in genomics research between developed and developing/resource-limited countries, which is likely to create benefits for all parties. To this end, developing countries will undoubtedly benefit from training opportunities, knowledge transfer, and expanding transnational networks, while developed countries are likely to benefit through comparative work and multicenter projects on families with rare diseases or unique clinical features (Fig. 1) [57].

The outcomes of the studies, outlined in the previous paragraphs, indicate that, as far as genomic medicine is concerned, developing countries may be resource-limited but are also potential-rich in producing data in various genomic medicine-related disciplines, from the perspective of public health genomics. Although this summary of examples depicting successful implementation of genomic medicine in resource-limited countries is far from complete, it sets a paradigm for replication in other countries, contributing towards not only acquiring more and better insights into the requirements to implement genomic medicine in these environments but also harmonizing the strategies and policies for the faster and smoother adoption of genomic medicine practices in the various national health-care systems.

Competing interests

KM is scientific advisor of the Golden Helix Foundation. AB, MTML, and GPP are members of the Scientific Advisory Committee of the Genomic Medicine Alliance. DAF is supported by research grants from Colciencias and VCTI-UAN. The authors declare that they have no competing interests.

Authors' contributions

KM and GPP conceived the theme of the article. KM, HAJ, DAF, PL, CLC, ZM, WC, MTML, AL, AB, BRA and GPP drafted the manuscript. All authors read and approved the final manuscript.

Acknowledgements

This article was encouraged by the Genomic Medicine Alliance Public Health Genomics Working Group.

Author details

[1]The Golden Helix Foundation, London, UK. [2]University of Maastricht, Maastricht, The Netherlands. [3]Department of Pathology, College of Medicine and Health Sciences, United Arab Emirates University, Al-Ain, United Arab Emirates. [4]Laboratory of NeuroPsychiatric Genetics, Biomedical Sciences Research Group, School of Medicine, Universidad Antonio Nariño, Bogotá, Colombia. [5]Unidad de Genética, Grupo GENIUROS, Escuela de Medicina y Ciencias de la Salud, Universidad del Rosario, Bogotá, Colombia. [6]Division of Human Genetics, Faculty of Health Sciences, University of Cape Town, Cape Town, South Africa. [7]Genome Quebec, Montreal, Canada. [8]Department of Pharmacology, Faculty of Medicine, University of Malaya, Kuala Lumpur, Malaysia. [9]Department of Pathology, Medical Genomic Center, Ramathibodi Hospital, Faculty of Medicine, Mahidol University, Bangkok, Thailand. [10]Laboratory for International Alliance on Genomic Research, RIKEN Center for Integrative Medical Sciences, Yokohama, Japan. [11]Institute of Biomedical Sciences, Academia Sinica, Taipei, Taiwan. [12]CICAB Clinical Research Center, Extremadura University Hospital and Medical School, Badajoz, Spain. [13]Department of Pharmacy, University of Patras School of Health Sciences, Patras, Greece.

References

1. McCarthy JJ, McLeod HL, Ginsburg GS. Genomic medicine: a decade of successes, challenges, and opportunities. Sci Transl Med. 2013;5(189):189sr4.
2. Mardis ER. A decade's perspective on DNA sequencing technology. Nature. 2011;470(7333):198–203.
3. Mitropoulos K, Johnson L, Vozikis A, Patrinos GP. Relevance of pharmacogenomics for developing countries in Europe. Drug Metabol Drug Interact. 2011;26(4):143–6.
4. Giardine B, Borg J, Higgs DR, Peterson KR, Philipsen S, Maglott D, et al. Systematic documentation and analysis of human genetic variation in hemoglobinopathies using the microattribution approach. Nat Genet. 2011;43(4):295–301.
5. Chung WH, Hung SI, Hong HS, Hsih MS, Yang LC, Ho HC, et al. Medical genetics: a marker for Stevens-Johnson syndrome. Nature. 2004;428(6982):486.
6. Hung SI, Chung WH, Liou LB, Chu CC, Lin M, Huang HP, et al. HLA-B*5801 allele as a genetic marker for severe cutaneous adverse reactions caused by allopurinol. Proc Natl Acad Sci USA. 2005;102(11):4134–9.
7. Chen P, Lin JJ, Lu CS, Ong CT, Hsieh PF, Yang CC, et al. Carbamazepine-induced toxic effects and HLA-B*1502 screening in Taiwan. N Engl J Med. 2011;364(12):1126–33.
8. Dalabira E, Viennas E, Daki E, Komianou A, Bartsakoulia M, Poulas K, et al. DruGeVar: an online resource triangulating drugs with genes and genomic biomarkers for clinical pharmacogenomics. Public Health Genomics. 2014;17(5-6):265–71.
9. Borchers AT, Lee JL, Naguwa SM, Cheema GS, Gershwin ME. Stevens-Johnson syndrome and toxic epidermal necrolysis. Autoimmun Rev. 2008;7(8):598–605.
10. Niemz A, Ferguson TM, Boyle DS. Point-of-care nucleic acid testing for infectious diseases. Trends Biotechnol. 2011;29(5):240–50.
11. Sirugo G, Hennig BJ, Adeyemo AA, Matimba A, Newport MJ, Ibrahim ME, et al. Genetic studies of African populations: an overview on disease susceptibility and response to vaccines and therapeutics. Hum Genet. 2008;123(6):557–98.
12. Dandara C, Swart M, Mpeta B, Wonkam A, Masimirembwa C. Cytochrome P450 pharmacogenetics in African populations: implications for public health. Expert Opin Drug Metab Toxicol. 2014;10(6):769–85.
13. Bayoumi RA, Nur-E-Kamal MS, Tadayyon M, Mohamed KK, Mahboob BH, Qureshi MM, et al. Molecular characterization of erythrocyte glucose-6-phosphate dehydrogenase deficiency in Al-Ain District, United Arab Emirates. Hum Hered. 1996;46(3):136–41.
14. Woolhouse NM, Qureshi MM, Bastaki SM, Patel M, Abdulrazzaq Y, Bayoumi RA. Polymorphic N-acetyltransferase (NAT2) genotyping of Emiratis. Pharmacogenetics. 1997;7(1):73–82.
15. Qumsieh RY, Ali BR, Abdulrazzaq YM, Osman O, Akawi NA, Bastaki SM. Identification of new alleles and the determination of alleles and genotypes frequencies at the CYP2D6 gene in Emiratis. PloS One. 2011;6(12):e28943.
16. Fortina P, Al Khaja N, Al Ali MT, Hamzeh AR, Nair P, Innocenti F, et al. Genomics into healthcare: the 5th Pan Arab Human Genetics Conference and 2013 Golden Helix Symposium. Hum Mutat. 2014;35(5):637–40.
17. Abu Dhabi HAA. Reporting adverse reaction. http://www.haad.ae/haad. Accessed 29-Mar-2015.
18. Mitropoulou C, Mai Y, van Schaik RH, Vozikis A, Patrinos GP. Stakeholder analysis in pharmacogenomics and genomic medicine in Greece. Public Health Genomics. 2014;17(5-6):280–6.

19. Reydon TA, Kampourakis K, Patrinos GP. Genetics, genomics and society: the responsibilities of scientists for science communication and education. Personalized Medicine. 2012;9(6):633–43.
20. Syurina E, Brankovic I, Probst-Hensch N, Brand A. Genome-based health literacy: a new challenge for public health genomics. Public Health Genomics. 2011;14(4-5):201–10.
21. Pisanu C, Tsermpini EE, Mavroidi E, Katsila T, Patrinos GP, Squassina A. Assessment of the pharmacogenomics educational environment in Southeast Europe. Public Health Genomics. 2014;17(5-6):272–9.
22. Mai Y, Mitropoulou C, Papadopoulou XE, Vozikis A, Cooper DN, van Schaik RH, et al. Critical appraisal of the views of healthcare professionals with respect to pharmacogenomics and personalized medicine in Greece. Personalized Medicine. 2014;11(1):15–26.
23. Palacios R, Collado-Vides J. Development of genomic sciences in Mexico: a good start and a long way to go. PLoS Comput Biol. 2007;3(9):1670–3.
24. Wonkam A, Njamnshi AK, Angwafo 3rd FF. Knowledge and attitudes concerning medical genetics amongst physicians and medical students in Cameroon (sub-Saharan Africa). Genet Med. 2006;8(6):331–8.
25. Wonkam A, Hurst S. A call for policy action in sub-Saharan Africa to rethink diagnostics for pregnancy affected by sickle cell disease: differential views of medical doctors, parents and adult patients predict value conflicts in Cameroon. OMICS. 2014;18(7):472–80.
26. Mercier S, Küry S, Shaboodien G, Houniet DT, Khumalo NP, Bou-Hanna C, et al. Mutations in FAM111B cause hereditary fibrosing poikiloderma with tendon contracture, myopathy, and pulmonary fibrosis. Am J Hum Genet. 2013;93(6):1100–7.
27. Mtatiro SN, Singh T, Rooks H, Mgaya J, Mariki H, Soka D, et al. Genome wide association study of fetal hemoglobin in sickle cell anemia in Tanzania. PloS One. 2014;9(11):e111464.
28. Wonkam A, Ngo Bitoungui VJ, Vorster AA, Ramesar R, Cooper RS, Tayo B, et al. Association of variants at BCL11A and HBS1L-MYB with hemoglobin F and hospitalization rates among sickle cell patients in Cameroon. PloS One. 2014;9(3):e92506.
29. Wonkam A. Letter to the editor regarding "GJB2, GJB6 or GJA1 genes should not be investigated in routine in non syndromic deafness in people of sub-Saharan African descent". Int J Pediatr Otorhinolaryngol. 2015;79(4):632–3.
30. Tekola Ayele F, Adeyemo A, Finan C, Hailu E, Sinnott P, Burlinson ND, et al. HLA class II locus and susceptibility to podoconiosis. N Engl J Med. 2012;366(13):1200–8.
31. Beighton P, Fieggen K, Wonkam A, Ramesar R, Greenberg J. UCT's contribution to medical genetics in Africa - from the past into the future. South African medical journal (Suid-Afrikaanse tydskrif vir geneeskunde). 2012;102(6):446–8.
32. Chaabouni-Bouhamed H. Tunisia: communities and community genetics. Community Genet. 2008;11(6):313–23.
33. El-Beshlawy A, El-Shekha A, Momtaz M, Said F, Hamdy M, Osman O, et al. Prenatal diagnosis for thalassaemia in Egypt: what changed parents' attitude? Prenat Diagn. 2012;32(8):777–82.
34. Wonkam A, Tekendo CN, Sama DJ, Zambo H, Dahoun S, Béna F, et al. Initiation of a medical genetics service in sub-Saharan Africa: experience of prenatal diagnosis in Cameroon. Eur J Med Genet. 2011;54(4):e399–404.
35. Pepper MS. Launch of the Southern African Human Genome Programme. South African medical journal (Suid-Afrikaanse tydskrif vir geneeskunde). 2011;101(5):287–8.
36. H3Africa Consortium, Rotimi C, Abayomi A, Abimiku A, Adabayeri VM, Adebamowo C, et al. Research capacity. Enabling the genomic revolution in Africa. Science. 2014;344(6190):1346–8.
37. Gurdasani D, Carstensen T, Tekola-Ayele F, Pagani L, Tachmazidou I, Hatzikotoulas K, et al. The African Genome Variation Project shapes medical genetics in Africa. Nature. 2015;517(7534):327–32.
38. Ruiz-Linares A, Adhikari K, Acuña-Alonzo V, Quinto-Sanchez M, Jaramillo C, Arias W, et al. Admixture in Latin America: geographic structure, phenotypic diversity and self-perception of ancestry based on 7,342 individuals. PLoS Genet. 2014;10(9):e1004572.
39. Jimenez-Sanchez G, Silva-Zolezzi I, Hidalgo A, March S. Genomic medicine in Mexico: initial steps and the road ahead. Genome Res. 2008;18(8):1191–8.
40. Silva-Zolezzi I, Hidalgo-Miranda A, Estrada-Gil J, Fernandez-Lopez JC, Uribe-Figueroa L, Contreras A, et al. Analysis of genomic diversity in Mexican Mestizo populations to develop genomic medicine in Mexico. Proc Natl Acad Sci USA. 2009;106(21):8611–6.
41. Moreno-Estrada A, Gignoux CR, Fernández-López JC, Zakharia F, Sikora M, Contreras AV, et al. The genetics of Mexico recapitulates Native American substructure and affects biomedical traits. Science. 2014;344(6189):1280–5.
42. Passos-Bueno MR, Bertola D, Horovitz DD, de Faria Ferraz VE, Brito LA. Genetics and genomics in Brazil: a promising future. Mol Genet Genomic Med. 2014;2(4):280–91.
43. Ortega-Recalde O, Vergara JI, Fonseca DJ, Ríos X, Mosquera H, Bermúdez OM, et al. Whole-exome sequencing enables rapid determination of xeroderma pigmentosum molecular etiology. PloS One. 2014;8(6):e64692.
44. Pinto WB, Oliveira AS, Souza PV. Whole exome sequencing identifies three recessive FIG 4-mutations in an apparently dominant pedigree with Charcot-Marie-Tooth disease. Neuromuscul Disord. 2015;25(4):359–60.
45. Benitez BA, Forero DA, Arboleda GH, Granados LA, Yunis JJ, Fernandez W, et al. Exploration of genetic susceptibility factors for Parkinson's disease in a South American sample. J Genet. 2010;89(2):229–32.
46. Hodges E, Xuan Z, Balija V, Kramer M, Molla MN, Smith SW, et al. Genome-wide in situ exon capture for selective resequencing. Nat Genet. 2007;39(12):1522–7.
47. Albert TJ, Molla MN, Muzny DM, Nazareth L, Wheeler D, Song X, et al. Direct selection of human genomic loci by microarray hybridization. Nat Methods. 2007;4(11):903–5.
48. Shendure J, Ji H. Next-generation DNA sequencing. Nat Biotechnol. 2008;26(10):1135–45.
49. Gnirke A, Melnikov A, Maguire J, Rogov P, LeProust EM, Brockman W, et al. Solution hybrid selection with ultra-long oligonucleotides for massively parallel targeted sequencing. Nat Biotechnol. 2009;27(2):182–9.
50. Diggle CP, Parry DA, Logan CV, Laissue P, Rivera C, Restrepo CM, et al. Prostaglandin transporter mutations cause pachydermoperiostosis with myelofibrosis. Hum Mutat. 2012;33(8):1175–81.
51. Prada CF, Laissue P. A high resolution map of mammalian X chromosome fragile regions assessed by large-scale comparative genomics. Mamm Genome. 2014;25(11-12):618–35.
52. Snyder SR, Mitropoulou C, Patrinos GP, Williams MS. Economic evaluation of pharmacogenomics: a value-based approach to pragmatic decision making in the face of complexity. Public Health Genomics. 2014;17(5-6):256–64.
53. Rattanavipapong W, Koopitakkajorn T, Praditsitthikorn N, Mahasirimongkol S, Teerawattananon Y. Economic evaluation of HLA-B*15:02 screening for carbamazepine-induced severe adverse drug reactions in Thailand. Epilepsia. 2013;54(9):1628–38.
54. Grosse SD. Assessing cost-effectiveness in healthcare: history of the $50,000 per QALY threshold. Expert Rev Pharmacoecon Outcomes Res. 2008;8(2):165–78.
55. Dong D, Sung C, Finkelstein EA. Cost-effectiveness of HLA-B*1502 genotyping in adult patients with newly diagnosed epilepsy in Singapore. Neurology. 2012;79(12):1259–67.
56. Mitropoulou C, Fragoulakis V, Bozina N, Vozikis A, Supe S, Bozina T, et al. Economic evaluation of pharmacogenomic-guided warfarin treatment for elderly Croatian atrial fibrillation patients with ischemic stroke. Pharmacogenomics. 2015;16(2):137–48.
57. Cooper DN, Brand A, Dolzan V, Fortina P, Innocenti F, Lee MT, et al. Bridging genomics research between developed and developing countries: the Genomic Medicine Alliance. Per Med. 2014;11(7):615–23.

4

Genomics in the renal clinic - translating nephrogenetics for clinical practice

Andrew Mallett[1,2,3*], Christopher Corney[1,2], Hugh McCarthy[4,5], Stephen I. Alexander[4,5,6] and Helen Healy[1,2]

Abstract

Genetic Renal Disease (GRD) presents to mainstream clinicians as a mixture of kidney-specific as well as multi-organ entities, many with highly variable phenotype-genotype relationships. The rapid increase in knowledge and reduced cost of sequencing translate to new and additional approaches to clinical care. Specifically, genomic technologies to test for known genes, the development of pathways to research potential new genes and the collection of registry data on patients with mutations allow better prediction of outcomes. The aim of such approaches is to maximise personal and health-system utility from genomics for those affected by nephrogenetic disorders.

Keywords: Nephrology, Genomics, Translation

Introduction

Chronic kidney disease (CKD) in paediatric and adult populations produces a significant burden of morbidity and mortality [1] and frequently has a genetic aetiology [2]. However, Genetic Renal Disease (GRD) itself represents a heterogeneous and poorly defined group of, often rare, disorders. GRD is the cause for 10 % of kidney disease in adult renal practice [3] and up to 10–15 % and 50 %, respectively, of adults and children commencing dialysis [4]. The emergence of genomic technologies presents opportunities for better delineation of these conditions and for further gene discovery, thus overcoming genetics exceptionalism to enable optimised clinical care and providing the opportunity to develop targeted therapies. To realise this potential for patients, families and their physicians, managing increasing volumes and complexity of genetic and clinical information requires a multifaceted novel approach.

Main text

Over the past decade, genomics and genomic technologies have resulted in a greater integration of genetics into healthcare [5]. Whilst sporadic renal genetics clinics (RGCs) have been established, there is little data on the specific models employed. RGCs attempt to provide a better way for patients and families with rare nephrogenetic diseases in accessing appropriate diagnostics, useful disease-specific information, genetic counselling, and highly specialised therapies in a centralised patient-focussed approach.

Currently, these clinics are located in tertiary hospitals, accessible to patients with rare/genetic diseases, with specialised nephrologists with genetic training and clinical geneticists, genetic counsellors, specialised nurses and allied health with whom to operate combined clinics. Additionally, RGCs need close contact with diagnostic laboratories and scientists. Such multidisciplinary clinics are increasingly necessary for delivering care in rare genetic disease [6]. Examples include ophthalmology, cardiology, oncology, hepatology, neurology and otolaryngology. These innovative clinical models have been encouraged as part of health service delivery reorganisation to deliver more patient-focussed care [7]. Successful models share in common an interaction between clinical geneticists, sub-specialists, genetic counsellors, speciality nursing staff and other allied health staff with ongoing collaborations with molecular geneticists and scientists. One challenge is a general lack of sub-specialised professional staff; however, targeted training and education are likely to overcome this in the medium-long term. Another challenge is patient transition

* Correspondence: Andrew.mallett@health.qld.gov.au
[1]Kidney Health Service & Conjoint Kidney Research Laboratory, Royal Brisbane and Women's Hospital, Butterfield Street, Herston, Brisbane, Qld 4029, Australia
[2]Centre for Kidney Disease Research, CKD.QLD and Centre for Chronic Disease, School of Medicine, The University of Queensland, Brisbane, Australia
Full list of author information is available at the end of the article

from paediatric to adult healthcare, which may be remedied by active involvement of paediatric nephrologists within the RGC in order to provide lifespan and whole family care. A third potential challenge is the pitfalls associated with genetic testing, including pre-symptomatic testing in at-risk individuals, prenatal diagnostics, non-paternity/maternity and medically actionable incidental findings in whole exomic or genomic sequencing. Within the RGC, patient consultation with clinical geneticists and genetic counsellors is ideally placed as a standard-of-care to minimise such risks whilst maximising patient benefit and support. Further, additional specialists are required for GRDs with extra-renal involvement, such as oncologists and endocrinologists for *WT1* disorders, metabolic physicians and neurologists for mitochondrial disorders and hepatologists and ophthalmologists for ciliopathies. Supportive medical administrators and molecular geneticists enhance the model further. An RGC should be no different, with natural implications for broader patient management such as medical interventions, therapies and genetic counselling.

GRDs are phenotypically diverse and attributed to growing numbers of known genes, with increasingly complex phenotype-genotype relationships. Genomics enables rapid diagnosis of mutations in known nephrogenes. This includes very efficient sequencing of many known genes simultaneously and effectively for ciliopathies [8], podocytopathies and glomerular disease [9, 10], complement dysregulopathies [11], congenital abnormalities of the kidney and urinary tract (CAKUT) [12], tubular disease and nephrocalcinosis/nephrolithiasis [13]. This may be via whole exome or genome sequencing, or targeted and prioritised gene panel screening of these. For several diagnoses, precise genetic diagnosis drives therapeutic decisions. Examples of this include steroid-resistant nephrotic syndrome where therapies with significant side-effect profiles are unlikely to be effective, Alport syndrome in which the early instigation of renin-angiotensin system blockade may delay renal dysfunction progression and atypical haemolytic uraemic syndrome in which some genotypes (*CFH*) are associated with more pressing requirements for eculizumab or combined liver-kidney transplantation whilst others (*C5, DGKE, MMACHC*) may confer altered responses to medical therapy. There are also indirect and surprising findings. For instance, where 12 genes are responsible for only 6 % of unselected paediatric CAKUT cases [12], 14 genes are causative for 15 % of similarly unselected nephrolithiasis/nephrocalcinosis [13]. Intriguingly, CAKUT is a common paediatric nephropathy of potentially and well-recognised genetic aetiology, where nephrolithiasis/nephrocalcinosis is a common adult renal presentation of potentially though "rare" genetic aetiology. Genomics is altering prevailing concepts of kidney disease, including diagnosis and therapy, whilst translating to changes in nephrological practice.

Amongst other applications, genomics has also opened the frontier to discovery of undescribed causative genes. A genomic approach provides a research pathway to discovery in those with individually rare undiagnosed GRDs. For example, the identification of a specific *LMX1B* mutation associated with a renal-limited rather than multisystem form of Nail-Patella syndrome [14] challenges classical phenotype-genotype relationships. Other examples include the findings of podocyte-related gene mutations in some patients with histological membranoproliferative glomerulonephritis [10], mutations in a ciliary gene (*TTC21B*) causing focal segmental glomerulosclerosis [15] and mutations in a recently described gene (*DGKE*) resulting in atypical haemolytic uraemic syndrome [16], membranoproliferative glomerulonephritis [17] and steroid-resistant nephrotic syndrome [10]. Similarly, the discovery of mutations in DNA damage repair genes (*ZNF423; CEP164*) causing nephronophthisis [18] expands pathophysiological understanding. Such advances have potential implications for future directed approaches to treatment, as these are likely to be underpinned by accurate understanding of disease pathogenesis. The autosomal recessive spectrum of nephronophthisis and related ciliopathies continues to present promising opportunity for gene discovery utilising genomic technologies [19–21], a necessary prequel to translational proteomics [22].

There are many specific examples of the rapidly expanding diagnostic success of massively parallel sequencing (MPS). An instance has been Autosomal Dominant Tubulointerstitial Kidney Disease, a subset of which was chronically refractory to MPS [23] though subsequently found to be due to specific *MUC1* mutations. Further, accurate genomic sequencing is notoriously difficult for Autosomal Dominant Polycystic Kidney Disease (*PKD1* and *PKD2* mutations) due to homology with pseudogenes [24]. This assumes significance as this is the most common potentially lethal monogenic inherited disease amongst humans. Whilst genetic approaches have overcome these obstacles for diagnostic purposes [25, 26], they highlight that genomic studies may not always adequately resolve specific GRDs and that one needs to be cognisant of technological limitations, including copy number variations [27], read depth, coverage of regions of interest, a relative lack of bioinformaticians in the healthcare system and incomplete knowledge. The utilisation of family-based bioinformatics, such as trios, in genomic studies for gene discovery and diagnosis [28] appears crucial, especially when a complex clinical phenotype has not been appreciated [29].

For many GRDs, only a fraction of the genetic causes is known. There are three major issues that dominate the application of new genetics to kidney disease. Firstly, the increasing heterogeneity of phenotypes linked to genes, secondly, many clinical phenotypes have numerous differing genetic and undiagnosed causes, and thirdly, frequent extra-renal organ involvement in GRDs. Whilst many genetic causes can be identified, variants of uncertain significance may be found. In such cases, intra-family segregation analysis or functional study of such variants in pre-clinical non-human, fibroblast, or autologous self-organising renal organoid model systems [30] may be utilised to clarify variant significance. Families and individuals in whom a genetic cause seems likely can then be directed into discovery programmes to illuminate their disease. Therefore, this increasingly variable and rapidly changing field now needs a co-ordinated team approach linking patients, clinicians and scientists. This may have health economic benefits within the context of increased uptake of emerging genomic technologies in the RGC, whilst due caution is required with regard to local legislative, regulatory, health funding and insurance environments.

A recent Norwegian population study suggests that the magnitude of undiagnosed GRD may be as large as diagnosed GRD [31]. These findings highlight the importance of epidemiological and registry studies as an adjunct to genomic diagnostics or discovery studies. Epidemiological investigation is critical to describe and target nephrogenetic conditions for investigation utilising genomic technologies. Particularly to prevent confusion when disease or genotype frequency estimations reported for single-centre or highly selected cohorts [32] have resulted in over-estimation. This becomes apparent when large multicenter cohorts are further examined [12] or when interrogation of such cohorts for highly defined phenotypes is undertaken [33].

Conclusions

In conclusion, an initial step for nephrogenetic clinical translation is to progress a conversation defining patient-centric priorities within a changing context of clinical care and genomic technologies. We postulate that this involves reconceptualising clinical interfaces, applying such genomics for clinical diagnosis of known nephrogenes, utilising genomics in research to discover new genetic aetiologies and furthering epidemiological investigation of GRD. The RGC is a proposed multidisciplinary construct potentially capable of incorporating and actioning such changes. The aim of such an approach is to maximise personal and health-system benefit from genomics for those affected by nephrogenetic disorders. This approach reflects the increasing likelihood for the explanation of the majority of inheritable causes for kidney disease and, in the future, defined and effective treatments.

Abbreviations

CAKUT: Congenital abnormalities of the kidney and urinary tract; GRD: Genetic Renal Disease; MPS: Massively parallel sequencing; RGC: Renal genetics clinic.

Competing interests

AM has received a travel grant and honorarium from Amgen. The other authors have no competing interests.

Authors' contributions

AM, CC, HM, HH, SA have made substantial contributions to the conception and have been involved in the drafting of the manuscript. All authors have given final approval of the final version to be published.

Author details

[1]Kidney Health Service & Conjoint Kidney Research Laboratory, Royal Brisbane and Women's Hospital, Butterfield Street, Herston, Brisbane, Qld 4029, Australia. [2]Centre for Kidney Disease Research, CKD.QLD and Centre for Chronic Disease, School of Medicine, The University of Queensland, Brisbane, Australia. [3]Centre for Rare Diseases Research, Institute for Molecular Bioscience, The University of Queensland, Brisbane, Australia. [4]Department of Paediatric Nephrology, Children's Hospital at Westmead, Sydney, Australia. [5]Centre for Kidney Research, University of Sydney, Sydney, Australia. [6]Discipline of Paediatrics and Child Health, University of Sydney, Sydney, Australia.

References

1. AIHW. End-stage kidney disease in Australia: total incidence 2003–2007. Canberra: Australian Institute of Health and Welfare; 2011.
2. Shaw C, Simms RJ, Pitcher D, Sandford R. Epidemiology of patients in England and Wales with autosomal dominant polycystic kidney disease and end-stage renal failure. Nephrol Dial Transplant. 2014;29(10):1910–8. doi:10.1093/ndt/gfu087.
3. Mallett A, Patel C, Salisbury A, Wang Z, Healy H, Hoy W. The prevalence and epidemiology of genetic renal disease amongst adults with chronic kidney disease in Australia. Orphanet J Rare Dis. 2014;9:98. doi:10.1186/1750-1172-9-98.
4. Fletcher J, McDonald S, Alexander SI. Australian and New Zealand Pediatric Nephrology Association. Prevalence of genetic renal disease in children. Pediatr Nephrol. 2013;28(2):251–6. doi:10.1007/s00467-012-2306-6.
5. Our inheritance, our future. Realising the potential of genetics in the NHS. UK: Department of Health; 2003.
6. Battista RN, Blancquaert I, Laberge AM, van Schendel N, Leduc N. Genetics in health care: an overview of current and emerging models. Public Health Genom. 2012;15(1):34–45. doi:10.1159/000328846.
7. Burton H, Wright CF, Zimmern R. A new strategic phase for genomic medicine in UK health services. Gen Med. 2009;1(10):93. doi:10.1186/gm93.
8. Gee HY, Otto EA, Hurd TW, Ashraf S, Chaki M, Cluckey A, et al. Whole-exome resequencing distinguishes cystic kidney diseases from phenocopies in renal ciliopathies. Kidney Int. 2014;85(4):880–7. doi:10.1038/ki.2013.450.
9. Moriniere V, Dahan K, Hilbert P, Lison M, Lebbah S, Topa A, et al. Improving mutation screening in familial hematuric nephropathies through next generation sequencing. J Am Soc Nephrol. 2014;25(12):2740–51. doi:10.1681/ASN.2013080912.
10. Sadowski CE, Lovric S, Ashraf S, Pabst WL, Gee HY, Kohl S et al. A single-gene cause in 29.5% of cases of steroid-resistant nephrotic syndrome. J Am Soc Nephrol. 2014. doi:10.1681/ASN.2014050489.
11. Bu F, Maga T, Meyer NC, Wang K, Thomas CP, Nester CM, et al. Comprehensive genetic analysis of complement and coagulation genes in atypical hemolytic uremic syndrome. J Am Soc Nephrol. 2014;25(1):55–64. doi:10.1681/ASN.2013050453.
12. Hwang DY, Dworschak GC, Kohl S, Saisawat P, Vivante A, Hilger AC, et al. Mutations in 12 known dominant disease-causing genes clarify many congenital anomalies of the kidney and urinary tract. Kidney Int. 2014;85(6):1429–33. doi:10.1038/ki.2013.508.
13. Halbritter J, Baum M, Hynes AM, Rice SJ, Thwaites DT, Gucev ZS, et al. Fourteen monogenic genes account for 15% of nephrolithiasis/nephrocalcinosis. J Am Soc Nephrol. 2014. doi:10.1681/ASN.2014040388.

14. Boyer O, Woerner S, Yang F, Oakeley EJ, Linghu B, Gribouval O, et al. LMX1B mutations cause hereditary FSGS without extrarenal involvement. J Am Soc Nephrol. 2013;24(8):1216–22. doi:10.1681/ASN.2013020171.
15. Huynh Cong E, Bizet AA, Boyer O, Woerner S, Gribouval O, Filhol E, et al. A homozygous missense mutation in the ciliary gene TTC21B causes familial FSGS. J Am Soc Nephrol. 2014;25(11):2435–43. doi:10.1681/ASN.2013101126.
16. Lemaire M, Fremeaux-Bacchi V, Schaefer F, Choi M, Tang WH, Le Quintrec M, et al. Recessive mutations in DGKE cause atypical hemolytic-uremic syndrome. Nat Genet. 2013;45(5):531–6. doi:10.1038/ng.2590.
17. Ozaltin F, Li B, Rauhauser A, An SW, Soylemezoglu O, Gonul II, et al. DGKE variants cause a glomerular microangiopathy that mimics membranoproliferative GN. J Am Soc Nephrol. 2013;24(3):377–84. doi:10.1681/ASN.2012090903.
18. Chaki M, Airik R, Ghosh AK, Giles RH, Chen R, Slaats GG, et al. Exome capture reveals ZNF423 and CEP164 mutations, linking renal ciliopathies to DNA damage response signaling. Cell. 2012;150(3):533–48. doi:10.1016/j.cell.2012.06.028.
19. Coussa RG, Otto EA, Gee HY, Arthurs P, Ren H, Lopez I, et al. WDR19: an ancient, retrograde, intraflagellar ciliary protein is mutated in autosomal recessive retinitis pigmentosa and in Senior-Loken syndrome. Clin Genet. 2013;84(2):150–9. doi:10.1111/cge.12196.
20. Failler M, Gee HY, Krug P, Joo K, Halbritter J, Belkacem L, et al. Mutations of CEP83 cause infantile nephronophthisis and intellectual disability. Am J Hum Genet. 2014;94(6):905–14. doi:10.1016/j.ajhg.2014.05.002.
21. Halbritter J, Bizet AA, Schmidts M, Porath JD, Braun DA, Gee HY, et al. Defects in the IFT-B component IFT172 cause Jeune and Mainzer-Saldino syndromes in humans. Am J Hum Genet. 2013;93(5):915–25. doi:10.1016/j.ajhg.2013.09.012.
22. Sang L, Miller JJ, Corbit KC, Giles RH, Brauer MJ, Otto EA, et al. Mapping the NPHP-JBTS-MKS protein network reveals ciliopathy disease genes and pathways. Cell. 2011;145(4):513–28. doi:10.1016/j.cell.2011.04.019.
23. Kirby A, Gnirke A, Jaffe DB, Baresova V, Pochet N, Blumenstiel B, et al. Mutations causing medullary cystic kidney disease type 1 lie in a large VNTR in MUC1 missed by massively parallel sequencing. Nat Genet. 2013;45(3):299–303. doi:10.1038/ng.2543.
24. Qi XP, Du ZF, Ma JM, Chen XL, Zhang Q, Fei J, et al. Genetic diagnosis of autosomal dominant polycystic kidney disease by targeted capture and next-generation sequencing: utility and limitations. Gene. 2013;516(1):93–100. doi:10.1016/j.gene.2012.12.060.
25. Ekici AB, Hackenbeck T, Moriniere V, Pannes A, Buettner M, Uebe S, et al. Renal fibrosis is the common feature of autosomal dominant tubulointerstitial kidney diseases caused by mutations in mucin 1 or uromodulin. Kidney Int. 2014;86(3):589–99. doi:10.1038/ki.2014.72.
26. Trujillano D, Bullich G, Ossowski S, Ballarin J, Torra R, Estivill X, et al. Diagnosis of autosomal dominant polycystic kidney disease using efficient PKD1 and PKD2 targeted next-generation sequencing. Mol Gen Gen Med. 2014;2(5):412–21. doi:10.1002/mgg3.82.
27. Sanna-Cherchi S, Kiryluk K, Burgess KE, Bodria M, Sampson MG, Hadley D, et al. Copy-number disorders are a common cause of congenital kidney malformations. Am J Hum Genet. 2012;91(6):987–97. doi:10.1016/j.ajhg.2012.10.007.
28. Gbadegesin RA, Hall G, Adeyemo A, Hanke N, Tossidou I, Burchette J, et al. Mutations in the gene that encodes the F-actin binding protein anillin cause FSGS. J Am Soc Nephrol. 2014;25(9):1991–2002. doi:10.1681/ASN.2013090976.
29. Wentworth JM, Lukic V, Bahlo M, Finlay M, Nguyen C, Morahan G, et al. Maturity-onset diabetes of the young type 5 in a family with diabetes and mild kidney disease diagnosed by whole exome sequencing. Inter Med J. 2014;44(11):1137–40. doi:10.1111/imj.12584.
30. Takasato M, Er PX, Becroft M, Vanslambrouck JM, Stanley EG, Elefanty AG, et al. Directing human embryonic stem cell differentiation towards a renal lineage generates a self-organizing kidney. Nat Cell Biol. 2014;16(1):118–26. doi:10.1038/ncb2894.
31. Skrunes R, Svarstad E, Reisaeter AV, Vikse BE. Familial clustering of ESRD in the Norwegian population. Clin J Am Soc Nephrol. 2014;9(10):1692–700. doi:10.2215/CJN.01680214.
32. Musetti C, Quaglia M, Mellone S, Pagani A, Fusco I, Monzani A, et al. Chronic renal failure of unknown origin is caused by HNF1B mutations in 9% of adult patients: a single centre cohort analysis. Nephrology. 2014;19(4):202–9. doi:10.1111/nep.12199.
33. Saisawat P, Tasic V, Vega-Warner V, Kehinde EO, Gunther B, Airik R, et al. Identification of two novel CAKUT-causing genes by massively parallel exon resequencing of candidate genes in patients with unilateral renal agenesis. Kidney Int. 2012;81(2):196–200. doi:10.1038/ki.2011.315.

5

Update of the human and mouse Fanconi anemia genes

Hongbin Dong[1], Daniel W. Nebert[2], Elspeth A. Bruford[3], David C. Thompson[4], Hans Joenje[5] and Vasilis Vasiliou[1*]

Abstract

Fanconi anemia (FA) is a recessively inherited disease manifesting developmental abnormalities, bone marrow failure, and increased risk of malignancies. Whereas FA has been studied for nearly 90 years, only in the last 20 years have increasing numbers of genes been implicated in the pathogenesis associated with this genetic disease. To date, 19 genes have been identified that encode Fanconi anemia complementation group proteins, all of which are named or aliased, using the root symbol "FANC." Fanconi anemia subtype (FANC) proteins function in a common DNA repair pathway called "the FA pathway," which is essential for maintaining genomic integrity. The various FANC mutant proteins contribute to distinct steps associated with FA pathogenesis. Herein, we provide a review update of the 19 human FANC and their mouse orthologs, an evolutionary perspective on the FANC genes, and the functional significance of the FA DNA repair pathway in association with clinical disorders. This is an example of a set of genes--known to exist in vertebrates, invertebrates, plants, and yeast--that are grouped together on the basis of shared biochemical and physiological functions, rather than evolutionary phylogeny, and have been named on this basis by the HUGO Gene Nomenclature Committee (HGNC).

Keywords: Fanconi anemia, Genes, Classification, Human, Mouse, Genome

Introduction

Fanconi anemia (FA) is an autosomal recessive disorder having an incidence of ~1/200,000–400,000 in most populations; the incidence is higher in Ashkenazi Jews (~1/30,000) and Afrikaners (~1/22,000) [1–4]. Most FA patients exhibit developmental abnormalities, developing early bone marrow failure and acute myelogenous leukemia (AML). Later, these patients display a higher risk of developing carcinomas of the head, neck, and anogenital region [5].

In recent decades, 19 human genes have been implicated in the causation of FA. These genes code for a group of proteins, viz. the Fanconi anemia subtype (FANC) proteins, which function cooperatively in a DNA damage recognition - and - repair pathway [6]. The FA pathway plays a crucial role in maintaining hematological homeostasis--particularly blood cell development and differentiation. FA is a congenital disease resulting from a somatic mutation in both alleles of the specific FANC gene; a notable exception is *FANCB* in which the mutation occurs on the X chromosome [7]. The primary causal factor in FA is generally thought to involve chromosomal instability in hematopoietic stem cells, a result of defective DNA repair caused by mutant FANC proteins [8, 9]. However, precise molecular mechanisms underlying the roles of specific FANC proteins (as well as their interactions with non-FANC proteins) in the FA pathway or other DNA damage repair pathways remain to be defined.

* Correspondence: vasilis.vasiliou@yale.edu
[1]Department of Environmental Health Sciences, Yale School of Public Health, 60 College St, New Haven, CT 06250, USA
Full list of author information is available at the end of the article

Genetics of FA: human FANC genes

FA was first reported in 1927 by Swiss pediatrician Guido Fanconi. After finding three siblings who suffered from complex physical defects relating to aplastic anemia, Dr. Fanconi described the intrinsic nature of the abnormalities as "panmyelopathy" and proposed that multiple genes were likely causing the underlying complexity of FA symptoms [10]. It was later recognized that a high degree of underlying genetic heterogeneity existed in this disease [11]. Sixty-five years after the initial FA case was reported, the first FANC gene (*FANCC*) was identified, following development of a complementation-cloning method [12]. This approach was subsequently used in identification of an additional four FANC genes [13–16]. Through the use of complementation cloning, positional cloning, protein association, and candidate-gene and whole-genome sequencing, 19 FANC genes have now been identified as being involved in the etiology of FA (Table 1). The FANC genes are phylogenetically unrelated and have been grouped together and named or aliased with the FANC root symbol, based on association of mutations in the encoded proteins having a FA-like disease phenotype in combination with cellular hypersensitivity to DNA cross-linking agents.

Information about most published FANC gene mutations is available on the public Fanconi Anemia Mutation Database (http://www.rockefeller.edu/fanconi/). Genetic studies have revealed that mutations in the *FANCA*, *FANCC*, and *FANCG* genes are most common and account for ~85 % of FA cases [5, 17]. The *FANCA* gene was the second FANC gene identified [13]. *FANCA* mutations account for nearly ~65 % of FA cases [18]. About 200 different mutated *FANCA* alleles, comprising almost all the known mutation types, have been reported to date. Large intragenic deletions appear to be the major form of mutations [18].

FANCC mutations account for ~14 % of FA cases [5]. Among all known mutants, 322delG and IVS4+4A>T occurring in exon 1 and intron 4, respectively, are the most commonly observed *FANCC* mutations [19, 20]. Deletion of a single G at base 322 (322delG) produces a truncated protein of 44 amino acids. The IVS4+4A>T mutation results in either deletion of the entire exon 4 or a 40-bp deletion leading to a frame-shift.

FANCG was found to be identical to the X-ray repair cross-complementing protein 9 (*XRCC9*) gene; the gene is named as *FANCG*, with XRCC9 as an alias for the DNA repair protein. *FANCG* mutations account for ~10 % of FA cases [5] and have been implicated as founder mutations in different populations. For instance, a deletion mutation at c.637_643delTACCGCC was found to be associated with 82 % of FA cases in black populations of Southern Africa [21]. Screening of 45 FA families in Japan showed that nine of the families carried a splice mutation of IVS3+1G>C, with three of these nine families also carrying a 1066C>T mutation. Haplotype analysis revealed IVS3+1G>C and 1066C>T to be associated with Japanese and Korean ethnicities [22], respectively.

Mutations in the *FANCB*, *FANCD1*, *FANCD2*, *FANCE*, and *FANCF* genes, combined, account for ~13 % of reported FA cases [5]. The *FANCB* gene is the only FANC gene not to be autosomal, but rather X-linked. Point mutations, small insertions, and large deletions in the *FANCB* gene have been reported. For instance, a frame-shift mutation in exon 8 and a 3314-bp deletion in exon 1 (that includes some of the promoter region of *FANCB*) were reported in cell lines derived from FA patients [7]. Most *FANCB* mutations result in truncation of the encoded protein [23].

FANCD1 is identical to the breast cancer susceptibility gene *BRCA2*; because the latter gene symbol was so extremely well-established, this gene is officially named *BRCA2* by the HGNC but has the alias of *FANCD1*. Studies reveal that FA-D1 patients have biallelic mutations in the *BRCA2* gene and express a truncated protein [24]. Heterozygotes in FA families (e.g., parents of FA patients) display increased risk of early-onset breast and ovarian cancers [25]. These findings connect FA and breast cancer, which share common mechanisms of defective DNA repair.

FANCD2 encodes a protein that plays a central role in the FA pathway of DNA repair. *FANCD2* mutations involving large deletions and/or single-base changes have been reported [26, 27]. In addition, specific *FANCD2* mutations (for example, c.458T>C and c.2715+1G>A) have been associated with T cell acute lymphoblastic leukemia (T-ALL) and testicular seminoma [26, 27].

Mutations in the *FANCE* and *FANCF* genes account for 5–8 % of reported FA cases [5, 17]. Multiple types of mutation have been reported for *FANCE*, including a 355C>T transition in exon 2 in the EUFA410 FA cell line and the IVS5-8G>A splice mutation in EUFA622 cells [16, 28]. Disease-associated mutations have been reported throughout the single coding exon of the *FANCF* gene. The most commonly seen *FANCF* mutations are short deletions, resulting in frame-shifts and premature termination of the protein [29].

Mutations in the remaining FA genes, *FANCI*, *BRIP1* (*FANCJ*), *FANCL*, *FANCM*, *PALB2* (*FANCN*), *RAD51C* (*FANCO*), *SLX4* (*FANCP*), *ERCC4* (*FANCQ*), *BRCA1* (*FANCS*), and the recently reported *RAD51*(*FANCR*) and *UBE2T* (*FANCT*), contribute to <5 % of FA cases, combined [5, 17]. Documented mutations in these eleven genes––in FA patients and/or FA subtype cell lines––include point mutations, nucleotide insertions, splice-site mutations, and mutations resulting in protein truncation. For example, biallelic mutations [30] and a 30-residue C-terminal protein truncation [31] were reported for *FANCI*.

BRIP1 (BRCA1-interacting protein C-terminal helicase 1) is the official gene symbol for *FANCJ*. Amino-acid substitutions in BRIP1/FANCJ, such as R251C, Q255H, and A349P, were found to be disease-causing [32, 33].

A dinucleotide insertion (c.755-756insAT) in *FANCL* [34], c.5569G>A transition in *FANCM* [35], and 3549C>G transition and 3549C>A transversion mutations in *PALB2*/*FANCN* [36] were reported in FA families. *PALB2* (partner and localizer of BRCA2) is the official gene symbol for *FANCN*. However, it should be noted that Lim et al.

Table 1 Human FANC genes

Gene symbol (NCBI gene ID)	Gene name	FANC symbol	Gene symbol synonyms	Chromosomal location	Ref seq RNA	Ref seq protein	Protein size (aa)
FANCA (2175)	Fanconi anemia complementation group A	*FANCA*	*FA, FA-H, FA1, FAA, FACA, FAH, FANCH*	16q24.3	NM_000135.2	NP_000126.2	1,455
FANCB (2187)	Fanconi anemia complementation group B	*FANCB*	*FA2, FAAP90, FAAP95, FAB, FACB*	Xp22.31	NM_001018113.1	NP_001018123.1	859
FANCC (2176)	Fanconi anemia complementation group C	*FANCC*	*RP11-80I15.2, FA3, FAC, FACC*	9q22.3	NM_000136.2	NP_000127.2	558
BRCA2 (675)	Breast cancer 2	*FANCD1*	*RP11-298P3.4, BRCC2, BROVCA2, FACD, FAD, FAD1, FANCD, GLM3, PNCA2, XRCC11*	13q12.13	NM_000059.3	NP_000050.2	3,418
FANCD2 (2177)	Fanconi anemia complementation group D2	*FANCD2*	*FA-D2, FA4, FACD, FAD, FAD2, FANCD*	3p25.3	NM_001018115.1	NP_001018125.1	1,451
FANCE (2178)	Fanconi anemia complementation group E	*FANCE*	*FACE, FAE*	6p21.22	NM_021922.2	NP_068741.1	536
FANCF (2188)	Fanconi anemia complementation group F	*FANCF*	*FAF*	11p15	NM_022725.3	NP_073562.1	374
FANCG (2189)	Fanconi anemia complementation group G	*FANCG*	*FAG, XRCC9*	9p13	NM_004629.1	NP_004620.1	622
FANCI (55215)	Fanconi anemia complementation group I	*FANCI*	*KIAA1794*	15q26.1	NM_001113378.	NP_001106849.1	1,328
BRIP1 (83990)	BRCA1 interacting protein C-terminal helicase 1	*FANCJ*	*BACH1, OF*	17q23.2	NM_032043.2	NP_114432.2	1,249
FANCL (55120)	Fanconi anemia complementation group L	*FANCL*	*FAAP43, PHF9, POG*	2p16.1	NM_001114636.1	NP_001108108.1	380
FANCM (57697)	Fanconi anemia complementation group M	*FANCM*	*FAAP250, KIAA1596*	14q21.3	NM_020937.2	NP_065988.1	2,048
PALB2 (79728)	Partner and localizer of BRCA2	*FANCN*	*PNCA3*	16p12	NM_024675.3	NP_078951.2	1,186
RAD51C (5889)	RAD51 paralog C	*FANCO*	*ROVCA3, R51H3, RAD51L2*	17q23	NM_002876.3	NP_002867.1	376
SLX4 (84464)	SLX4 structure-specific endonuclease subunit	*FANCP*	*BTBD12, MUS312*	16p13.3	NM_032444.2	NP_115820.2	1,834
ERCC4 (2072)	Excision repair cross-complementation group 4	*FANCQ*	*RAD1, XPF, ERCC11*	16p13.12	NM_005236.2	NP_005227.1	916
RAD51 (5888)	RAD51 recombinase	*FANCR*	*BRCC5, HRAD51, HsRad51, HsT16930, MRMV2A, RECA*	15q15.1	NM_001164269.1	NP_001157741.1	340
BRCA1 (672)	Breast cancer 1	*FANCS*	*BRCAI, BRCC1, BROVCA1, IRIS, PNCA4, PPP1R53, PSCP, RNF53*	17q21.31	NM_007294.3	NP_009225.1	1863
UBE2T (29089)	Ubiquitin- conjugating enzyme E2T	*FANCT*	*HSPC150*	1q32.1	NM_014176.3	NP_054895.1	197

found individuals in the Finnish population who were homozygous for *FANCM* loss-of-function mutations but appeared to have no reported FA phenotype [37], casting doubt over the pathogenicity of this gene in FA.

RAD51C (RAD51 paralog C) is the official gene symbol for the *FANCO* gene. Meindl et al. reported 14 *RAD51C/FANCO* mutations--which included single-base-pair insertions, splice-site mutations, and sequence alterations [38]. *SLX4* (SLX4 structure-specific endonuclease subunit) and *ERCC4* (excision-repair cross-complementation group 4) are the official gene symbols for *FANCP* and *FANCQ*, respectively. Biallelic mutations in the *SLX4/FANCP* and *ERCC4/FANCQ* genes have been documented to cause FA subtypes [39–41].

BRCA1 (breast cancer 1, early onset) has recently been identified as the 17th FANC gene and assigned the *FANCS* synonym [42]. Despite knowing that the BRCA1 protein cooperates in the FA pathway through forming a complex with several FANC proteins at DNA repair loci [43], *BRCA1* was previously precluded from being assigned as a FA gene due to the lack of reported biallelic *BRCA1* mutations in patients. However, recently, two cases of individuals harboring biallelic deleterious *BRCA1* mutations were reported [42, 44]. Detailed phenotypic and cellular characterization of one patient provided lines of evidence supporting the hypothesis that biallelic *BRCA1* (*FANCS*) mutations cause a new Fanconi anemia subtype associated with increased breast and ovarian cancer susceptibility [42].

Most recently, researchers have identified two new genes, mutations of which cause FA-like symptoms. The RAD51 gene encodes a key recombinase essential for homologous recombination of DNA during double strand break repair [45]. RAD51 is a mammalian homologue of the bacterial DNA repair protein RecA. A novel heterozygous mutation (T131P) in RAD51 was identified in a FA-like patient [46]. Expression of this dominant-negative mutant RAD51 in the patient's cell line disrupted interstrand cross-link (ICL) repair but spared homologous recombination [46]. The authors proposed that RAD51 plays an ICL-repair-specific function through protection of nascent DNA strands from excessive processing at the ICL sites; this function may be regulated by BRCA2/FANCD1 [46]. The *UBE2T* gene encodes an ubiquitin-conjugating enzyme E2T that was already known to act in the FA pathway [47, 48]. Two unrelated individuals were found with biallelic *UBE2T* missense mutations that rendered the UBE2T protein unable to interact with FANCL [48]. The *RAD51* and *UBE2T* genes have now been given the aliases *FANCR* and *FANCT*, respectively.

Evolution of *FANC* genes

It was originally thought that the FA DNA repair pathway was restricted to vertebrates. However, counterparts of several FA proteins have been discovered in lower eukaryotes, including sea squirt (*C. intestinalis*) [49], fly [50-52], worm [53-55], and yeast [56, 57], as well as in plants [58]. Nevertheless, it appears that the majority of lower eukaryotes possess a simplified FA pathway (Fig. 1) consisting of FANCL, FANCM, UBE2T, FANCD2, FANCI, BRCA2, BRIP1, RAD51C, SLX4, ERCC4, and RAD51. These FA proteins represent two components

Genus, species	FA core complex									D2/I complex		FA effector proteins							
Homo sapiens	A	B	C	E	F	G	L	M	T	D2	I	D1	J	N	O	P	Q	R	S
Mus musculus	A	B	C	E	F	G	L	M	T	D2	I	D1	J	N	O	P	Q	R	S
Gallus gallus	A	B	C	E	F	G	L	M	T	D2	I	D1	J	N	O	P	Q	R	S
Xenopus laevis	A	B	C	E	F	G	L	M	T	D2	I	D1	J	N	O	P	Q	R	S
Danio rerio	A	B	C	E	F	G	L	M	T	D2	I	D1	J	N	O	P	Q	R	
Ciona intestinalis							L	M		D2	I		J		O	P	Q	R	
Drosophila melanogaster							L	M	T	D2	I				O		Q	R	
Caenorhabditis elegans									T	D2	I		J		O	P	Q	R	
Saccharomyces cerevisiae								M	T				J		O	P	Q	R	
Arabidopsis thaliana				E			L	M	T	D2	I	D1	J		O		Q	R	

Fig. 1 Overview of FA pathway genes identified in eukaryotic lineages. Representative species include mammals (*Homo sapiens, Mus musculus, and Gallus gallus*), amphibian (African clawed toad, *Xenopus laevis*), fish (zebrafish, *Danio rerio*), sea squirt (*Ciona intestinalis*), insect (*Drosophila melanogaster*), worm (*Caenorhabditis elegans*), yeast (*Saccharomyces cerevisiae*), and plant (*Arabidopsis thaliana*). *FANC* genes are grouped into three classes. Group I includes nine genes that encode proteins that form the FA core complex; group II encodes FANCD2 and FANCI that form the D2/I complex; group III comprises eight genes that encode FA effector proteins that function downstream of D2/I complex. Lower eukaryotes tend to be missing orthologues of the FA core complex genes. *A = FANCA, B = FANCB, C = FANCC, D2 = FANCD2, E = FANCE, F = FANCF, G = FANCG, I = FANCI, L = FANCL, M = FANCM, D1 = BRCA2/FANCD1, J = BRIP1/FANCJ, N = PALB2/FANCN, O = RAD51C/FANCO, P = SLX4/FANCP, Q = ERCC4/*FANCQ/*XPF, R = RAD51/FANCR, S = BRCA1/FANCS, T = UBE2T/FANCT*. If we extend this gene family update to include prokaryotes, it might be noted that, whereas no orthologs of any of the 19 eukaryotic *FANC* genes exist in prokaryote genomes, RAD51 (as a nineteenth FANC member in living organisms) qualifies as a homologue of bacterial RecA

of the FA core complex, the D2/I complex, and most of the FA downstream effector proteins (*vide infra*).

What appear to have evolved later in the ancestral animal kingdom are most of the FA core complex proteins (Fig. 1). In addition to the 19 human FANC genes, two pseudogenes of the *FANCD2* gene have been annotated in the human genome, *FANCD2P1* (gene ID 100421239) and *FANCD2P2* (gene ID 101929530).

Comparative genomic analysis revealed genes of the FA pathway to be conserved among vertebrate genomes [49, 59]. A single ortholog of each of the 19 human FANC genes has been identified in other vertebrates--including rodents, chicken, *Xenopus*, and zebrafish (Fig. 1). However, the zebrafish genome has no *BRCA1* orthologue, suggesting that the entire vertebrate FA gene network had not been completely formed after the land-animal/sea-animal split.

In the mouse genome, 19 *Fanc* genes have been mapped to 13 chromosomes (Table 2). Mouse FANC proteins share 50–85 % sequence identity with their corresponding human orthologs. Transgenic knockout mouse lines have been generated for many *Fanc* genes [60-68]. In general, cells derived from *Fanc*(–/–) knockout mice recapitulate the phenotypes of human FA patient cells, whereas these mice only partially reproduce the clinical features of FA patients.

FANC complementation group proteins that cause the FA disorder

FA is characterized primarily by progressive bone marrow dysfunction and sensitivity to DNA cross-linking agents [5, 17]. This congenital disease results from loss-of-function of any of the 19 FANC genes, thereby revealing the essential roles of FANC proteins in maintaining chromosomal stability of hematopoietic stem cells. As noted above, more than 95 % of FA cases are attributed to mutations in known FANC genes [5]. In a few FA cases, genetic contributions remain unclassified. The unique clinical phenotype associated with *FANC* gene mutations implies that proteins encoded by these genes function in a common cellular pathway. This pathway, known as the FA/BRCA DNA repair pathway, functions pivotally in preserving genomic homeostasis in response to specific types of DNA damage [6].

In a proposed model of the FA/BRCA DNA repair pathway (Fig. 2) [5, 17], eight FANC proteins--FANCA, FANCB, FANCC, FANCE, FANCF, FANCG, FANCL, and FANCM--plus three FA-associated proteins, FAAP20, FAAP24, and FAAP100, form the nuclear FA core complex. Fanconi anemia core complex associated proteins (FAAP) are functionally equivalent to FANC proteins, except that, thus far, no FA patients have been found whose disease phenotype could be ascribed to mutations in a FAAP-encoding gene. The FA core complex functions to receive upstream signals in response to DNA damage, through phosphorylation of multiple FA core units. The activated FA core complex binds the enzyme UBE2T (FANCT) via the putative plant homeodomain (PHD) zinc finger of the FANCL subunit, and then mono-ubiquitinates the FANCD2/I complex. This then translocates to DNA damage sites and recruits eight downstream FA effector proteins, i.e., BRCA1, BRCA2, BRIP1, PALB2, RAD51C, SLX4, ERCC4, RAD51, plus other DNA repair molecules, to DNA damage sites.

Distinct roles of FA proteins in the FA core complex and FANCD2/I complex have been suggested. FANCE contributes to core complex integrity--by promoting nuclear accumulation of FANCC protein and FANCA—-FANCC complex formation and directly targeting FANCD2 for ubiquitination [69]. Phe-522, at the highly conserved carboxyl terminus of FANCE, was found to be a critical residue for mediating mono-ubiquitination of the FANCD2/I complex [70]. FANCL is an E3 ubiquitin ligase containing three WD40 repeats and a PHD zinc finger motif. These account for protein-protein interactions and recruitment of UBE2T (FANCT), respectively [71], both of which function importantly in FANCD2 mono-ubiquitination. FANCM in the FA core complex was reported to possess endonuclease and DNA helicase domains and is believed to function in translocation of the FA core complex along DNA [51]. FANCD2 mono-ubiquitination is essential for FA pathway-mediated DNA repair. However, the specific role of FANCD2 in the repair process remains unknown. A higher frequency of telomere dysfunction-induced foci (TIFs) and telomere sister-chromatid exchanges (T-SCE) was observed in primary cells derived from FA patients carrying a mutated *FANCD2* gene [72], suggesting its involvement in telomere regulation.

Of the 19 FANC proteins, some have been previously identified as part of different DNA damage repair pathways that may interact with the FA pathway [73, 74]. For example, FANCA has been reported to interact with DNA repair-associated proteins, such as the endonuclease ERCC4 and the ATP-dependent helicase SMARCA4 [75, 76]. In addition, FANCA mutant cells (derived from FA patients) exhibit defective mitochondrial respiration and impaired ATP production [77]. In human embryonic kidney (HEK 293T) cells, FANCA was found to influence centrosome integrity by way of its capacity to interact with NIMA-related kinase 2 (NEK2) [78].

FA pathway combats genomic instability

One of the hallmarks of FA is hypersensitivity of cells from FA patients to the clastogenic and cytostatic effects of DNA cross-linking agents such as diepoxybutane (DEB) and mitomycin C (MMC) [5, 17]. In particular,

Table 2 Mouse Fanc genes

Gene symbol (NCBI gene ID)	Gene name	FANC symbol	Gene symbol synonyms	Chromosome location	Ref seq RNA	Ref seq protein	Protein size (aa)
Fanca (14087)	Fanconi anemia complementation group A	*Fanca*	*AW208693, Faca*	8	NM_016925.3	NP_058621.2	1,439
Fancb (237211)	Fanconi anemia complementation group B	*Fancb*	*RP23-32J17.2, BC022692*	X	NM_001146081.1	NP_001139553.1	853
Fancc (14088)	Fanconi anemia complementation group C	*Fancc*	*Facc*	13	NM_001042673.2	NP_001036138.1	558
Brca2 (12190)	Breast cancer 2	*Fancd1*	*Rab163*	5	NM_001081001.2	NP_001074470.1	3,329
Fancd2 (211651)	Fanconi anemia complementation group D2	*Fancd2*	*2410150007Rik, Au015151, Bb137857, Fad2, Fa4, Facd, Fad, Fancd*	6	NM_001033244.3	NP_001028416.2	3,329
Fance (72775)	Fanconi anemia complementation group E	*Fance*	*Rp24-68J3.2, 2810451d06Rik, Ai415634, Aw209126*	17	NM_001163819.1	NP_001157291.1	1,437
Fancf (100040608)	Fanconi anemia complementation group F	*Fancf*	*A730016a17*	7	NM_001115087.1	NP_001108559.1	343
Fancg (60534)	Fanconi anemia complementation group G	*Fancg*	*Rp23-124l1.6, Au041407, Xrcc9*	4	NM_001163233.	NP_001156705.1	616
Fanci (208836)	Fanconi anemia complementation group I	*Fanci*	None	7	NM_145946.2	NP_666058.2	1,329
Brip1 (237911)	BRCA1 interacting protein C-terminal helicase 1	*Fancj*	*Rp23-36p4.3, 3110009N10Rik, 8030460j03Rik, Bach1, Facj, Of*	11	NM_178309.2	NP_840094.1	1,174
Fancl (67030)	Fanconi anemia complementation group L	*Fancl*	*2010322C19Rik, AW554273, B230118H11Rik, gcd, Phf9, Pog*	11	NM_0253923.3	NP_080199.1	375
Fancm (104806)	Fanconi anemia complementation group M	*Fancm*	*Ai427100, C730036b14Rik, D12ertd364e*	12	XM_006515344.1	XP_006515407.1	2,021
Palb2 (558923)	Partner and localizer of BRCA2	*Fancn*	*si:ch211-14k19.9*	7	XM_001919731.5	XP_001919766.3	1,104
Rad51c (114714)	RAD51 homologue C	*Fanco*	*RP23-209O5.3, R51H3, Rad51l2*	11	NM_001291440.1	NP_001278369.1	384
Slx4 (850826)	SLX4 structure-specific endonuclease subunit homologue (S. cerevisiae)	*Fancp*	*Rai256635, Ai426760, Btbd12, D16bwg1016e*	16	NM_177472.5	NP_803423.2	1,565
Ercc4 (50505)	Excision repair cross-complementing rodent repair deficiency, complementation group 4	*Fancq*	*Ai606920, Xpf*	16	NM_015769.2	NP_056584.2	917
Rad51 (19361)	RAD51 recombinase	*Fancr*	*AV304093a, Reca*	2	NM_011234.4	NP_035364.1	339
Brca1 (12189)	Breast cancer 1	*Fancs*	None	11	NM_009764.3	NP_033894.3	1812
Ube2t (67196)	Ubiquitin-conjugating enzyme E2T (putative)	*Fanct*	*2700084L22Rik*	1	NM_026024.3	NP_080300.1	204

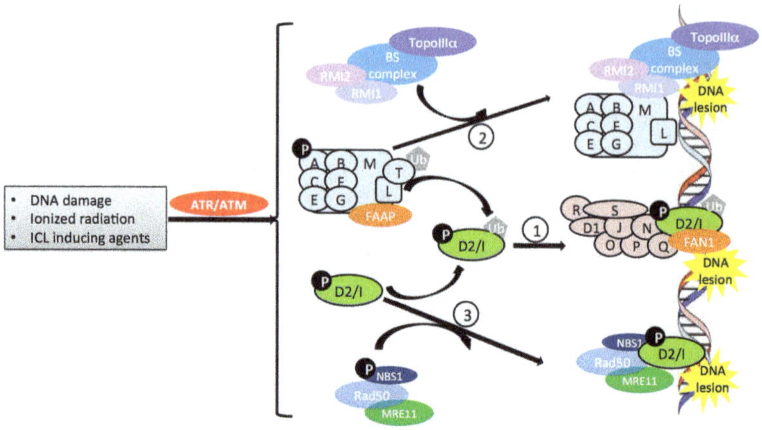

Fig. 2 FA/BRCA pathway and crosstalk between FA and other DNA repair pathways. In response to upstream DNA damage signaling (such as phosphorylation by ATR/ATM), in the FA/BRCA pathway [1], the FA core complex forms––comprising FANCA (*A*), FANCB (*B*), FANCC (*C*), FANCE (*E*), FANCF (*F*), FANCG (*G*), FANCM (*M*), and FANCL (*L*) proteins, plus FAAP20, FAAP24, and FAAP100 (*FAAP*). This core complex binds UBE2T(T) via FANCL, which then activates FANCD2/I dimers through mono-ubiquitination. The activated FANCD2/I (D2/I) complex then translocates to DNA - damage sites and recruits downstream FA effector proteins––including BRCA1 (S), BRCA2 (D1), RAD51 (R), BRIP1 (J), PALB2 (N), RAD51C (O), SLX4 (P), and ERCC4 (Q), plus other DNA repair molecules (such as FAN1) to the lesion site to repair damage. In the FANCM/BS pathway [2], the FA core complex binds to the BS complex by way of interactions between FANCM-RMI1 and TopoIIIα of the BS complex and translocates to the lesion site. In the FANCD2/ATM pathway [3], in response to ionizing radiation or ICL-inducing agents, FANCD2 is phosphorylated by ATM and co-localizes with the NMR complex to repair DNA damage or cause S-phase arrest. *ICL* interstrand cross-links, *ATR* ataxia-telangiectasia-Ser/Thr-protein kinase, *ATM* ataxia telangiectasia mutated kinase, *FAAP* FA-associated proteins, *FAN1* FA-associated nuclease-1, *BS* Bloom's syndrome protein, *RMI1/2* RecQ-mediated genomic instability protein 1/2, *TopoIIIα* topoisomerase IIIα, *NMR* the NBS1/MRE11/RAD50 complex

DNA ICLs are highly cytotoxic and difficult to repair because these affect both strands of the DNA helix [79]. The FA/BRCA DNA damage-response pathway is a complex network that functions to remove ICLs through the coordinated actions of FANC proteins––plus other non-FANC proteins such as FAAPs and FANCD2/I-associated nuclease-1 (FAN1) [5, 17].

From an evolutionary point of view, the complete FA pathway is conserved in higher eukaryotes as an efficient pathway to manage ICLs [59]. In this model (Fig. 2), the FA core complex, comprising eight FANC proteins and three FAAPs, forms in response to DNA - damage signaling. The assembled FA core complex binds the ubiquitin-conjugating enzyme UBE2T via the FANCL subunit, which then activates the FANCD2/I complex via mono-ubiquitination at the K561 residue of FANCD2. The ubiquitinated FANCD2/I complex translocates to sites of DNA damage following binding with BRCA1/2 and RAD51, which ultimately triggers DNA repair.

Extensive crosstalk occurs between the FA/BRCA pathway and other DNA repair pathways. FANCD2-deficient cells are hypersensitive to ionizing radiation [80]. In these cells, the FANCD2 mutant cannot be efficiently phosphorylated by the Ser/Thr kinase ATM, resulting in a defect in the ionizing radiation-inducible S-phase checkpoint. FANCD2 was found to initiate S-phase arrest, in response to ionizing radiation, by interacting with ATM-phosphorylated nibrin of the MRE11–RAD50-NBN/NBS1 (MRN) complex [81, 82]. In response to ICL agents such as mitomycin C (MMC), phosphorylated FANCD2 co-localizes with the MRN complex at the DNA damage sites. This FANCD2/ATM pathway operates independently of the FANCD2/BRCA pathway because FANCD2 mono-ubiquitination-mediated formation of nuclear foci is not affected in ATM-deficient (*ATM(−/−)*) cells. In addition, a non-ubiquitinated mutant K561R of FANCD2 has no effect on FANCD2 phosphorylation, following ionizing radiation. FANCM was reported to interact with the Bloom syndrome (BS) complex using its highly conserved protein-protein interaction motifs, MM1 and MM2 [83]. The BS complex binds to the FA core complex by means of MM1-mediated FANCM-FANCF interaction and MM2-mediated interaction between FANCM, RecQ-mediated genomic instability 1 (RMI1), and topoisomerase IIIα (TOP3A) of the BS complex. This FANCM-mediated FA-BS crosstalk is required for MMC resistance of cells.

FA and cancer

A high risk of carcinogenesis, particularly in hematopoietic and squamous cells, is another characteristic phenotype in FA patients, due to loss-of-function of FA proteins. FA-related malignancies vary between organs and cell types and in ages of onset and frequencies. Statistical analysis of 1300 identified FA cases revealed the highest frequency to be leukemia (9 %), followed by myelodysplastic syndrome (MDS) (7 %), solid tumors (5 %), and liver tumors (3 %) [84].

Using the International Fanconi Anemia Registry (IFAR) database to analyze 397 FA patients carrying *FANCC* mutations (specifically the IVS4 splice mutation in intron 4, 322delG or Q13X in exon 1 and R548X or L554P in exon 14) revealed that IVS4 and exon-14 mutations were highly correlated with severe congenital malformations and early onset of hematologic disorders at a median age of 2.7 and 2.1 years, respectively. Patients with exon-1 322delG or Q13X mutations exhibited mild congenital malformations and later onset of hematologic disease (median age 7.6 years) [85]. The IVS4 mutation caused distinct phenotypes in patients of Ashkenazi Jewish ancestry; interestingly, Japanese carriers display no significant clinical abnormality [86]. Patients carrying biallelic mutations in *FANCD1* demonstrate an early-onset leukemia (median age 2.2 years), compared with 13.4 years in other FA patients [87]. Increased risk of esophageal squamous cell carcinoma (ESCC) was reported to be associated with mutations in *FANCD2*, *FANCE*, *FANCL*, and *FANCA* in patients from an Iranian population [88]. Screening of germline DNA in 421 pancreatic cancer cases showed that, besides homozygote-associated cancer formation, heterozygous *FANCC* mutations were associated with increased susceptibility to pancreatic cancer [89]. A *BRIP1* mutation (c.2040_2041insTT), found at an allelic frequency of 0.41 % in an Icelandic cohort of 323,000 samples, was found to confer an elevated risk of ovarian cancer and is associated with an overall decrease of 3.6 years in lifespan--due to all cancers [90].

Summary

Many of the currently identified 19 FA proteins have already been characterized with respect to their relative roles in FA etiology and FA-associated neoplasm. However, our understanding of the full range of molecular actions of these important and intriguing proteins remains to be clarified. For example, the specific role of individual FA protein members and their interaction with non-FA pathways in response to DNA damage are not fully understood. Reported cases of certain heterozygous *FANC* mutations, resulting in altered FA proteins, that predispose some individuals to cancer might involve non-FA mechanisms in specific organ or cell types. The observation that a specific *FANC* mutation can induce a different phenotype, depending on each patient's specific genetic background, suggests that non-FA factor(s), or unidentified FA proteins, might also be participating in cancer risk. Further investigation of FA proteins should provide valuable insights into understanding molecular mechanisms involved in maintaining genomic integrity.

Finally, it should be mentioned that almost all previous Human Genomics "Nomenclature Update" reviews have emphasized gene nomenclature based on evolutionary divergence from an original ancestral gene. In the case of the *FANC* gene group--or "family"--we show here that the HGNC-approved classification of these 19 genes is based on a common phenotype resulting from a shared biochemical or physiological functions, rather than evolutionary divergence and, as such, this is not a classical "gene family."

Competing interests

The authors declare that they have no competing interests.

Authors' contributions

VV and DWN proposed and oversaw the analyses; HD and VV drafted the manuscript; EAB drafted the gene nomenclature sections; EAB, DCT, HJ, DWN and VV edited the manuscript. All authors read and approved the final manuscript.

Acknowledgements

We thank our colleagues for valuable discussions during the course of writing this review and careful readings of this manuscript. This work was supported in part by NIH grants AA022057 and AA021724 (V.V.), U41HG003345 (E.A.B.) and P30 ES006096 (D.W.N.) and Wellcome Trust grant 099129/Z/12/Z (E.A.B).

Author details

[1]Department of Environmental Health Sciences, Yale School of Public Health, 60 College St, New Haven, CT 06250, USA. [2]Department of Environmental Health and Center for Environmental Genetics, University Cincinnati Medical Center, Cincinnati, OH 45267-0056, USA. [3]HUGO Gene Nomenclature Committee (HGNC), European Bioinformatics Institute (EMBL-EBI), European Molecular Biology Laboratory, Hinxton CB10 1SD, UK. [4]Department of Clinical Practice, University of Colorado Denver, Aurora, CO 80045, USA. [5]Department of Clinical Genetics and the Cancer Center Amsterdam/VUmc Institute for Cancer and Immunology, VU University Medical Center, NL-1081 BT Amsterdam, The Netherlands.

References

1. Mathew CG. Fanconi anaemia genes and susceptibility to cancer. Oncogene. 2006;25(43):5875–84.
2. Barankin B, Metelitsa AI, Schloss EH, Wasel NR. Skin disorders in Ashkenazi Jews: a review. Int J Dermatol. 2005;44(8):630–5.
3. Tipping AJ, Pearson T, Morgan NV, Gibson RA, Kuyt LP, Havenga C, et al. Molecular and genealogical evidence for a founder effect in Fanconi anemia families of the Afrikaner population of South Africa. Proc Natl Acad Sci U S A. 2001;98(10):5734–9.
4. Whitney MA, Jakobs P, Kaback M, Moses RE, Grompe M. The Ashkenazi Jewish Fanconi anemia mutation: incidence among patients and carrier frequency in the at-risk population. Hum Mutat. 1994;3(4):339–41.
5. Alter BP, and Kupfer G (1993–2015) Fanconi Anemia. In: Pagon RA, Adam MP, Ardinger HH, Wallace SE, Amemiya A, Bean LJH, Bird TD, Dolan CR, Fong CT, Smith RJH, Stephens K, editors. GeneReviews® [Internet]. Seattle (WA): University of Washington, Seattle. Available From http://www.ncbi.nlm.nih.gov/books/NBK1401/ Access date February 7, 2013.
6. Wang LC, Gautier J. The Fanconi anemia pathway and ICL repair: implications for cancer therapy. Crit Rev Biochem Mol Biol. 2010;45(5):424–39.
7. Meetei AR, Levitus M, Xue Y, Medhurst AL, Zwaan M, Ling C, et al. X-linked inheritance of Fanconi anemia complementation group B. Nat Genet. 2004;36(11):1219–24.
8. Yung SK, Tilgner K, Ledran MH, Habibollah S, Neganova I, Singhapol C, et al. Brief report: human pluripotent stem cell models of Fanconi anemia deficiency reveal an important role for Fanconi anemia proteins in cellular reprogramming and survival of hematopoietic progenitors. Stem Cells. 2013;31(5):1022–9.
9. Alter BP. Fanconi anemia and the development of leukemia. Best Pract Res Clin Haematol. 2014;27(3–4):214–21.
10. Lobitz S, Velleuer E. Guido Fanconi (1892–1979): a jack of all trades. Nat Rev Cancer. 2006;6(11):893–8.

11. Rogers KJ, Fu W, Akey JM, Monnat Jr RJ. Global and disease-associated genetic variation in the human Fanconi anemia gene family. Hum Mol Genet. 2014;23(25):6815–25.
12. Strathdee CA, Gavish H, Shannon WR, Buchwald M. Cloning of cDNAs for Fanconi's anaemia by functional complementation. Nature. 1992;356(6372): 763–7.
13. Lo Ten Foe JR, Rooimans MA, Bosnoyan-Collins L, Alon N, Wijker M, Parker L, et al. Expression cloning of a cDNA for the major Fanconi anaemia gene, FAA. Nat Genet. 1996;14(3):320–3.
14. de Winter JP, Waisfisz Q, Rooimans MA, van Berkel CG, Bosnoyan-Collins L, Alon N, et al. The Fanconi anaemia group G gene *FANCG* is identical with XRCC9. Nat Genet. 1998;20(3):281–3.
15. de Winter JP, Rooimans MA, van Der WL, van Berkel CG, Alon N, Bosnoyan-Collins L, et al. The Fanconi anaemia gene *FANCF* encodes a novel protein with homology to ROM. Nat Genet. 2000;24(1):15–6.
16. de Winter JP, Leveille F, van Berkel CG, Rooimans MA, van Der WL, Steltenpool J, et al. Isolation of a cDNA representing the Fanconi anemia complementation group E gene. Am J Hum Genet. 2000;67(5):1306–8.
17. Schneider M, Chandler K, Tischkowitz M, Meyer S. Fanconi anaemia: genetics, molecular biology, and cancer--implications for clinical management in children and adults. Clin Genet. 2014;88(1):13–24.
18. Solomon PJ, Margaret P, Rajendran R, Ramalingam R, Menezes GA, Shirley AS, et al. A case report and literature review of Fanconi Anemia (FA) diagnosed by genetic testing. Ital J Pediatr. 2015;41:38.
19. Pang Q, Christianson TA, Keeble W, Diaz J, Faulkner GR, Reifsteck C, et al. The Fanconi anemia complementation group C gene product: structural evidence of multifunctionality. Blood. 2001;98(5):1392–401.
20. Kutler DI, Auerbach AD. Fanconi anemia in Ashkenazi Jews. Fam Cancer. 2004;3(3–4):241–8.
21. Yagasaki H, Oda T, Adachi D, Nakajima T, Nakahata T, Asano S, et al. Two common founder mutations of the Fanconi anemia group G gene *FANCG/XRCC9* in the Japanese population. Hum Mutat. 2003;21(5):555.
22. Park J, Chung NG, Chae H, Kim M, Lee S, Kim Y, et al. FANCA and FANCG are the major Fanconi anemia genes in the Korean population. Clin Genet. 2013;84(3):271–5.
23. Moldovan GL, D'Andrea AD. How the Fanconi anemia pathway guards the genome. Annu Rev Genet. 2009;43:223–49.
24. Howlett NG, Taniguchi T, Olson S, Cox B, Waisfisz Q, De Die-Smulders C, et al. Biallelic inactivation of *BRCA2* in Fanconi anemia. Science. 2002;297(5581):606–9.
25. Petrucelli N, Daly MB, Feldman GL. Hereditary breast and ovarian cancer due to mutations in *BRCA1* and *BRCA2*. Genet Med. 2010;12(5):245–59.
26. Smetsers S, Muter J, Bristow C, Patel L, Chandler K, Bonney D, et al. Heterozygote *FANCD2* mutations associated with childhood T Cell ALL and testicular seminoma. Fam Cancer. 2012;11(4):661–5.
27. Flynn EK, Kamat A, Lach FP, Donovan FX, Kimble DC, Narisu N, et al. Comprehensive analysis of pathogenic deletion variants in Fanconi anemia genes. Hum Mutat. 2014;35(11):1342–53.
28. Waisfisz Q, Saar K, Morgan NV, Altay C, Leegwater PA, de Winter JP, et al. The Fanconi anemia group E gene, *FANCE*, maps to chromosome 6p. Am J Hum Genet. 1999;64(5):1400–5.
29. Gille JJ, Floor K, Kerkhoven L, Ameziane N, Joenje H, de Winter JP. Diagnosis of Fanconi anemia: mutation analysis by multiplex ligation-dependent probe amplification and PCR-based Sanger sequencing. Anemia. 2012;2012: 603253.
30. Sims AE, Spiteri E, Sims III RJ, Arita AG, Lach FP, Landers T, et al. FANCI is a second monoubiquitinated member of the Fanconi anemia pathway. Nat Struct Mol Biol. 2007;14(6):564–7.
31. Colnaghi L, Jones MJ, Cotto-Rios XM, Schindler D, Hanenberg H, Huang TT. Patient-derived C-terminal mutation of *FANCI* causes protein mislocalization and reveals putative EDGE motif function in DNA repair. Blood. 2011;117(7): 2247–56.
32. Wu Y, Sommers JA, Suhasini AN, Leonard T, Deakyne JS, Mazin AV, et al. Fanconi anemia group J mutation abolishes its DNA repair function by uncoupling DNA translocation from helicase activity or disruption of protein-DNA complexes. Blood. 2010;116(19):3780–91.
33. Guo M, Vidhyasagar V, Ding H, Wu Y. Insight into the roles of helicase motif Ia by characterizing Fanconi anemia group J protein (FANCJ) patient mutations. J Biol Chem. 2014;289(15):10551–65.
34. Ameziane N, Sie D, Dentro S, Ariyurek Y, Kerkhoven L, Joenje H, et al. Diagnosis of Fanconi anemia: mutation analysis by next-generation sequencing. Anemia. 2012;2012:132856.
35. Garcia MJ, Fernandez V, Osorio A, Barroso A, Fernandez F, Urioste M, et al. Mutational analysis of *FANCL*, *FANCM* and the recently identified *FANCI* suggests that among the 13 known Fanconi anemia genes, only *FANCD1/BRCA2* plays a major role in high-risk breast cancer predisposition. Carcinogenesis. 2009;30(11):1898–902.
36. Reid S, Schindler D, Hanenberg H, Barker K, Hanks S, Kalb R, et al. Biallelic mutations in *PALB2* cause Fanconi anemia subtype FA-N and predispose to childhood cancer. Nat Genet. 2007;39(2):162–4.
37. Lim ET, Wurtz P, Havulinna AS, Palta P, Tukiainen T, Rehnstrom K, et al. Distribution and medical impact of loss-of-function variants in the Finnish founder population. PLoS Genet. 2014;10(7):e1004494.
38. Meindl A, Hellebrand H, Wiek C, Erven V, Wappenschmidt B, Niederacher D, et al. Germline mutations in breast and ovarian cancer pedigrees establish *RAD51C* as a human cancer susceptibility gene. Nat Genet. 2010;42(5):410–4.
39. Kim Y, Lach FP, Desetty R, Hanenberg H, Auerbach AD, Smogorzewska A. Mutations of the *SLX4* gene in Fanconi anemia. Nat Genet. 2011;43(2):142–6.
40. de Garibay GR, Diaz A, Gavina B, Romero A, Garre P, Vega A, et al. Low prevalence of *SLX4* loss-of-function mutations in non-*BRCA1/2* breast and/or ovarian cancer families. Eur J Hum Genet. 2013;21(8):883–6.
41. Bogliolo M, Schuster B, Stoepker C, Derkunt B, Su Y, Raams A, et al. Mutations in *ERCC4*, encoding the DNA-repair endonuclease XPF, cause Fanconi anemia. Am J Hum Genet. 2013;92(5):800–6.
42. Sawyer SL, Tian L, Kahkonen M, Schwartzentruber J, Kircher M, Majewski J, et al. Biallelic mutations in *BRCA1* cause a new Fanconi anemia subtype. Cancer Discov. 2015;5(2):135–42.
43. Stecklein SR, Jensen RA. Identifying and exploiting defects in the Fanconi anemia/BRCA pathway in oncology. Transl Res. 2012;160(3):178–97.
44. Domchek SM, Tang J, Stopfer J, Lilli DR, Hamel N, Tischkowitz M, et al. Biallelic deleterious *BRCA1* mutations in a woman with early-onset ovarian cancer. Cancer Discov. 2013;3(4):399–405.
45. Jasin M, Rothstein R. Repair of strand breaks by homologous recombination. Cold Spring Harb Perspect Biol. 2013;5(11):a012740.
46. Wang AT, Kim T, Wagner JE, Conti BA, Lach FP, Huang AL, et al. A dominant mutation in human *RAD51* reveals its function in DNA interstrand crosslink repair independent of homologous recombination. Mol Cell. 2015;59(3):478–90.
47. Machida YJ, Machida Y, Chen Y, Gurtan AM, Kupfer GM, D'Andrea AD, et al. UBE2T is the E2 in the Fanconi anemia pathway and undergoes negative autoregulation. Mol Cell. 2006;23(4):589–96.
48. Hira A, Yoshida K, Sato K, Okuno Y, Shiraishi Y, Chiba K, et al. Mutations in the gene encoding the E2 conjugating enzyme UBE2T cause Fanconi anemia. Am J Hum Genet. 2015;96(6):1001–7.
49. Titus TA, Selvig DR, Qin B, Wilson C, Starks AM, Roe BA, et al. The Fanconi anemia gene network is conserved from zebrafish to human. Gene. 2006;371(2):211–23.
50. Marek LR, Bale AE. Drosophila homologs of FANCD2 and FANCL function in DNA repair. DNA Repair (Amst). 2006;5(11):1317–26.
51. Meetei AR, Medhurst AL, Ling C, Xue Y, Singh TR, Bier P, et al. A human ortholog of archaeal DNA repair protein Hef is defective in Fanconi anemia complementation group M. Nat Genet. 2005;37(9):958–63.
52. Lo T, Pellegrini L, Venkitaraman AR, Blundell TL. Sequence fingerprints in BRCA2 and RAD51: implications for DNA repair and cancer. DNA Repair (Amst). 2003;2(9):1015–28.
53. Petalcorin MI, Sandall J, Wigley DB, Boulton SJ. CeBRC-2 stimulates D-loop formation by RAD-51 and promotes DNA single-strand annealing. J Mol Biol. 2006;361(2):231–42.
54. Collis SJ, Barber LJ, Ward JD, Martin JS, Boulton SJ. *C. elegans* FANCD2 responds to replication stress and functions in interstrand cross-link repair. DNA Repair (Amst). 2006;5(11):1398–406.
55. Youds JL, Barber LJ, Ward JD, Collis SJ, O'Neil NJ, Boulton SJ, et al. DOG-1 is the *Caenorhabditis elegans* BRIP1/FANCJ homologue and functions in interstrand cross-link repair. Mol Cell Biol. 2008;28(5):1470–9.
56. Daee DL, Myung K. Fanconi-like crosslink repair in yeast. Genome Integr. 2012;3(1):7.
57. Ward TA, Dudasova Z, Sarkar S, Bhide MR, Vlasakova D, Chovanec M, et al. Components of a Fanconi-like pathway control Pso2-independent DNA interstrand crosslink repair in yeast. PLoS Genet. 2012;8(8):e1002884.
58. Knoll A, Higgins JD, Seeliger K, Reha SJ, Dangel NJ, Bauknecht M, et al. The Fanconi anemia ortholog FANCM ensures ordered homologous recombination in both somatic and meiotic cells in *Arabidopsis*. Plant Cell. 2012;24(4):1448–64.

59. Zhang XY, Langenick J, Traynor D, Babu MM, Kay RR, Patel KJ. Xpf and not the Fanconi anaemia proteins or Rev3 accounts for the extreme resistance to cisplatin in *Dictyostelium discoideum*. PLoS Genet. 2009;5(9):e1000645.
60. Houghtaling S, Timmers C, Noll M, Finegold MJ, Jones SN, Meyn MS, et al. Epithelial cancer in Fanconi anemia complementation group D2 (*Fancd2*) knockout mice. Genes Dev. 2003;17(16):2021–35.
61. Whitney MA, Royle G, Low MJ, Kelly MA, Axthelm MK, Reifsteck C, et al. Germ cell defects and hematopoietic hypersensitivity to gamma-interferon in mice with a targeted disruption of the Fanconi anemia C gene. Blood. 1996;88(1):49–58.
62. Hakem R, de la Pompa JL, Mak TW. Developmental studies of *Brca1* and *Brca2* knock-out mice. J Mammary Gland Biol Neoplasia. 1998;3(4):431–45.
63. Cheng NC, van de Vrugt HJ, van der Valk MA, Oostra AB, Krimpenfort P, de VY, et al. Mice with a targeted disruption of the Fanconi anemia homolog *Fanca*. Hum Mol Genet. 2000;9:1805–11.
64. Yang Y, Kuang Y, De Montes OR, Hays T, Moreau L, Lu N, et al. Targeted disruption of the murine Fanconi anemia gene, *Fancg/Xrcc9*. Blood. 2001;98(12):3435–40.
65. Wong JC, Alon N, Mckerlie C, Huang JR, Meyn MS, Buchwald M. Targeted disruption of exons 1 to 6 of the Fanconi Anemia group A gene leads to growth retardation, strain-specific microphthalmia, meiotic defects and primordial germ cell hypoplasia. Hum Mol Genet. 2003;12(16):2063–76.
66. Bakker ST, van de Vrugt HJ, Rooimans MA, Oostra AB, Steltenpool J, Delzenne-Goette E, et al. Fancm-deficient mice reveal unique features of Fanconi anemia complementation group M. Hum Mol Genet. 2009;18(18): 3484–95.
67. Bouwman P, Drost R, Klijn C, Pieterse M, van der Gulden H, Song JY, et al. Loss of p53 partially rescues embryonic development of *Palb2* knockout mice but does not foster haploinsufficiency of *Palb2* in tumour suppression. J Pathol. 2011;224(1):10–21.
68. Bakker ST, van de Vrugt HJ, Visser JA, Delzenne-Goette E, van der Wal A, Berns MA, et al. Fancf-deficient mice are prone to develop ovarian tumours. J Pathol. 2012;226(1):28–39.
69. Taniguchi T, D'Andrea AD. The Fanconi anemia protein, FANCE, promotes the nuclear accumulation of FANCC. Blood. 2002;100(7):2457–62.
70. Polito D, Cukras S, Wang X, Spence P, Moreau L, D'Andrea AD, et al. The carboxyl terminus of FANCE recruits FANCD2 to the Fanconi Anemia (FA) E3 ligase complex to promote the FA DNA repair pathway. J Biol Chem. 2014;289(10):7003–10.
71. Gurtan AM, Stuckert P, D'Andrea AD. The WD40 repeats of FANCL are required for Fanconi anemia core complex assembly. J Biol Chem. 2006; 281(16):10896–905.
72. Joksic I, Vujic D, Guc-Scekic M, Leskovac A, Petrovic S, Ojani M, et al. Dysfunctional telomeres in primary cells from Fanconi anemia *FANCD2* patients. Genome Integr. 2012;3(1):6.
73. Garaycoechea JI, Patel KJ. Why does the bone marrow fail in Fanconi anemia? Blood. 2014;123(1):26–34.
74. Howard SM, Yanez DA, Stark JM. DNA damage response factors from diverse pathways, including DNA crosslink repair, mediate alternative end joining. PLoS Genet. 2015;11(1):e1004943.
75. Otsuki T, Furukawa Y, Ikeda K, Endo H, Yamashita T, Shinohara A, et al. Fanconi anemia protein, FANCA, associates with BRG1, a component of the human SWI/SNF complex. Hum Mol Genet. 2001;10(23):2651–60.
76. Sridharan D, Brown M, Lambert WC, McMahon LW, Lambert MW. Nonerythroid alpha II spectrin is required for recruitment of FANCA and XPF to nuclear foci induced by DNA interstrand cross-links. J Cell Sci. 2003;116(Pt 5):823–35.
77. Ravera S, Vaccaro D, Cuccarolo P, Columbaro M, Capanni C, Bartolucci M, et al. Mitochondrial respiratory chain Complex I defects in Fanconi anemia complementation group A. Biochimie. 2013;95(10):1828–37.
78. Kim S, Hwang SK, Lee M, Kwak H, Son K, Yang J, et al. Fanconi anemia complementation group A (FANCA) localizes to centrosomes and functions in the maintenance of centrosome integrity. Int J Biochem Cell Biol. 2013;45(9):1953–61.
79. Scharer OD. DNA interstrand crosslinks: natural and drug-induced DNA adducts that induce unique cellular responses. Chembiochem. 2005;6(1):27–32.
80. Castillo P, Bogliolo M, Surralles J. Coordinated action of the Fanconi anemia and ataxia telangiectasia pathways in response to oxidative damage. DNA Repair (Amst). 2011;10(5):518–25.
81. Taniguchi T, Garcia-Higuera I, Xu B, Andreassen PR, Gregory RC, Kim ST, et al. Convergence of theFanconi anemia and ataxia telangiectasia signaling pathways. Cell. 2002;109(4):459–72.
82. Nakanishi K, Taniguchi T, Ranganathan V, New HV, Moreau LA, Stotsky M, et al. Interaction of FANCD2 and NBS1 in the DNA damage response. Nat Cell Biol. 2002;4(12):913–20.
83. Deans AJ, West SC. FANCM connects the genome instability disorders Bloom's syndrome and Fanconi anemia. Mol Cell. 2009;36(6):943–53.
84. Alter BP. Cancer in Fanconi anemia, 1927–2001. Cancer. 2003;97(2):425–40.
85. Gillio AP, Verlander PC, Batish SD, Giampietro PF, Auerbach AD. Phenotypic consequences of mutations in the Fanconi anemia *FANCC* gene: an International Fanconi Anemia Registry study. Blood. 1997;90(1):105–10.
86. Futaki M, Yamashita T, Yagasaki H, Toda T, Yabe M, Kato S, et al. The IVS4 + 4 A to T mutation of the Fanconi anemia gene *FANCC* is not associated with a severe phenotype in Japanese patients. Blood. 2000;95(4):1493–8.
87. Wagner JE, Tolar J, Levran O, Scholl T, Deffenbaugh A, Satagopan J, et al. Germline mutations in *BRCA2*: shared genetic susceptibility to breast cancer, early onset leukemia, and Fanconi anemia. Blood. 2004;103(8):3226–9.
88. Akbari MR, Malekzadeh R, Lepage P, Roquis D, Sadjadi AR, Aghcheli K, et al. Mutations in Fanconi anemia genes and the risk of esophageal cancer. Hum Genet. 2011;129(5):573–82.
89. Couch FJ, Johnson MR, Rabe K, Boardman L, McWilliams R, de AM, et al. Germ line Fanconi anemia complementation group C mutations and pancreatic cancer. Cancer Res. 2005;65(2):383–6.
90. Rafnar T, Gudbjartsson DF, Sulem P, Jonasdottir A, Sigurdsson A, Jonasdottir A, et al. Mutations in *BRIP1* confer high risk of ovarian cancer. Nat Genet. 2011;43(11):1104–7.

6

Association of six CpG-SNPs in the inflammation-related genes with coronary heart disease

Xiaomin Chen[1], Xiaoying Chen[3], Yan Xu[3], William Yang[2], Nan Wu[1,3], Huadan Ye[3], Jack Y. Yang[5], Qingxiao Hong[3], Yanfei Xin[4], Mary Qu Yang[5], Youping Deng[6,7] and Shiwei Duan[3*]

Abstract

Background: Chronic inflammation has been widely considered to be the major risk factor of coronary heart disease (CHD). The goal of our study was to explore the possible association with CHD for inflammation-related single nucleotide polymorphisms (SNPs) involved in cytosine-phosphate-guanine (CpG) dinucleotides. A total of 784 CHD patients and 739 non-CHD controls were recruited from Zhejiang Province, China. Using the Sequenom MassARRAY platform, we measured the genotypes of six inflammation-related CpG-SNPs, including *IL1B* rs16944, *IL1R2* rs2071008, *PLA2G7* rs9395208, *FAM5C* rs12732361, *CD40* rs1800686, and *CD36* rs2065666). Allele and genotype frequencies were compared between CHD and non-CHD individuals using the CLUMP22 software with 10,000 Monte Carlo simulations.

Results: Allelic tests showed that *PLA2G7* rs9395208 and *CD40* rs1800686 were significantly associated with CHD. Moreover, *IL1B* rs16944, *PLA2G7* rs9395208, and *CD40* rs1800686 were shown to be associated with CHD under the dominant model. Further gender-based subgroup tests showed that one SNP (*CD40* rs1800686) and two SNPs (*FAM5C* rs12732361 and *CD36* rs2065666) were associated with CHD in females and males, respectively. And the age-based subgroup tests indicated that *PLA2G7* rs9395208, *IL1B* rs16944, and *CD40* rs1800686 were associated with CHD among individuals younger than 55, younger than 65, and over 65, respectively.

Conclusions: In conclusion, all the six inflammation-related CpG-SNPs (rs16944, rs2071008, rs12732361, rs2065666, rs9395208, and rs1800686) were associated with CHD in the combined or subgroup tests, suggesting an important role of inflammation in the risk of CHD.

Keywords: Coronary heart disease, Inflammation, Promoter, CpG-SNP, Polymorphism

Background

Coronary heart disease (CHD) is considered to be the leading cause of mortality and morbidity in the elderly [1]. CHD has emerged as a serious burden to human health [2]. Both genetic and environmental factors were shown to play an important role in the development of CHD [3]. Environmental factors, including smoking and dietary changes, were found to be associated with CHD [4]. Heritable factors were estimated to contribute to 30–60 % of the variation in the risk of CHD [3]. In addition, the incidence of CHD was generally higher in men than in women regardless of their menopause type [5]. Therefore, further exploration of the interactive mechanism between genes and environment is much more significant and helpful for specific diagnosis [6].

Increasing amount of evidence has indicated that inflammation is responsible for CHD [7, 8]. Many inflammation-related genes are found to be associated with risk of CHD [9, 10]. Interleukin 1, beta gene (*IL1B*) encodes the cytokine which exerts a wide range of inflammatory activities [11]. Genetic association between *IL1B* and CHD has been previously found [12]. Interleukin 1 receptor, type II (*IL1R2*) encodes a cytokine receptor that belongs to the interleukin 1 receptor family [13]. Notably, *IL1R2* is recognized as a general factor in

* Correspondence: duanshiwei@nbu.edu.cn
[3]School of Medicine, Ningbo University, Ningbo, Zhejiang 315211, China
Full list of author information is available at the end of the article

inflammatory response [14]. Phospholipase A2, group VII (*PLA2G7*) gene encodes a kind of secreted enzyme [15], and patients with high *PLA2G7* expression was found to have an increased risk of cardiovascular diseases [16]. Gene polymorphisms in family with sequence similarity 5, member C (*FAM5C*) gene were shown to be associated with an increased risk of acute myocardial infarction [17], and elevated FAM5C levels were found in atherosclerotic plaques and coronary artery endothelium [18]. *CD40* encodes a cell surface receptor that plays a pivotal role in macrophage activation and parasite immunity [19], and *CD40* could up-regulate prime macrophages through a proinflammatory program in recent studies [19]. *CD36* encodes a platelet receptor glycoprotein involved in different biological processes such as inflammation, atherosclerosis, and platelet activation [20]. The association between monocyte/macrophage *CD36* and atherosclerosis has been found in the previous studies [21].

Single nucleotide polymorphisms (SNPs) can change biological properties of the encoded protein and affect gene expression levels in an allele-specific manner (24450106). Due to the mutability of cytosine-phosphate-guanine (CpG) dinucleotides, CpG-SNPs, as an important class of cis-regulatory polymorphisms, connect genetic variation to the individual variability of the epigenome [22]. CpG-SNPs in the promoter regions had been found to be associated with multiple diseases, including type 2 diabetes [23], breast cancer [24], schizophrenia [25], and epithelial ovarian cancer [26]. In light of previous studies, we aimed to evaluate whether the six inflammation-related gene CpG-SNPs could contribute to the risk of CHD.

Results and discussion

Genotypic and allelic tests were performed for a total of six CpG-SNPs between CHD and non-CHD individuals (Table 1). According to the most recent human assembly, hg38/GRCh38, five CpG-SNPs (*FAM5C* rs12732361, *IL1R2* rs2071008, *IL1B* rs16944, *CD40* rs1800686, and *CD36* rs2065666) were located upstream of the corresponding transcription start sites (47, 178, 387, 508, and 659 bp, respectively). The remaining one (*PLA2G7* rs9395208) was located in the 111 bp downstream of transcription start sites.

As shown in Table 2, the genotype distributions of all the six SNPs in the non-CHD controls met Hardy-Weinberg equilibrium (HWE). Our results showed that *PLA2G7* rs9395208 and *CD40* rs1800686 were significantly associated with CHD on the allele level. The frequency of allele rs9395208-G was significantly lower in the case group than in the control (84.7 versus 87.3 %; $P = 0.04$, OR = 0.806, 95 % CI = 0.657–0.991). Meanwhile, a higher rs1800686-G frequency showed in the cases than in controls (69.4 versus 65.4 %; $P = 0.02$; OR = 1.198, 95 % CI = 1.029–0.394). No significant difference was observed on the genotype level for all the CpG-SNPs ($P > 0.05$).

Gender disparities widely existed in the prevalence of CHD [27], and female CHD patients aged 40 or older have 10 % greater risk of death than the males [27]. Hence, we performed a gender-based subgroup analysis

Table 1 The list of genotyping primers for six CpG-SNPs

Gene	SNP	Primers	Sequence (5′ to 3′)
IL1B	rs16944	1st PCR primer	ACGTTGGATGAGAGGCTCCTGCAATTGACA
		2nd primer	ACGTTGGATGCTGTCTGTATTGAGGGTGTG
		Extend primer	GGGGTGGGTGCTGTTCTCTGCCTC
IL1R2	rs2071008	1st PCR primer	ACGTTGGATGGAAAAATCCATGCAGCCTCC
		2nd primer	ACGTTGGATGTGGTGGCTGACTTTCCAAGG
		Extend primer	TGGGAAGAAGCAAGCACCCC
PLA2G7	rs9395208	1st PCR primer	ACGTTGGATGTGGACCCGCGGTTAACTTAG
		2nd primer	ACGTTGGATGATCAGGTCTGCGGAAAGGAG
		Extend primer	GCATTGCCTGGCTCT
FAM5C	rs12732361	1st PCR primer	ACGTTGGATGTTACACAGAGAGCCACGAAC
		2nd primer	ACGTTGGATGAGGATCACCACGAATCACCC
		Extend primer	GAAACCCCCACCATTCCCCA
CD40	rs1800686	1st PCR primer	ACGTTGGATGATGGATGGGAAGTTGAGACG
		2nd primer	ACGTTGGATGCCCAACTCAGAATTTCGCTC
		Extend primer	GTCGCTTTCAAAGGAAATTCCCT
CD36	rs2065666	1st PCR primer	ACGTTGGATGCTCTGAAGATATAATGACAAG
		2nd primer	ACGTTGGATGCAGTTTCTCTGTTCACTTCG
		Extend primer	CGTTCACTTCGTTTTAGTATAGAATTA

Table 2 Comparisons of genotype and allele frequencies between cases and controls

SNP	Groups	Genotype (counts)			χ^2	*P* (*df* = 2)	HWE *P* value[a]	Allele (counts)		χ^2	*P* (*df* = 1)	OR (95 % CI)
IL1B rs16944		GG	AG	AA				G	A			
	Cases	220	380	176			0.627	820	732			
	Controls	173	379	180	4.387	0.112	0.335	725	739	3.310	0.069	1.142 (0.990–1.317)
IL1R2 rs2071008		GG	GT	TT				G	T			
	Cases	434	285	65			0.064	1153	415			
	Controls	417	275	46	2.382	0.304	0.941	1109	367	1.020	0.313	0.919 (0.781–1.082)
PLA2G7 rs9395208		GG	GC	CC				G	C			
	Cases	565	198	21			0.468	1328	240			
	Controls	568	154	17	4.603	0.100	0.095	1290	188	4.210	0.040	0.806 (0.657–0.991)
FAM5C rs12732361		GG	AG	AA				G	A			
	Cases	492	242	49			0.011	1226	340			
	Controls	431	254	52	3.022	0.221	0.088	1116	358	2.850	0.091	1.157 (0.977–1.370)
CD40 rs1800686		GG	AG	AA				G	A			
	Cases	378	332	74			0.929	1088	480			
	Controls	317	333	89	5.411	0.067	0.914	967	511	5.440	0.020	1.198 (1.029–1.394)
CD36 rs2065666		GG	GC	CC				G	C			
	Cases	439	288	56			0.356	1166	400			
	Controls	411	282	43	1.24	0.538	0.555	1104	368	0.120	0.729	0.972 (0.825–1.145)

[a]*HWE* Hardy-Weinberg equilibrium; *P* value <0.05 was considered a departure from HWE

to detect the difference both in genotype and allele frequencies (Table 3). It showed significant associations of *FAM5C* rs12732361 and *CD36* rs2065666 with CHD in males on the allele level ($P = 0.03$, OR = 1.266, 95 % CI = 1.022–1.568; $P = 0.04$, OR = 0.806, 95 % CI = 0.652–0.996, respectively). Meanwhile, *CD40* rs1800686 was shown to be significantly associated with CHD in females ($P = 0.02$, OR = 1.347, 95 % CI = 1.043–1.740 by allele).

Age is another well-known risk factor in the development and prognosis of CHD [28], and there were over 70 % of coronary-related deaths occurred in the people older than 70 in North America and Western Europe [28]. Therefore, we further evaluated the genotype and allele frequencies in different age subgroups (Table 3). For the individuals younger than 55, the frequencies of both rs16944-G and rs2071008-G alleles were significantly lower in case group than in control group ($P = 0.01$, OR = 1.422, 95 % CI = 1.077–1.877; $P = 0.04$, OR = 0.733, 95 % CI = 0.538–1.000, respectively). For the individuals with age between 55 and 65 years old, rs16944 was associated with CHD on both genotype and allele levels ($\chi^2 = 6.15$, $P = 0.04$ by genotype; $P = 0.03$, OR = 1.299, 95 % CI = 1.022–1.653 by allele). Among the individuals older than 55, rs1800686 was also shown to be associated with CHD on both genotype and allele levels (genotype: $\chi^2 = 9.44$, $P = 0.009$; allele: $P = 0.003$; OR = 1.456, 95 % CI = 1.132–1.8740).

Additionally, we have conducted a comparison under the dominant and recessive inheritance models between cases and controls (Table 3). In the dominant model, significant associations among rs16944, rs9395208 and rs1800686 with CHD were observed. The rs16944-A and rs1800686-A alleles were risk factors for CHD (rs16944: $P = 0.03$, OR = 1.279, 95 % CI = 1.015–1.611; rs1800686: $P = 0.04$, OR = 1.239, 95 % CI = 1.013–1.517). The rs9395208-C allele was a protective factor for CHD ($P = 0.03$, OR = 0.777, 95 % CI = 0.616–0.979). Meanwhile, all the six CpG-SNPs showed no significant association with CHD in the recessive model.

Besides, a post hoc power analysis showed that our association study had strong power (93.9–94.1 %) to detect significant association of the six CpG-SNPs under an OR of 1.3.

The present study performed a comprehensive analysis of association between six CpG-SNPs (*IL1B* rs16944, *IL1R2* rs2071008, *PLA2G7* rs9395208, *FAM5C* rs12732361, *CD40* rs1800686, and *CD36* rs2065666) and CHD. At the allelic level, *CD40* rs1800686-G was found to be a risk factor, while *PLA2G7* rs9395208-G was found to be a protective factor. Moreover, all the CpG-SNPs were significantly associated with the risk of CHD in the combined or subgroup analyses.

Inflammation represents an important feature in the process of atherosclerosis, which can form, destabilize, and rupture atherosclerotic plaques, finally causing CHD [29]. Over the years, researchers have found some inflammatory factors related to the pathogenesis and prognosis of CHD, such as *CLOCK* SNP rs4580704 [30], *ICAM-1*

Table 3 A list of SNPs associated with CHD in the subgroup tests

Gene	SNP	Model or subgroup	Group	Genotype or allele (counts)	χ^2	P (*df*)	OR (95 % CI)
IL1B	rs16944	Dominant	Cases	GG/GA + AA (220/556)	4.350	0.037 (1)	1.279 (1.015–1.611)
			Controls	GG/GA + AA (173/559)			
IL1B	rs16944	≤55 years of age	Cases	G/A (236/236)	6.190	0.013 (1)	1.422 (1.077–1.877)
			Controls	G/A (292/248)			
IL1B	rs16944	55–65 years of age	Cases	GG/GA/AA (79/134/57)	6.147	0.046 (2)	
			Controls	GG/GA/AA (53/145/66)			
IL1B	rs16944	55–65 years of age	Cases	G/A (292/248)	4.560	0.033 (1)	1.299 (1.022–1.653)
			Cases	G/A (251/277)			
IL1R2	rs2071008	≤55 years of age	Controls	G/T (254/106)	3.860	0.049 (1)	0.733 (0.538–1.000)
			Cases	G/T (366/112)			
PLA2G7	rs9395208	Dominant	Cases	GG/GC + CC (565/219)	4.590	0.032 (1)	0.777 (0.616–0.979)
			Controls	GG/GC + CC (568/171)			
PLA2G7	rs9395208	≤55 years of age	Cases	G/C (295/65)	5.750	0.016 (1)	0.627 (0.427–0.920)
			Controls	G/C (420/58)			
FAM5C	rs12732361	Male	Cases	G/C (849/225)	4.660	0.031 (1)	1.266 (1.022–1.568)
			Controls	G/C (629/211)			
CD40	rs1800686	Female	Cases	G/A (354/138)	5.230	0.022 (1)	1.347 (1.043–1.740)
			Controls	G/A (417/219)			
CD40	rs1800686	Dominant	Cases	GG/GA + AA (378/406)	4.340	0.037 (1)	1.239 (1.013–1.517)
			Controls	GG/GA + AA (317/422)			
CD40	rs1800686	≥65 years of age	Cases	GG/GA/AA (163/146/24)	9.437	0.009 (2)	
			Controls	GG/GA/AA (90/109/32)			
CD40	rs1800686	≥65 years of age	Cases	G/A (472/194)	8.600	0.0034 (1)	1.456 (1.132–1.874)
			Controls	G/A (289/173)			
CD36	rs2065666	Male	Cases	G/C (790/286)	4.000	0.046 (1)	0.806 (0.652–0.996)
			Controls	G/C (641/187)			

SNP rs281432 [31], and *NFKB1* SNP rs28362491 [32]. Some of these inflammation-related genes were expected to be drug targets for the control and treatment of CHD. Meanwhile, we hypothesized that hereditable methylation could be associated with CHD. Because of low minor allele frequency or weak haplotype associations, genome-wide searches for genetic risk factors for CHD have in general not investigated the CpG-SNPs. Our previous work [33] indicated that CpG-SNPs of the thrombotic pathway genes contributed to the risk of CHD, which suggested a clue for investigating the contributions of the inflammation-related CpG-SNPs to the susceptibility to CHD.

PLA2G7 gene encodes a secreted enzyme whose activity is associated with CHD [34]. *PLA2G7* functions as a biomarker of plaque inflammation and stability [35]. Several *PLA2G7* SNPs (e.g., rs7756935, rs1805017, and rs13210554) have been reported on the susceptibility to CHD [35, 36]. Here, we discovered a significant association of *PLA2G7* CpG-SNP rs9395208 with CHD, even in the individuals aged ≤55, providing additional evidence of age dimorphism in the risk of CHD. Additionally, Jiang et al. [15] have reported that the correlation between *PLA2G7* methylation and CHD risk in females is independent of age, smoking, diabetes, and hypertension, which indicated a close relationship between *PLA2G7* and hereditable methylation in the pathogenic mechanism of CHD.

The contribution of *CD40* rs1800686 is another main finding in the current study. *CD40* is considered to determine T cell responses to antigen presentation and B cells immunoglobulin isotype switching, which plays a key role in the inflammatory and prothrombotic processes by bonding with CD40 ligand (CD40L) in atherosclerosis [37]. Previous study provided evidence of association of *CD40* rs1883832 with an overall increased risk of CHD in Chinese population [38]. In the current study, a similar result was drawn that *CD40* rs1800686-A allele contributed to CHD risk. Age and gender are considered as two independent risk factors in CHD [28, 39]. Subsequent subgroup analysis identified age and gender differences existed in the rs1800686, which revealed an age- and gender-based mechanism on the genetic variations.

As a scavenger receptor, CD36 is not only involved in the metabolism of lipids but also plays an important role in the adhesion of negatively charged macromolecules [40]. CD36 is widely expressed in cells and tissues including microvascular endothelial cells, monocytes, and macrophages [41]. Previous study implied that increased CD36 expression level could reflect the severity of coronary artery atherosclerosis [42]. Several *CD36* SNPs (e.g., rs5956, rs3173798, and rs3211892) have been reported to be associated with CHD [42]. Here, we detected a significant protection role of *CD36* CpG-SNP rs2065666 G carries in CHD male patients. Our data suggested a possible molecular mechanism through which SNP could influence a phenotype.

Interleukins (IL-1B and IL1R2) were shown to play a role in the inflammatory response, and they lead to the development of atherosclerotic plaques [43, 44]. Recently, gender dimorphism was observed in the association of *IL-1B* polymorphism with CHD [45]. We find no significant difference on *IL-1B* rs16944 allele or genotype level by gender subgroup analysis. However, age-based subgroup tests showed that *IL-1B* rs16944-G was a risk factor of CHD in younger population, while *IL1R2* rs2071008-G was a protective factor. Further validation study or functional analysis of these variants is needed in the future.

Increased expression of FAM5C may be induced by inflammatory stimuli [17]. This case-control study observed significant associations between *FAM5C* rs12732361 polymorphisms and CHD only in males. Due to a lack of CHD study on *FAM5C*, more investigations are needed to validate our results.

There are also limitations in the current study. The findings of our study are limited to a small population with documented CHD and cannot be generalized to the population at large. Although we found positive results in the current study, the power effect might be reduced by strict multiple adjustment or subgroup analyses. Therefore, larger sample size and other ethnic populations are required to be investigated.

Conclusions

In conclusion, our case-control study suggested that the six inflammation-related CpG-SNPs were significantly associated with the risk of CHD in the combined or the subgroup samples. Moreover, our results also revealed that *IL1B* rs16944, *PLA2G7* rs9395208, and *CD40* rs1800686 had a significant contribution to the risk of CHD under the dominant model.

Methods

Sample collection

A total of 784 CHD patients and 739 healthy controls were collected from Ningbo First Hospital of Ningbo University between May 2008 and April 2015 in Zhejiang province, China. CHD patients and non-CHD controls were defined as described before [33, 46]. Patients with congenital heart disease, cardiomyopathy, liver disease, and renal disease were excluded. Blood samples were collected in 3.2 % citrate sodium-treated tubes and processed in the central clinical laboratory of the hospital. All the participants provided written informed consent form under a protocol approved by the Medical Ethics Committees of Ningbo First Hospital and Ningbo University.

SNP selection and genotyping

The selected CpG-SNPs are on the promoter of inflammation-related genes. Meanwhile, the minor allele frequencies of the selected CpG-SNPs are over 10 % in HapMap HCB population. CpG-SNPs with design problems or failed assays were excluded. Finally, six CpG-SNPs in inflammation-related genes were included in the current study. DNA extraction and quantification were described as previously [33, 46]. The polymerase chain reaction (PCR) amplification was performed on the GeneAmp® PCR System 9700 (Applied Biosystems, Foster City, CA, USA), and the genotyping was performed on the MassARRAY iPLEX® assay platform (Sequenom, San Diego, CA, USA). The sequences of the amplification and extension primers for the six CpG-SNPs were shown in Table 1.

Statistical analyses

Genotype and allele frequencies of the polymorphisms between cases and controls were calculated by the CLUMP22 software with 10,000 Monte Carlo simulations [47]. The distribution of Hardy-Weinberg equilibrium (HWE) was tested using the Arlequin program (version 3.5, Bern, Switzerland), and $P > 0.05$ was considered to be in HWE. Power analysis was performed using the Power and Sample Size Calculation software (v3.0.43). A two-tailed $P < 0.05$ was considered statistically significant.

Competing interests

The authors declare that they have no competing interests.

Authors' contributions

XMC, SWD, and MQY conceived and designed the experiments. XYC, YX, NW, HDY, QXH, and YPD performed the experiments. XYC, HDY, and WY analyzed the data. JYY and YFX contributed reagents/materials/analysis tools. XYC and YX wrote the paper. XMC, XYC, and YX contributed equally to this work. All authors read and approved the final manuscript.

Declarations

The research and publication was supported by the grants from the National Natural Science Foundation of China (31100919, 81371469), Zhejiang Provincial Natural Science Foundation (LR13H020003), Ningbo City Medical Science and Technology projects (2014A20), and K. C. Wong Magna Fund in Ningbo University. This article has been published as part of *Human Genomics* volume 10 Supplement

2, 2016: from genes to systems genomics: human genomics. The full contents of the supplement are available online at http://humgenomics.biomedcentral.com/articles/supplements/volume-10-supplement-2.

Author details
[1]Cardiovascular Center of Ningbo First Hospital, Ningbo University, Ningbo, Zhejiang 315010, China. [2]Texas Advanced Computing Center, University of Texas at Austin, 10100 Burnet Road (R8700), Austin, TX 78758-4497, USA. [3]School of Medicine, Ningbo University, Ningbo, Zhejiang 315211, China. [4]Center of Safety Evaluation, Zhejiang Academy of Medical Sciences, Hangzhou, Zhejiang 310007, China. [5]MidSouth Bioinformatics Center, Department of Information Science, George Washington Donaghey College of Engineering and Information Science, and Joint Bioinformatics Graduate Program, University of Arkansas at Little Rock and University of Arkansas for Medical Sciences, 2881 S. University Ave, Little Rock, AR 72204, USA. [6]Medical College, Wuhan University of Science and Technology, Wuhan 430064, China. [7]Department of Internal Medicine and Biochemistry, Rush University Medical Center, Chicago, IL 60612, USA.

References

1. Lauer MS. Advancing cardiovascular research. Chest. 2012;141:500–5.
2. Beatty AL, Ku IA, Bibbins-Domingo K, Christenson RH, DeFilippi CR, Ganz P, et al. Traditional risk factors versus biomarkers for prediction of secondary events in patients with stable coronary heart disease: from the heart and soul study. J Am Heart Assoc. 2015;4. doi:10.1161/JAHA.114.001646.
3. Mega JL, Stitziel NO, Smith JG, Chasman DI, Caulfield MJ, Devlin JJ, et al. Genetic risk, coronary heart disease events, and the clinical benefit of statin therapy: an analysis of primary and secondary prevention trials. Lancet. 2015;385:2264–71.
4. Dalen JE, Alpert JS, Goldberg RJ, Weinstein RS. The epidemic of the 20(th) century: coronary heart disease. Am J Med. 2014;127:807–12.
5. Kim C, Cushman M, Khodneva Y, Lisabeth LD, Judd S, Kleindorfer DO, et al. Risk of incident coronary heart disease events in men compared to women by menopause type and race. J Am Heart Assoc. 2015;4. doi:10.1161/JAHA.115.001881.
6. Xiaoying C, Huadan Y, Qingxiao H, Annan Z, Linlin T, Shiwei D. The effects of DNA methylation on the homeostasis in vascular diseases. Yi Chuan. 2015;37:221–32.
7. Ross R. Atherosclerosis—an inflammatory disease. N Engl J Med. 1999;340:115–26.
8. Rothenbacher D, Kleiner A, Koenig W, Primatesta P, Breitling LP, Brenner H. Relationship between inflammatory cytokines and uric acid levels with adverse cardiovascular outcomes in patients with stable coronary heart disease. PLoS One. 2012;7:e45907.
9. Gigante B, Strawbridge RJ, Velasquez IM, Golabkesh Z, Silveira A, Goel A, et al. Analysis of the role of interleukin 6 receptor haplotypes in the regulation of circulating levels of inflammatory biomarkers and risk of coronary heart disease. PLoS One. 2015;10:e0119980.
10. Li L, He M, Zhou L, Miao X, Wu F, Huang S, et al. A solute carrier family 22 member 3 variant rs3088442 G→A associated with coronary heart disease inhibits lipopolysaccharide-induced inflammatory response. J Biol Chem. 2015;290:5328–40.
11. Stahelova A, Mrazek F, Smizansky M, Petrek M, Gallo J. Variation in the IL1B, TNF and IL6 genes and individual susceptibility to prosthetic joint infection. BMC Immunol. 2012;13:25.
12. Zhang YM, Zhong LJ, He BX, Li WC, Nie J, Wang X, et al. The correlation between polymorphism at position -511C/T in the promoter region of interleukin 1B and the severity of coronary heart disease. Zhonghua Yi Xue Yi Chuan Xue Za Zhi. 2006;23:86–8.
13. Palomo J, Dietrich D, Martin P, Palmer G, Gabay C. The interleukin (IL)-1 cytokine family—balance between agonists and antagonists in inflammatory diseases. Cytokine. 2015;76:25–37.
14. Garlanda C, Riva F, Bonavita E, Mantovani A. Negative regulatory receptors of the IL-1 family. Semin Immunol. 2013;25:408–15.
15. Jiang D, Zheng D, Wang L, Huang Y, Liu H, Xu L, et al. Elevated PLA2G7 gene promoter methylation as a gender-specific marker of aging increases the risk of coronary heart disease in females. PLoS One. 2013;8:e59752.
16. Vainio P, Lehtinen L, Mirtti T, Hilvo M, Seppanen-Laakso T, Virtanen J, et al. Phospholipase PLA2G7, associated with aggressive prostate cancer, promotes prostate cancer cell migration and invasion and is inhibited by statins. Oncotarget. 2011;2:1176–90.
17. Sato J, Kinugasa M, Satomi-Kobayashi S, Hatakeyama K, Knox AJ, Asada Y, et al. Family with sequence similarity 5, member C (FAM5C) increases leukocyte adhesion molecules in vascular endothelial cells: implication in vascular inflammation. PLoS One. 2014;9:e107236.
18. Kim CW, Song H, Kumar S, Nam D, Kwon HS, Chang KH, et al. Anti-inflammatory and antiatherogenic role of BMP receptor II in endothelial cells. Arterioscler Thromb Vasc Biol. 2013;33:1350–9.
19. Morgado P, Sudarshana DM, Gov L, Harker KS, Lam T, Casali P, et al. Type II toxoplasma gondii induction of CD40 on infected macrophages enhances interleukin-12 responses. Infect Immun. 2014;82:4047–55.
20. Petta S, Handberg A, Marchesini G, Camma C, Di Marco V, Cabibi D, et al. High sCD36 plasma level is associated with steatosis and its severity in patients with genotype 1 chronic hepatitis C. J Viral Hepat. 2013;20:174–82.
21. Collot-Teixeira S, Martin J, McDermott-Roe C, Poston R, McGregor JL. CD36 and macrophages in atherosclerosis. Cardiovasc Res. 2007;75:468–77.
22. Shoemaker R, Deng J, Wang W, Zhang K. Allele-specific methylation is prevalent and is contributed by CpG-SNPs in the human genome. Genome Res. 2010;20:883–9.
23. Dayeh TA, Olsson AH, Volkov P, Almgren P, Ronn T, Ling C. Identification of CpG-SNPs associated with type 2 diabetes and differential DNA methylation in human pancreatic islets. Diabetologia. 2013;56:1036–46.
24. Harlid S, Ivarsson MI, Butt S, Hussain S, Grzybowska E, Eyfjord JE, et al. A candidate CpG SNP approach identifies a breast cancer associated ESR1-SNP. Int J Cancer. 2011;129:1689–98.
25. Bani-Fatemi A, Goncalves VF, Zai C, de Souza R, Le Foll B, Kennedy JL, et al. Analysis of CpG SNPs in 34 genes: association test with suicide attempt in schizophrenia. Schizophr Res. 2013;147:262–8.
26. Koestler DC, Chalise P, Cicek MS, Cunningham JM, Armasu S, Larson MC, et al. Integrative genomic analysis identifies epigenetic marks that mediate genetic risk for epithelial ovarian cancer. BMC Med Genomics. 2014;7:8.
27. Cline JL, Beckie TM. The relationships between FAM5C SNP (rs10920501) variability and metabolic syndrome and inflammation in women with coronary heart disease. Biol Res Nurs. 2013;15:160–6.
28. Che JJ, Shao YX, Li GP. Association between rs1049673 polymorphism in CD36 and premature coronary heart disease. Genet Mol Res. 2014;13:7708–17.
29. Hoffmeister A, Rothenbacher D, Bazner U, Frohlich M, Brenner H, Hombach V, et al. Role of novel markers of inflammation in patients with stable coronary heart disease. Am J Cardiol. 2001;87:262–6.
30. Gomez-Delgado F, Garcia-Rios A, Alcala-Diaz JF, Rangel-Zuniga O, Delgado-Lista J, Yubero-Serrano EM, et al. Chronic consumption of a low-fat diet improves cardiometabolic risk factors according to the CLOCK gene in patients with coronary heart disease. Mol Nutr Food Res. 2015;59:2556–64.
31. Chou CH, Ueng KC, Liu YF, Wu CH, Yang SF, Wang PH. Impact of intercellular adhesion molecule-1 genetic polymorphisms on coronary artery disease susceptibility in Taiwanese subjects. Int J Med Sci. 2015;12:510–6.
32. Lai HM, Li XM, Yang YN, Ma YT, Xu R, Pan S, et al. Genetic variation in NFKB1 and NFKBIA and susceptibility to coronary artery disease in a Chinese Uygur population. PLoS One. 2015;10:e0129144.
33. Ye H, Zhou A, Hong Q, Chen X, Xin Y, Tang L, et al. Association of seven thrombotic pathway gene CpG-SNPs with coronary heart disease. Biomed Pharmacother. 2015;72:98–102.
34. Vittos O, Toana B, Vittos A, Moldoveanu E. Lipoprotein-associated phospholipase A2 (Lp-PLA2): a review of its role and significance as a cardiovascular biomarker. Biomarkers. 2012;17:289–302.
35. Xu L, Zhou J, Huang S, Huang Y, Le Y, Jiang D, et al. An association study between genetic polymorphisms related to lipoprotein-associated phospholipase A(2) and coronary heart disease. Exp Ther Med. 2013;5:742–50.
36. Hou L, Chen S, Yu H, Lu X, Chen J, Wang L, et al. Associations of PLA2G7 gene polymorphisms with plasma lipoprotein-associated phospholipase A2 activity and coronary heart disease in a Chinese Han population: the Beijing atherosclerosis study. Hum Genet. 2009;125:11–20.
37. Blanco-Colio LM, Martin-Ventura JL, de Teresa E, Farsang C, Gaw A, Gensini G, et al. Atorvastatin decreases elevated soluble CD40L in subjects at high cardiovascular risk. Atorvastatin on inflammatory markers study: a substudy of ACTFAST. Kidney Int Suppl. 2008:S60-3. doi:10.1038/ki.2008.514.
38. Yun Y, Ma C, Ma X. The SNP rs1883832 in CD40 gene and risk of atherosclerosis in Chinese population: a meta-analysis. PLoS One. 2014;9:e97289.
39. European Heart Rhythm A, European Association for Cardio-Thoracic S, Camm AJ, Kirchhof P, Lip GY, Schotten U, et al. Guidelines for the

management of atrial fibrillation: the Task Force for the Management of Atrial Fibrillation of the European Society of Cardiology (ESC). Europace. 2010;12:1360–420.

40. Zhang S, Wang W, Li J, Cheng K, Zhou J, Zhu D, et al. Behavioral characterization of CD36 knockout mice with SHIRPA primary screen. Behav Brain Res. 2015;299:90–6.
41. Ramos-Arellano LE, Munoz-Valle JF, De la Cruz-Mosso U, Salgado-Bernabe AB, Castro-Alarcon N, Parra-Rojas I. Circulating CD36 and oxLDL levels are associated with cardiovascular risk factors in young subjects. BMC Cardiovasc Disord. 2014;14:54.
42. Zhang Y, Ling ZY, Deng SB, Du HA, Yin YH, Yuan J, et al. Associations between CD36 gene polymorphisms and susceptibility to coronary artery heart disease. Braz J Med Biol Res. 2014;47:895–903.
43. He F, Teng X, Gu H, Liu H, Zhou Z, Zhao Y, et al. Interleukin-6 receptor rs7529229 T/C polymorphism is associated with left main coronary artery disease phenotype in a Chinese population. Int J Mol Sci. 2014;15:5623–33.
44. McGeachie M, Ramoni RL, Mychaleckyj JC, Furie KL, Dreyfuss JM, Liu Y, et al. Integrative predictive model of coronary artery calcification in atherosclerosis. Circulation. 2009;120:2448–54.
45. Qi X, Bai F, You C, Guo X, Shi L, Hu Z. High-resolution melting technology for detecting genetic polymorphisms of IL-1beta and IL-1Ra in patients with coronary artery disease. Xi Bao Yu Fen Zi Mian Yi Xue Za Zhi. 2015;31:816–20.
46. Xu L, Chen X, Ye H, Hong Q, Xu M, Duan S. Association of four CpG-SNPs in the vascular-related genes with coronary heart disease. Biomed Pharmacother. 2015;70:80–3.
47. Huang Y, Zhou J, Ye H, Xu L, Le Y, Yang X, et al. Relationship between chemokine (C-X-C motif) ligand 12 gene variant (rs1746048) and coronary heart disease: case-control study and meta-analysis. Gene. 2013;521:38–44.

7

AMD and the alternative complement pathway: genetics and functional implications

Perciliz L. Tan[1,2], Catherine Bowes Rickman[3,2] and Nicholas Katsanis[1,2*]

Abstract

Age-related macular degeneration (AMD) is an ocular neurodegenerative disorder and is the leading cause of legal blindness in Western societies, with a prevalence of up to 8 % over the age of 60, which continues to increase with age. AMD is characterized by the progressive breakdown of the macula (the central region of the retina), resulting in the loss of central vision including visual acuity. While its molecular etiology remains unclear, advances in genetics and genomics have illuminated the genetic architecture of the disease and have generated attractive pathomechanistic hypotheses. Here, we review the genetic architecture of AMD, considering the contribution of both common and rare alleles to susceptibility, and we explore the possible mechanistic links between photoreceptor degeneration and the alternative complement pathway, a cascade that has emerged as the most potent genetic driver of this disorder.

Background

Age-related macular degeneration is the third leading cause of vision loss worldwide. It is a late-onset disease with a complex etiology. Major risk factors contributing to susceptibility include age, family history, and smoking [1–3]. The earliest clinical manifestations of age-related macular degeneration (AMD) are focal deposits of debris, termed drusen, which are also considered to be a normal part of aging, present almost ubiquitously in the eyes of healthy individuals over the age of 50. Progression into the spectrum of pathological consequences begins with excessive accumulation of drusen in the central retina during the early/intermediate stages of AMD, followed by localized inflammation, and ultimately neurodegeneration in the macula that characterizes advanced stages of AMD.

Combining epidemiological and genetic approaches has enabled the identification of environmental and genetic contributors to AMD, both of which have tracked with technological advances in conceptual and practical statistical and genomic tools. Linkage of an AMD locus to 1q32 [4, 5], and the genome-wide association at the complement factor H (*CFH*) locus [6] led to the identification of the first common genome-wide significant risk variant, Y402H, that has upon sequencing in ethnic stratified cohorts revealed differential frequencies ranging from 5 % in East Asian populations to 35 % in European populations [7, 8]. This discovery propagated numerous genetics and genomic studies that have contributed to our understanding of the pathomechanisms contributing to AMD. Notably, the subsequent association of common and rare alleles at or near several additional complement genes (*CFH, C2/CFB, C3, CFI,* and *C9)* has had a significant impact of the formation of pathomechanistic hypotheses, with the cumulative evidence both from human genetics but also from histopathological studies highlighting a major role of the alternative complement pathway as a driver of AMD [9–21]. Here, we synthesize genetic evidence from rare- and common-allele studies in AMD, and we discuss the emergent picture of the genetic architecture of this atypical complex trait. Moreover, benefiting from the discovery of likely potent coding mutations in genes encoding complement components, we explore how these mutations might impede specific functions and discuss the potential contribution of aspects of this pathway to AMD pathogenesis.

* Correspondence: Nicholas.Katsanis@duke.edu
[1]Center for Human Disease Modeling, Duke University Medical Center, Durham, NC 27710, USA
[2]Department of Cell Biology, Duke University Medical Center, Durham, NC 27710, USA
Full list of author information is available at the end of the article

AMD histopathology

The retina is composed of five major layers: the neurosensory retina; the retinal pigment epithelium (RPE); Bruch's membrane (BM); the choriocapillaris; and the choroid (Fig. 1). The sensory cells of the neural retina are the photoreceptors (rods and cones), which through phototransduction convert light into electrical signals. Adjacent to the photoreceptors is the RPE, a part of the blood-ocular barrier and has numerous functions, including photoreceptor outer segment phagocytosis; regulation of the transportation nutrients; and cytokine secretion [22]. Lining the basal side of the RPE is BM, which is a pentalaminar extracellular matrix (ECM) consisting of elastin semipermeable barrier between inner and outer collagenous zones that provides connective tissue-based structural support and transport of waste from photoreceptors and RPE to the choroid and nutrients from the choroid to the RPE. The outermost layer of BM is composed of the basement membrane of the choriocapillaris, a fenestrated capillary bed that together with the choroid, a highly vascularized, pigmented tissue, are responsible for supplying the high metabolic demands of oxygen and nutrients to the outer retina [23].

During the natural process of aging, the human eye undergoes physiological changes that include changes in the distribution of photoreceptors (30 % loss of rod photoreceptors [24]); thickening of BM [25]; and accumulation of sub-RPE debris, including drusen [22, 26–29]. Drusen are composed of esterified cholesterol, phospholipids, lipofuscin, inflammatory components (e.g., complement), and other intra- and extraocular degenerative materials [30, 31]. They are classified according to their appearance, with inert, "hard" drusen being small with well-demarcated borders in contrast to the generally pathogenic "soft" drusen that lack distinct borders and can range in size from <63 to >124 μm in diameter, the larger diameters coinciding with disease progression [32].

The clinical pathology of AMD has been described extensively [3, 33]. It involves the progressive degeneration of the macula, a small, pigmented area at the center of the retina that has the densest concentration of photoreceptors and is responsible for visual acuity. Damage to the macula results in loss of central vision. Initial indications of AMD are seen as focal hyperpigmentation of the RPE and accumulation of sub-RPE deposits, including drusen, both between BM and the RPE and within the RPE itself [34, 35].

Even though the degeneration of rods and cones does define the end-stage of the disorder, AMD is not a primary disease of the photoreceptor; most of the candidate processes, biochemical pathways, and molecules exert their effects primarily on the RPE-choroid complex [36].

AMD subtypes

The anatomical histopathology and clinical progression contribute to the clinical definition of four major AMD subtypes as categorized by the Age-Related Eye Disease Study (AREDS) severity scale grading system [37]: 1. Early AMD; 2. Intermediate AMD; 3. Advanced non-neovascular ("Dry" or geographic atrophy) AMD; and 4. Advanced neovascular ("Wet" or exudative) AMD [32, 38, 39]. Early AMD features few small (<63 μm) or medium-sized drusen (63–124 μm) and pigmentary abnormalities in the RPE, resulting in either mild visual impairment (blurred vision or decreased contrast sensitivity) or can be asymptomatic. The progression from early to intermediate AMD is hallmarked by the appearance of at least one large druse (>125 μm), along with numerous medium-size drusen. This pathology can progress to one of the two advanced forms of AMD: Dry AMD

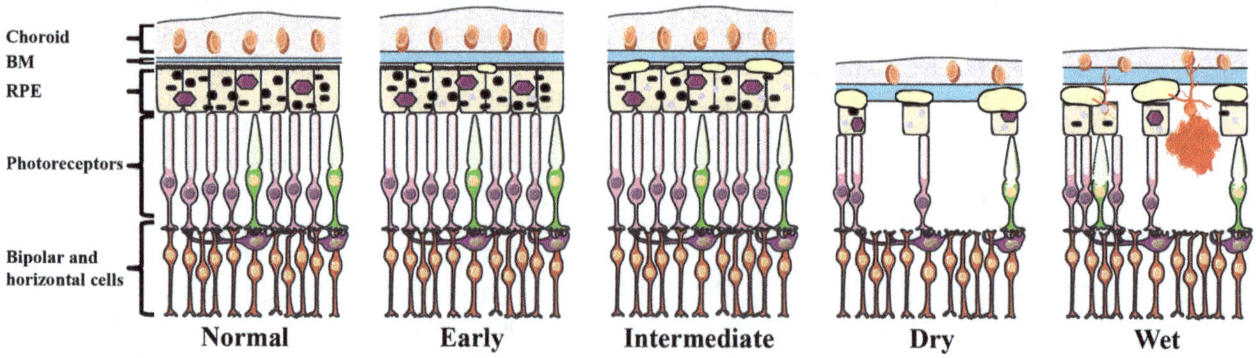

Fig. 1 Illustration of the anatomical retinal pathology associated with the various AMD subtypes. Diagram of the outer layers of the human central retina in normal and in AMD. As the disease progresses, Bruch's membrane (BM) increases in thickness. Early AMD is associated with small drusen and retinal pigmented epithelium (RPE) pigment abnormalities. As the disease progresses to the intermediate form, additional drusen are observed. In the two late forms of AMD (Dry and Wet), there is extensive drusen and photoreceptor cell death, with atrophy of the RPE and choroid in the Dry form and choroidal neovascularization (CNV), hemorrhaging, and RPE detachment in the Wet form. In all forms, the underlying circuitry including the horizontal and bipolar cells remains intact initially. This figure was prepared using Servier Medical Art (http://www.servier.com/Powerpoint-image-bank)

(non-neovascular), characterized by presence of drusen and atrophy of the RPE and choroid; or Wet AMD (neovascular), defined by newly formed vessels (choroidal neovascular membranes (CNV)) and RPE detachment. While occurring gradually in the Dry form versus suddenly/profoundly in the Wet form, the end result of both of these processes leads to photoreceptor cell death and vision loss (Fig. 1, Table 1).

Genetics of AMD: common variants versus rare variants

AMD exemplifies complex disorders: natural history and epidemiological studies have highlighted a prominent environmental role in disease risk with factors such as smoking resulting in a relative risk (RR) of >2, diet and obesity (RR > 2), nutritional supplements (odds ratio (OR) ~0.6) all contributing to pathogenicity [40]. In addition, family- and population-based studies have also highlighted that AMD carries a significant genetic burden, demonstrating >45 % concordance found in monozygotic and dizygotic twins as well as a recurrence-risk ratio between three to six times greater in siblings than in the general population [41–46].

In many ways, the dissection of the genetic basis of AMD has been an early beneficiary of advances in genetic and genomic technologies, wherein the development of both analytic platforms (genotyping, sequencing) as well as statistical methods, have found early application in this field.

Before our ability to query the genome in toto, complex trait studies focused on more traditional tools such as linkage and candidate gene association studies. Utilizing the latter, AMD was shown to be associated with two genes, *ABCA4* (ATP-binding cassette subfamily A member 4) and *APOE* (apolipoprotein E), both of which only confer a minor risk contribution to AMD. *ABCA4* is a causal gene for Stargardt disease, a retinopathy whose clinical symptoms overlap with AMD [47, 48]; *APOE* is a gene associated with Alzheimer's disease (AD), a neurological degenerative disorder, whose pathology overlaps with AMD [49]. Nonetheless, and despite this initial discovery, the candidate gene approach was largely unsuccessful in identifying genetic contributors to AMD. This was due in part to limited cohort sizes, imperfect statistical methodologies, and unclear pathomechanisms hindering the ability to define candidate genes and in part due to our lack of appreciation of the extensive rare and common variation carried in human genomes [50–52].

In the era following the completion of the human genome project and the International HapMap Project, traditional family-based studies retained utility, as exemplified by the family-based linkage mapping of an AMD locus on 1q25-q31 and on 10q26 [4, 53]. However, transformative genetic progress in AMD was driven by the common-allele hypothesis explored through genome-wide association studies (GWAS) [6, 54]. Remarkably, modest GWAS analysis on 96 cases and 50 controls yielded a genome-wide significant signal ($P < 10^{-7}$) on 1q32 of a common single nucleotide polymorphism (SNP) on a gene encoding *CFH* that revealed a polymorphism in linkage disequilibrium, Y402H, that has proven to be a common, predisposing allele that confers a two- to sevenfold increased risk for developing AMD [6, 9, 55, 56].

Table 1 Characteristics of AMD Clinical Subtypes (based on AREDS)

		AMD Subtype			
		Early	Intermediate	Advanced Dry/ Geographic Atrophy	Advanced Neovascular/ Exudative/Wet
Clinical Features	Drusen	Few small (<63 μm) or medium sized (63–124 μm)	Numerous medium (63–124 μm) + at least 1 large (>125 μm) sized	Extensive medium (63–124 μm) + large (>125 μm) sized	Extensive medium (63–124 μm) + large (>125 μm) sized
	Bruch's membrane	Thickening	Thickening	Thickening	Thickening
	Retinal pigment epithelium	Pigmentary abnormalities	Pigmentary abnormalities; atrophy excluding fovea	Atrophy including fovea/macula	Detachment
	Choroid/ choriocapillaris	Decreased vascular density	Decreased vascular density	Atrophy	Choroidal neovascularization; hemorrhage; leak fluid
	Neural retina	None	Photoreceptor thinning above drusen	Photoreceptor cell death	Photoreceptor detachment and cell death
	Impairment/ outcome	Mild visual impairment (blurred vision or decreased contrast sensitivity) or asymptomatic	Mild visual impairment (blurred spots in central vision or decreased contrast sensitivity) or asymptomatic	Blurred central vision; gradual vision loss	Sudden/profound vision loss

Soon after the identification of the *CFH* locus, another modestly sized GWAS performed on 96 cases and 130 controls yielded a genome-wide significant signal on 10q26, another primary locus for AMD that contains the candidate genes *ARMS2/HTRA1* (age-related maculopathy susceptibility 2/HtrA serine peptidase 1) coding for a protein of unknown function and a serine protease, respectively [54, 57]. Thereafter, additional GWAS studies with progressively increasing cohort size led to the identification of more associated loci but generally resulted in diminishing returns with many of the loci having a minor contribution to AMD (Table 2).

The associated loci discovered also germinated targeted sequencing strategies with a goal of identifying rare variants that might (a) provide direct causal evidence for the gene(s) in associated regions; (b) improve our measure of the overall risk of such genes to AMD pathogenesis; and (c) inform the direction of effect. Targeted high-throughput sequencing in combination with genotyping of the *CFH* locus led to the identification of a highly penetrant, rare variant R1210C which was shown to be associated with advanced AMD and to potentially result in disease onset 6 years earlier [58]. Similarly, in a smaller discovery cohort of 84 unrelated AMD patients, another penetrant, rare missense mutation in complement factor I (*CFI*), was unveiled, encoding G119R. This allele confers high risk to AMD (OR = 22.2), with patients with the heterozygous mutation having lower FI serum concentration [19].

With a goal of identifying elusive rare variants, a larger targeted exon sequencing study was undertaken in 2013, in which all exons of the 681 genes mapping at or close to all the AMD reported loci were sequenced in 1676 cases, 745 controls, and 36 siblings with discordant disease status [59]. This study combined sequencing-based genotypes, with the exome chip genome-wide genotyping data, with SNP genotyping to uncover K155Q (OR = 2.8) in the complement component C3 gene (*C3)* and P167S (OR = 2.2) in *C9* as contributors to AMD disease pathophysiology. Importantly, the study also showed an overall increase in the burden of rare variants in cases compared to controls. Much of that signal originated from specific genes, such as *CFI* (7.8 % in cases compared to 2.3 % in controls). However, the data suggested that there were variants in additional genes that were likely involved but could not be powered sufficiently to show association for specific alleles [59]. More recent studies have involved a targeted capture enriched for

Table 2 Past genome-wide association studies of AMD

Discovered gene/locus	Method	# Cases/Controls	OR	Reference
CFH	Affymetrix GeneChip Mapping 100K Set of microarrays	96/50	4.6–7.4	[6]
HTRA1/LOC387715	Affymetrix GeneChip Mapping 100K Set of microarrays	99/131	1.66–11.14	[54]
LIPC	Affymetrix SNP 6.0 GeneChip and Sequenom	979/1709	0.82	[124]
CETP	Affymetrix SNP 6.0 GeneChip and Sequenom	979/1709	1.15	[124]
TIMP3	Illumina Human370 Bead Chips and Illumina Infinium II assay	2157/1150	0.63	[125]
SKIV2L	Affymetrix SNP 5.0 GeneChip	1896/1866	0.54	[126]
MYRIP	Affymetrix SNP 5.0 GeneChip	1896/1866	0.86	[126]
TNFRSF10A/LOC389641	Illumina Human610-Quad BeadChip and Illumina HumanHap550v3 BeadChip	1536/18894	0.73	[127]
FRK/COL10A1	Affymetrix SNP 6.0 GeneChip and Illumina HumanCNV370v1 Bead Array	2594/4134	0.87	[128]
VEFGA	Affymetrix SNP 6.0 GeneChip and Illumina HumanCNV370v1 Bead Array	2594/4134	1.15	[128]
COL8A1/FILIP1L	Meta-analysis of GWAS	>17000/>60000	1.23	[129]
APOE	Meta-analysis of GWAS	>17000/>60000		[129]
IER3/DDR1	Meta-analysis of GWAS	>17000/>60000	1.16	[129]
SLC16A8	Meta-analysis of GWAS	>17000/>60000	1.15	[129]
TGFBR1	Meta-analysis of GWAS	>17000/>60000	1.13	[129]
RAD51B	Meta-analysis of GWAS	>17000/>60000	1.11	[129]
ADAMTS9/MIR548A2	Meta-analysis of GWAS	>17000/>60000	1.1	[129]
B3GALTL	Meta-analysis of GWAS	>17000/>60000	1.1	[129]

Meta-analysis genotyping method/platforms include Illumina HumanHap300, Human610-Quad, HumanHapCNV370, or HumanCNV370v1 BeadChips, Affymetrix 250K Nspl, Illumina Human670-QuadCustom chip, Illumina 660-Quadv1A, Illumina 610-Quad, Illumina Infinium HumanHap300K, HumanHap550v1, or Human-Hap550v3 BeadChip, Illumina Infinium II HumanHap550, Affymetrix GeneChip Human Mapping 250k Styl Array, Affymetrix 6.0 or 1M complement components that led to discovery of enrichment of rare variants in *CFH* in AMD patients [60] as well as the largest AMD GWAS study to date that examined >12 million variants in 16,144 patients and 17,832 controls [61]. This study leads to the identification of 52 common and rare variants across 34 loci, 16 of which reached genome-wide significance for the first time [61]. Taken together, these studies highlight two key points. First, they showed that, for AMD, a blend of rare and common alleles can contribute substantially to the disease burden and, as accepted by evolutionary theory, coding alleles of major functional effect can have a much larger contribution to susceptibility. Second, however, was the more sobering observation that AMD is quite different from most other common traits studied to date. A few exceptions notwithstanding, the genetic architecture of AMD has intimated the presence of a few genes in which common, modestly penetrant alleles account for a significant fraction of the genetic burden, with rare coding variants in the same genes providing both causal evidence and adding further to the population burden [6, 58, 62, 63]. When juxtaposed with the >1000 GWAS executed for a variety of traits, this landscape has, for the most part, been confined to this disorder. The reason for this is unclear. These observations might underscore a "winner's curse" of the first major complex trait's GWAS successes. More importantly, they raise the possibility that the biochemical underpinnings of AMD might be fundamentally different from other complex traits and that understanding the reasons for such differences might inform our approach to both genetic discovery and therapeutic design.

Also contrasting other GWAS approaches in other diseases, a significant fraction of the susceptibility signal in AMD has mapped to, or near, genes encoding components of the complement cascade, although this is not the sole pathway implicated. Overall, the genes and alleles thought to confer significant susceptibility to AMD pathology can be clustered broadly into five major pathways (Table 3): (a) the inflammation and immune response, (b) lipid metabolism and transport, (c) extracellular matrix and cell adhesion, (d) angiogenesis, and (e) cellular stress responses. Among these, risk assessment analysis for either common or rare alleles has highlighted in genes encoding complement pathway components. The common variants near six complement genes, *CFH, C2/CFB, C3, CFI,* and *C9* together, account for almost 60 % of the AMD genetic risk [36]. Notably, for the rare alleles found in sufficient recurrent rates to empower meaningful studies, the individual risk to AMD is sharply higher and appears as if they are almost Mendelian, as observed in the case of *CFI* [19].

A pathogenic route to AMD: alternative complement pathway

One of the leading candidates for predisposition to AMD is the inflammatory pathogenesis theory, which hypothesizes dysregulation of the immune response, specifically complement system [6, 9, 12, 14, 15, 20, 55, 56, 64–68]. Reports dating back to 1875 have hypothesized that macular lesions were due to inflammation and that disciform degeneration were associated with choroidal inflammation [69]. Since then multiple components of the complement pathway have been linked to AMD and its pathological consequences [15, 16, 30, 64, 70, 71]. The complement system is a specialized part of innate immunity that can respond to antigen-antibody complexes (classical pathway) or bacterial mannose groups (lectin pathway) and can also be active in a low-level continuous state (alternative pathway (AP)), to allow for an immediate amplified response [72]. All complement pathways culminate in the creation of the membrane attack complex (MAC) for cell lysis and organismal defense.

AMD is not the first human genetic disorder associated with AP complement dysfunction. A number of disorders are thought to be the result of excessive AP activation, including membranoproliferative glomerulonephritis type II (MPGN type II); atypical hemolytic uremic syndrome (aHUS); and paroxysmal nocturnal hemoglobinuria (PNH, a rare form of hemolytic anemia). Of note, MPGN type II, which is characterized by renal disease and low serum C3 levels, is also associated with complete FH deficiency, arguing for a mechanistic similarity between MPGN and AMD [55, 73]. Similarly, aHUS has been associated with low FH levels in addition to low C3 levels and has mutations in several AP components, however, at a unique haplotype compared to AMD and MPGN [73]. PNH is caused by mutations in phosphatidylinositol glycan-complementation class A (PIGA) that is essential in the establishment of glycophosphatidylinositol anchors. Two known inhibitors of AP activation are glycolipid-anchored proteins that are required for the regulation at the C3 convertase step and MAC assembly [74].

Dysregulation of the AP specifically is currently thought to underlie AMD. Several lines of supporting evidence include (1) the presence of complement components in the choriocapillaris and the retina, especially in drusen [14–16, 75]; (2) increased MAC in the choriocapillaris of AMD patients [18]; and (3) the genetic association of *C2, C3, CFB, CFI,* and the regulator of complement activation (RCA) gene cluster on 1q32 (which includes *CFH* and *CFHR1-5*) with AMD [9–13, 17, 19–21]. However, the effects of variation within the components of the AP on AMD pathogenicity is largely unknown.

Table 3 Genes associated with AMD that cluster into five major pathways

Inflammation and immune response				Cell stress response			
C2	Complement component 2	HLA-C	Major histocompatibility complex, class I, C	ABCA4	ATP-binding cassette subfamily A member 4	HTRA1	HtrA serine peptidase 1
C3	Complement component 3	IL8	Interleukin B	ACE	Angiotensin I converting enzyme 1	RORA	RAR-related orphan receptor alpha
CFB	Complement factor B	MMP9	Matrix metallopeptidase 9	APOE	Apoliporotein E	SOD2	Superoxide dismutase 2, mitochondrial
CFH	Complement factor H	PLEKHA1	Pleckstrin homology domain containing, family A member 1	ARMS2	Age-related maculopathy susceptibility 2	TF	Transferrin
CFD	Complement factor D	RORA	RAR-related orphan receptor alpha	CST3	Cystatin C	TLR3	Toll-like receptor 3
CFHR1-5	Complement factor H-related 1-5	SERPING1	Serpin peptidase inhibitor, clade G, member 1	CX3CR1	Chemokine receptor 1	TLR4	Toll-like receptor 4
CFI	Complement factor I	TLR3	Toll-like receptor 3	CYP24A1	Cytochrome P450, family 24, subfamily A peptide 1	VLDLR	Very low-density lipoprotein receptor
C9	Complement component 9	TLR4	Toll-like receptor 4	GSTM1	Glutathione S-transferase mu 1	TNFRSF10A/ LOC389641	Tumor necrosis factor receptor superfamily, member 10a
CX3CR1	Chemokine receptor 1	VLDLR	Very low-density lipoprotein receptor	GSTP1	Glutathione S-transferase pi 1	IER3	Immediate early response 3
F13B	Coagulation factor XIII, B polypeptide	VTN	Vitronectin	GSTT1	Glutathione S-transferase tau 1	TGFBR1	Transforming growth factor, beta receptor 1
Lipid metabolism and transport				**Extracellular matrix and cell adhesion**			
ABCA1	ATP-binding cassette, subfamily A, member 1	FADS1-3	Fatty acid desaturases 1-3	ACE	Angiotensin 1 converting enzyme 1	ROBO1	Roundabout, axon guidance receptor, homolog 1
ABCA4	ATP-binding cassette, subfamily A, member 4	LIPC	Hepatic lipase	ARMS2	Age-related maculopathy susceptibility 2	TIMP3	Tissue inhibitor of metalloproteinase 3
APOE	Apolipoprotein E	LPL	Lipoprotein lipases	ADAMTS9	ADAM metallopeptidase with trhombospondin type 1 motif, 9	MMP19	Matrix metallopeptidase 19
CETP	Cholesteryl ester transfer protein, plasma	LRP6	Low-density lipoprotein receptor-related protein 6	COL8A1	Collagen, type VIII, alpha 1	PCOLCE	Procollagen c-endopeptidase enhancer
CFHR1-5	Complement factor H-related 1-5	RORA	RAR-related orphan receptor alpha	COL10A1	Collagen, type X, alpha 1	VTN	Vitronectin
CYP24A1	Cytochrome P450, family 24, subfamily A peptide 1	VLDLR	Very low-density lipoprotein receptor	CST3	Cystatin C	ABCA7	ATP-binding cassette, cubfamily A, member 7
ELOVL4	ELVL fatty acid elongase 4	PLTP	Phospholipid transfer protein	CX3CR1	Chemokine receptor 1	ACTG1	Actin gamma 1
Angiogenesis				F13B	Coagulation factor XIII, B polypeptide	BCAR1	Breast cancer anti-estrogen resistance 1
ACE	Angiotensin I converting enzyme 1	LRP6	Low-density lipoprotein receptor-related protein 6	FBLN5	Fibulin 5	COL4A4	Collagen, type IV, alpha 4
COL10A1	Collagen, type X, alpha 1	MMP9	Matrix metallopeptidase 9	HMCN1	Hemicentin	ITGA7	Integrin, alpha 7
COL8A1	Collagen, type VIII, alpha 1	RORA	RAR-related orphan receptor alpha	HTRA1	HtrA serine peptidase 1	MYL2	Myosin, light chain 2, regulatory, cardiac, slow
CST3	Cystatin C	SERPINF1	Serpin peptidase inhibitor, clade F	MMP9	Matrix metallopeptidase 1		
FBLN5	Fibulin 5	TIMP3	Tissue inhibitor of metalloproteinase 3				

Table 3 Genes associated with AMD that cluster into five major pathways *(Continued)*

GDF6	Growth differentiation factor 6	VEGFA	Vascular endothelial growth factor A
HTRA1	HtrA serine peptidase 1	VLDLR	Very low-density lipoprotein receptor
IL8	Interleukin 8		

AMD is associated with activators of alternative pathway components

Low levels of constitutive complement activation via the AP allows for immediate immune response. It involves the central molecule of all three arms of the complement pathway, C3. In the AP, C3, is activated in two ways (Fig. 2): (1) it is either cleaved by convertases/plasma proteases to generate C3b or (2) a small portion is hydrolyzed spontaneously to $C3_{H2O}$ establishing a continuous "tick-over" ready for immediate C3b deposition on pathogens for target opsonization [76–79]. Factor B (FB) binds to $C3_{H2O}$ or C3b and the complex is cleaved by the plasma protease factor D (FD) forming the essential C3 convertase (C3bBb or $C3_{H2O}$Bb), leading to an amplification loop that cleaves and assembles C3 to C3b to C3bBb continuously. The accumulation of C3b leads to C3b binding to C3bBb, thereby creating a new enzyme, the C5 convertase (C3bBbC3b) that cleaves C5 to C5a (an anaphylatoxin and chemoattractant) and C5b, a component of the lytic pore which combines with C6–C9 to form the membrane attack complex (MAC) resulting in cell lysis [72].

The AP has the unique characteristic of being able to be activated spontaneously, allowing for an immediate immune response, which must be tightly regulated to prevent excessive activation. Intrinsically, the AP has two major negative regulators encoded by *CFH* and *CFI*. *CFH* is the soluble inhibitor of the complement cascade and encodes a secreted glycoprotein, FH that acts as cofactor for FI mediated cleavage of C3b as well as accelerating decay of the C3bBb convertase.

Many cells also express membrane-associated AP regulators that hinder the C3 amplification loop and/or prevent the deposition/accumulation of C3b on self-tissue. These membrane-associated proteins include membrane cofactor protein (MCP), decay-accelerating factor (DAF), and complement receptor 1 (CR1) all of which are encoded by genes located within the *RCA* gene cluster on 1q32 [80]. MCP and CR1 have cofactor activity for CFI, while CR1 along with DAF have decay acceleration activity. Differential expression of *MCP* has been linked to AMD and upon the addition of an environmental stimulus such as smoking, a risk factor of AMD, both MCP and DAF are down regulated [81, 82]. Both activating and inhibiting components have been reported to harbor variants that potentially have functional impacts on the AP (Table 4), with an increase in overall mutational burden being reported in *CFH* and *CFI* in AMD patients [60, 83]. These perturbations of the components themselves or of their ability to interact with other AP components typically result in uncontrolled AP activation.

Pathogenic outcomes of the AP

Advanced age is the only risk factor common to all AMD patients. During the aging process, the physiological changes include redistribution of the photoreceptors, thickening of BM, and accumulation of debris in the eye in conjunction with environmental factors and genetic variation contribute to cascading dysfunction of physiological pathways such as lipid transport, angiogenesis, stress response, and ECM remodeling [24–26]. In turn, disruption of each of these pathways can lead to an inflammatory and an AP immune response ultimately culminating in cell death [72]. Each of these pathways has been hypothesized to alter components of the retina [36, 84] affecting the interdependence of the photoreceptors, RPE, BM, and choriocapillaris making it challenging to understand the model for AMD pathogenesis.

During the early stages of AMD, sub-RPE deposit formation (drusen and soft basal linear deposits) between the RPE and BM occurs and is also thought to be the main site of immune complex formation in AMD. While containing over 40 % lipids, other components of sub-RPE deposits include TIMP3 (TIMP metallopeptidase inhibitor 3), which plays a role in ECM maintenance and remodeling [85, 86]; amyloid beta (Aβ) that is produced either systemically or from the RPE and is proangiogenic and a known activator of complement [87]; apolipoproteins, which are also generated systemically and by the RPE [88]); and CFH and other complement components [30].

Lipid accumulation, similar to that seen in atherosclerosis, can increase choroidal vessel resistance preventing the choriocapillaris from properly clearing additional lipoproteins from the RPE and BM [89]. The accumulation of lipoproteins along with Aβ lead to the formation of a lipid "wall" external to the RPE [90, 91] that is the precursor to basal linear deposits that forms between the RPE basement membrane and the inner collagenous zone of BM [92]. The accumulated, peroxidizable lipoproteins are oxidized contributing to RPE damage [93].

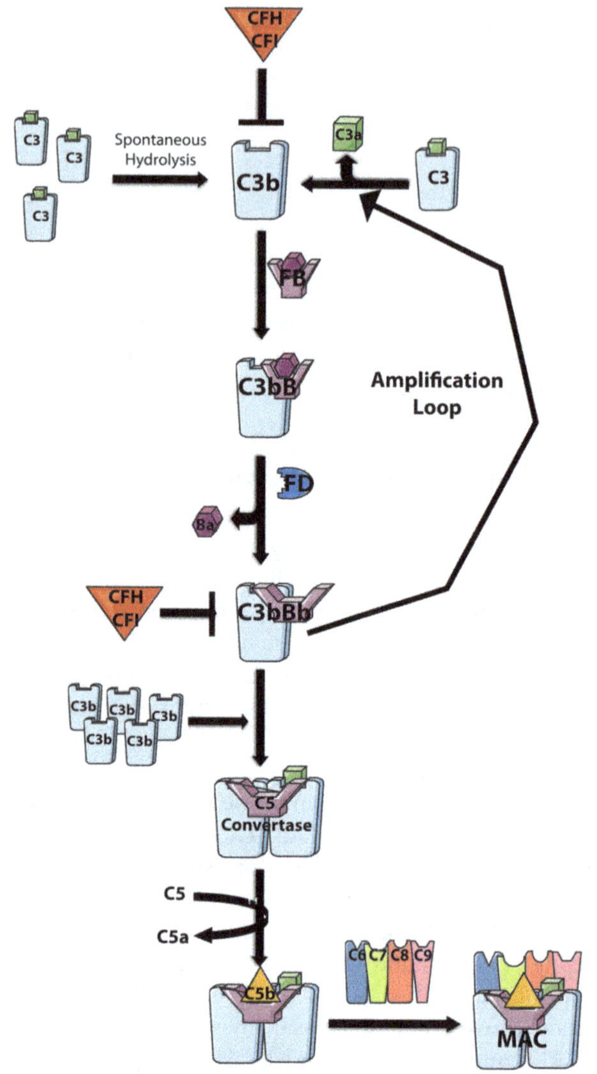

Fig. 2 The alternative complement pathway and the formation of the C3 convertase. In the AP, the generation of C3b can occur by either spontaneous hydrolysis of C3 ("tick-over" allowing for continuous low-level activation) or by plasma proteolytic cleavage all allowing for immediate C3b deposition. C3b forms the C3 convertase upon binding to FB and cleavage by FD resulting in an amplification loop producing additional C3b to stimulate a large immune response. C3b additionally binds to the C3 convertase leading to the formation of the C5 convertase initiating the terminal pathway and the establishment of the MAC. This figure was prepared using Servier Medical Art (http://www.servier.com/Powerpoint-image-bank)

Additionally, one byproduct of lipid peroxidation product is malondialdehyde (MDA), a marker for oxidative stress that contributes to RPE dysfunction [94] and a binding partner to CFH, allowing for an endogenous anti-inflammatory mediated response to this pro-inflammatory byproduct [95]. Similar to MDA, another cholesterol oxidation product having pro-inflammatory effects is 7-ketocholesterol (7KCh), which has been associated with cytotoxicity and has been shown to interact with retinal microglia, possibly promoting choroidal neovascularization [96] [97]. Further, these oxidized low-density lipoproteins can bind C-reactive protein initiating an inflammatory response leading to complement activation [98, 99]. Supplementing evidence has also been reported that complement activation leads to the recruitment of mononuclear phagocytes that contribute to RPE pathology in AMD [100]. All points that support immune system activation as a consequence of pathologic lipid accumulation.

The majority of complement is synthesized primarily by the liver and is delivered through circulation; however, some local tissues are also able to synthesize complement components, specifically the RPE and choroid [55]. Upon factors such as aging, oxidative stress (including cigarette smoke which that has been reported in vitro to activate C3 [101]), and lipid accumulation, increased AP activation in the RPE, which is thought to be the site of primary dysfunction in AMD, is primed for genetic predispositions to onset disease progression [14, 75, 101]. Upon AP activation, initiation of the terminal pathway ensues, forming MAC in BM and the choriocapillaris contributing to compromised function of the tight interaction of the RPE-BM-choroid complex [18].

Additional clues and emerging thoughts on pathogenic contributions to complex disease

There have been multiple insights implicating complement components in the pathobiology of AMD including genetic associations and accumulation of complement components in sub-RPE deposits of patient retinas [30, 102]. With common variants accounting for 65 % of the heritability of AMD, the search for rare variant contributors has only recently been undertaken through the advances of next generation sequencing [40]. Rare variants of C3, CFH, CFI, and C9 that have thus far been associated with AMD have been shown to play a role in either the complement pathway, to have an impact on the mutational load, or to hold the promise of putative future therapeutic targets [19, 58, 59, 63, 65]. However, a leading limitation in understanding disease outcome has been the lack of comprehension of the functional impact of the genetic contributors themselves. By combining the common variant common disease and rare variant common disease hypotheses [103–105], the idea of mutational burden emerges as a prognostic/diagnostic alternative for AMD, as exemplified by both common and rare variants in AP inhibitors leading to pathogenic dysregulated AP activity (Table 4). The latter highlights the necessity to functionally assess the role of a variant(s) in a gene(s) in order to more explicitly understand AMD pathogenesis. This highlights the need for development of animal models which are currently in development, for example, a transgenic mouse model expressing the human normal (Y402)

Table 4 AP complement variants

Gene	Variant	Position	OR	Common/Rare	Domain	Variant domain effect	Effect on AP	Ref
C3	R102G	19:6718387	1.7–2.6	Common	Macroglobulin 1	Decreased binding efficiency of C3b to its inhibitor CFH decreasing CFH's cofactor activity	Increased AP	[20, 65]
C3	P314L	19:6713262	1.5	Common	Macroglobulin 3	Decreased binding efficiency of C3b to its inhibitor CFH decreasing CFH's cofactor activity	Increased AP	[65]
C3	K155Q	19:6718146	2.8–3.8	Rare	Macroglobulin 2	Reduces binding to FH and C3b proteolytic cleavage by CFI	Increase C3 convertase production	[59, 65]
CFB	R32Q	6:31914180	0.32	Common	Ba	Reduced affinity for C3b and reduced hemolytic activity	Decrease formation of C3 convertase; reduced AP	[130]
CFB	L9H	6:31914024	0.37	Common	Signal peptide	Affects secretion of CFB	Decrease formation of C3 convertase; reduced AP	[12]
CFH	Y402H	1:196659291	2.45–5.57	Common	Complement control protein 7	Affects binding to GAG heparin sulfate, sialic acid, and C-reactive protein	Reduces ability of CFH to degrade C3: increased AP	[131]
CFH	R1210C	1:196716375	23.11	Rare	Complement control protein 20	Defective binding to C3b, C3d, and heparin	Impaired CFH attachment to host surfaces; reduces AP regulation	[58]
CFH	R53C	1:196642206		Rare	Complement control protein 1	Reduced accelerating activity for AP C3 convertase	Altered CFH-mediated cofactor activity or decay-accelerating activity; increased AP	[63]
CFH	D90G	1:196643011		Rare	Complement control protein 2	Alters CFI cofactor activity	Decreased cofactor-mediated inactivation; increased AP	[63]
CFH	I62V	1:196642233	1.95–2.79	Common	Complement control protein 2	Binds more efficiently to C3b	Enhanced cofactor activity and increased formation of iC3b; reduced AP	[63]
CFH	N1050Y	1:196712596	0.4	Common	Complement control protein 18	Possibly affects GAG and sialic acid binding	Increased AP	[62]
CFHR1/3	CFHR1/3del		0.29	Common	n/a	n/a	Reduces cofactor activity for CFI and inhibits C5 convertase; reduced AP	[13] [132–135]
CFI	G119R	4:110685820	22.2	Rare	Scavenger receptor cysteine-rich	Perturbs interdomain packing and stability of CFI	Diminished ability to degrade C3b; increased formation of C5 convertase; increased AP	[19]
CFI	G188A	4:110682768		Rare	Scavenger receptor cysteine-rich	Perturbs interdomain packing and stability of CFI	Diminished ability to degrade C3b; increased formation of C5 convertase; increased AP	[19]
C9	P167S	5:39331894	2.2	Rare	Membrane attack complex/perforin	Alters oligomerization and possibly inhibits C9's lytic activity	Affects binding with CD59; alters pore formation	[59]

and AMD-risk associated (Y402H) variants of FH has recently been described [106].

Familial aggregation is observed in most complex disease since there is greater likelihood of sharing disease-predisposing genotypes; however, non-genetic factors can contribute to discordant phenotypes [40]. In an effort to understand disease phenotypic outcomes, most studies have started by trying to identify causal variants. The identification of susceptibility variants is hindered by numerous confounding factors that have to be acknowledged to gain insight into disease mechanism. (1) Excluding a few cases such as AD and AMD, the vast majority of common variants exhibit a modest effect therefore large cohorts are required to power the findings [107, 108]. (2) Rare, disease-causing mutations, while numerous, are rarely observed in the general population [60, 83, 109, 110]. (3) SNP association of a locus does not imply that the causal variant itself is a SNP, as observed in Crohn's disease where the causal mutations is a deletion upstream of the promoter [111]. (4) Multiple distinct alleles either common, rare, or both, can be present at a single locus [58, 112]. 5) Allele frequencies vary among ethnic groups, as not only observed in AMD but also described in Hirschsprung's disease in which the causal variant has a minor allele frequency (MAF) ranging from 0.01 to 0.45 depending on the population [113]. (6) Causality due to non-coding variants is difficult to establish, similar to what was observed in coronary artery disease [114–116]. (7) Similar to pathways functioning in multiple processes, variants can also be pleiotropic, with their effect being dependent on the genetic content in which they are identified [117]. 8) Genes with causal variants identified need to be further studied for additional variation that could contribute to disease, as was seen in the case when delving deeper into *CFH* and *CFI* in AMD [19, 58]. (9) Structural variation cannot be ignored, as was observed in the case of Bardet-Biedl Syndrome in which copy number variations lead to disease progression (unpublished data). (10) Environmental factors can modify genetic effects and phenotypic outcomes [2, 101, 118].

Conclusions

Genetics has aided in the understanding of the complex, multifactorial nature of AMD. However, with modest signals differentiating the Dry versus Wet advanced forms of AMD, genetics has not revealed a strong predictive value on phenotypic severity or progression. Despite the long road of discovery that lies ahead, various lines of evidence linking the AP to AMD disease pathogenesis including (a) clinical phenotypes that associate with deficiencies of AP regulators [119]; (b) linkage of SNPs in AP components to disease risk [11, 120]; and (c) the functional analysis of individual AP components in the establishment of clinical phenotypes observed in both mouse and zebrafish models [74]. With numerous mouse models recapitulating at least 10 distinct human disorders, such as rheumatoid arthritis, traumatic brain injury, and AMD, the effects of AP on development and homeostasis have been established, making it clear that dysregulation/dysfunction of the process of innate immunity plays a contributory role in disease outcome [74]. Predominant functional assays for measuring the impact of variation on the complement pathway have been hemolytic and enzyme immunoassays [59, 121–123]; focus should and has begun to be placed on additional in vivo model systems to further understand the roles of AP disease contributors in a more systemic context [100, 106].

Abbreviations

7KCh: 7-ketocholesterol; ABCA4: ATP-binding cassette subfamily A member 4; AD: Alzheimer's disease; aHUS: atypical hemolytic uremic syndrome; AMD: age-related macular degeneration; AP: alternative pathway; APOE: apolipoprotein E; AREDS: Age-Related Eye Disease Study; ARMS2: age-related maculopathy susceptibility 2; Aβ: amyloid beta; BM: Bruch's membrane; C2: complement component 2; C3: complement component 3; C9: complement component 9; CFB or FB: complement factor B; CFH or FH: complement factor H; CFI or FI: complement factor I; CNV: choroidal neovascular membranes; CR1: complement receptor 1; DAF: decay-accelerating factor; ECM: extracellular matrix; FD: complement factor D; GWAS: genome-wide association studies; HTRA1: HtrA serine peptidase 1; MAC: membrane attack complex; MAF: minor allele frequency; MCP: membrane cofactor protein; MDA: malondialdehyde; MPGN: membranoproliferative glomerulonephritis; OR: odds ratio; PIGA: phosphatidylinositol glycan-complement class A; PNH: paroxysmal nocturnal Hemoglobinuria; RCA: regulator of complement activation; RPE: retinal pigment epithelium; RR: relative risk; SNP: single nucleotide polymorphism; TIMP3: TIMP metallopeptidase inhibitor 3.

Acknowledgements

We thank Allison Ashley-Koch, Maria Kousi, and Erik Madsen for their thoughtful comments on the manuscript.

Authors' contributions

The manuscript was written by PLT. All authors critically revised the manuscript. All authors read and approved the final manuscript.

Competing interests

The authors declare that they have no competing interests.

Author details

[1]Center for Human Disease Modeling, Duke University Medical Center, Durham, NC 27710, USA. [2]Department of Cell Biology, Duke University Medical Center, Durham, NC 27710, USA. [3]Department of Ophthalmology, Duke Eye Center, Duke University, Durham, NC 27710, USA.

References

1. Klein R, Peto T, Bird A, Vannewkirk MR. The epidemiology of age-related macular degeneration. Am J Ophthalmol. 2004;137:486–95. doi: 10.1016/j.ajo.2003.11.069.
2. Thornton J et al. Smoking and age-related macular degeneration: a review of association. Eye (Lond). 2005;19:935–44. doi:10.1038/sj.eye.6701978.
3. Young RW. Pathophysiology of age-related macular degeneration. Surv Ophthalmol. 1987;31:291–306.
4. Weeks DE et al. Age-related maculopathy: a genomewide scan with continued evidence of susceptibility loci within the 1q31, 10q26, and 17q25 regions. Am J Hum Genet. 2004;75:174–89. doi:10.1086/422476.

5. Weeks DE et al. Age-related maculopathy: an expanded genome-wide scan with evidence of susceptibility loci within the 1q31 and 17q25 regions. Am J Ophthalmol. 2001;132:682–92.
6. Klein RJ et al. Complement factor H polymorphism in age-related macular degeneration. Science (New York, NY). 2005;308:385–9. doi:10.1126/science.1109557.
7. Kondo N, Bessho H, Honda S, Negi A. Complement factor H Y402H variant and risk of age-related macular degeneration in Asians: a systematic review and meta-analysis. Ophthalmology. 2011;118:339–44. doi:10.1016/j.ophtha.2010.06.040.
8. Thakkinstian A et al. Systematic review and meta-analysis of the association between complement factor H Y402H polymorphisms and age-related macular degeneration. Hum Mol Genet. 2006;15:2784–90. doi:10.1093/hmg/ddl220.
9. Edwards AO et al. Complement factor H polymorphism and age-related macular degeneration. Science (New York, NY). 2005;308:421–4. doi:10.1126/science.1110189.
10. Ennis S, Gibson J, Cree AJ, Collins A, Lotery AJ. Support for the involvement of complement factor I in age-related macular degeneration. Eur J Hum Genet. 2010;18:15–6. doi:10.1038/ejhg.2009.113.
11. Fagerness JA et al. Variation near complement factor I is associated with risk of advanced AMD. Eur J Hum Genet. 2009;17:100–4. doi:10.1038/ejhg.2008.140.
12. Gold B et al. Variation in factor B (BF) and complement component 2 (C2) genes is associated with age-related macular degeneration. Nat Genet. 2006;38:458–62. doi:10.1038/ng1750.
13. Hageman GS et al. Extended haplotypes in the complement factor H (CFH) and CFH-related (CFHR) family of genes protect against age-related macular degeneration: characterization, ethnic distribution and evolutionary implications. Ann Med. 2006;38:592–604.
14. Hageman GS et al. An integrated hypothesis that considers drusen as biomarkers of immune-mediated processes at the RPE-Bruch's membrane interface in aging and age-related macular degeneration. Prog Retin Eye Res. 2001;20:705–32.
15. Johnson LV, Leitner WP, Staples MK, Anderson DH. Complement activation and inflammatory processes in Drusen formation and age related macular degeneration. Exp Eye Res. 2001;73:887–96. doi:10.1006/exer.2001.1094.
16. Johnson LV, Ozaki S, Staples MK, Erickson PA, Anderson DH. A potential role for immune complex pathogenesis in drusen formation. Exp Eye Res. 2000;70:441–9. doi:10.1006/exer.1999.0798.
17. Li M et al. CFH haplotypes without the Y402H coding variant show strong association with susceptibility to age-related macular degeneration. Nat Genet. 2006;38:1049–54. doi:10.1038/ng1871.
18. Mullins RF et al. The membrane attack complex in aging human choriocapillaris: relationship to macular degeneration and choroidal thinning. Am J Pathol. 2014;184:3142–53. doi:10.1016/j.ajpath.2014.07.017.
19. van de Ven JP et al. A functional variant in the CFI gene confers a high risk of age-related macular degeneration. Nat Genet. 2013;45:813–7. doi:10.1038/ng.2640.
20. Yates JR et al. Complement C3 variant and the risk of age-related macular degeneration. N Engl J Med. 2007;357:553–61. doi:10.1056/NEJMoa072618.
21. Zhan X et al. Identification of a rare coding variant in complement 3 associated with age-related macular degeneration. Nat Genet. 2013;45:1375–9. doi:10.1038/ng.2758.
22. Strauss O. The retinal pigment epithelium in visual function. Physiol Rev. 2005;85:845–81. doi:10.1152/physrev.00021.2004.
23. Lutty GA et al. Development of the human choriocapillaris. Eye (Lond). 2010;24:408–15. doi:10.1038/eye.2009.318.
24. Curcio CA, Owsley C, Jackson GR. Spare the rods, save the cones in aging and age-related maculopathy. Invest Ophthalmol Vis Sci. 2000;41:2015–8.
25. Feeney-Burns L, Ellersieck MR. Age-related changes in the ultrastructure of Bruch's membrane. Am J Ophthalmol. 1985;100:686–97.
26. Curcio CA, Millican CL, Bailey T, Kruth HS. Accumulation of cholesterol with age in human Bruch's membrane. Invest Ophthalmol Vis Sci. 2001;42:265–74.
27. Delori FC, Goger DG, Dorey CK. Age-related accumulation and spatial distribution of lipofuscin in RPE of normal subjects. Invest Ophthalmol Vis Sci. 2001;42:1855–66.
28. Eldred GE, Miller GV, Stark WS, Feeney-Burns L. Lipofuscin: resolution of discrepant fluorescence data. Science (New York, NY). 1982;216:757–9.
29. Moreira EF, Larrayoz IM, Lee JW, Rodriguez IR. 7-Ketocholesterol is present in lipid deposits in the primate retina: potential implication in the induction of VEGF and CNV formation. Invest Ophthalmol Vis Sci. 2009;50:523–32. doi:10.1167/iovs.08-2373.
30. Mullins RF, Russell SR, Anderson DH, Hageman GS. Drusen associated with aging and age-related macular degeneration contain proteins common to extracellular deposits associated with atherosclerosis, elastosis, amyloidosis, and dense deposit disease. Faseb J. 2000;14:835–46.
31. Russell SR, Mullins RF, Schneider BL, Hageman GS. Location, substructure, and composition of basal laminar drusen compared with drusen associated with aging and age-related macular degeneration. Am J Ophthalmol. 2000;129:205–14.
32. Jager RD, Mieler WF, Miller JW. Age-related macular degeneration. N Engl J Med. 2008;358:2606–17. doi:10.1056/NEJMra0801537.
33. Sarks SH. Ageing and degeneration in the macular region: a clinico-pathological study. Br J Ophthalmol. 1976;60:324–41.
34. Sarks SH, Arnold JJ, Killingsworth MC, Sarks JP. Early drusen formation in the normal and aging eye and their relation to age related maculopathy: a clinicopathological study. Br J Ophthalmol. 1999;83:358–68.
35. Spraul CW, Grossniklaus HE. Characteristics of Drusen and Bruch's membrane in postmortem eyes with age-related macular degeneration. Arch Ophthal. 1997;115:267–73.
36. Fritsche LG et al. Age-related macular degeneration: genetics and biology coming together. Annu Rev Genomics Hum Genet. 2014;15:151–71. doi:10.1146/annurev-genom-090413-025610.
37. Group, A.-R. E. D. S. R. Risk factors associated with age-related macular degeneration. A case-control study in the Age-Related Eye Disease Study: Age-Related Eye Disease Study report number 3. Ophthalmology. 2000;107:2224–32.
38. Davis MD et al. The Age-Related Eye Disease Study severity scale for age-related macular degeneration: AREDS report no. 17. Arch Ophthal. 2005;123:1484–98. doi:10.1001/archopht.123.11.1484.
39. Ferris FL et al. A simplified severity scale for age-related macular degeneration: AREDS report no. 18. Arch Ophthal. 2005;123:1570–4. doi:10.1001/archopht.123.11.1570.
40. Sobrin L, Seddon JM. Nature and nurture- genes and environment- predict onset and progression of macular degeneration. Prog Retin Eye Res. 2014;40:1–15. doi:10.1016/j.preteyeres.2013.12.004.
41. Hammond CJ et al. Genetic influence on early age-related maculopathy: a twin study. Ophthalmology. 2002;109:730–6.
42. Klaver CC et al. Genetic risk of age-related maculopathy. Population-based familial aggregation study. Arch Ophthal. 1998;116:1646–51.
43. Klein ML, Mauldin WM, Stoumbos VD. Heredity and age-related macular degeneration. Observations in monozygotic twins. Arch Ophthal. 1994;112:932–7.
44. Meyers SM, Greene T, Gutman FA. A twin study of age-related macular degeneration. Am J Ophthalmol. 1995;120:757–66.
45. Seddon JM, Ajani UA, Mitchell BD. Familial aggregation of age-related maculopathy. Am J Ophthalmol. 1997;123:199–206.
46. Seddon JM, Cote J, Page WF, Aggen SH, Neale MC. The US twin study of age-related macular degeneration: relative roles of genetic and environmental influences. Arch Ophthal. 2005;123:321–7. doi:10.1001/archopht.123.3.321.
47. Allikmets R et al. Mutation of the Stargardt disease gene (ABCR) in age-related macular degeneration. Science (New York, NY). 1997;277:1805–7.
48. Zhang K et al. The ABCR gene in recessive and dominant Stargardt diseases: a genetic pathway in macular degeneration. Genomics. 1999;60:234–7. doi:10.1006/geno.1999.5896.
49. Klaver CC et al. Genetic association of apolipoprotein E with age-related macular degeneration. Am J Hum Genet. 1998;63:200–6. doi:10.1086/301901.
50. Flint J, Mackay TF. Genetic architecture of quantitative traits in mice, flies, and humans. Genome Res. 2009;19:723–33. doi:10.1101/gr.086660.108.
51. Risch N, Merikangas K. The future of genetic studies of complex human diseases. Science (New York, NY). 1996;273:1516–7.
52. Peter I, Seddon JM. Genetic epidemiology: successes and challenges of genome-wide association studies using the example of age-related macular degeneration. Am J Ophthalmol. 2010;150:450–452.e452. doi:10.1016/j.ajo.2010.06.012.
53. Majewski J et al. Age-related macular degeneration—a genome scan in extended families. Am J Hum Genet. 2003;73:540–50. doi:10.1086/377701.

54. Dewan A et al. HTRA1 promoter polymorphism in wet age-related macular degeneration. Science (New York, NY). 2006;314:989–92. doi:10.1126/science.1133807.
55. Hageman GS et al. A common haplotype in the complement regulatory gene factor H (HF1/CFH) predisposes individuals to age-related macular degeneration. Proc Natl Acad Sci U S A. 2005;102:7227–32. doi:10.1073/pnas.0501536102.
56. Haines JL et al. Complement factor H variant increases the risk of age-related macular degeneration. Science (New York, NY). 2005;308:419–21. doi:10.1126/science.1110359.
57. Rivera A et al. Hypothetical LOC387715 is a second major susceptibility gene for age-related macular degeneration, contributing independently of complement factor H to disease risk. Hum Mol Genet. 2005;14:3227–36. doi:10.1093/hmg/ddi353.
58. Raychaudhuri S et al. A rare penetrant mutation in CFH confers high risk of age-related macular degeneration. Nat Genet. 2011;43:1232–6. doi:10.1038/ng.976.
59. Seddon JM et al. Rare variants in CFI, C3 and C9 are associated with high risk of advanced age-related macular degeneration. Nat Genet. 2013;45:1366–70. doi:10.1038/ng.2741.
60. Triebwasser MP et al. Rare variants in the functional domains of complement factor H are associated with age-related macular degeneration. Invest Ophthalmol Vis Sci. 2015;56:6873–8. doi:10.1167/iovs.15-17432.
61. Fritsche LG et al. A large genome-wide association study of age-related macular degeneration highlights contributions of rare and common variants. Nat Genet. 2016;48:134–43. doi:10.1038/ng.3448.
62. Boon CJ et al. Basal laminar drusen caused by compound heterozygous variants in the CFH gene. Am J Hum Genet. 2008;82:516–23. doi:10.1016/j.ajhg.2007.11.007.
63. Yu Y et al. Whole-exome sequencing identifies rare, functional CFH variants in families with macular degeneration. Hum Mol Genet. 2014;23:5283–93. doi:10.1093/hmg/ddu226.
64. Anderson DH, Mullins RF, Hageman GS, Johnson LV. A role for local inflammation in the formation of drusen in the aging eye. Am J Ophthalmol. 2002;134:411–31.
65. Despriet DD et al. Complement component C3 and risk of age-related macular degeneration. Ophthalmology. 2009;116:474–480.e472. doi:10.1016/j.ophtha.2008.09.055.
66. Maller JB et al. Variation in complement factor 3 is associated with risk of age-related macular degeneration. Nat Genet. 2007;39:1200–1. doi:10.1038/ng2131.
67. Jakobsdottir J, Conley YP, Weeks DE, Ferrell RE, Gorin MB. C2 and CFB genes in age-related maculopathy and joint action with CFH and LOC387715 genes. PLoS One. 2008;3:e2199. doi:10.1371/journal.pone.0002199.
68. Park KH, Fridley BL, Ryu E, Tosakulwong N, Edwards AO. Complement component 3 (C3) haplotypes and risk of advanced age-related macular degeneration. Invest Ophthalmol Vis Sci. 2009;50:3386–93. doi:10.1167/iovs.08-3231.
69. Pagenstecher, H. a. G., C. Atlas der Pathologischen Anatomie des Augapfels. CW Kreidel, Wiesbaden (1875).
70. Hanssen R. Zur anatomie der scheibenformigen degeneration der netzhaumitte. *Z. Augenh.* 1930. 360-368.
71. Penfold PL, Killingsworth MC, Sarks SH. Senile macular degeneration: the involvement of immunocompetent cells. Graefes Arch Clin Exp Ophthalmol. 1985;223:69–76.
72. Ricklin D, Hajishengallis G, Yang K, Lambris JD. Complement: a key system for immune surveillance and homeostasis. Nat Immunol. 2010;11:785–97. doi:10.1038/ni.1923.
73. Pickering MC et al. Spontaneous hemolytic uremic syndrome triggered by complement factor H lacking surface recognition domains. J Exp Med. 2007;204:1249–56. doi:10.1084/jem.20070301.
74. Holers VM. The spectrum of complement alternative pathway-mediated diseases. Immunol Rev. 2008;223:300–16. doi:10.1111/j.1600-065X.2008.00641.x.
75. Anderson DH et al. The pivotal role of the complement system in aging and age-related macular degeneration: hypothesis re-visited. Prog Retin Eye Res. 2010;29:95–112. doi:10.1016/j.preteyeres.2009.11.003.
76. Pangburn MK, Schreiber RD, Muller-Eberhard HJ. Formation of the initial C3 convertase of the alternative complement pathway. Acquisition of C3b-like activities by spontaneous hydrolysis of the putative thioester in native C3. J Exp Med. 1981;154:856–67.
77. Pangburn MK, Muller-Eberhard HJ. Initiation of the alternative complement pathway due to spontaneous hydrolysis of the thioester of C3. Ann N Y Acad Sci. 1983;421:291–8.
78. Bexborn F, Andersson PO, Chen H, Nilsson B, Ekdahl KN. The tick-over theory revisited: formation and regulation of the soluble alternative complement C3 convertase (C3(H2O)Bb). Mol Immunol. 2008;45:2370–9. doi:10.1016/j.molimm.2007.11.003.
79. Lachmann PJ, Halbwachs L. The influence of C3b inactivator (KAF) concentration on the ability of serum to support complement activation. Clin Exp Immunol. 1975;21:109–14.
80. Pardo-Manuel de Villena F, Heine-Suner D, Rodriguez de Cordoba S. Ordering of the human regulator of complement activation gene cluster on 1q32 by two-colour FISH. Cytogenet Cell Genet. 1996;72:339–41.
81. Fett AL, Hermann MM, Muether PS, Kirchhof B, Fauser S. Immunohistochemical localization of complement regulatory proteins in the human retina. Histol Histopathol. 2012;27:357–64.
82. Wang L et al. Nrf2 signaling modulates cigarette smoke-induced complement activation in retinal pigmented epithelial cells. Free Radic Biol Med. 2014;70:155–66. doi:10.1016/j.freeradbiomed.2014.01.015.
83. Kavanagh, D. et al. Rare genetic variants in the CFI gene are associated with advanced age-related macular degeneration and commonly result in reduced serum factor I levels. Hum Mol Genet. 2015. doi:10.1093/hmg/ddv091.
84. Miller JW. Age-related macular degeneration revisited—piecing the puzzle: the LXIX Edward Jackson memorial lecture. Am J Ophthalmol. 2013;155:1–35 e13. doi:10.1016/j.ajo.2012.10.018.
85. Fariss RN, Apte SS, Olsen BR, Iwata K, Milam AH. Tissue inhibitor of metalloproteinases-3 is a component of Bruch's membrane of the eye. Am J Pathol. 1997;150:323–8.
86. Kamei M, Hollyfield JG. TIMP-3 in Bruch's membrane: changes during aging and in age-related macular degeneration. Invest Ophthalmol Vis Sci. 1999;40:2367–75.
87. Yoshida T et al. The potential role of amyloid beta in the pathogenesis of age-related macular degeneration. J Clin Invest. 2005;115:2793–800. doi:10.1172/jci24635.
88. Anderson DH et al. Local cellular sources of apolipoprotein E in the human retina and retinal pigmented epithelium: implications for the process of drusen formation. Am J Ophthalmol. 2001;131:767–81.
89. Friedman E. A hemodynamic model of the pathogenesis of age-related macular degeneration. Am J Ophthalmol. 1997;124:677–82.
90. Ruberti JW et al. Quick-freeze/deep-etch visualization of age-related lipid accumulation in Bruch's membrane. Invest Ophthalmol Vis Sci. 2003;44:1753–9.
91. Curcio CA, Johnson M, Rudolf M, Huang JD. The oil spill in ageing Bruch membrane. Br J Ophthalmol. 2011;95:1638–45. doi:10.1136/bjophthalmol-2011-300344.
92. Curcio CA, Johnson M, Huang JD, Rudolf M. Aging, age-related macular degeneration, and the response-to-retention of apolipoprotein B-containing lipoproteins. Prog Retin Eye Res. 2009;28:393–422. doi:10.1016/j.preteyeres.2009.08.001.
93. Gordiyenko N et al. RPE cells internalize low-density lipoprotein (LDL) and oxidized LDL (oxLDL) in large quantities in vitro and in vivo. Invest Ophthalmol Vis Sci. 2004;45:2822–9. doi:10.1167/iovs.04-0074.
94. Kaemmerer E, Schutt F, Krohne TU, Holz FG, Kopitz J. Effects of lipid peroxidation-related protein modifications on RPE lysosomal functions and POS phagocytosis. Invest Ophthalmol Vis Sci. 2007;48:1342–7. doi:10.1167/iovs.06-0549.
95. Weismann D et al. Complement factor H binds malondialdehyde epitopes and protects from oxidative stress. Nature. 2011;478:76–81. doi:10.1038/nature10449.
96. Indaram M et al. 7-Ketocholesterol increases retinal microglial migration, activation, and angiogenicity: a potential pathogenic mechanism underlying age-related macular degeneration. Sci Rep. 2015;5:9144. doi:10.1038/srep09144.
97. Rodriguez IR, Alam S, Lee JW. Cytotoxicity of oxidized low-density lipoprotein in cultured RPE cells is dependent on the formation of 7-ketocholesterol. Invest Ophthalmol Vis Sci. 2004;45:2830–7. doi:10.1167/iovs.04-0075.
98. Chang MK, Binder CJ, Torzewski M, Witztum JL. C-reactive protein binds to both oxidized LDL and apoptotic cells through recognition of a common ligand: Phosphorylcholine of oxidized phospholipids. Proc Natl Acad Sci U S A. 2002;99:13043–8. doi:10.1073/pnas.192399699.

99. Rodriguez IR, Larrayoz IM. Cholesterol oxidation in the retina: implications of 7KCh formation in chronic inflammation and age-related macular degeneration. J Lipid Res. 2010;51:2847–62. doi:10.1194/jlr.R004820.
100. Toomey CB, Kelly U, Saban DR, Bowes Rickman C. Regulation of age-related macular degeneration-like pathology by complement factor H. Proc Natl Acad Sci U S A. 2015;112:E3040–9. doi:10.1073/pnas.1424391112.
101. Kew RR, Ghebrehiwet B, Janoff A. Cigarette smoke can activate the alternative pathway of complement in vitro by modifying the third component of complement. J Clin Invest. 1985;75:1000–7. doi:10.1172/jci111760.
102. Gass JD. Drusen and disciform macular detachment and degeneration. Arch Ophthal. 1973;90:206–17.
103. Cirulli ET, Goldstein DB. Uncovering the roles of rare variants in common disease through whole-genome sequencing. Nat Rev Genet. 2010;11:415–25. doi:10.1038/nrg2779.
104. Reich DE, Lander ES. On the allelic spectrum of human disease. Trends Genet. 2001;17:502–10.
105. Schork NJ, Murray SS, Frazer KA, Topol EJ. Common vs. rare allele hypotheses for complex diseases. Curr Opin Genet Dev. 2009;19:212–9. doi:10.1016/j.gde.2009.04.010.
106. Ding JD et al. Expression of human complement factor H prevents age-related macular degeneration-like retina damage and kidney abnormalities in aged Cfh knockout mice. Am J Pathol. 2015;185:29–42. doi:10.1016/j.ajpath.2014.08.026.
107. Genome-wide association study of 14,000 cases of seven common diseases and 3,000 shared controls. Nature. 2007. 447, 661-678. doi:10.1038/nature05911.
108. Zeggini E et al. Meta-analysis of genome-wide association data and large-scale replication identifies additional susceptibility loci for type 2 diabetes. Nat Genet. 2008;40:638–45. doi:10.1038/ng.120.
109. Cohen JC et al. Multiple rare alleles contribute to low plasma levels of HDL cholesterol. Science (New York, NY). 2004;305:869–72. doi:10.1126/science.1099870.
110. Ji W et al. Rare independent mutations in renal salt handling genes contribute to blood pressure variation. Nat Genet. 2008;40:592–9. doi:10.1038/ng.118.
111. McCarroll SA et al. Deletion polymorphism upstream of IRGM associated with altered IRGM expression and Crohn's disease. Nat Genet. 2008;40:1107–12. doi:10.1038/ng.215.
112. Schulte EC et al. Targeted resequencing and systematic in vivo functional testing identifies rare variants in MEIS1 as significant contributors to restless legs syndrome. Am J Hum Genet. 2014;95:85–95. doi:10.1016/j.ajhg.2014.06.005.
113. Emison ES et al. A common sex-dependent mutation in a RET enhancer underlies Hirschsprung disease risk. Nature. 2005;434:857–63. doi:10.1038/naturc03467.
114. Helgadottir A et al. A common variant on chromosome 9p21 affects the risk of myocardial infarction. Science (New York, NY). 2007;316:1491–3. doi:10.1126/science.1142842.
115. McPherson R et al. A common allele on chromosome 9 associated with coronary heart disease. Science (New York, NY). 2007;316:1488–91. doi:10.1126/science.1142447.
116. Samani NJ et al. Genomewide association analysis of coronary artery disease. N Engl J Med. 2007;357:443–53. doi:10.1056/NEJMoa072366.
117. Jordan DM et al. Identification of cis-suppression of human disease mutations by comparative genomics. Nature. 2015;524:225–9. doi:10.1038/nature14497.
118. Hobbs RP, Bernstein PS. Nutrient supplementation for age-related macular degeneration, cataract, and dry eye. J Ophthalmic Vis Res. 2014;9:487–93. doi:10.4103/2008-322X.150829.
119. Botto M et al. Complement in human diseases: lessons from complement deficiencies. Mol Immunol. 2009;46:2774–83. doi:10.1016/j.molimm.2009.04.029.
120. Fisher SA et al. Meta-analysis of genome scans of age-related macular degeneration. Hum Mol Genet. 2005;14:2257–64. doi:10.1093/hmg/ddi230.
121. Nilsson UR, Nilsson B. Simplified assays of hemolytic activity of the classical and alternative complement pathways. J Immunol Methods. 1984;72:49–59.
122. Tortajada A et al. C3 glomerulopathy-associated CFHR1 mutation alters FHR oligomerization and complement regulation. J Clin Invest. 2013;123:2434–46. doi:10.1172/jci68280.
123. Yoshida Y et al. A novel quantitative hemolytic assay coupled with restriction fragment length polymorphisms analysis enabled early diagnosis of atypical hemolytic uremic syndrome and identified unique predisposing mutations in Japan. PLoS One. 2015;10:e0124655. doi:10.1371/journal.pone.0124655.
124. Neale BM, et al. Genome-wide association study of advanced age-related macular degeneration identifies a role of the hepatic lipase gene (LIPC). Proc Natl Acad Sci USA. 2010;107:7395-7400. doi:10.1073/pnas.0912019107.
125. Chen W, et al. Genetic variants near TIMP3 and high-density lipoprotein-associated loci influence susceptibility to age-related macular degeneration. Proc Natl Acad Sci USA. 2010;107:7401-6. doi:10.1073/pnas.0912702107.
126. Kopplin LJ, et al. Genome-wide association identifies SKIV2L and MYRIP as protective factors for age-related macular degeneration. Genes and immunity. 2010;11:609–21. doi:10.1038/gene.2010.39.
127. Arakawa S, et al. Genome-wide association study identifies two susceptibility loci for exudative agerelated macular degeneration in the Japanese population. Nat Genet. 2011;43:1001–4. doi:10.1038/ng.938.
128. Yu Y, et al. Common variants near FRK/COL10A1 and VEGFA are associated with advanced agerelated macular degeneration. Hum Mol Genet. 2011;20:3699-709. doi:10.1093/hmg/ddr270.
129. Fritsche LG, et al. Seven new loci associated with age-related macular degeneration. Nat Genet. 2013;45:433-439. 439e431–432, doi:10.1038/ng.2578.
130. Montes T, Tortajada A, Morgan BP, Rodriguez de Cordoba S, Harris, CL. Functional basis of protection against age-related macular degeneration conferred by a common polymorphism in complement factor B. Proc Natl Acad Sci USA. 2009;106:4366–71. doi:10.1073/pnas.0812584106.
131. Herbert AP, et al. Structure shows that a glycosaminoglycan and protein recognition site in factor H is perturbed by age-related macular degeneration-linked single nucleotide polymorphism. The Journal of biological chemistry. 2007;282:18960–8. doi:10.1074/jbc.M609636200.
132. Eberhardt HU, et al. Human factor H-related protein 2 (CFHR2) regulates complement activation. PLoS One. 2013;8:e78617. doi:10.1371/journal.pone.0078617.
133. Fritsche LG, et al. An imbalance of human complement regulatory proteins CFHR1, CFHR3 and factor H influences risk for age-related macular degeneration (AMD). Hum Mol Genet. 2010;19:4694–704. doi:10.1093/hmg/ddq399.
134. Hughes AE, et al. A common CFH haplotype, with deletion of CFHR1 and CFHR3, is associated with lower risk of age-related macular degeneration. Nat Genet. 2006;38:1173–7. doi:10.1038/ng1890.
135. Spencer KL, et al. Deletion of CFHR3 and CFHR1 genes in age-related macular degeneration. Hum Mol Genet. 2008;17:971–7. doi:10.1093/hmg/ddm369.

8

Mutation analysis of the *COL1A1* and *COL1A2* genes in Vietnamese patients with osteogenesis imperfecta

Binh Ho Duy[1,2,3*], Lidiia Zhytnik[2], Katre Maasalu[2,3], Ivo Kändla[5], Ele Prans[5], Ene Reimann[5], Aare Märtson[2,3] and Sulev Kõks[4,5]

Abstract

Background: The genetics of osteogenesis imperfecta (OI) have not been studied in a Vietnamese population before. We performed mutational analysis of the *COL1A1* and *COL1A2* genes in 91 unrelated OI patients of Vietnamese origin. We then systematically characterized the mutation profiles of these two genes which are most commonly related to OI.

Methods: Genomic DNA was extracted from EDTA-preserved blood according to standard high-salt extraction methods. Sequence analysis and pathogenic variant identification was performed with Mutation Surveyor DNA variant analysis software. Prediction of the pathogenicity of mutations was conducted using Alamut Visual software. The presence of variants was checked against Dalgleish's osteogenesis imperfecta mutation database.

Results: The sample consisted of 91 unrelated osteogenesis imperfecta patients. We identified 54 patients with *COL1A1/2* pathogenic variants; 33 with *COL1A1* and 21 with *COL1A2*. Two patients had multiple pathogenic variants. Seventeen novel *COL1A1* and 10 novel *COL1A2* variants were identified. The majority of identified *COL1A1/2* pathogenic variants occurred in a glycine substitution (36/56, 64.3 %), usually serine (23/36, 63.9 %). We found two pathogenic variants of the *COL1A1* gene c.2461G > A (p.Gly821Ser) in four unrelated patients and one, c.2005G > A (p.Ala669Thr), in two unrelated patients.

Conclusion: Our data showed a lower number of collagen OI pathogenic variants in Vietnamese patients compared to reported rates for Asian populations. The OI mutational profile of the Vietnamese population is unique and related to the presence of a high number of recessive mutations in non-collagenous OI genes. Further analysis of OI patients negative for collagen mutations, is required.

Keywords: Osteogenesis imperfecta, Collagen type I, Bone fragility, Sanger sequencing

Background

Osteogenesis imperfecta (OI) is associated with high genetic heterogeneity. To date, mutations in 16 different genes have been found to cause OI phenotypes of varying severity [1]. About 90 % of the mutations are related to alterations in the *COL1A1* and *COL1A2* genes, located at chromosome 17q21.33 and 7q21.3, respectively [2, 3]. These genes code for the α1/α2 chains of type 1 collagen [1, 4]. It was hypothesized that due to the presence of two α1 and one α2 chains in the procollagen triple helix, the *COL1A1* is more susceptible to mutation, as more α1 chains are implemented in the collagen fibrils. *COL1A1* gene mutations are more pathogenic and cause OI more often than *COL1A2* gene mutations. One third of glycine (Gly) substitutions in the *COL1A1* gene are lethal, whereas only 1/5 of Gly pathogenic variants in the *COL1A2* gene are fatal [5]. The collagen primary structure differs with an obligatory presence of Gly residues, the smallest amino acid, in every third position of an α chain, composing $(Gly\text{-}X\text{-}Y)_n$ repetitions, where X and Y are random amino acids [6]. The substitution of

* Correspondence: binhthuybi@yahoo.com
[1]Hue University of Medicine and Pharmacy, Hue University, 06 Ngo Quyen, Hue city 530000, Vietnam
[2]Department of Traumatology and Orthopaedics, University of Tartu, Puusepa 8, 51014 Tartu, Estonia
Full list of author information is available at the end of the article

Gly positioned in the center of the triple helix by a different amino acid would prevent interchain hydrogen bond formation between the NH-group of Gly and the CO-group in the X-position of a neighboring chain. Moreover, substitution of Gly residues with branched nonpolar or charged amino acids changes the helix to bulky and unstructured [5]. In this way, helix strength and stability decrease, which are crucially important for protein function [6–8].

Type 1 collagen is one of the most abundant proteins in the human body. It is a structural component of the bone, skin, tendons, cornea, and blood vessel walls and other connective tissues [4]. OI is generally caused by qualitative or quantitative collagen type I defects [9]. More than 2500 OI mutations have been found in type I collagen genes, which can cause a wide range of OI phenotypes that range in severity from mild to severe [10, 11] (http://www.le.ac.uk/ge/collagen/). Previous studies have shown that *COL1A1/2* mutations account for up to 85–90 % of all OI causative mutations, whereas only 10–15 % of OI mutations occur in non-collagenous genes [2, 11, 12]. While in more recent studies, many new genetic causes have been described, the mutations in the *COL1A1/2* genes remain a common origin of OI [1, 10]. However, there is a lack of systematic information regarding the mutational characteristics of OI patients. In addition, the genetics of Vietnamese OI patients has not been studied before. Our main aim with the current study was to perform mutational analysis of the *COL1A1* and *COL1A2* genes among unrelated OI patients of Vietnamese origin. We applied a systematic approach to characterizing the mutation profiles of these two genes.

Materials and methods

The study was conducted in accordance with the Helsinki Declaration and received approval from the ethical review board of Hue University Hospital (approval no. 75/CN-BVYD) and the Ethical Review Committee on Human Research of the University of Tartu (permit no. 221/M-34). Patients were selected from the Vietnamese database of osteogenesis imperfecta patients. The database includes information on 146 OI patients from 120 OI families and also about their healthy family members. A total of 91 unrelated OI patients were included in the study. Informed written consent from the patients or their legal representatives was obtained prior to inclusion to the study. Investigators then contacted patients in order to conduct an interview, perform a clinical examination, and collect blood samples, including blood samples from parents, siblings, and close relatives. Genomic DNA was extracted from EDTA-preserved blood according to standard high-salt extraction methods, stored at −80 °C, and analyzed at the University of Tartu, Estonia.

DNA samples were amplified using a polymerase chain reaction (PCR) with 25 specially designed primer pairs covering the 5′ UTR and 3′ UTR regions and 51 exons of the *COL1A1* gene; 36 primer pairs covering the 5′ UTR and 3′ UTR regions and 52 exons of the *COL1A2* gene. The PCR reaction was performed in a total volume of 20 µl, which included 4 µl of 5× HOT FIREPol® Blend Master Mix Ready to Load with 7.5 mM $MgCl_2$ (Solis BioDyne, Estonia), 1 µl each of forward and reverse primer (5 pmol), and 1 µl of gDNA (50 ng). PCR reaction was performed with a Thermal Cycler (Applied Biosystems, USA) PCR machine. The PCR *touchdown* program was used as follows for the reaction of amplification:

1 = 95.0°; 15:00 min
2 = 95.0°; 0:25 min
3 = 64.0°; 0:30 min
4 = 72.0°; 0:40 min
5 = go to 2.4 times
6 = 95.0°; 0:25 min
7 = 62.0°; 0:30 min
8 = 72.0°; 0:40 min
9 = go to 6.30 times
10 = 72.0°; 5:00 min
11 = 6.0°; forever

Amplified PCR products were electrophoresed through a 1.5 % agarose gel, to control the quality of fragments. The PCR products then purified with exonuclease I and shrimp alkaline phosphatase (Thermo Fisher Scientific, USA). Sanger sequencing reactions were performed on the purified PCR fragments using a BigDye® Terminator v3.1 Cycle Sequencing Kit (Applied Biosystems, USA). Reactions were processed on the ABI3730xl instrument.

Sequence reads were analyzed using Applied Biosystems' Sequence Scanner v1.0 and aligned to the human reference genome Local Reference Genomic sequence LGR_1 and GR_2. Raw sequencing data are available from authors upon request. Sequence analysis and pathogenic variant identification were performed with Mutation Surveyor DNA variant analysis software (Softgenetics, USA). Prediction of mutation's pathogenicity was performed using Alamut Visual software (Interactive Biosoftware, France). Variants were checked against the osteogenesis imperfecta mutation database (http://www.le.ac.uk/ge/collagen/). The pathogenicity of the pathogenic variants was predicted with SIFT score [13].

Results

We studied 42 female and 49 male OI patients. To characterize the OI patients' clinical features, all participants underwent clinical and physical examinations, and their medical records were reviewed. Cases were described according to the Sillence classification (types I–IV) [14].

Fifty-four patients were found to have *COL1A1/2* mutations, 33 with *COL1A1* and 21 with *COL1A2*; this equated to 36.3 and 23.1 % of patients, respectively, totaling 59.4 % of the studied OI cases exhibiting collagen type I mutations. Thirty-four pathogenic variants in the *COL1A1* gene (missense = 23, nonsense = 4, splice site = 7) and 22 pathogenic variants in the *COL1A2* gene (missense = 21, splice site = 1) were identified (patients VN01 and VN47 were carriers of double pathogenic variants in both the *COL1A1/2* genes) (Fig. 1; Tables 1 and 2). According to Dalgliesh database, 17 *COL1A1* and 10 *COL1A2* variants have not been reported before (Tables 1 and 2). De novo mutations were observed in 50 % (17/34) of *COL1A1* variants and 45.5 % (10/22) of *COL1A2* variants. All mutations were highly pathogenic, with a SIFT score of 0.0 and rarely 0.1, and located in regions of high conservation.

Discussion

In our study, we performed mutational analysis of 91 Vietnamese patients clinically diagnosed with OI (types I–IV). Thirty-three patients had 34 pathogenic variants of the *COL1A1* gene, and 21 patients had 22 pathogenic variants of the *COL1A2* gene, equating to a total of 54/91 (59.4 %) patients with *COL1A1/2* pathogenic variants. Previous studies have indicated that nearly 90 % of all OI mutations appear in the *COL1A1* and *COL1A2* genes [12, 15]. However, reported collagen type I mutational rates vary between different populations from 58 to 96 % [16–18].

We identified the substitution of Gly residuals in 17 out of 23 missense *COL1A1* mutations and 19 of 21 missense *COL1A2* pathogenic variants. Gly substitutions composed 36/56 (64.3 %) of *COL1A1/2* pathogenic variants. It has been hypothesized that the majority of the clinically severe forms of OI are caused by Gly missense mutations [17, 18]. However, there may exist a complex relationship between OI pathogenic variant and OI severity, whereby genetic, epigenetic, and environmental factors altogether affect the phenotype [19, 20].

Our research showed that out of 36 glycine substitutions, serine was the most prevalent (23/36; 63.9 %), followed by valine (4/36; 11.1 %), and cysteine and aspartic acid (3/36 cases each). Previous studies have suggested that glycine substitutions by cysteine often cause a greater severity of OI phenotype, and glycine substitutions by arginine were often fatal [21]. However, there are alternative reports that also suggest serine is the most common substitutional residue of Gly (72 % among Chinese OI patients) [18]. Aspartic acid substituted Gly in 40 % of Taiwanese OI patients [22]. The cause of variation in amino acid substitutions among populations of different geographical regions is still unclear.

In our research, intronic variants were represented by seven splice site mutations; other research has reported intronic variants among 7/56 of Chinese OI patients [18]. These mutations may cause exon skipping, intronic inclusion, and activation of cryptic sites [23]. In addition, analyses identified two nonsense mutations located in exons 52 and 37. Nonsense and splice site mutations are associated with haploinsufficiency, and as a result, quantitative collagen type I defects and a mild–moderate OI phenotype (type I/IV).

Patients VN01, VN34, VN40, and VN49 had the same heterozygous mutation: c.2461G > A (p.Gly821Ser) in

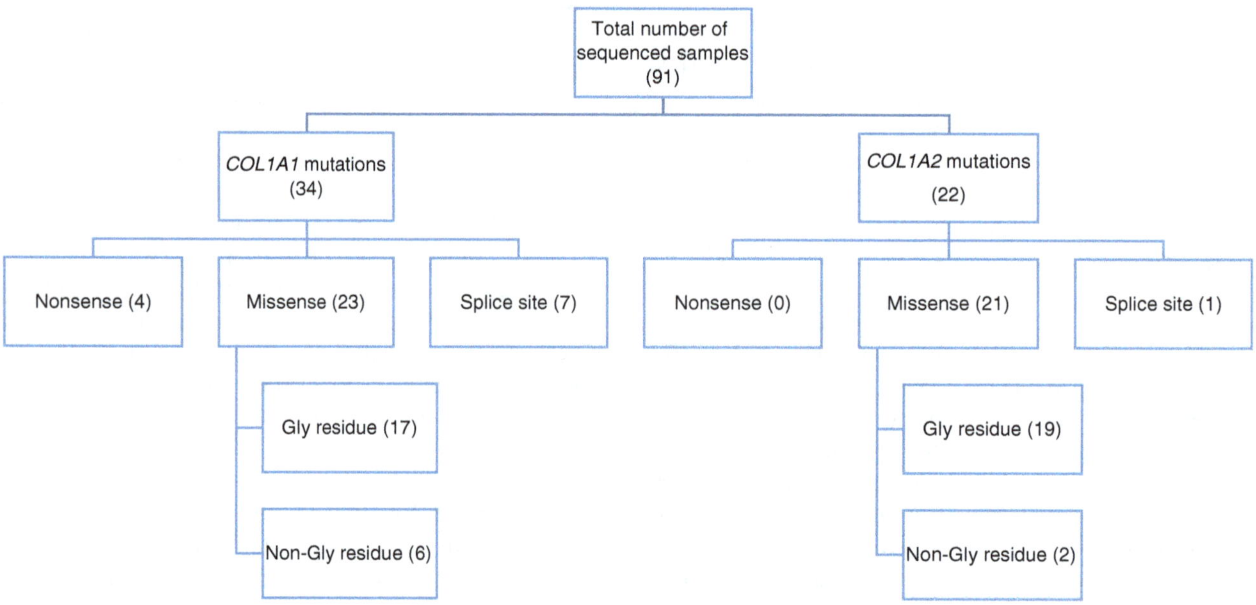

Fig. 1 Type I collagen OI mutations present among the studied Vietnamese OI patients

Table 1 *COL1A1* mutations in unrelated Vietnamese OI patients

No	Patient ID	COL1A1 mutation	Exon	Mutation type	Protein alteration	Sillence OI type
1	VN01	c.2461G > GA	Exon 37	Missense	p.Gly821Ser	I
		c.2005G > GA*	Exon 30	Missense	p.Ala669Thr,	
2	VN02	c.1200 + 1G > GT*	Intron 18	Splice site	–	I
3	VN05	c.1072delC, het*	Exon 17	Frameshift	p.Glu358Lysfs*26	III
4	VN13	c.4391 T > C	Exon 52	Missense	p.Leu1464Pro	I
5	VN18	c.103 + 2 T > TC*	Intron 1	Splice site	–	IV
6	VN21	c.4352dupA, het.*	Exon 52	Nonsense Frameshift	p.Asp1451Glufs*100	IV
7	VN26	c.3226G > GA	Exon 45	Missense	p.Gly1076Ser	IV
8	VN34	c.2461G > GA	Exon 37	Missense	p.Gly821Ser,	IV
9	VN38	c.959G > GA*	Exon 15	Missense	p.Gly320Asp	IV
10	VN39	c.630delG, het*	Exon 8	Frameshift	p.Glu210Aspfs*3	III
11	VN40	c.2461G > GA	Exon 37	Missense	p.Gly821Ser	IV
12	VN41	c.1102G > GA	Exon 17	Missense	p.Gly368Ser	IV
13	VN49	c.2461G > GA	Exon 37	Missense	p.Gly821Ser	IV
14	VN50	c.932G > GT*	Exon 14	Missense	p.Gly311Val	III
15	VN51	c.949G > GA*	Exon 14	Missense	p.Gly317Ser	IV
16	VN52	c.2523delT, het.	Exon 37	Frameshift Nonsense	p.Gly842Alafs*266	I
17	VN58	c.2236-2A > AG*	Intron 32	Splice site	-	I
18	VN66	c.2596G > AG*	Exon 38	Missense	p.Gly866Ser	III
19	VN68	c.2299G > GA	Exon 33/34	Missense	p.Gly767Ser	I
20	VN70	c.2281G > GA*	Exon 33/34	Missense	p.Gly761Ser	IV
21	VN71	c.1002 + 2 T > C	Intron 15	Splice site	–	IV
22	VN72	c.1165G > GT	Exon 18	Missense	p.Gly389Cys	I
23	VN76	c.1165G > GA	Exon 18	Missense	p.Gly389Ser	III
24	VN78	c.3766G > GA	Exon 49	Missense	p.Ala1256Thr	I
25	VN86	c.977G > AG	Exon 15	Missense	p.Gly326Asp	I
26	VN88	c.2005G > GA*	Exon 30	Missense	p.Ala669Thr	IV
27	VN89	c.2005G > GA*	Exon 30	Missense	p.Ala669Thr	IV
28	VN91	c.1299 + 1G > C	Intron 19	Splice site	–	IV
29	VN92	c.2299G > GA	Exon 33/34	Missense	p.Gly767Ser	III
30	VN95	c.590G > GA	Exon 8	Missense	p.Gly197Asp	I
31	VN99	c.103 + 2 T > TC*	Intron 1	Splice site	–	I
32	VN104	c.3369 + 1G > GC*	Intron 46	Splice site	–	I
33	VN106	c.1350G > GC*	Exon 20	Missense	p.Glu450Asp	III

Mutations unreported in the Dalgliesh's OI database are marked with an *asterisk* (*). In the case of heterozygous mutation, both the wild type and mutated alleles are indicated after an *arrow* (>)

exon 37 of the *COL1A1* gene. With respect to clinical severity, these patients showed nearly the same manifestations (clinical types I and IV). However, previous studies have described OI patients with different clinical features, despite their being carriers of the c.2461G > A mutation. Current data highlights the complexity of OI genotype–phenotype correlations. It is not yet possible to predict disorder severity based only on mutational analysis data.

Families VN88 and VN89 shared the same heterozygous *COL1A1* c.2005G > A (p.Ala669Thr) pathogenic variant in exon 30. Two patients had the same pathogenic variant and level of OI severity (type IV). Similar cases of variant reoccurance have been described before by Zhang et al. and Lee et al. in both *COL1A1/2* genes [17, 18]. However, OI pathogenic variants are usually unique and rarely repeated among different families [17].

Table 2 *COL1A2* mutations in unrelated Vietnamese OI patients

	Patient ID	COL1A2 mutation	Exon	Mutation type	Protein alteration	Sillence OI type
1	VN09	c.3305G > GT	Exon 49	Missense	p.Gly1102 > Val	I
2	VN23	c.2261G > GT*	Exon 37	Missense	p.Gly754Val	III
3	VN25	c.1072G > GT	Exon 37	Missense	p.Gly358Ser	I
4	VN29	c.1630G > GA*	Exon 28	Missense	p.Gly544Ser	IV
5	VN45	c.1090G > GA	Exon 21	Missense	p.Gly364Ser	III
6	VN47	c.3034G > GA	Exon 46	Missense	p.Gly1012Ser	IV
		c.2569C > CA	Exon 41	Missense	p.Pro857Thr	
7	VN48	c.1451G > GA	Exon 25	Missense	p.Gly484Glu	IV
8	VN56	c.1729G > GA*	Exon 30	Missense	p.Gly577Ser	III
9	VN60	c.1009G > GA	Exon 19	Missense	p.Gly337Ser	IV
10	VN62	c.1378G > GA	Exon 24	Missense	p.Gly460Ser	IV
11	VN64	c.1964G > GT*	Exon 32	Missense	p.Gly655Val	IV
12	VN65	c.1981G > GC*	Exon 33	Missense	p.Gly661Ser	III
13	VN69	c.874G > GA	Exon 17	Missense	p.Gly292Ser	III
14	VN81	c.982G > GA	Exon 19	Missense	p.Gly328Ser	III
15	VN82	c.2503G > GA	Exon 40	Missense	p.Gly835Ser	III
16	VN83	c.792 + 1G > GA	Exon 16	Splice site	-	III
17	VN84	c.2791G > GA*	Exon 43	Missense	p.Gly931Arg	IV
18	VN85	c.838G > GT*	Exon 17	Missense	p.Gly280Cys	IV
19	VN87	c.2791G > GA*	Exon 43	Missense	p.Gly931Arg	IV
20	VN96	c.892G > GT*	Exon 18	Missense	p.Gly298Cys	III
21	VN97	c.2538G > GT*	Exon 40	Missense	p.Lys846Asp	I

Mutations unreported in the Dalgliesh's OI database are marked with an *asterisk* (*). In the case of heterozygous mutation, both the wild type and mutated alleles are indicated after an *arrow* (>)

Genetic analysis revealed the presence of two heterozygous *COL1A1* mutations: exon 37 c.2461G > A (p.Gly821Ser) and exon 30 c.2005G > A (p.Ala669Thr) in patient VN01. Both pathogenic variants were shared by other unrelated patients among our study cohort. Patient VN47 had two heterozygous *COL1A2* pathogenic variants: exon 46 c.3034G > GA (p.Gly1012Ser) and exon 41 c.2569C > CA (p.Pro857Thr). Takagi et al. reported one case of severe OI (types II–III) due to a double substitution of glycine residues in the *COL1A2* gene (p.Gly208Glu and p.Gly235Asp), located on the same allele [24]. Our patients had only one substituted Gly residue in the *COL1A1* gene and a mild phenotype (VN01) and moderate phenotype (VN47) based on the clinic examination.

Of the 56 mutations found during our research, 17 *COL1A1* and 10 *COL1A2* variants (27/56 pathogenic variants; 48.2 %) were not present in Dalgleish's OI mutation database (Tables 1 and 2) [https://oi.gene.le.ac.uk/home.php?select_db=COL1A1; https://oi.gene.le.ac.uk/home.php?select_db=COL1A2]. The percentage of new variants among our patients was higher than in previous studies [16, 22, 25, 26]. The novelty of the pathogenic variants highlights the originality of the genetic epidemiology of the Vietnamese OI population. Half of Vietnamese OI patients are carriers of rare recessive non-collagenous OI pathogenic variants, which will be further identified with the whole exome sequencing analysis and reported in a future paper.

According to our data, more OI causative pathogenic variants occurred in the *COL1A1* gene than the *COL1A2* gene. Mutation hotspots were observed in intron 1; exons 8, 14–15, 17–20, 30, 33, 34, 37, and 52 of the *COL1A1* gene; and exons 17–49 of the *COL1A2* gene (Fig. 2). Products of the *COL1A1/2* gene consisted of signal peptide, N-terminal propeptide, collagen alpha I/II chain triple helical domain, and C-terminal propeptide (COLFI). COLFI controls procollagen intracellular assembly and the extracellular assembly of collagen fibrils. Mutation hotspots were situated in the regions that tolerate amino acid substitutions, and pathogenic variant resulted in an altered protein, but the organisms were still able to survive. Gaps in the mutation map connected to regions with crucial functions can however lead to fatal alterations [5, 27].

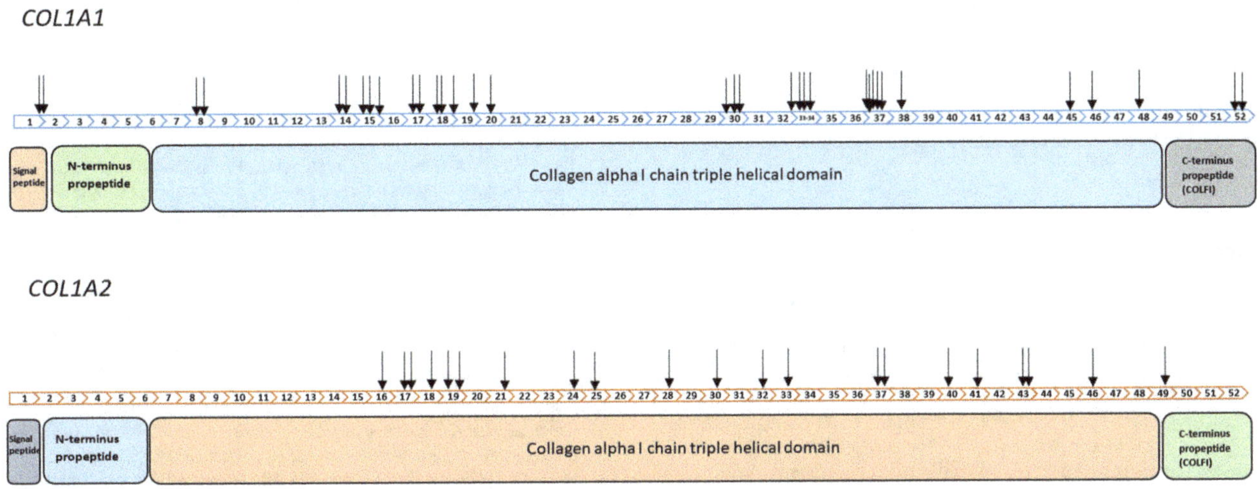

Fig. 2 Diagram of the *COL1A1* and *COL1A2* exons, with identified mutations and corresponding to protein product domains

Sequencing primers for the performed Sanger sequencing of the *COL1A1* and *COL1A2* genes in patients with clinical signs of osteogenesis imperfecta were designed far from intron-exon splice sites, which allowed the identifying of splice site, missense, frameshift, and nonsense mutations in the exons of the *COL1A1/2* genes. The gold standard of sequencing, the Sanger method, has an accuracy of approximately 99.9 % [28]. However, it has limitations in identifying whole genes and exon duplications and deletions. Therefore, the number of *COL1A1/2* pathogenic variants in the studied OI patients might have been underestimated.

We must also take into consideration that the percentage of collagen pathogenic variants among osteogenesis imperfecta patients may vary between studies due to their different sample sizes. However, we cannot exclude the possibility that the Vietnamese population has lower rates of collagenous OI pathogenic variants, and a unique OI mutational profile with higher levels of rare non-collagenous pathogenic variants, compared to other populations.

Conclusion

In the current study, we conducted mutational analysis of the *COL1A1* and *COL1A2* genes among 91 Vietnamese patients with osteogenesis imperfecta. After sequencing of the *COL1A1* and *COL1A2* genes, we found 56 mutations in 54 patients (59.4 % of patients). Our data showed a lower number of collagen OI pathogenic variants in these Vietnamese patients compared to reported rates for other Asian OI populations. The OI mutational profile of the Vietnamese population is likely unique and is related to the presence of a high number of recessive mutations in non-collagenous OI genes. Further analysis of patients negative for collagen OI mutations is needed in order to reveal unidentified OI genotypes from the sample.

Abbreviations

3′ UTR, 3′ untranslated region; 5′ UTR, 5′ untranslated region; COLFI, fibrillary collagen C-terminal domain; EDTA, ethylenediaminetetraacetic acid; gDNA, genomic DNA; OI, osteogenesis imperfecta; PCR, polymerase chain reaction

Acknowledgements

We would like to thank the following people and organizations for their help and support with data collection: The Vietnamese National Hospital of Pediatrics; Hanoi OI Center; OI Booming Diamond Center in Ho Chi Minh City; Hue University Hospital; and The University of Tartu. This research would not have been possible without the support, teaching, and cooperation of the Department of Traumatology and Orthopaedics and Department of Pathophysiology of University of Tartu.

Funding

This work was supported by institutional research funding IUT20-46 of the Estonian Ministry of Education and Research and the European Union's European Regional Development Fund Programme "Supporting international cooperation in R&D" projects "EVMED" and "DIOXMED." The research leading to these results has received funding from the European Union's Seventh Framework Programme (FP7/2007-2013) under grant agreement no. 602398.

Authors' contributions

HDB conceived the study, participated in its design, interacted with the patients, coordinated the blood sample collection, and drafted the manuscript. LZ, IK, EP, SK, ER carried out the genetic studies, performed the data analysis, and helped to draft the manuscript. KM participated in its design, interacted with the patients, coordinated the blood sample collection, and helped to draft the manuscript. SK and AM participated in the design of the study, coordinated the data interpretation and statistical analysis and helped to draft the manuscript. All authors read and approved the final manuscript.

Competing interests

The authors declare that they have no competing interests.

Consent for publication

Not applicable.

Author details
[1]Hue University of Medicine and Pharmacy, Hue University, 06 Ngo Quyen, Hue city 530000, Vietnam. [2]Department of Traumatology and Orthopaedics, University of Tartu, Puusepa 8, 51014 Tartu, Estonia. [3]Clinic of Traumatology and Orthopaedics, Tartu University Hospital, Puusepa 8, 51014 Tartu, Estonia. [4]Centre of Translational Medicine, University of Tartu, Ravila 14a, Tartu 50411, Estonia. [5]Department of Pathophysiology, University of Tartu, Ravila 19, Tartu 50411, Estonia.

References

1. Van Dijk FS, Sillence DO. Osteogenesis imperfecta: clinical diagnosis, nomenclature and severity assessment. Am J Med Genet A. 2014;164A:1470–81.
2. van Dijk FS, Byers PH, Dalgleish R, et al. EMQN best practice guidelines for the laboratory diagnosis of osteogenesis imperfecta. Eur J Hum Genet. 2012;20:11–19.
3. Rauch F, Glorieux F. Osteogenesis imperfecta. Lancet. 2004;363(9418):1377–85.
4. Pokidysheva E, Mizuno K, Bächinger HP. The collagen folding machinery: Biosynthesis and post-translational modifications of collagens. In: Jay R. Shapiro, Peter H. Byers, Francis H. Glorieux, Paul D. Sponseller, editors. Osteogenesis imperfecta a translational approach to brittle bone disease. London: Elsevier; 2014. p.57–70.
5. Marini JC, Forlino A, Cabral WA, Barnes AM, San Antonio JD, Milgrom S, et al. Consortium for osteogenesis imperfecta mutations in the helical domain of type I collagen: regions rich in lethal mutations align with collagen binding sites for integrins and proteoglycans. Hum Mutat. 2007;28:209–21.
6. Gelse K. Collagens—structure, function, and biosynthesis. Adv Drug Deliv Rev. 2003;55:1531–46.
7. Kadler KE, Holmes DF, Trotter JA, Chapman JA. Collagen fibril formation. J Biochem. 1996;316:1–11.
8. Makareeva E, Leikin S. Collagen structure, folding and function. In: Jay R. Shapiro, Peter H. Byers, Francis H. Glorieux, Paul D. Sponseller, editors. Osteogenesis Imperfecta. A translational approach to brittle bone disease. London: Elsevier; 2014. p.71–84.
9. Marini J, Smith SM. Osteogenesis Imperfecta MDText.com, Inc. 2015.
10. Zukowsky K, Editor CS. Osteogenesis Imperfecta types I–XI. 2014;1–7.
11. Basel D, Steiner RD. Osteogenesis imperfecta: recent findings shed new light on this once well-understood condition. Genet Med. 2009;11:375–85.
12. Pollitt R, McMahon R, Nunn J, Bamford R, Afifi A, Bishop N, et al. Mutation analysis of COL1A1 and COL1A2 in patients diagnosed with osteogenesis imperfecta type I-IV. Hum Mutat. 2006;27:716.
13. Kumar P, Henikoff S, Ng PC. Predicting the effects of coding non-synonymous variants on protein function using the SIFT algorithm. Nat Protoc. 2009;4:1073–81.
14. Sillence DO, Senn A, Danks DM. Genetic heterogeneity in osteogenesis imperfecta. J Med Genet. 1979;16:101–16.
15. Shaker JL, Albert C, Fritz J, Harris G. Recent developments in osteogenesis imperfecta F1000Res. 2015;4:681. doi:10.12688/f1000research.6398.1.
16. Stephen J, Shukla A, Dalal A, Girisha KM, Shah H, Gupta N, et al. Mutation spectrum of *COL1A1* and *COL1A2* genes in Indian patients with osteogenesis imperfecta. Am J Med Genet Part A. 2014;164:1482–9.
17. Lee K-S, Song H-R, Cho T-J, Kim HJ, Lee T-M, Jin H-S, et al. Mutational spectrum of type I collagen genes in Korean patients with osteogenesis imperfecta. Hum Mutat. 2006;27:599.
18. Zhang Z-L, Zhang H, Ke Y, Yue H, Xiao W-J, Yu J-B, et al. The identification of novel mutations in COL1A1, COL1A2, and LEPRE1 genes in Chinese patients with osteogenesis imperfecta. J Bone Miner Metab. 2012;30:69–77.
19. Roughley PJ, Rauch F, Glorieux FH. Osteogenesis imperfecta—clinical and molecular diversity. Eur Cell Mater. 2003;5:41–7. discussion 47.
20. Kataoka K, Ogura E, Hasegawa K, Inoue M, Seino Y, et al. Mutations in type I collagen genes in Japanese osteogenesis imperfecta patients. Pediatr Int. 2007;49:564–9.
21. Cole WG, Chow CW, Rogers JG, Bateman JF. The clinical features of three babies with osteogenesis imperfecta resulting from the substitution of glycine by arginine in the pro alpha 1(I) chain of type I procollagen. J Med Genet. 1990;27:228–35.
22. Lin H-Y, Chuang C-K, Su Y-N, Chen M-R, Chiu H-C, Niu D-M, et al. Genotype and phenotype analysis of Taiwanese patients with osteogenesis imperfecta. Orphanet J Rare Dis. 2015;10:152.
23. Kuivaniemi H, Tromp G, Prockop DJ. Mutations in fibrillar collagens (types I, II, III, and XI), fibril-associated collagen (type IX), and network-forming collagen (type X) cause a spectrum of diseases of bone, cartilage, and blood vessels. Hum Mutat. 1997;9:300–15.
24. Takagi M, Kouwaki M, Kawase K, Shinohara H, Hasegawa Y, Yamada T, et al. Severe osteogenesis imperfecta caused by double glycine substitutions near the amino-terminal triple helical region in COL1A2. Am J Med Genet Part A. 2015;167:2851–4.
25. Yang Z, Ke ZF, Zeng C, Wang Z, Shi HJ, Wang LT. Mutation characteristics in type I collagen genes in Chinese patients with osteogenesis imperfecta. Genet Mol Res. 2011;10:177–85.
26. Ward LM, Lalic L, Roughley PJ, Glorieux FH. Thirty-three novel COL1A1 and COL1A2 mutations in patients with osteogenesis imperfecta types I-IV. Hum Mutat. 2001;17:434.
27. Sweeney SM, Orgel JP, Fertala A, McAuliffe JD, Turner KR, Di Lullo GA, et al. Candidate cell and matrix interaction domains on the collagen fibril, the predominant protein of vertebrates. J Biol Chem. 2008;283:21187–97.
28. Sanger F, Nicklen S, Coulson AR. DNA sequencing with chain-terminating inhibitors. Proc Natl Acad Sci U S A. 1977;74:5463–7.

9

Major influence of repetitive elements on disease-associated copy number variants (CNVs)

Ana R. Cardoso[1,2,3], Manuela Oliveira[1,2,3], Antonio Amorim[1,2,3] and Luisa Azevedo[1,2,3*]

Abstract

Copy number variants (CNVs) are important contributors to the human pathogenic genetic diversity as demonstrated by a number of cases reported in the literature. The high homology between repetitive elements may guide genomic stability which will give rise to CNVs either by non-allelic homologous recombination (NAHR) or non-homologous end joining (NHEJ). Here, we present a short guide based on previously documented cases of disease-associated CNVs in order to provide a general view on the impact of repeated elements on the stability of the genomic sequence and consequently in the origin of the human pathogenic variome.

Keywords: Copy number variants (CNVs), Genetic diseases, Genomic structural variation, Low copy repeats, Retrotransposons, LINE, SINE, Non-allelic homologous recombination (NAHR)

Background

Copy number variants (CNVs) are structural genomic markers (insertions or deletions) ranging in size from 1 kb to several megabytes for each copy. They are categorized as copy number polymorphisms (CNPs) when multiple allelic states exist in the population or as rare copy number variants when they are found to be associated with genetic diseases (pathogenic copy number variants) [1, 2]. The origin of each repeated element of the CNV is influenced by the local genomic architecture which includes the presence of repetitive sequences within or flanking the repeated segment [3–7]. These repeated sequences drive non-allelic homologous recombination (NAHR) events which result in recurrent insertions and deletions with similar sequence sizes and clustered breakpoints [3, 6, 8] or non-homologous end joining (NHEJ) events that result in non-recurrent rearrangements that vary in terms of their size and breakpoint location [3, 6, 9]. Although several studies have been demonstrating the contribution of structural variants to the genome architecture, few have specifically focused the influence of repeated sequences at breakpoint locations. With the aim to draw attention to these unstable regions and to establish their role in CNVs, we collated a number of cases of CNV-associated disorders proven to have been generated by low and high copy number repeats which may have influenced the degree of stability of the genomic sequence.

Low copy repeats and their influence on pathogenic CNV formation

Low copy repeats (LCRs) are homologous sequences of ≥1 kb in length which are found in many copies throughout the genome since they are generated by duplication events [3, 10]. Large LCRs (>10 kb) with high sequence homology promote non-allelic homologous recombination (NAHR) [3–6, 10–12] and the misalignment of directly oriented sister chromatids carrying the LCR may promoted NAHR thereby generating both duplications and deletions [4, 5] which in turn give rise to copy number variation. A schematic representation of this process is shown in Fig. 1.

Certain properties of the LCRs such as homology length, sequence similarity, and distance, serve to influence the frequency of NAHR events [3, 6, 12] (Fig. 1). As recently reviewed by Carvalho and Lupski [3], the NAHR

* Correspondence: lazevedo@ipatimup.pt
[1]Instituto de Investigação e Inovação em Saúde, Universidade do Porto, Rua Alfredo Allen 208, 4200-135 Porto, Portugal
[2]IPATIMUP-Institute of Molecular Pathology and Immunology, University of Porto, Rua Júlio Amaral de Carvalho 45, 4200-135 Porto, Portugal
Full list of author information is available at the end of the article

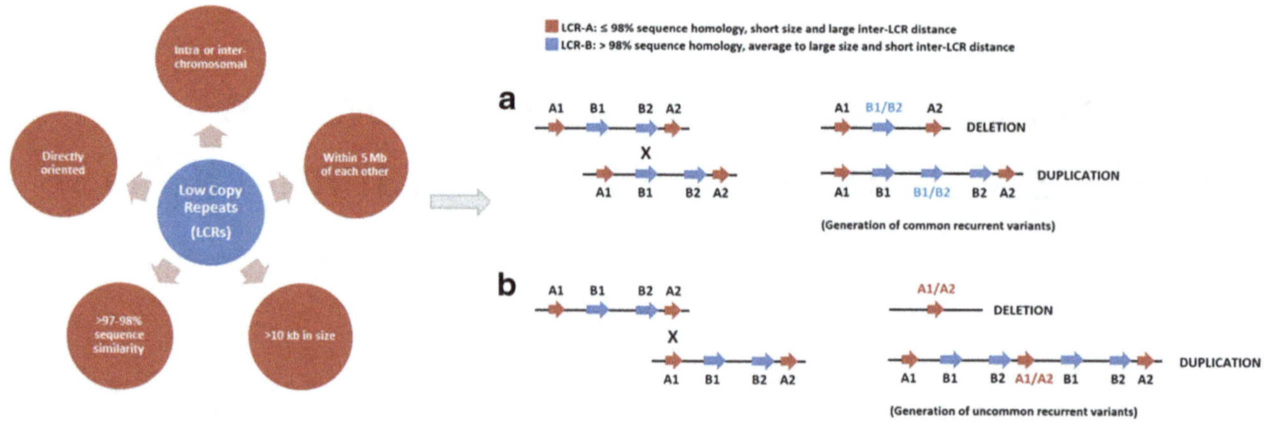

Fig. 1 Optimal LCRs features for the occurrence of NAHR events that result in CNV formation. Distinct LCR pairs with counter features such as homology, size, and inter-LCR distance influence NAHR rate and lead to the formation of common recurrent (**a**) or rare recurrent (**b**) copy number variants. Adapted from [3, 6, 12]

rate varies according to the length of the LCR sequence, the distance between distinct LCR sequences and the DNA sequence. The NAHR rate is, therefore, positively correlated with the LCR length but is inversely proportional to the distance between distinct LCRs [3, 9]. Since there is a high homology between distinct LCR sequences proximal to copy number variation regions; there is also an increased predisposition to NAHR events in these genomic regions [3, 4, 6, 9, 12].

A considerable number of disease-associated CNVs generated by LCRs have been documented and reviewed in previous works (e.g. [3, 6]), but for the purposes of this paper, we have only collated cases for which the specific repetitive element was found at the breakpoints of the structural variant and not those for which the causality of the repeats elements was only suggested. The resulting set is presented in Table 1. For example, a complex array of LCRs spanning a 4-Mb region around the X-linked *MECP2* gene was associated with unique duplications ranging in size from 200 kb to 2.2 Mb in developmentally delayed males [13]. Duplications and deletions affecting the *PLP1* gene causing Pelizaeus-Merzbacher disease (OMIM #312080) are also associated with a specific LCR (LCR-PMD A/B pair) within a 3-Mb region flanking the gene in which a multitude of LCRs are located [14]. LCRs are also frequent at the 2q11-q21.1 locus [11], where recurrent deletions of the *NPHP1* gene (2q13) have been associated with nephronophthisis 1 (OMIM #256100). A 0.3-Mb copy number gain was detected in three X-linked intellectual disability (XLID) families and one sporadic patient [15]. The region overlapped the *GDI1* gene, an important XLID-associated

Table 1 Repetitive elements detected at the breakpoints of CNVs associated with clinical phenotypes

Phenotype	Critical genes	Type of variant	Locus	Repetitive element involved	Ref.
MECP2 duplication syndrome	*MECP2, L1CAM*	Dup	Xq28	Several LCR-MECP2s pairs	[3, 6, 13, 44–46]
Rett syndrome	*MECP2*	Del	Xq28	Several LCR-MECP2 pairs	[6]
Neurofibromatosis type I	*NF1*	Del	17q11.2	NF1-REPs A/B/C	[3, 6]
Nephronophthisis	*NPHP1*	Del	2q13	Several LCR pairs	[11, 47–49]
Mental retardation, X-linked 41 (MRX41)	*GDI1*	Dup/Trip	Xq28	LCR-K1/L2 pair	[15]
Angelman and Prader-Willi syndromes	*UBE3A*	Del	15q11-q13	END-repeats (LCRs)	[6, 50]
Smith-Magenis syndrome	*RAI1* and *PMP22*	Del	17p11.2	SMS-REPs (LCRs)	[3, 6, 18]
Williams-Beuren syndrome	28 dosage-sensitive genes	Dup/Tripe/Del	7q11.23	A/B/C LCR blocks	[3, 6, 51]
15q13.1 microdeletion syndrome	*CHRNA7*	Dup/Trip	15q13.3	BP3/4/5	[3, 6, 52, 53]
3q29 microduplication or microdeletion syndrome	*DLG1, PAK2*	Dup/Del	3q29	A/B/C LCR blocks	[3, 54, 55]
Pelizaeus-Merzbacher disease	*PLP1*	Dup/Del	Xq22	LCR-PMD A/B pair	[3, 6, 14]
DiGeorge syndrome/velo-cardio facial syndrome	*COMT, TBX1*	Del	22q11.2	8 specific LCR22 repeats	[6, 17, 40]
Charcot-Marie-Tooth type 1A	*PMP22*	Dup	17p12	CMTA1-Reps (LCRs)	[3, 6, 37, 38]

gene highly expressed in the brain. The aberration was located in Xq28, a locus that includes other intellectual disability genes and that is frequently associated with recombination events caused by proximal LCRs (e.g., LCR K1/L2). The Angelman syndrome (AS) (OMIM #105830) and Prader-Willi syndrome (PWS) (OMIM #176270) are caused by recurrent 4-Mb deletions at the 15q11-q13 locus. The deleted region is flanked by LCRs [6] and accounts for 70 % of cases of AS and 70–75 % of cases of PWS [16]. The Smith-Magenis syndrome (SMS) (OMIM #182290) results from recurrent deletions of 3.7 Mb at 17p11.2 which account for more than 70 % of cases; about 25 % of affected individuals harbor deletions ranging from 1.5–9 Mb [6, 17]. The deletions are flanked by 200-kb highly homologous LCRs that play a role in generating meiotic NAHR events [16]. These deletions encompass the *RAI1* gene, which is critical in organ and neuronal development—patients with larger deletions manifest a more severe phenotype when the dosage-sensitive gene *PMP22* is deleted [18].

Retrotransposons (high copy repeats) and their influence on pathogenic CNVs

Interspersed repeats are the most common type of high copy repeats, covering about 44 % of the human genome [4]. Retrotransposons account for the majority of transposable elements [5, 7, 19]. These are mobile elements that through reverse transcription have the ability to integrate into different regions [7, 19]. Long interspersed nuclear elements (LINEs), short interspersed nuclear elements (SINEs), and retrovirus-like elements (LTR transposons) are the three major categories of mammalian retrotransposons (Table 2).

Among LINEs, L1 is the most abundant element, typically of 6–8 kb in length, with the ability to increase genomic instability through NAHR events [4]. It is known that about 83 % of the human genome is prone to LINE-LINE recombination events that contribute to genomic instability and can give rise to unbalanced structural variants [20].

Alu elements are the most common SINEs and have been associated with NAHR events that lead to pathogenic duplications and deletions [3, 4, 21, 22]. Table 3 presents examples of high copy repeats that have been detected at the breakpoints of disease-associated CNVs.

Borun and colleagues [23] reported the presence of CNV breakpoints within Alu elements in the *STK11* gene which lead to the Peutz-Jeghers syndrome (OMIM #175200), where CNVs account for 30 % of cases. The 17p13.3 locus is enriched in copy number variations associated with genomic disorders, such as the Miller-Dieker syndrome (17p13.3 deletion syndrome) (OMIM #247200) and its reciprocal 17p13.3 duplication syndrome (OMIM #613215) [24]. The breakpoints of the reported CNVs at this locus are highly enriched in Alu elements, which mediate these junctions through an Alu-Alu mechanism. About 70 % of CNVs found in the *SPAST* gene have been associated with Alu recombination events [25]. Local Alu-rich architecture predisposes to the formation of pathogenic structural rearrangements associated with spastic paraplegia (OMIM #182601). An extra copy of the *LMNB1* gene at the 5q23 locus has been previously associated with autosomal dominant adult-onset demyelinating leukodystrophy (ADLD) (OMIM #169500). The analysis of twenty ADLD-affected families revealed sixteen duplications ranging from 128 to 475 kb in size, all of them spanning the *LMNB1* gene [26]. The centromeric region of the critical gene is enriched with SINE elements, particularly Alus. Alu-mediated recombination events were also found to be linked to pathogenic deletions at the *OTC* gene [27], a urea cycle gene for which a significant number of structural variants are known [28]. NAHR events between Alu repeats are also strongly correlated with the birth of structural rearrangements at the Alu-rich *BRCA1* locus [29] which is associated with breast cancer. Duplications (220 to 394 kb) and a triplication (1.61 to 2.04 Mb) of the *SNCA* gene located at 4q21 locus have been implicated in autosomal dominant Parkinson's disease (PD1 and PD4) (OMIM #168601, #605543). The phenotypic severity is consistent with a gene dosage effect [6]. Regarding recessive PD (OMIM #600116), about one third of pathogenic variants associated with the *PRKN* gene are CNVs occurring between exon 2 and exon 5, which may therefore be considered to be a

Table 2 Main characteristics of the most abundant retrotransposons [4, 5, 7, 19]

	Retrotransposons (interspersed repeats)—44 % human genome		
	Non-long terminal repeat (LTR)		Long terminal repeat (LTR)
Repetitive element	Long interspersed nuclear repeats (LINEs)	Short interspersed nuclear repeats (SINEs)	Endogenous retroviruses (ERV)
Genomic coverage	20 %	11 %	8 %
Features	• L1 is the most abundant class • Autonomous transposons • Reverse transcriptase (RT) encoded by LINE-1	• Alu is the most abundant class • Dependent on LINEs transposable machinery • Mobile polymerase III promoter • 100–400 bp in length	• Reduced transposable activity • Presence of *gag* and *pol* viral genes

Table 3 High copy repeats detected at the breakpoints of CNVs associated with clinical phenotypes

Phenotype	Critical genes	Type of variant	Locus	Repetitive elements involved	Ref.
Peutz-Jeghers syndrome	*STK11*	Del	19p13.3	Several AluY/AluY pairs	[23]
Spastic paraplegia 4	*SPAST, SLC30A6*	Dup/Del	2p22.3	Several Alu pairs	[25]
OTC deficiency	*OTC*	Del	Xp11.4	AluSx/AluSq pair	[27, 56]
Miller-Dieker syndrome and 17p13.3 duplication syndrome	*LIS1*	Del	17p13.3	Several Alu pairs	[6, 24]
Breast cancer	*BRCA1*	Del	17q21.31	AluSx/AluSc pair	[29, 57]
Autosomal dominant adult-onset demyelinating leukodystrophy (ADLD)	*LMNB1*	Dup/Trip	5q23.2	LIPA3 LINE repeats AluYA/AluYB pair	[26]
Azoospermia	*AZFa*	Del	Yq11	HERV15 A/B proviruses	[34, 58]
Mental retardation, X-linked 60 (MRX60)	*OPHN1*	Del	Xq12	AluY/AluY pair	[35]
Pelizaeus-Merzbacher disease	*PLP1*	Del	Xq22	AluSq/AluSx pair	[3, 6, 59]
DiGeorge syndrome/velo-cardio facial syndrome	*COMT, TBX1*	Del	22q11.2	Unclassified Alu/Alu pair	[6, 17, 40]
Charcot-Marie-Tooth type 1A	*PMP22*	Dup	17p12	AluY/AluY pair AluSg/AluSg pair	[39]
Williams-Beuren syndrome	28 dosage-sensitive genes	Dup/Del	7q11.23	AluS subfamily elements	[36]
Parkinson's disease	*SNCA*	Dup/Trip	4q21	Several Alu pairs	[32]

recombination hotspot [30, 31]. Ross and colleagues [32] reported the presence of Alu and LINE1 elements at the *SNCA* locus that may contribute to the genomic instability at this locus.

Human endogenous retroviruses (HERVs) represent about 4.9 % of the human genome [4]. Sequences with about 95 % sequence similarity were previously associated with NAHR events and recurrent CNVs, some of which with pathogenic implications [3, 33]. For example, the occurrence of NAHR between a particular set of HERV elements flanking the male fertility *AZFa* locus in the Y chromosome is strongly associated with pathogenic deletions associated with male infertility (OMIM #400042, #415000) [4, 34].

Pathogenic copy number variants associated with both LCRs and retrotransposons

The breakpoints of some disease-associated CNVs have been reported to be caused by more than one type of repetitive elements which indicates that the same phenotype involves both low copy and high copy repeats that affect the stability of a target gene. Bergmann and colleagues [35] conducted a family study in which five brothers shared the same phenotypic pattern that included intellectual disability. The analysis of the OPHN1 locus (Xq12) revealed the presence of a 17.6-kb intronic deletion and the breakpoints spanning the deletion revealed two highly homologous Alu repeats and additional repetitive sequences (interspersed and simple repeats).

A recurrent deletion of 1.6 to 1.8 Mb (>95 % of the patients) at the 7q11.23 locus causes the Williams-Beuren syndrome (OMIM #194050) [6]. Genes within this region are dosage-sensitive and the recurrently deleted region encompasses a total of 28 genes. This locus is characterized by highly homologous flanking LCRs that contribute to NAHR events [6]. Antonell and colleagues [36] reported the presence of Alu elements at the junctions of large duplicated blocks in 7q11.23 suggesting the influence of these retrotransposons in the generation of large LCRs.

Heterozygous duplication and reciprocal deletions of a 1.4–1.5-Mb segment at the 17p12 locus have been previously linked with the Charcot-Marie-Tooth type 1A syndrome (CMT1A) (OMIM #118220). About 70 % of CMT1A patients have a recurrent duplication of the dosage-sensitive PMP22 locus and the NAHR event that gave rise to this copy number variation was mediated by LCRs [3, 6, 37, 38]. A study by Zhang and colleagues [39] revealed the presence of SINEs (Alu elements) and LINEs (L1 and L2) as well as LCRs within the breakpoints of rare non-recurrent deletions and duplications at the CMT1A locus.

About 96 % of the DiGeorge syndrome (DGS) (OMIM #188400)- and velo-cardio-facial syndrome (VCFS) (OMIM #192430)-affected patients harbor a 1.5–3 Mb deletion at the 22q11.2 locus that includes 24 to 30 genes [16]. The breakpoints of the common recurrent deletions at this locus are associated with LCRs [17] and one Alu sequence [40]. Both the deletions and duplications at this locus are generated by NAHR events between the repeated regions flanking the CNV, specifically the low copy repeat known as LCR22 [41]. Furthermore, 20–25 % of individuals who harbor this deletion also show signs of schizophrenia, mood disorders, and other behavioral alterations [41].

Conclusions

Although the majority of genetic diseases are caused by non-structural variants (e.g. [42, 43], an increasing number of causative mutations have been associated with CNVs and these cases were the focus of this short review. Low copy repeats and retrotransposons are the major contributors to CNV formation. Recurrent CNVs are mainly directed by NAHR events that occur between highly homologous LCR sequences. In terms of non-recurrent CNVs, NHEJ (among other molecular mechanisms [3]) generally occurs between sequences with a degree of homology lower than that observed between distinct LCRs. The diversity of breakpoint junctions of non-recurrent variants renders the establishment of phenotype-genotype relationships less reliable because the sequence that is deleted or duplicated in each patient is different and the affected region may also involve other genes. This review focused on disease-associated CNVs in order to show that although numerous cases of instability driven by repeated sequences around the affected locus (or loci) have been documented, we are still far from understanding all the phenotypic complexities associated with these unbalanced variants, mainly because the number of reported cases is still too small to draw general conclusions. Finally, it is important to mention that collated data, such as those presented in this paper, pertaining to the pathogenic structural variome are expected to drive future studies with the aim of establishing a map of unstable genomic hotspots which promises to be useful in the context of clinical genetic testing where the determination of the molecular basis of Mendelian and complex diseases (e.g., cancer) is of paramount importance.

Abbreviations

CNV: Copy number variant; LCR: Low copy repeat; CNP: Copy number polymorphism; LINE: Long interspersed nuclear repeat; SINE: Short interspersed nuclear repeat; LTR: Long terminal repeat; NAHR: Non-allelic homologous recombination; NHEJ: Non-homologous end joining; XLID: X-linked intellectual disability

Acknowledgements

Not applicable.

Funding

IPATIMUP integrates the i3S Research Unit, which is partially supported by FCT, the Portuguese Foundation for Science and Technology. This work is funded by FEDER funds through the Operational Programme for Competitiveness Factors - COMPETE and National Funds through the FCT-Foundation for Science and Technology, under the projects "PEst-C/SAU/LA0003/2013".

M. Oliveira (SFRH/BPD/66071/2009) was supported by FCT fellowships funded by POPH-QREN - Promotion of Scientific Employment, the European Social Fund, and National Funds of the Ministry of Education and Science.

Authors' contributions

ARC performed literature search. ARC and LA drafted the manuscript. MO and AA discussed the data and performed critical revisions to the manuscript. All authors read and approved the final manuscript.

Competing interests

The authors declare that they have no competing interests.

Consent for publication

Not applicable.

Author details

[1]Instituto de Investigação e Inovação em Saúde, Universidade do Porto, Rua Alfredo Allen 208, 4200-135 Porto, Portugal. [2]IPATIMUP-Institute of Molecular Pathology and Immunology, University of Porto, Rua Júlio Amaral de Carvalho 45, 4200-135 Porto, Portugal. [3]Department of Biology, Faculty of Sciences, University of Porto, Rua do Campo Alegre S/N, 4169-007 Porto, Portugal.

References

1. Itsara A, Cooper GM, Baker C, Girirajan S, Li J, Absher D, et al. Population analysis of large copy number variants and hotspots of human genetic disease. Am J Hum Genet. 2009;84(2):148–61.
2. Henrichsen CN, Chaignat E, Reymond A. Copy number variants, diseases and gene expression. Hum Mol Genet. 2009;18(R1):R1–8.
3. Carvalho CM, Lupski JR. Mechanisms underlying structural variant formation in genomic disorders. Nat Rev Genet. 2016;17(4):224–38.
4. Chen L, Zhou W, Zhang L, Zhang F. Genome architecture and its roles in human copy number variation. Genomics Inform. 2014;12(4):136–44.
5. Jobling MA, Hollox E, Hurles M, Kivisild T, Tyler-Smith C. Human evolutionary genetics: origins, peoples and disease. 2nd ed. New York: Garland Science; 2014.
6. Lee JA, Lupski JR. Genomic rearrangements and gene copy-number alterations as a cause of nervous system disorders. Neuron. 2006;52(1):103–21.
7. Strachan T, Read A. Human Molecular Genetics. 4th ed. New York:Garland Science; 2011.
8. Gu W, Zhang F, Lupski JR. Mechanisms for human genomic rearrangements. Pathogenetics. 2008;1(1):4.
9. Liu P, Lacaria M, Zhang F, Withers M, Hastings PJ, Lupski JR. Frequency of nonallelic homologous recombination is correlated with length of homology: evidence that ectopic synapsis precedes ectopic crossing-over. Am J Hum Genet. 2011;89(4):580–8.
10. Potier MC, Golfier G, Eichler EE. Chromosome-specific repeats (Low-copy Repeats). In:eLS. Chichester: Wiley; 2007.
11. Dittwald P, Gambin T, Szafranski P, Li J, Amato S, Divon MY, et al. NAHR-mediated copy-number variants in a clinical population: mechanistic insights into both genomic disorders and Mendelizing traits. Genome Res. 2013;23(9):1395–409.
12. Peng Z, Zhou W, Fu W, Du R, Jin L, Zhang F. Correlation between frequency of non-allelic homologous recombination and homology properties: evidence from homology-mediated CNV mutations in the human genome. Hum Mol Genet. 2015;24(5):1225–33.
13. del Gaudio D, Fang P, Scaglia F, Ward PA, Craigen WJ, Glaze DG, et al. Increased MECP2 gene copy number as the result of genomic duplication in neurodevelopmentally delayed males. Genet Med. 2006;8(12):784–92.
14. Lee JA, Inoue K, Cheung SW, Shaw CA, Stankiewicz P, Lupski JR. Role of genomic architecture in PLP1 duplication causing Pelizaeus-Merzbacher disease. Hum Mol Genet. 2006;15(14):2250–65.

15. Vandewalle J, Van Esch H, Govaerts K, Verbeeck J, Zweier C, Madrigal I, et al. Dosage-dependent severity of the phenotype in patients with mental retardation due to a recurrent copy-number gain at Xq28 mediated by an unusual recombination. Am J Hum Genet. 2009;85(6):809–22.
16. Firth HV, Richards SM, Bevan AP, Clayton S, Corpas M, Rajan D, et al. DECIPHER: Database of Chromosomal Imbalance and Phenotype in Humans Using Ensembl Resources. Am J Hum Genet. 2009;84(4):524–33.
17. Shaikh TH, Kurahashi H, Saitta SC, O'Hare AM, Hu P, Roe BA, et al. Chromosome 22-specific low copy repeats and the 22q11.2 deletion syndrome: genomic organization and deletion endpoint analysis. Hum Mol Genet. 2000;9(4):489–501.
18. Madduri N, Peters SU, Voigt RG, Llorente AM, Lupski JR, Potocki L. Cognitive and adaptive behavior profiles in Smith-Magenis syndrome. J Dev Behav Pediatr. 2006;27(3):188–92.
19. Smit AF. The origin of interspersed repeats in the human genome. Curr Opin Genet Dev. 1996;6(6):743–8.
20. Startek M, Szafranski P, Gambin T, Campbell IM, Hixson P, Shaw CA, et al. Genome-wide analyses of LINE-LINE-mediated nonallelic homologous recombination. Nucleic Acids Res. 2015;43(4):2188–98.
21. Batzer MA, Deininger PL. Alu repeats and human genomic diversity. Nat Rev Genet. 2002;3(5):370–9.
22. Teixeira-Silva A, Silva RM, Carneiro J, Amorim A, Azevedo L. The role of recombination in the origin and evolution of Alu subfamilies. PloS one. 2013;8(6):e64884.
23. Borun P, De Rosa M, Nedoszytko B, Walkowiak J, Plawski A. Specific Alu elements involved in a significant percentage of copy number variations of the STK11 gene in patients with Peutz-Jeghers syndrome. Fam Cancer. 2015;14(3):455–61.
24. Gu S, Yuan B, Campbell IM, Beck CR, Carvalho CM, Nagamani SC, et al. Alu-mediated diverse and complex pathogenic copy-number variants within human chromosome 17 at p13.3. Hum Mol Genet. 2015;24(14):4061–77.
25. Boone PM, Yuan B, Campbell IM, Scull JC, Withers MA, Baggett BC, et al. The Alu-rich genomic architecture of SPAST predisposes to diverse and functionally distinct disease-associated CNV alleles. Am J Hum Genet. 2014;95(2):143–61.
26. Giorgio E, Rolyan H, Kropp L, Chakka AB, Yatsenko S, Di Gregorio E, et al. Analysis of LMNB1 duplications in autosomal dominant leukodystrophy provides insights into duplication mechanisms and allele-specific expression. Hum Mutat. 2013;34(8):1160–71.
27. Quental R, Azevedo L, Rubio V, Diogo L, Amorim A. Molecular mechanisms underlying large genomic deletions in ornithine transcarbamylase (OTC) gene. Clin Genet. 2009;75(5):457–64.
28. Azevedo L, Stolnaja L, Tietzeova E, Hrebicek M, Hruba E, Vilarinho L, et al. New polymorphic sites within ornithine transcarbamylase gene: population genetics studies and implications for diagnosis. Mol Genet Metab. 2003; 78(2):152–7.
29. Ewald IP, Ribeiro PL, Palmero EI, Cossio SL, Giugliani R, Ashton-Prolla P. Genomic rearrangements in BRCA1 and BRCA2: a literature review. Genet Mol Biol. 2009;32(3):437–46.
30. Toft M, Ross OA. Copy number variation in Parkinson's disease. Genome Med. 2010;2(9):62.
31. Hedrich K, Eskelson C, Wilmot B, Marder K, Harris J, Garrels J, et al. Distribution, type, and origin of Parkin mutations: review and case studies. Mov Disord. 2004;19(10):1146–57.
32. Ross OA, Braithwaite AT, Skipper LM, Kachergus J, Hulihan MM, Middleton FA, et al. Genomic investigation of alpha-synuclein multiplication and parkinsonism. Ann Neurol. 2008;63(6):743–50.
33. Campbell IM, Gambin T, Dittwald P, Beck CR, Shuvarikov A, Hixson P, et al. Human endogenous retroviral elements promote genome instability via non-allelic homologous recombination. BMC Biol. 2014;12:74.
34. Bosch E, Jobling MA. Duplications of the AZFa region of the human Y chromosome are mediated by homologous recombination between HERVs and are compatible with male fertility. Hum Mol Genet. 2003;12(3):341–7.
35. Bergmann C, Zerres K, Senderek J, Rudnik-Schoneborn S, Eggermann T, Hausler M, et al. Oligophrenin 1 (OPHN1) gene mutation causes syndromic X-linked mental retardation with epilepsy, rostral ventricular enlargement and cerebellar hypoplasia. Brain. 2003;126(Pt 7):1537–44.
36. Antonell A, de Luis O, Domingo-Roura X, Perez-Jurado LA. Evolutionary mechanisms shaping the genomic structure of the Williams-Beuren syndrome chromosomal region at human 7q11.23. Genome Res. 2005;15(9):1179–88.
37. Pentao L, Wise CA, Chinault AC, Patel PI, Lupski JR. Charcot-Marie-Tooth type 1A duplication appears to arise from recombination at repeat sequences flanking the 1.5 Mb monomer unit. Nat Genet. 1992;2(4):292–300.
38. Weterman MA, van Ruissen F, de Wissel M, Bordewijk L, Samijn JP, van der Pol WL, et al. Copy number variation upstream of PMP22 in Charcot-Marie-Tooth disease. Eur J Hum Genet. 2010;18(4):421–8.
39. Zhang F, Seeman P, Liu P, Weterman MA, Gonzaga-Jauregui C, Towne CF, et al. Mechanisms for nonrecurrent genomic rearrangements associated with CMT1A or HNPP: rare CNVs as a cause for missing heritability. Am J Hum Genet. 2010;86(6):892–903.
40. Uddin RK, Zhang Y, Siu VM, Fan YS, O'Reilly RL, Rao J, et al. Breakpoint Associated with a novel 2.3 Mb deletion in the VCFS region of 22q11 and the role of Alu (SINE) in recurring microdeletions. BMC Med Genet. 2006;7:18.
41. Shishido E, Aleksic B, Ozaki N. Copy-number variation in the pathogenesis of autism spectrum disorder. Psychiatry Clin Neurosci. 2014;68(2):85–95.
42. Ferreira F, Esteves S, Almeida LS, Gaspar A, da Costa CD, Janeiro P, et al. Trimethylaminuria (fish odor syndrome): genotype characterization among Portuguese patients. Gene. 2013;527(1):366–70.
43. Quelhas D, Quental R, Vilarinho L, Amorim A, Azevedo L. Congenital disorder of glycosylation type Ia: searching for the origin of common mutations in PMM2. Ann Hum Genet. 2007;71(Pt 3):348–53.
44. Van Esch H. MECP2 duplication syndrome. Mol Syndromol. 2012;2(3-5):128–36.
45. Bauters M, Van Esch H, Friez MJ, Boespflug-Tanguy O, Zenker M, Vianna-Morgante AM, et al. Nonrecurrent MECP2 duplications mediated by genomic architecture-driven DNA breaks and break-induced replication repair. Genome Res. 2008;18(6):847–58.
46. Carvalho CM, Zhang F, Liu P, Patel A, Sahoo T, Bacino CA, et al. Complex rearrangements in patients with duplications of MECP2 can occur by fork stalling and template switching. Hum Mol Genet. 2009;18(12):2188–203.
47. Saunier S, Calado J, Benessy F, Silbermann F, Heilig R, Weissenbach J, et al. Characterization of the NPHP1 locus: mutational mechanism involved in deletions in familial juvenile nephronophthisis. Am J Hum Genet. 2000; 66(3):778–89.
48. Yuan B, Liu P, Gupta A, Beck CR, Tejomurtula A, Campbell IM, et al. Comparative genomic analyses of the human NPHP1 locus reveal complex genomic architecture and its regional evolution in primates. PLoS Genet. 2015;11(12):e1005686.
49. Konrad M, Saunier S, Heidet L, Silbermann F, Benessy F, Calado J, et al. Large homozygous deletions of the 2q13 region are a major cause of juvenile nephronophthisis. Hum Mol Genet. 1996;5(3):367–71.
50. Amos-Landgraf JM, Ji Y, Gottlieb W, Depinet T, Wandstrat AE, Cassidy SB, et al. Chromosome breakage in the Prader-Willi and Angelman syndromes involves recombination between large, transcribed repeats at proximal and distal breakpoints. Am J Hum Genet. 1999;65(2):370–86.
51. Bayes M, Magano LF, Rivera N, Flores R, Perez Jurado LA. Mutational mechanisms of Williams-Beuren syndrome deletions. Am J Hum Genet. 2003;73(1):131–51.
52. Willatt L, Cox J, Barber J, Cabanas ED, Collins A, Donnai D, et al. 3q29 microdeletion syndrome: clinical and molecular characterization of a new syndrome. Am J Hum Genet. 2005;77(1):154–60.
53. Ballif BC, Theisen A, Coppinger J, Gowans GC, Hersh JH, Madan-Khetarpal S, et al. Expanding the clinical phenotype of the 3q29 microdeletion syndrome and characterization of the reciprocal microduplication. Mol Cytogenet. 2008;1:8.
54. Soler-Alfonso C, Carvalho CM, Ge J, Roney EK, Bader PI, Kolodziejska KE, et al. CHRNA7 triplication associated with cognitive impairment and neuropsychiatric phenotypes in a three-generation pedigree. Eur J Hum Genet. 2014;22(9):1071–6.
55. Sharp AJ, Mefford HC, Li K, Baker C, Skinner C, Stevenson RE, et al. A recurrent 15q13.3 microdeletion syndrome associated with mental retardation and seizures. Nat Genet. 2008;40(3):322–8.
56. Shchelochkov OA, Li FY, Geraghty MT, Gallagher RC, Van Hove JL, Lichter-Konecki U, et al. High-frequency detection of deletions and variable rearrangements at the ornithine transcarbamylase (OTC) locus by oligonucleotide array CGH. Mol Genet Metab. 2009;96(3):97–105.
57. Mazoyer S. Genomic rearrangements in the BRCA1 and BRCA2 genes. Hum Mutat. 2005;25(5):415–22.
58. Sun C, Skaletsky H, Rozen S, Gromoll J, Nieschlag E, Oates R, et al. Deletion of azoospermia factor a (AZFa) region of human Y chromosome caused by recombination between HERV15 proviruses. Hum Mol Genet. 2000;9(15):2291–6.
59. Inoue K, Osaka H, Thurston VC, Clarke JT, Yoneyama A, Rosenbarker L, et al. Genomic rearrangements resulting in PLP1 deletion occur by nonhomologous end joining and cause different dysmyelinating phenotypes in males and females. Am J Hum Genet. 2002;71(4):838–53.

10

Novel genetic risk variants for pediatric celiac disease

Angeliki Balasopoulou[1†], Biljana Stanković[2†], Angeliki Panagiotara[1], Gordana Nikčevic[2], Brock A. Peters[3,4], Anne John[5], Effrosyni Mendrinou[1], Apostolos Stratopoulos[1], Aigli Ioanna Legaki[1], Vasiliki Stathakopoulou[1], Aristoniki Tsolia[1], Nikolaos Govaris[1], Sofia Govari[1], Zoi Zagoriti[1], Konstantinos Poulas[1], Maria Kanariou[6], Nikki Constantinidou[6], Maro Krini[7], Kleopatra Spanou[6], Nedeljko Radlovic[8], Bassam R. Ali[5], Joseph Borg[9], Radoje Drmanac[3,4], George Chrousos[7], Sonja Pavlovic[2], Eleftheria Roma[7], Branka Zukic[2], George P. Patrinos[1,5] and Theodora Katsila[1*]

Abstract

Background: Celiac disease is a complex chronic immune-mediated disorder of the small intestine. Today, the pathobiology of the disease is unclear, perplexing differential diagnosis, patient stratification, and decision-making in the clinic.

Methods: Herein, we adopted a next-generation sequencing approach in a celiac disease trio of Greek descent to identify all genomic variants with the potential of celiac disease predisposition.

Results: Analysis revealed six genomic variants of prime interest: *SLC9A4* c.1919G>A, *KIAA1109* c.2933T>C and c.4268_4269delCCinsTA, *HoxB6* c.668C>A, *HoxD12* c.418G>A, and *NCK2* c.745_746delAAinsG, from which *NCK2* c.745_746delAAinsG is novel. Data validation in pediatric celiac disease patients of Greek ($n = 109$) and Serbian ($n = 73$) descent and their healthy counterparts ($n = 111$ and $n = 32$, respectively) indicated that *HoxD12* c.418G>A is more prevalent in celiac disease patients in the Serbian population ($P < 0.01$), while *NCK2* c.745_746delAAinsG is less prevalent in celiac disease patients rather than healthy individuals of Greek descent ($P = 0.03$). *SLC9A4* c.1919G>A and *KIAA1109* c.2933T>C and c.4268_4269delCCinsTA were more abundant in patients; nevertheless, they failed to show statistical significance.

Conclusions: The next-generation sequencing-based family genomics approach described herein may serve as a paradigm towards the identification of novel functional variants with the aim of understanding complex disease pathobiology.

Keywords: Celiac disease, Genomic variants, Family genomics, Next-generation sequencing, Disease predisposition

Background

Celiac disease is a complex chronic immune-mediated disorder of the small intestine. Today, the pathobiology of the disease is unclear, perplexing differential diagnosis, patient stratification, and decision-making in the clinic. Genetics has been reported to play a key role. The *HLA-DQ2* gene is identified in up to 95 % of celiac disease patients, while most of the remaining patients have the *HLA-DQ8* gene. Notwithstanding, the Chinese and Japanese populations (devoid of *HLA-DQ2*) are not expected to develop the disease, yet this is not true for the individuals with the *HLA-DQ8* gene. Celiac disease is also associated with an extended ancestral haplotype that is defined by class I and II *HLA*s (*A*, *B*, *DR*, *DQ*). Notably, *HLA-DQ2* and/or *HLA-DQ8* expression is necessary but not sufficient for disease development. Thus, other genes are anticipated to be involved. Indeed, genome-wide association studies (GWAS) have revealed 26 non-*HLA* genetic loci-associated celiac disease and other autoimmune or chronic immune

* Correspondence: thkatsila@upatras.gr
†Equal contributors
1Department of Pharmacy, School of Health Sciences, University of Patras, University Campus, Rion, 265 04 Patras, Greece
Full list of author information is available at the end of the article

disorders (diabetes mellitus type I, rheumatoid arthritis) [1, 2]. In 2008 to 2011, several new celiac disease risk loci have been identified [3–5], bringing the number of known loci (including the *HLA* one) to 40 and indicating genes and gene regulatory elements of paramount importance. In 2015, five new genetic loci were identified, being independent of *HLA-DQA1* and *HLA-DQB1* and associated with celiac disease predisposition [6].

Although a genetic component has been described, disease occurrence has been also associated with environmental factors and gut microbiome. In all cases, gluten has been identified as the environmental trigger of the disease, leading to the stimulation of gluten-specific T cells. Differential diagnosis is still a major issue. Although a gold standard diagnostic approach has been defined (endoscopy with biopsy of the small intestine coupled to positive disease serology), several pathological conditions have been reported sharing similar mucosal transformations with celiac disease as well as other autoimmune disorders (thyroid disease, Addison disease, autoimmune liver disease, Sjögren syndrome) that occur ten times more frequently in celiac disease patients often masking celiac disease symptoms. Disease management options are restricted to a gluten-free lifestyle, which ultimately fails to protect patients from disease symptoms due to its chronic nature. Can we delineate individual variability towards differential diagnosis? Can we highlight the disease mechanisms in question to assist disease management?

So far, findings account for 49 % of the genetic basis of the disease. As in other immune-mediated diseases, genetic predisposition to celiac disease remains unresolved as we still need to explain the remaining major fraction of heritability, including rare as well as additional common risk variants. Causal variants and genes still need to be identified and/or more finely localized. In this context, the Immunochip Consortium was developed to explore comprehensive datasets containing common, low-frequency, and rare variants in related diseases (autoimmune thyroid disease, ankylosing spondylitis, Crohn disease, celiac disease, IgA deficiency, multiple sclerosis, primary biliary cirrhosis, psoriasis, rheumatoid arthritis, systemic lupus erythematosus, type 1 diabetes mellitus, and ulcerative colitis) [7].

As expected, the advent of technology and, in particular, next-generation sequencing has provided unprecedented opportunities to delineate disease pathobiology as well as inter-individual differences [8, 9]. Herein, we propose a multi-step next-generation sequencing-based family genomics approach, piloted in a celiac disease trio of Greek descent to identify novel genomic variants of functional significance with the aim of understanding disease pathobiology.

Methods

Case selection, DNA isolation, and whole-genome sequencing

A seven-member Greek family has been recruited (informed consents have been obtained), and a trio analysis (III-1, III-2, IV-3) has been performed using the celiac disease model (Additional file 1: Figure S1). A family-based design was employed rather than a population-based design, as the former is generally considered to be robust against population admixture and stratification and may yield both within- and between-family information [10]. Genomic DNA isolation was performed from saliva using the Oragene collection kit (DNA Genotek, Ontario, Canada) (Serbian cohort) and peripheral blood using an automated system (MagNA Pure Compact, Roche, Basel, Switzerland) (Greek cohort). Whole-genome sequencing was performed using Complete Genomics' (CA, USA) DNA nanoarray platform [11]. DNA sequencing coverage was 110×. Only high-quality call variants were included in the analysis (>93 %). Genomes were aligned with the hg19 reference genome.

Bioinformatics and in silico analyses

Next-generation sequencing data (Complete Genomics Inc., CA) were analyzed using Ingenuity Variant Analysis version 3.1.2 (Ingenuity® Systems, www.ingenuity.com). This is a well-established software that identifies associations between phenotypes, defined by the user by classification of the tested individuals, and variants in the sequenced genome. Upon classification of the family members by phenotype (celiac vs. normal), a number of variants were listed; the output was filtered into a smaller variant list upon classification of the family members by those being celiac patients vs. those who were healthy and known not to be celiac disease subjects. The genetic model used for this comparison was of an autosomal dominant model, since it traces the genetic inheritance from mother (III-2) to daughter (IV-3) in a highly penetrant form. A total of 263 genes followed an autosomal dominant pattern, and 227 variants were identified in the genetic model. Out of these, 6 genes and 7 variants were identified in the biological/phenotype pattern of celiac disease, due to either the past association of the genes considered or via the biological significance as determined by the IVA software.

Due to the large amount of variants which are normally present in the genome, even when excluding intronic sequences, several filtering steps are used in data analysis to include only the genes which are likely to be causative in the final output connected with just the disease of interest, in this case—celiac disease. All variants were filtered according to the analysis required, using custom scripts and Complete Genomics Analysis Tools

(CGA™ Tools). The filtering cascade utilized in the present data analysis is as follows:

1. Confidence: Only variants with call quality at least 20.0 in cases or at least 20.0 in controls (i.e., 99 % call accuracy) were included.
2. Common variants: All variants observed to have an allele frequency ≥3.0 % of the genomes in the 1000 genomes project OR ≥3.0 % of the public Complete Genomics genomes OR ≥3.0 % of the NHLBI ESP exomes were excluded.
3. Predicted deleterious: Only variants that are experimentally observed to be associated with a phenotype (Pathogenic, Possibly Pathogenic, Unknown Significance OR established gain of function in the literature OR gene fusions OR inferred activating mutations by Ingenuity OR predicted gain of function by BSIFT OR in a microRNA binding site OR Frameshift, in-frame indel, or stop codon change OR Missense and not predicted to be innocuous by SIFT OR disrupt splice site up to 2.0 bases into intron OR deleterious to a microRNA OR structural variant) were kept.
4. Genetic analysis: Only variants with the following genotype characteristics were kept: associated with gain of function OR heterozygous_alt OR haploinsufficient OR heterozygous OR homozygous OR heterozygous_amb OR compound_heterozygous OR hemizygous AND occur in at least 2 of the case samples at the gene level in the Case samples AND not which are associated with gain of function OR heterozygous_alt OR haploinsufficient OR heterozygous OR homozygous OR heterozygous_amb OR compound_heterozygous OR hemizygous AND occur in at least 1 of the control samples at the variant level in the control samples.
5. Biological context: Only variants that are within 1 hop (direct targets) of upstream regulators or downstream regulatory targets of such genes and that are known or predicted to affect celiac disease.

Variants of interest were annotated with Annovar in Galaxy [12] and compared with NCBI dbSNP build 137 (http://www.ncbi.nlm.nih.gov/projects/SNP/snp_summary.cgi), 69 reference genomes from Complete Genomes (http://www.completegenomics.com/publicdata/69Genomes/), and GWAS (http://www.genome.gov/gwastudies) to determine their novelty or otherwise. To obtain a list of variants of potential functional significance, we employed protein variation effect analyzer (PROVEAN) v1.1.3 (PROVEAN human genome variants tool) that provides both scale-invariant feature transform (SIFT) [13] and PROVEAN [14] predictions for a given list of human genome variants as well as accessory information (dbSNP rs IDs, gene description, PFAM domain, GO terms, etc.). PROVEAN is able to make predictions for any type of protein sequence alteration, including single or multiple amino acid substitutions, deletions, and insertions [15]. Additionally, Variant Effect Predictor [16] and RegulomeDB [8] were employed to allow further data interrogation.

Downstream molecular analysis

Selected variants were subsequently validated in pediatric celiac disease patients of Greek ($n = 109$) [17] and Serbian ($n = 73$) [18] descent and their healthy counterparts ($n = 111$ and $n = 32$, respectively). The diagnosis of celiac disease was based on the criteria of the European Society for Paediatric Gastroenterology, Hepatology and Nutrition (ESPGHAN) [19]. For children diagnosed prior to 1990, the "Interlaken criteria" were applied. The Ethics Committee of University Children's Hospital, University of Belgrade, and the Review Board of "Aghia Sophia" Children's Hospital have approved the study.

Amplification was carried out according to the KAPA2G Fast HotStart protocol (KAPABIOSYSTEMS, MA, USA); detailed information per SNP amplification conditions is available upon request. For *SLC9A4* c.1919G>A, an allele-specific polymerase chain reaction (PCR) assay was developed (two alternative reverse primers hybridizing exclusively either to the wild-type or the mutant allele). For *NCK2* c.745_746delAAinsG, PCR products were subjected to *XcmI* (New England Biolabs, MA, USA) restriction endonuclease analysis at 37 °C for 1.15 h and subsequent enzyme deactivation (65 °C, 20 min). Restriction fragments were visualized by 3 % agarose gel electrophoresis following ethidium bromide or Midori Green staining. For *HoxD12* c.418G>A, *HoxB6* c.668C>A, and *KIAA1109* c.2933T>C and c.4268_4269delCCinsTA, a PCR-based conventional Sanger resequencing approach was employed. Capillary electrophoresis was performed on the ABI Prism 3130xl DNA Analyzer (Applied Biosystems). Sanger sequencing was also employed to ensure PCR-RFLP and allele-specific PCR method verification.

Statistical analysis

Herein, a thorough statistical review and analysis has been attempted, having always in mind that we used the celiac disease model (trio analysis) as a reason to conduct a more refined approach in searching/genotyping the resulted variants in a selective population of celiac disease of Greek and Serbian descent. We tested for deviations from HWE using the chi-square goodness of fit test and principal component analysis. Considering that the χ^2 approximation can be poor when there are low genotype counts, a Fisher exact test (R genetics package) was also used, as it does not rely on the χ^2 approximation [20]. Tests were

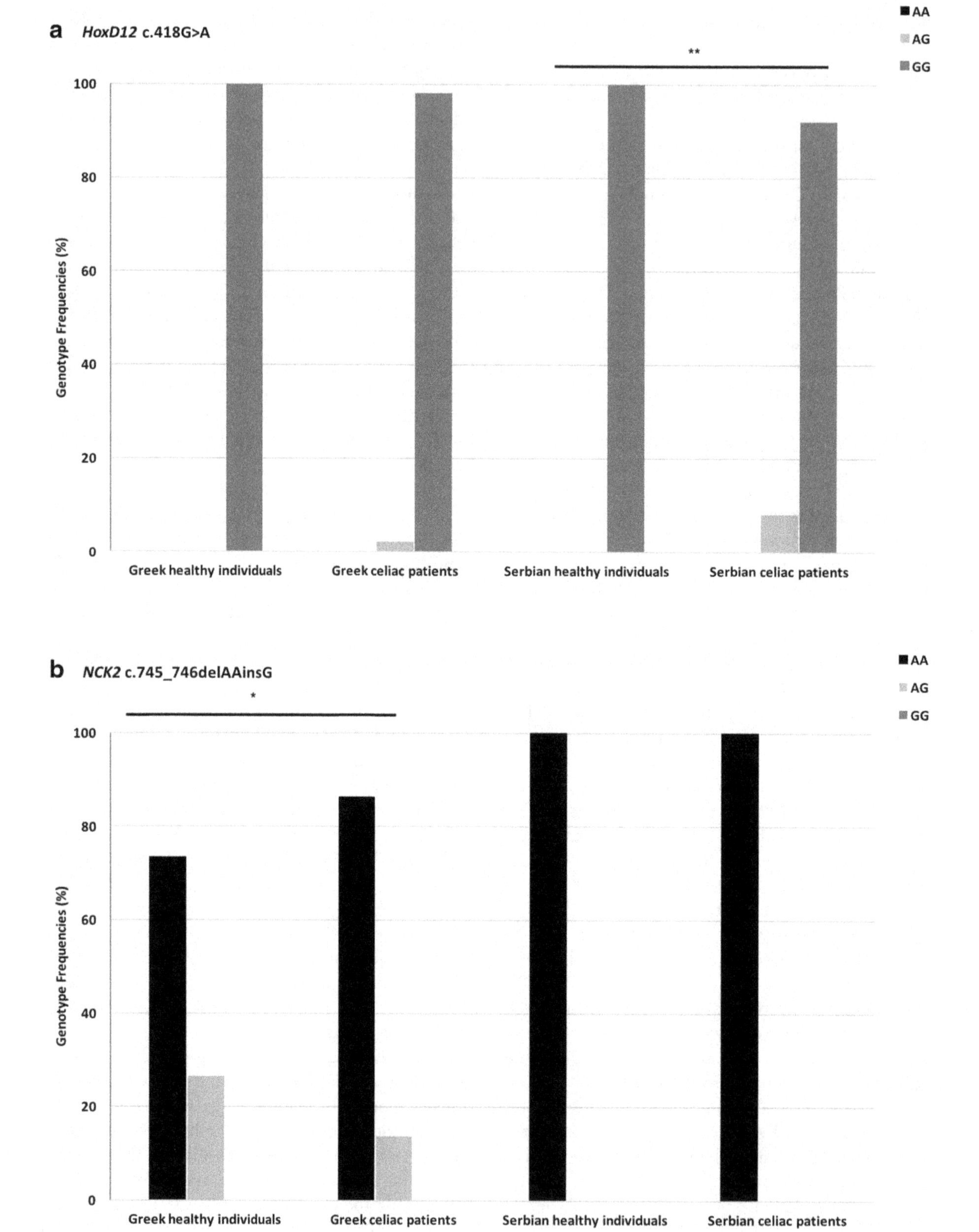

Fig. 1 Distribution of newly identified risk variants in Greek and Serbian populations. **a** *HoxD12* c.418G>A is more abundant in pediatric celiac disease patients of Greek and Serbian descent, reaching statistical significance ($^{**}P < 0.01$) in the Serbian population. **b** *NCK2* c.745_746delAAinsG is more abundant in healthy individuals of Greek and Serbian descent, reaching statistical significance ($^{*}P = 0.03$) in the Greek population

performed as two-tailed, and differences were considered statistically significant when $P < 0.05$. Focusing on case-control phenotypes, we tested the null hypothesis of no association between rows and columns of the 2×3 matrix that contains the counts of the three genotypes (the two homozygotes and the heterozygote) among cases and controls. Again, a Fisher exact test was preferred (to evaluate genotype and allele frequencies), as it is computationally more demanding, but it is easily implemented in R. We also performed the Armitage test (Monte Carlo method; it obtains results that are closer to an exact test, since the classical Cochran-Armitage trend test is based on approximation) [20].

Results and discussion

Whole-genome sequencing analysis of trio reveals newly identified genetic risk variants for pediatric celiac disease

Our multi-step next-generation sequencing-based family genomics approach revealed six genomic variants of prime interest: *SLC9A4* c.1919G>A, *HoxD12* c.418G>A, *KIAA1109* c.2933T>C and c.4268_4269delCCinsTA, *HoxB6* c.668C>A, and *NCK2* c.745_746delAAinsG. Susceptibility to celiac disease (CELIAC6) and to autoimmunity (AIS5) has been previously mapped to the 4q27 region, within a linkage disequilibrium block encompassing *KIAA1109*, *TENR*, *IL2*, and *IL21* genes [21]. So far, the most significant linkage outside the *HLA* region refers to rs13119723 ($P = 2.0 \times 10^{-7}$ in the *KIAA1109* gene on chromosome 4q27). Zhernakova and coworkers [2] hypothesized that the *KIAA1109/TENR/IL2/IL21* susceptibility region reported by van Heel and coworkers [21] might represent a general risk locus for multiple autoimmune diseases. Even though several CELIAC6 genomic variants have been reported [1, 2, 4, 21], this is the first time such a disease association is revealed for *KIAA1109* c.2933T>C and c.4268_4269delCCinsTA. *SLC9A4* c.1919G>A, *HoxD12* c.418G>A, *HoxB6* c.668C>A, and *NCK2* c.745_746delAAinsG are also reported for the first time as celiac disease risk variants (Fig. 1).

NCK2 c.745_746delAAinsG has not been annotated in either dbSNP or the 1000 Genomes Project/exome variant server data, and hence, it may be considered to be novel. *NCK2* codes for Human Nck2 (hNck2), a 380-residue adapter protein consisting of three SH3 domains and one SH2 domain. Nck2 plays a pivotal role in connecting and integrating signaling networks constituted by transmembrane receptors, such as ephrinB and effectors critical for cytoskeletal dynamics and remodeling [22–25]. A transient Nck2/PINCH-1 association process has been also reported that may trigger rapid focal adhesion turnover during integrin signaling, mediating cell shape change and migration [26, 27]. We showed that the novel variant identified herein results in a single amino acid change (p.K249E), being this exact amino acid that is reported of fundamental importance during the abovementioned Nck2 SH3 domain protein-protein interactions (Fig. 2a) [22, 26, 27]. p.K249E could severely alter this network of polar interactions and affect the interaction between the two proteins (Fig. 2b). In 2014, Nadalutti et al. [28] observed that celiac patient IgA antibodies disturb the extracellular protein cross-linking function of transglutaminase 2, thus altering cell-extracellular matrix interactions and thereby affecting endothelial cell adhesion, polarization, and motility.

In silico analyses

To ascertain whether the variants of interest have functional significance, in silico analysis was performed using

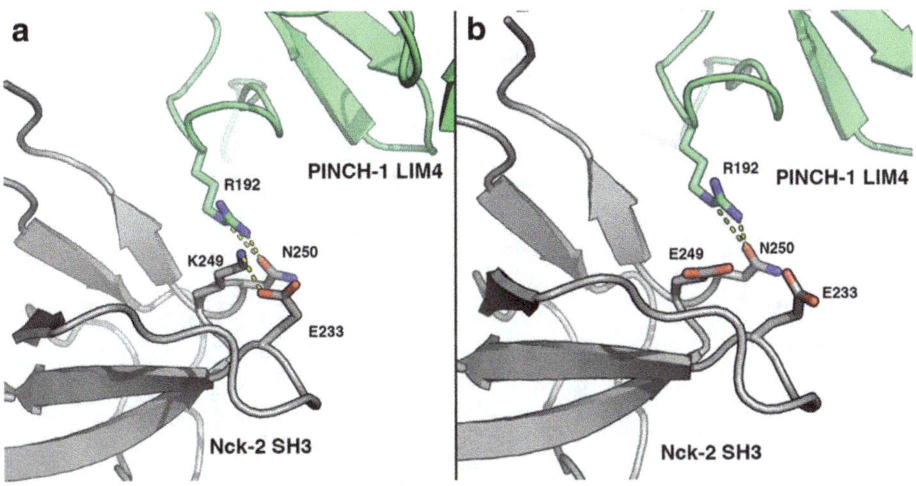

Fig. 2 **a** View of the SH3-3/LIM4 binding interface as previously shown by NMR spectroscopy [26]. The Nck2 DH3 domain interface is shown in *gray* and the PINCH-1 LIM4 domain in *green*. K249 interacts with E233 and is part of a network connecting R192 of LIM4 and N250 of SH3. **b** Structural model of the mutant p.K249E and the potential effect in the interactions between SH3 and LIM4

Table 1 In silico analyses outcome of the six variants of prime interest identified in the family trio

HUGO gene symbol	HGVS description of variant	AA position	Reference residue	Alternative residue	PROVEAN prediction			SIFT prediction		Variant effect predictor			
					Variation type	Score	Prediction	Score	Prediction	Consequence	Impact	PolyPhen	LoFtool
SLC9A4	c.1919G>A	640	R	K	Single AA change	−0.67	Neutral	0.140	Tolerated	Frameshift variant	High	–	0.911
NCK2	c.745_746delAAinsG	249	K	E	Single AA change	−1.97	Neutral	0.010	Damaging	Frameshift variant	High	–	0.223
HOXD12	c.418G>A	140	A	T	Single AA change	−0.01	Neutral	0.201	Tolerated	Frameshift variant	High	–	0.432
KIAA1109	c.2933T>C	978	I	T	Single AA change	−0.25	Neutral	0.187	Tolerated	Frameshift variant	High	–	0.845
	c.4268_4269delCCinsTA	1423	T	I	Single AA change	−1.22	Neutral	0.108	Tolerated	Missense variant	Moderate	Benign (0.031)	0.845
HOXB6	c.668C>A	223	A	D	Single AA change	−.029	Neutral	0.230	Tolerated	Frameshift variant	High	–	–

Source: PROVEAN v1.1.3 (PROVEAN human genome variants tool, http://provean.jcvi.org/genome_submit_2.php?species=human) and Variant Effect Predictor (http://grch37.ensembl.org/Homo_sapiens/Tools/VEP). Assembly: GRCh37. PROVEAN introduces a delta alignment score based on the reference and variant versions of a protein query sequence with respect to sequence homologs (NCBI NR protein database through BLAST, http://www.ncbi.nlm.nih.gov/). The default score threshold was set at −2.5 for binary classification (deleterious <−2.5 vs. neutral > −2.5). Similarly, (through PSI-BLAST, http://blast.ncbi.nlm.nih.gov/Blast.cgi?CMD=Web&PAGE=Proteins&PROGRAM=blastp&RUN_PSIBLAST=on), SIFT (http://sift.jcvi.org/) may be applied to naturally occurring non-synonymous variants. SIFT score ranges from 0 to 1. A SIFT score of ≤0.05 corresponds to a "damaging" prediction, whereas a SIFT score >0.05 predicts that the variant is likely to be "tolerated." VEP; Consequence—consequence type of this variation, Impact—a subjective classification of the severity of the variant consequence (high: the variant is assumed to have disruptive impact in the protein, probably causing protein truncation or loss of function or triggering nonsense mediated decay, moderate: a non-disruptive variant that might change protein effectiveness, low: assumed to be mostly harmless or unlikely to change protein behavior, modifier: usually non-coding variants affecting non-coding genes, where predictions are difficult or there is no evidence of impact), PolyPhen—the PolyPhen prediction and/or score, LoFtool—provides a per-gene rank of genic intolerance and consequent susceptibility to disease based on the ratio of loss of function (LoF) to synonymous mutations in ExAC data

Table 2 Genotyping data of celiac disease pediatric patients of Greek and Serbian descent and healthy individuals

Population groups	Genotype frequency (%)											
	HoxB6 c.668C>A			*SLC9A4* c.1919G>A			*KIAA1109* c.2933T>C			*KIAA1109* c.4268_4269delCCinsTA		
	TT	GG	GT	AA	GG	AG	TT	CC	CT	CC/CC	TA/TA	CC/TA
Healthy individuals of Greek descent	0	100	0	0	96	4	86	1	13	100	0	0
Patients of Greek descent	0	100	0	0	93	7	81	2	16	98	0	2
Healthy individuals of Serbian descent	0	100	0	0	97	3	80	0	20	100	0	0
Patients of Serbian descent	0	100	0	0	93	7	81	0	19	100	0	0

In both Greek and Serbian patients, *SLC9A4* c.1919G>A and *KIAA1109* c.2933T>C and c.4268_4269delCCinsTA were more abundant in patients; nevertheless, they failed to show statistical significance, possibly due to a small sample size

the SIFT and PROVEAN algorithms [13, 14], as well as Variant Effect Predictor [16] and Regulome DB [8]. As summarized in Table 1, analyses yielded that all variants share an effect to protein structure, which in the case of *NCK2* c.745_746delAAinsG is considered to be damaging. Regulome DB questioned a possible role of the variants of interest in terms of transcription factor binding sites, chromatin states, eQTLs, differentially methylated regions, validated functional SNPs and DNase sensitivity. All variants had minimum or no impact (Additional file 2: Table S1).

Replication analyses

Replication analyses were carried out in two cohorts to account for population differences. We found that *NCK2* c.745_746delAAinsG is a novel variant that is more abundant in healthy individuals, reaching statistical significance ($P = 0.03$) in the Greek population. Moreover, *HoxD12* c.418G>A, a frameshift variant, was more abundant in pediatric celiac disease patients, reaching statistical significance ($P < 0.01$) in the Serbian population. When celiac disease risk assessment is considered, it is important to note that apart from genotype data, records related to family history along with gender and country of residence should not be disregarded [29]. In both Greek and Serbian patients, *SLC9A4* c.1919G>A and *KIAA1109* c.2933T>C and c.4268_4269delCCinsTA were more abundant in patients; nevertheless, they failed to show statistical significance, possibly due to small sample sizes. All the studied variants satisfied the Hardy-Weinberg equilibrium. All variants were verified as non-frequent ones in agreement with PROVEAN's scoring scheme, separating disease-associated variants from common ones [14]. Genotype frequencies (%) are summarized in Fig. 1 and Table 2.

Conclusions

In relation to disease diagnosis and prognosis, data interpretation requires an understanding of the variation in risk-associated variants. In celiac disease, in particular, this knowledge is still largely lacking. As whole-genome and/or whole-exome sequencing approaches begin to be employed in clinical care, the understanding of detected sequence variations on diagnosis (and prognosis) is still not a trivial undertaking. We envisage that the clinical implementation of next-generation sequencing will play a crucial role in delineating inter-individual variability and identification of novel variants towards improved therapeutic modalities. Herein, we propose a multi-step next-generation sequencing-based family genomics approach, similar to our previous conducted cancer genomics study [30], but piloted towards a complex genetic disease, such as celiac disease, to analyze a family trio of Greek descent to identify novel genomic variants of functional significance with the aim of understanding complex disease pathobiology. Recently, we have outlined the paradigm of pharmacometabolomics-aided pharmacogenomics in autoimmune diseases to address the interplay of genomic and environmental influences with information technologies to facilitate data analysis as well as sense- and decision-making on the basis of synergy between artificial and human intelligence. We propose that better-informed, rapid, and cost-effective "omics" studies need the implementation of holistic and multidisciplinary approaches [31].

Acknowledgements
Not applicable

Funding
This study was funded by the European Commission (RD-CONNECT; FP7-304555) research grant to GPP.

Authors' contributions
TK and GPP conceived and designed the study. AB, AP, BS, GN, AJ, EM, AS, AIL, VS, AT, NG, SG, ZZ, MK, MK, KS, and TK carried out the PCR-based conventional Sanger resequencing approach. BAP and RD supervised the next-generation sequencing analyses. TK carried out the in silico analyses. BRA, NC, ER, JB, KP, GC, BZ, NR, RD, SP, TK, and GPP drafted the manuscript. All authors read and approved the final manuscript.

Competing interests
The authors declare the following competing interests: BAP and RD are employees of the Complete Genomics Inc. (Mountain View, CA, USA).

Consent for publication
Not applicable

Author details
[1]Department of Pharmacy, School of Health Sciences, University of Patras, University Campus, Rion, 265 04 Patras, Greece. [2]Institute of Molecular Genetics and Genetic Engineering, University of Belgrade, Belgrade, Serbia. [3]Complete Genomics Inc., Mountain View, CA, USA. [4]BGI Shenzhen, Shenzhen 51803, People's Republic of China. [5]Department of Pathology, College of Medicine and Health Sciences, United Arab Emirates University, Al Ain, United Arab Emirates. [6]Department of Immunology and Histocompatibility, "Aghia Sophia" Children's Hospital, Athens, Greece. [7]First Department of Pediatrics, National and Kapodistrian University of Athens Medical School, Athens, Greece. [8]Department of Gastroenterology and Nutrition, University Children's Hospital, Medical Faculty, University of Belgrade, Belgrade, Serbia. [9]Department of Applied Biomedical Science, Faculty of Health Sciences, University of Malta, Msida, Malta.

References

1. Burton PR, et al. Genome-wide association study of 14,000 cases of seven common diseases and 3,000 shared controls. Nature. 2007;447(7145):661–78.
2. Zhernakova A, et al. Meta-analysis of genome-wide association studies in celiac disease and rheumatoid arthritis identifies fourteen non-HLA shared loci. PLoS Genet. 2011;7(2):e1002004.
3. Hunt KA, et al. Novel celiac disease genetic determinants related to the immune response. Nat Genet. 2008;40(4):395–402.
4. Romanos J, et al. Six new coeliac disease loci replicated in an Italian population confirm association with coeliac disease. J Med Genet. 2009; 46(1):60–3.
5. Trynka G, et al. Dense genotyping identifies and localizes multiple common and rare variant association signals in celiac disease. Nat Genet. 2011;43(12): 1193–201.
6. Gutierrez-Achury J, et al. Fine-mapping in the MHC region accounts for 18 % additional genetic risk for celiac disease. Nat Genet. 2015;47(6):577–8.
7. Cortes A, Brown MA. Promise and pitfalls of the Immunochip. Arthritis Res Ther. 2011;13(1):1.
8. Boyle AP, et al. Annotation of functional variation in personal genomes using RegulomeDB. Genome Res. 2012;22(9):1790–7.
9. Mizzi C, et al. Personalized pharmacogenomics profiling using whole-genome sequencing. Pharmacogenomics. 2014;15(9):1223–34.
10. Laird NM, Lange C. Family-based designs in the age of large-scale gene-association studies. Nat Rev Genet. 2006;7(5):385–94.
11. Drmanac R, et al. Human genome sequencing using unchained base reads on self-assembling DNA nanoarrays. Science. 2010;327(5961):78–81.
12. Hiltemann S, et al. CGtag: complete genomics toolkit and annotation in a cloud-based Galaxy. GigaScience. 2014;3:1.
13. Kumar P, Henikoff S, Ng PC. Predicting the effects of coding non-synonymous variants on protein function using the SIFT algorithm. Nat Protoc. 2009;4(8):1073–81.
14. Choi Y, et al. Predicting the functional effect of amino acid substitutions and indels. PLoS One. 2012;7(10):e46688.
15. Boycott KM, et al. Rare-disease genetics in the era of next-generation sequencing: discovery to translation. Nat Rev Genet. 2013;14(10):681–91.
16. McLaren W, et al. Deriving the consequences of genomic variants with the Ensembl API and SNP Effect Predictor. Bioinformatics. 2010;26(16):2069–70.
17. Krini M, et al. HLA class II high-resolution genotyping in Greek children with celiac disease and impact on disease susceptibility. Pediatr Res. 2012;72(6):625–30.
18. Stanković B, et al. HLA genotyping in pediatric celiac disease patients. Bosn J Basic Med Sci. 2014;14(3):171.
19. Walker-Smith J, et al. Revised criteria for diagnosis of coeliac disease. Report of working group of ESPGAN. Arch Dis Child. 1990;65:909–11.
20. Balding DJ. A tutorial on statistical methods for population association studies. Nat Rev Genet. 2006;7(10):781–91.
21. van Heel DA, et al. A genome-wide association study for celiac disease identifies risk variants in the region harboring IL2 and IL21. Nat Genet. 2007;39(7):827–9.
22. Liu J, et al. Structural insight into the binding diversity between the human Nck2 SH3 domains and proline-rich proteins. Biochemistry. 2006;45(23):7171–84.
23. Mayer BJ. SH3 domains: complexity in moderation. J Cell Sci. 2001;114(7):1253–63.
24. Koytiger G, et al. Phosphotyrosine signaling proteins that drive oncogenesis tend to be highly interconnected. Mol Cell Proteomics. 2013;12(5):1204–13.
25. Ran X, Song J. Structural insight into the binding diversity between the Tyr-phosphorylated human ephrinBs and Nck2 SH2 domain. J Biol Chem. 2005; 280(19):19205–12.
26. Vaynberg J, et al. Structure of an ultraweak protein-protein complex and its crucial role in regulation of cell morphology and motility. Mol Cell. 2005; 17(4):513–23.
27. Velyvis A, et al. Structural and functional insights into PINCH LIM4 domain-mediated integrin signaling. Nat Struct Mol Biol. 2003;10(7):558–64.
28. Nadalutti CA, et al. Celiac disease patient IgA antibodies induce endothelial adhesion and cell polarization defects via extracellular transglutaminase 2. Cell Mol Life Sci. 2014;71(7):1315–26.
29. Liu E, et al. Risk of pediatric celiac disease according to HLA haplotype and country. N Engl J Med. 2014;371(1):42–9.
30. Karageorgos I, et al. Identification of cancer predisposition variants in apparently healthy individuals using a next-generation sequencing-based family genomics approach. Hum Genomics. 2015;9(1):1.
31. Katsila T, et al. Pharmacometabolomics-aided pharmacogenomics in autoimmune disease. EBioMedicine. 2016;5:40–5.

11

Development and validation of a variant detection workflow for *BRCA1* and *BRCA2* genes and its clinical application based on the Ion Torrent technology

Ana Lígia Buzolin, Caroline Mônaco Moreira, Patricia Rossi Sacramento, Andre Yuji Oku, Alexandre Ricardo dos Santos Fornari, David Santos Marco Antonio, Caio Robledo D Angioli Costa Quaio, Wagner Rosa Baratela and Miguel Mitne-Neto*

Abstract

Background: Breast cancer is the most common among women worldwide, and ovarian cancer is the most difficult gynecological tumor to diagnose and with the lowest chance of cure. Mutations in *BRCA1* and *BRCA2* genes increase the risk of ovarian cancer by 60% and breast cancer by up to 80% in women. Molecular tests allow a better orientation for patients carrying these mutations, affecting prophylaxis, treatment, and genetic counseling.

Results: Here, we evaluated the performance of a panel for *BRCA1* and *BRCA2*, using the Ion Torrent PGM (Life Technologies) platform in a customized workflow and multiplex ligation-dependent probe amplification for detection of mutations, insertions, and deletions in these genes. We validated the panel with 26 samples previously analyzed by Myriad Genetics Laboratory, and our workflow showed 95.6% sensitivity and 100% agreement with Myriad reports, with 85% sensitivity on the positive control sample from NIST. We also screened 68 clinical samples and found 22 distinct mutations.

Conclusions: The selection of a robust methodology for sample preparation and sequencing, together with bioinformatics tools optimized for the data analysis, enabled the development of a very sensitive test with high reproducibility. We also highlight the need to explore the limitations of the NGS technique and the strategies to overcome them in a clinically confident manner.

Keywords: Cancer, Breast, Ovarian, Ion Torrent, BRCA

Background

Breast cancer is the most common among women worldwide, accounting for about 25% of new cases each year. Overall, there were 1.67 million new cases of breast cancer in 2012 and 522,000 deaths, with most of them being women [1]. Ovarian cancer, although infrequent, is the most difficult gynecological tumor to diagnose with the lowest chance of cure, accounting for 239,000 cases and 152,000 deaths in 2012 [1, 2].

A family history of breast and ovarian cancer is an important risk factor for the onset of the disease. *BRCA1* and *BRCA2* are genes that produce tumor-suppressing proteins. These proteins help the repair of damaged DNA and therefore play an essential role in ensuring the stability of the genetic material of cells. Together, *BRCA1* and *BRCA2* account for about 20 to 25% of cases of hereditary breast cancer and 15% of cases of ovarian cancer [3]. Specific germline mutations in these genes increase the risk of breast and ovarian cancer in women and are associated with an increased risk to develop other types of cancers. Women carrying mutations in *BRCA1* or *BRCA2* show up to 80% of increased risk for developing breast cancer, while men present up to 6%. For ovarian cancer, the risk is up to 50% [4–6].

* Correspondence: miguel.mitne@grupofleury.com.br
Research and Development, Fleury Group, Av. General Valdomiro de Lima, 508, São Paulo/SP 04344-070, Brazil

Molecular tests that are able to identify such mutations have a great impact on healthcare, since they allow a better orientation for patients, affecting prophylaxis, treatment, and genetic counseling. Women who tested positive for any of these genes can take steps to prevent the disease, as the realization of screenings before the recommended age for the general population, increasing the chance of detecting cancer at an initial stage. It is also possible to carry out a prophylactic mastectomy for risk reduction and even chemopreventive treatment, consisting in the use of natural or synthetic chemical agents to reverse, suppress, or prevent carcinogenic progression [7, 8].

From the technical perspective, the challenges of *BRCA1* and *BRCA2* mutation identification are the long genic extension and the clinical interpretation for each of the identified mutations. To overcome the technical challenges in terms of efficiency and turnaround time, the use of next-generation sequencing techniques have been adopted by diagnostic laboratories worldwide [9–11]. Here, we evaluated the performance of a panel for detecting *BRCA1* and *BRCA2* mutations, using the Ion Torrent PGM platform (Life Technologies) in a customized workflow. Accuracy tests were performed by using 26 samples that were previously analyzed by Myriad Genetic Laboratory and a reference sample from the National Institute for Standards and Technology (NIST). The pipeline that we created was able to identify all the pathogenic and variant of unknown significance (VUS) variants in both genes, reported by the reference laboratory and 85% of the variants present in the NIST sample, but all of them were benign. Using this workflow, we screened 68 clinical samples and found 22 distinct variants. Our data show that the present workflow is robust and is reliable for diagnostic procedures. Additionally, the generation of distinct databases for admixed populations, as the one studied here, and its comparison with other cohorts is an important step for the correct variant pathogenicity interpretation. Moreover, we explore the limitations of the technique and present strategies to overcome them in a clinically confident manner.

Methods

Validation

Sample selection and DNA extraction

Twenty-six blood samples were collected in two ethylenediaminetetraacetic acid (EDTA) vials. For each of them, one vial was sent to Myriad Genetic Laboratories as part of our diagnostic routine and the other was kept in Fleury Group. Samples were renumbered and anonymized so the donor could not be tracked.

DNA extraction from the whole EDTA blood was performed on QiaSymphony (Qiagen). DNA and amplicon quantification was based on Qubit 2.0 fluorometer (Life Technologies) using dsDNA BR Assay kit.

The reference sample NA12878, purchased from National Institute for Standards and Technology (NIST), was also used for the validation.

Strategies for capture and library preparation

In order to capture the entire coding region of both genes, we tested two capture strategies. In the first one, we designed 100 pairs of primers to amplify the target region (Additional file 1: Table S1), containing a total of 18,947 base pairs. These primers contained universal tag sequences, which allowed the amplification of the target region and insertion of barcodes and adaptors in a single PCR reaction. The primer design also allowed their use in Sanger sequencing.

A second capture strategy was based on the Ion AmpliSeq BRCA1 and BRCA2 panel (Ion Torrent) and was used to generate target amplicon libraries. This panel contains 167 primer pairs in 3 primer pools and is designed for 100% amplicon coverage of all targeted coding exons and exon–intron boundaries. Briefly, 20 ng of DNA was amplified by PCR in three distinct reactions of 10 μL using the Ion AmpliSeq primer pools and Ion AmpliSeq HiFi master mix (Ion AmpliSeq kit version 2.0). The resulting amplicons were pooled, and 20 μL was transferred to a new tube and treated with FuPa reagent to partially digest primer sequences and phosphorylate the amplicons. The amplicons were then ligated to adapters from the Ion Xpress barcoded adapters 1–16 kit. After ligation, the libraries were purified using Agencourt Ampure XP Beads and equalized to 100 pM with the Ion Library Equalizer kit according to the manufacturer's instructions (Life Technologies).

Emulsion PCR and sequencing

Multiplexed barcoded libraries were amplified by emulsion PCR on ion sphere particles (ISPs) using the Ion PGM Hi-Q OT2 Kit according to the manufacturer's instructions (Life Technologies). Positive-templated ISPs were biotinylated during the emulsion PCR process followed by enrichment with Dynabeads MyOne streptavidin C1 beads (Life Technologies). Ion 314 and 316 chips were used to sequence four and eight samples, respectively. Sequencing was performed on an Ion PGM System (Ion Torrent) using the Ion PGM Hi-Q Sequencing kit according to the manufacturer's instructions.

Bioinformatics

Torrent Suite software version 4.4 was used to demultiplex barcoded reads and to generate run metrics, including chip loading efficiency, coverage analysis, total read counts, and quality. A visual quality assessment of reads was performed with FastQC. The FASTQ files were used either in the Variant Caller plugin from the Torrent Suite 4.4 package or in the CLC Genomics Workbench 8.0 (CLCbio, Boston, MA). We designed a pipeline optimized for the Ion AmpliSeq BRCA1 and BRCA2 panel (Fig. 1), consisting of six main steps:

1. Trimming of 5 bp from the reads' 3′ end to avoid mapping of low-quality regions and exclusion of short reads (<15 bp) and reads end with a Phred score (Q value) <20.
2. Read mapping against UCSC hg19 (http://hgdownload.soe.ucsc.edu/goldenPath/hg19/bigZips, last accessed April 04, 2016) using default cost values for mismatches (2) and indels (3) and minimum reference similarity (80%). A mapping report and a .bam file were generated as outputs.
3. Read mapping was also performed against a reference containing all the amplicon sequences from the panels, so that the mean coverage could be assessed for each amplicon individually.
4. Variant calling was performed restricted to the target regions defined in the bed file. Bidirectional presence of variant alleles was required in a concordance of at least 5% between forward and reverse reads. The minimum coverage cut off was 10× with variant allele frequencies (VAFs) of 20%. Variant calls were filtered with a minimum average base quality of 16 (Phred Score), which removed all variants having alleles with an average base quality of less than the given threshold, even if they are in a region within a high overall quality and passed the first trimming step. This threshold increases sensitivity and lowers the number of variants called in homopolymer regions.
5. The variants were annotated with the COSMIC database and the Variant Effect Predictor (VEP) from Ensembl (http://grch37.ensembl.org/Homo_sapiens/Tools/VEP). The clinical significance of the variants was annotated with ClinVar database (http://www.ncbi.nlm.nih.gov/clinvar/) which contains publicly available information of the Sharing Clinical Reports Project, an initiative of diagnosis centers worldwide that submitted the variants of BRCA1/2 reported by Myriad Genetics since 2006. ClinVar also contains the variants from Breast Cancer Information Core (BIC, NIH), so it is

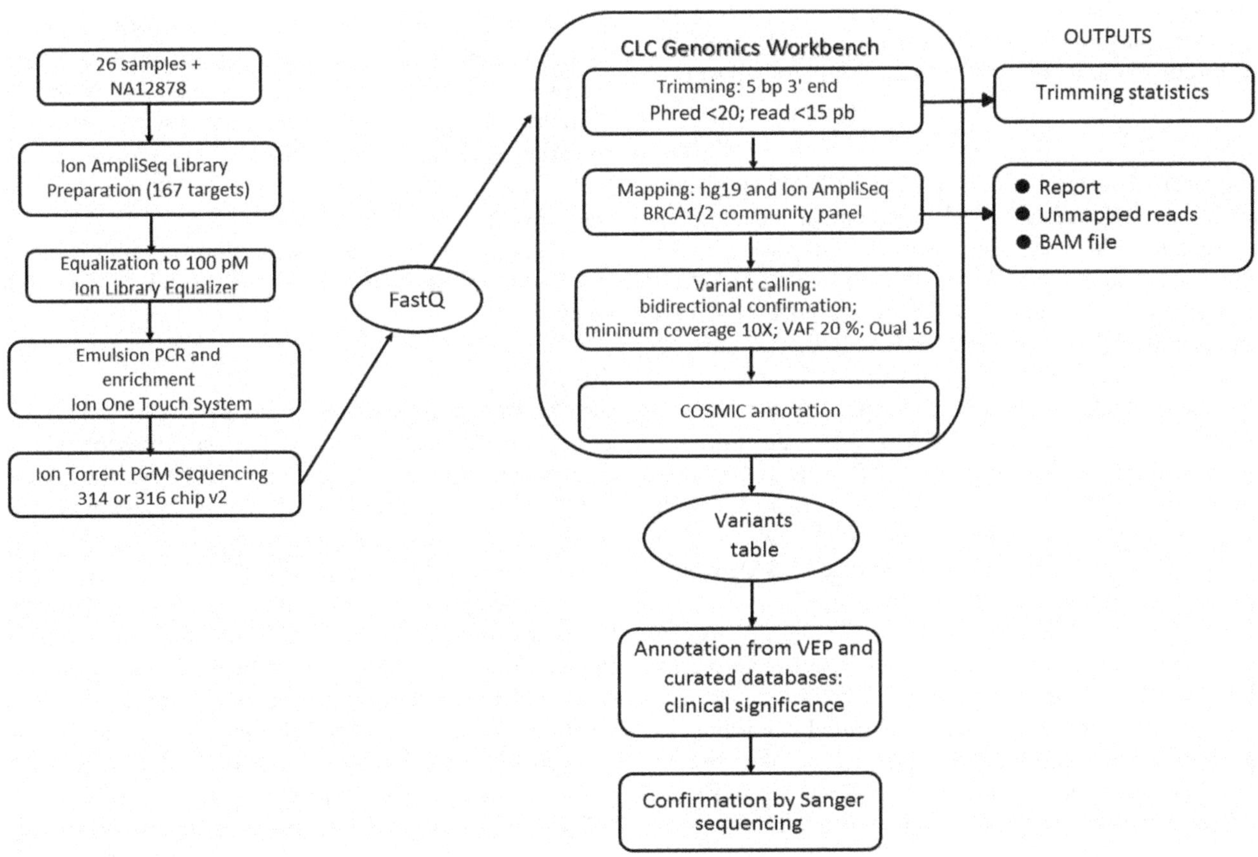

Fig 1 Workflow for processing and analysis of samples in the validation design. *PGM* personal genome machine, *VAF* variant allele frequency, *BAM* bam file, *VEP* variant effect predictor

the most complete public-curated database of BRCA1/2 variants. Fleury's database, consisting of past exams sent to Myriad, and Arup BRCA1/2 mutation database (http://arup.utah.edu/database/BRCA/) were also checked for variants not previously found.

A total of seven runs were performed in different days, accounting for 48 sequencings of the 26 samples. These assays comprehend inter- and intra-assay evaluations (Additional File 2: Table S2).

Confirmation by Sanger sequencing

All the identified variants were confirmed by bidirectional Sanger sequencing. The regions containing the variants were amplified using the above described primers for the first strategy. Amplification reactions were performed in a Veriti thermocycler (Applied Biosystems) using the enzyme AmpliTaq Gold DNA Polymerase (Applied Biosystems). PCR products were confirmed by 2% agarose gel and purified with the ExoSAP-IT enzyme (Affymetrix). The sequencing reactions were performed with BigDye Terminator v3.1 Cycle, and the capillary electrophoresis was carried out on ABI 3130xl equipment. Data analysis and comparison to reference was made in CLCbio Workbench software. The sensitivity of the sequencing by next-generation sequencing (NGS) was calculated by true positive ratio (confirmed by Sanger) and total positive.

MLPA

In order to follow the proper *BRCA1* and *BRCA2* evaluation workflow, we validated a multiplex ligation-dependent probe amplification (MLPA) assay, using 11 samples selected as described above. MLPA commercial kits from MRC-Holland for *BRCA1* and *BRCA2* were used here. Tests were performed in duplicate and at different days to evaluate the intra- and inter-assay reproducibility. We used 100 ng of DNA from each sample, three reference samples (which had no duplications and/or deletions), a negative control containing only ATE buffer (the same used in sample dilution), and a positive control for each gene. For the positive control of *BRCA1*, we used a sample purchased from Coriell Institute (USA), which presents the mutation 1294del40 in exon 11.

For the positive control of *BRCA2*, we amplified exon 9 and used the PCR product diluted proportionately in a sample without prior changes in order to simulate a duplication. The procedures were performed according to the manufacturer's instructions. The steps of denaturation, hybridization, binding, and PCR were performed in Veriti thermocycler (Applied Biosystems). The analysis of fragments was performed on ABI 3130xl sequencer and the data generated were imported and analyzed in Coffalyser.Net software.

Validation process and analytical assessment

Target regions containing variants detected in the Ion AmpliSeq panel were analyzed by Sanger sequencing. Thus, these variants were used for checking NGS accuracy on the patient's samples. Sensitivity was calculated as the relationship between true positive/total positives.

We also compared our results with Myriad reports to verify the agreement in the variant's classification between both exams. Myriad processes the test using HiSeq 2500 (Illumina) and classifies the variants through its proprietary pipeline (https://myriad.com/). Myriad's reports contain only VUS or pathogenic/likely pathogenic mutations, and other variants are not reported. For this reason, specificity could not be calculated.

To compare the NA12878 sample results obtained in our sequencing, we selected variants of the standard.vcf file for this sample (available at: ftp://ftp-trace.ncbi.nlm.nih.gov/giab/ftp/release/NA12878_HG001/NISTv3.2/) contained in the target intervals of Ion AmpliSeq panel BRCA1/2.

Additional sample evaluation

Based on the Ampliseq campture strategy, we analyzed 68 samples having a history of either mammary or ovarian cancer, which were sent to our service in order to evaluate the presence of *BRCA1* or *BRCA2* mutations. Variant classification followed the above described process. MLPA was performed for all the 68 samples. In order to guarantee the quality of the analysis, regions with <20× coverage were Sanger sequenced. Every pathogenic and VUS variants detected by the NGS workflow were also confirmed by Sanger sequencing.

The graphic of mutation distribution was built using the cBioPortal website (http://www.cbioportal.org/mutation_mapper.jsp).

Results

Development and validation process

The *in-house*-designed primer strategy presented a reduction of about 5× in the capture costs, when compared to the commercial available one. It was possible to cover the entire target region; however, there was a great coverage variability; while some amplicons presented 20× on average, others showed 1500× (data not shown). Since this variability could risk the following analysis, this method was set aside. Even being discarded for routine application, this strategy brought the advantage of creating a bank of validated primers, which can be used to sequence and confirm any *BRCA1* and *BRCA2* regions through Sanger sequencing.

The Ion Torrent PGM sequencings, based on the commercial available capture strategy, generated an average of 2.8 million reads with a mean size of 135 bp (based on the seven runs). The coverage analysis performed with the plugin Coverage Analysis from Torrent Suite v4.4 software showed that the target regions (167 amplicons) had 100% coverage (Fig. 2). Using 4 samples per 314 chips, the average coverage was 425×, with more than 95% of the bases with a coverage of at least 100× and 98.88% at least 20×. The template preparation showed values of polyclonal ranging from 28 to 42%.

Variant calling

During the validation process, we found 42 unique variants in the patients' samples (Table 1). Considering the complete sampling set, there were 574 variants, also accounting the reproducibility tests. The result obtained from the confirmation by capillary sequencing detected 25 false positives including 10 different variants with 8 in homopolymer regions (Additional File 3: Table S3). The variants reported by the reference laboratory (Myriad Genetics) were considered true positives variants and could be identified by our strategy, including a confirmation by Sanger.

Regarding the NA12878 sample from NIST, we identified 17 from the 20 variants (85%) contained in the vcf file filtered for Ion AmpliSeq regions. The three uncalled variants were present in endpoints of the target amplicons (5′ or 3′) located in exon–intron boundaries, and do not represent clinically significant variants.

Variant calling comparison

Using the in-house-developed bioinformatics pipeline, we could reach a variant calling sensitivity of 95.64%. The inter- and intra-assay evaluation, comprehended by 10 duplicates, 4 triplicates, and 1 quadruplicate showed high concordance in the variant calls, as demonstrated by the reproducibility of the test. The reproducibility rate within the NGS sequencing was 94.17%, but the errors only happened due to false positives. When we sequenced the target regions by Sanger, we excluded all the false positives and obtained 100% reproducibility for the true positive variants. The sensitivity observed separately for SNVs, insertions, and deletions using the in-house pipeline is summarized in Table 2.

As a comparison, we used the Variant Caller plugin available in the Torrent Suite v4.4 software (recommended by the supplier). The last one has a pipeline developed and optimized for the specific analysis of the Ion AmpliSeq panel *BRCA1*/*BRCA2*; however, the reached sensitivity was 94.03%, with the identification of 587 variants, with 35 of them being false positives (Table 3).

Regarding the reports from Myriad Genetic Laboratories, there was 100% agreement between the results *for mutation identification*. After comparing with databases, four mutations were classified as pathogenic and three as VUS (variants of unknown significance), as shown in Table 3.

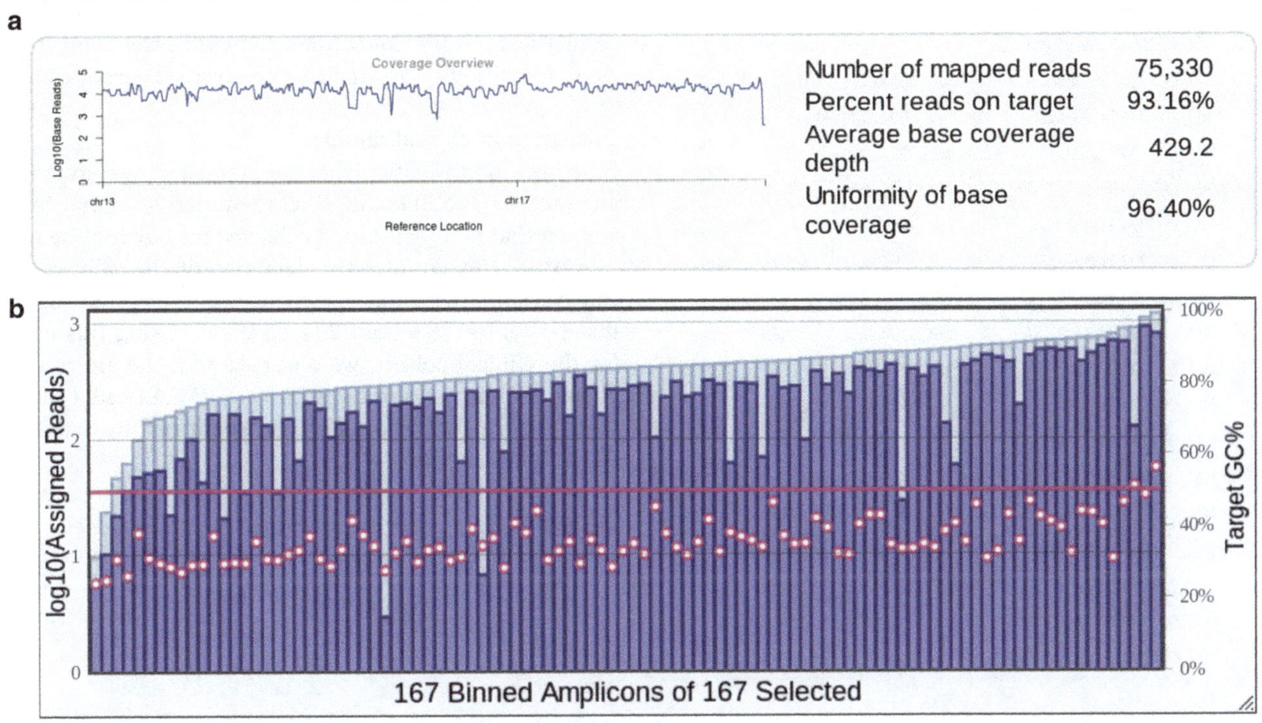

Fig 2 Coverage analysis report generated by Coverage Analysis plugin. **a** Coverage overview from the alignment regions of *BRCA1* (chr17) and *BRCA2* (chr13). **b** Reads distribution on the 167 targets of the Ion AmpliSeq *BRCA1/2* panel, overlayed with target GC content for each read. Representative data from one of the samples sequenced in this validation

Table 1 *BRCA1* and *BRCA2* variants in the 26 validation samples

Gene	HGVSc (hg19)	HGVSp
BRCA2	NM_000059.3:c.-26G>A	-
	NM_000059.3:c.425+67A>C	-
	NM_000059.3:c.681+56C>T	-
	NM_000059.3:c.865A>C	NP_000050.2:p.Asn289His
	NM_000059.3:c.1365A>G	NM_000059.3:c.1365A>G(p.Ser455=)
	NM_000059.3:c.1910-74T>C	-
	NM_000059.3:c.1910-51G>T	-
	NM_000059.3:c.2229T>C	NM_000059.3:c.2229T>C(p.His743=)
	NM_000059.3:c.2971A>G	NP_000050.2:p.Asn991Asp
	NM_000059.3:c.3396A>G	NM_000059.3:c.3396A>G(p.Lys1132=)
	NM_000059.3:c.3807T>C	NM_000059.3:c.3807T>C(p.Val1269=)
	NM_000059.3:c.4563A>G	NM_000059.3:c.4563ᵃ>G(p.Leu1521=)
	NM_000059.3:c.4585G>A	NP_000050.2:p.Gly1529Arg
	NM_000059.3:c.5744C>T	NP_000050.2:p.Thr1915Met
	NM_000059.3:c.6100C>T	NP_000050.2:p.Arg2034Cys
	NM_000059.3:c.6322C>T	NP_000050.2:p.Arg2108Cys
	NM_000059.3:c.6513G>C	NM_000059.3:c.6513G>C(p.Val2171=)
	*NM_000059.3:c.6988A>G	NP_000050.2:p.Ile2330Val
	NM_000059.3:c.7008-62A>G	-
	NM_000059.3:c.7242A>G	NM_000059.3:c.7242A>G(p.Ser2414=)
	NM_000059.3:c.7397T>C	NP_000050.2:p.Val2466Ala
	NM_000059.3:c.7806-14T>C	-
	NM_000059.3:c.8482A>G	NP_000050.2:p.Ile2828Val
	NM_000059.3:c.8518A>G	NP_000050.2:p.Ile2840Val
	NM_000059.3:c.8755-66T>C	-
BRCA1	NM_007294.3:c.5266dupC	NP_009225.1:p.Gln1756ProfsTer74
	NM_007294.3:c.5095C>T	NP_009225.1:p.Arg1699Trp
	NM_007294.3:c.4837A>G	NP_009225.1:p.Ser1613Gly
	NM_007294.3:c.4535G>T	NP_009225.1:p.Ser1512Ile
	NM_007294.3:c.4308T>C	NM_007294.3:c.4308T>C(p.Ser1436)
	NM_007294.3:c.3916_3917delTT	NP_009225.1:p.Leu1306AspfsTer23
	NM_007294.3:c.3548A>G	NP_009225.1:p.Lys1183Arg
	NM_007294.3:c.3119G>A	NP_009225.1:p.Ser1040Asn
	NM_007294.3:c.3113A>G	NP_009225.1:p.Glu1038Gly
	NM_007294.3:c.2612C>T	NP_009225.1:p.Pro871Leu
	NM_007294.3:c.2311T>C	NM_007294.3:c.2311T>C(p.Leu771)
	NM_007294.3:c.2082C>T	NM_007294.3:c.2082C>T(p.Ser694)
	NM_007294.3:c.2077G>A	NP_009225.1:p.Asp693Asn
	NM_007294.3:c.1067A>G	NP_009225.1:p.Gln356Arg
	NM_007294.3:c.736T>G	NP_009225.1:p.Leu246Val
	NM_007294.3:c.442-34C>T	-
	NM_007294.3:c.-19-115T>C	-

Myriad did not send us the entire list of variants, with the report being composed solely by the pathogenic and VUS variants. For this reason, the specificity compared to Myriad results could not be calculated (Table 4).

Table 2 Comparison of the variant call sensitivity between SNVs, insertions, and deletions with the *in-house pipeline*

	SNVs	Insertion	Deletion
Variants found	539	22	13
False positives	0	15	10
Sensibility	100%	31.8%	23.07%

MLPA

All samples met the quality criteria evaluated in the Coffalyser.Net software including FRSS (fragment run separation score) and FMRS (fragment MLPA reaction score), and all expected probes were detected (48 for *BRCA1* and 44 for *BRCA2*). The samples analyzed showed no deletions and/or duplications detected by MLPA in the *BRCA1* and *BRCA2* genes, which is in agreement with the results of sequencing and the reports sent by Myriad. Interestingly, one of the samples showed a decrease in fluorescence referring to one of the *BRCA2* probes. By analyzing the sequence, we observe the presence of the mutation c.6988A>G, located exactly in the hybridization probe region, which explains the signal decrease.

Both the deletion of 40 bp in exon 11 of the *BRCA1* and the duplication of exon 9 in *BRCA2*, which were used as positive controls, were correctly identified. All results were 100% concordant between inter- and intra-assay repetitions, showing that the test is reproducible.

Evaluation of clinical samples

Based on the validation that we performed, we sought to analyze the *BRCA1* and *BRCA2* mutation status in 68 women that had their blood collected for our routine test.

In order to guarantee the detection of clinically significant variants, we Sanger sequenced the targeted regions that presented less than 20× coverage. Using this cutoff for the clinical cohort, we observed that the entire exon 20 and the final end of exon 23 from *BRCA2* had a similar poor performance and had to be confirmed by Sanger in 90% of our samples.

Table 3 Comparison of the variant call sensitivity between the Variant Caller plugin and the pipeline developed in-house

	In-house pipeline	Variant Caller Ion Torrent Suite
Variants found	574	587
False positives	25	35
Sensitivity	95.64%	94.03%
Reproducibility (NGS only)	94.17%	94.71%
Reproducibility (NGS+Sanger)	100%	100%

Table 4 Variants called in agreement with Myriad results

Variants	Clinical significance	Number of samples
BRCA1 c.5266dupC	Pathogenic	2
BRAC1 c.5095C>T	Pathogenic	1
BRCA1 c.3916_3917del	Pathogenic	1
BRCA2 c.6988A>G	VUS	1
BRCA2 c.8482A>G	VUS	1
BRCA2 c.8518A>G	VUS	1

Over these 68 samples, we found a total of 22 variants in the *BRCA1* and 49 in the *BRCA2* gene. No alterations on MLPA were found in any of the samples. Fifty-seven variants were classified as benign, and 14 were either pathogenic or VUS (Table 5), with great majority being identified in *BRCA2*. Mutations in *BRCA1* were mapped in the N- and C-terminal, while *BRCA2* variants had a more homogeneous distribution, with a slightly clusterization near the OB3 domain coding region (Fig. 3). All of 14 variants were tested by Sanger sequencing and confirmed by the orthogonal approach.

Discussion

Here, we evaluated strategies for *BRCA1* and *BRCA2* mutation detection, through Ion Torrent PGM NGS platform, and found that a commercial panel for capturing the coding *BRCA1* and *BRCA2* regions (Ampliseq BRCA1/BRCA2) is robust and meets the clinical requirements for diagnostic. This panel proved to be efficient, covering all exons and a part of the introns. However, there is a limitation in terms of performance, since there is great variability in amplification efficiency of the 167 targets, reflecting a variable final coverage of the sequencing run. Thus, a high value of mean coverage is essential to ensure that even regions of lower efficiency in the PCR are represented in a minimum cutoff in the sequencing data. This situation was especially evidenced in our clinical cohort, with the need of Sanger sequencing for some hot spot areas that consistently presented a poor coverage (<20×).

The comparison between the workflow that we designed on CLC Workbench software and the Variant Caller from Torrent Suite v4.4 software showed that the last one presents an increased amount of false positives, with reduced sensitivity. Even with the optimization of the bioinformatics parameters used in our pipeline, which improved the quality of mapping and variant calling, our in-house pipeline has a high false positive rate (4.3%), which is due mostly to homopolymers regions. This has been previously reported by other authors [12–14] and highlights the need for orthogonal confirmations. Having this scenario, we opted for the confirmation of every pathogenic or variant of unknown significance through Sanger sequencing in our clinical analysis test. Despite having a higher processing cost, this strategy reduces the chance of losing clinically important variants.

The accuracy tests were performed with basis in the Myriad Genetics Laboratory reports and the NA12878 (NIST) evaluation. The first comparison showed 100% accuracy, since all the mutations reported by Myriad could be identified in our test and were also validated by Sanger sequencing. This data shows that our test is reliable, since Myriad is a reference when dealing with mutations in *BRCA1* and *BRCA2*. Furthermore, intra- and inter-assays demonstrated that the test is reproducible. It was not possible to obtain specificity values for the test because we do not have information of all the

Table 5 Summary of the main variants found in this clinical cohort

Gene	Mutation	Classification	Type
BRCA1 (NM_007294.3)	c.441+2T>A	Pathogenic	Intronic (splice donor variant)
	c.68_69delAG: p.Glu23Valfs*17	Pathogenic	Frameshift
	c.5365G>T: p.Ala1789Ser	VUS	Missense
BRCA2 (NM_000059.3)	c.4965C>: p.Y1655*	Pathogenic	Nonsense
	c.8878C>T: p.Gln2960*	Pathogenic	Nonsense
	c.9382C>T: p.Arg3128*	Pathogenic	Nonsense
	c.1813dupA: p.Ile605Asnfs*11	Pathogenic	Frameshift
	c.9004G>A: p.Glu3002Lys	Pathogenic	Missense
	c.8850G>T: p.Lys2950Asn	VUS	Missense
	c.5729A>T: p.Asn1910Ile	VUS	Missense
	c.7469T>C: p.Ile2490Thr	VUS	Missense
	c.956A>C: p.Asn319Thr	VUS	Missense
	c.3262C>T: p.Pro1088Ser	VUS	Missense
	c.4183G>T: p.Ala1395Ser	VUS	Missense

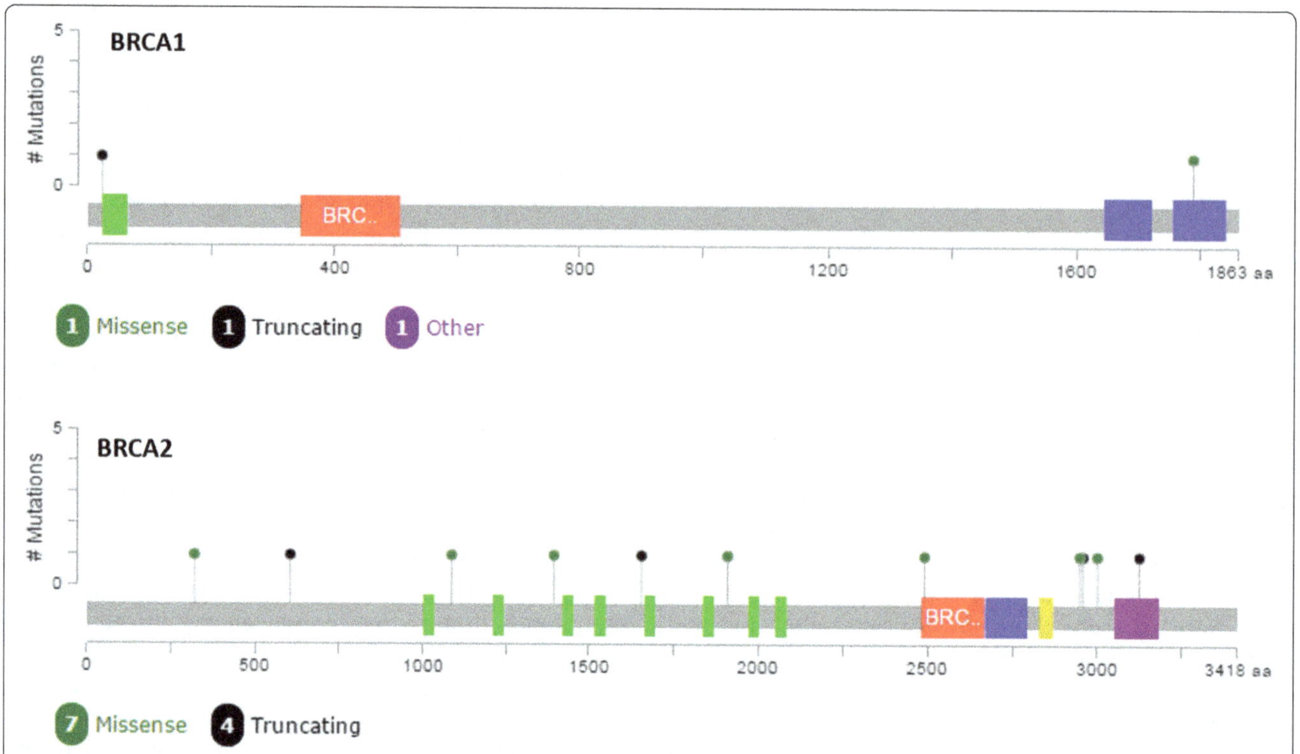

Fig 3 Distribution of the *BRCA1* and *BRCA2* mutations identified in the clinical cohort. The c.441+2T>A variant was not mapped, since it is an intronic variant.

variants in the samples that were sent to Myriad. Additionally, it is important to highlight that in the regions analyzed by Sanger sequencing for variants confirmation, we found no other changes than those observed by NGS.

The second comparison, using the sample NA12878 reference, found that our workflow failed to find three variants. However, when analyzing the read mappings, we observed that these variants are located in the endpoints of the target amplicons (5′ or 3′), regions usually with low-quality bases in exon–intron boundaries, with low mapping quality, and that do not contain clinically significant variants.

MLPA tests also showed high reproducibility, with concordant results between repetitions and the detection of any changes expected in the positive controls. One sample showed reduced fluorescence signal for one of the *BRCA2* probes, since this variant was present in the exact site of hybridization, which generated an equivocal result for the presence of a deletion. This observation is important to demonstrate that the results of sequencing and MLPA are complementary and that the thorough analysis and interpretation of data by qualified professionals is essential for diagnosis.

During this validation process and the evaluation of the 68 clinical samples, we were also able to join a huge amount of data from different databases. Using publicly available data and the insertion of *BRCA1* and *BRCA2* variants that were previously reported by Myriad Genetics Laboratory during our more than 10-year sent out test, turned possible to produce a very robust database with over 9000 variants that can be used for the interpretation of each identified variant. This is of special interest, since one of the most critical points of this workflow is the definition between a pathogenic mutation and a benign variant. Additionally, the generation of specific databases is important for populations like the one we have in Brazil due to its admixture, with different representations of African, European, and Native American variant frequencies [15]. It is interesting to note a slight clusterization of *BRCA2* variants near the OB3 domain.

Conclusion

The workflow for the complete analysis of *BRCA1* and *BRCA2* genes has proved to be highly efficient and accurate for the detection of point mutations and indels by NGS with the Ion Torrent PGM system, in addition to large insertions and deletions with MLPA technique. The selection of a robust methodology for sample preparation and sequencing, together with bioinformatics tools optimized for the data analysis, enabled the development of a very sensitive test with high reproducibility. We also highlight the need to explore the limitations of the NGS technique and the strategies to overcome them in a clinically confident manner.

Acknowledgements
We thank Fleury Group (São Paulo, Brazil) for supporting this research, including the materials and the development infrastructure.

Funding
Not applicable.

Authors' contributions
MMN conceived and designed the study and gave all the scientific assessment. ALB designed the primers, prepared the libraries, and performed the sequencings and data analysis. AYO and DSMA helped with the workflow design and development of a database search tool. ARSF helped with the NGS and Sanger sequencings. PRS and CMM did the DNA extractions and processed the clinical samples. WRB and CRDAC provided the medical assessment for the products' development. ALB and MMN prepared the manuscript. All authors read and approved the final manuscript.

Consent for publication
Not applicable.

Competing interests
The authors declare that they have no competing interests.

References

1. Ferlay J, Soerjomataram I, Dikshit R, Eser S, Mahters C, Rebelo M, Parkin D M, Forman D, Bray F. Cancer incidence and mortality worldwide: sources, methods and major patterns in GLOBOCAN 2012. International Journal Of Cancer. 2014; doi:10.1002/ijc.29210.
2. Cramer D W. The Epidemiology of Endometrial and Ovarian Cancer. Hematology/oncology Clinics Of North America. 2012; doi:10.1016/j.hoc.2011.10.009.
3. Pal T, Permuth-Wey J, Betts J A, Krischer J P, Fiorica J, Arango H, LaPolla J, Hoffman M, Martino M A, Wakeley K, Wilbanks G, Nicosia S, Cantor A, Stuphen R. BRCA1 and BRCA2 mutations account for a large proportion of ovarian carcinoma cases. Cancer. 2005; doi:10.1002/cncr.21536.
4. NIH, BRCA1 and BRCA2: Cancer Risk and Genetic Testing. 2016. http://www.cancer.gov/about-cancer/causes-prevention/genetics/brca-fact-sheet#r5. Accessed 04 Apr 2016.
5. O'Donovan P J, Livingston D M. BRCA1 and BRCA2: breast/ovarian cancer susceptibility gene products and participants in DNA double-strand break repair. Carcinogenesis. 2010; doi:10.1093/carcin/bgq069.
6. Roy R, Chun J, Powell S N. BRCA1 and BRCA2: different roles in a common pathway of genome protection. Nature Reviews Cancer. 2011; doi:10.1038/nrc3181.
7. Aebi S, Davidson T, Gruber G, Cardoso F, ESMO Guidelines Working Group. Primary breast cancer: ESMO Clinical Practice Guidelines for diagnosis, treatment and follow-up. Annals of Oncology. 2011; doi:10.1093/annonc/mdr371.
8. Bozovic-Spasojevic I, Azambuja E, McCaskill-Stevens W, Dinh P, Cardoso F. Chemoprevention for breast cancer. Cancer Treatment Reviews. 2012; doi:10.1016/j.ctrv.2011.07.005.
9. Feliubadaló L, Lopez-Doriga A, Castellsagué E, del Valle J, Menéndez M, Tornero E, Montes E, Cuesta R, Gómez C, Campos O, Pineda M, González S, Moreno V, Brunet J, Blanco I, Serra E, Capellá G, Lázaro C. Next-generation sequencing meets genetic diagnostics: development of a comprehensive workflow for the analysis of BRCA1 and BRCA2 genes. Eur J Hum Genet. 2012; doi:10.1038/ejhg.2012.270.
10. Spurdle A B, Healey S, Devereau A, Hogervorst F B L, Monteiro A N A, Nathanson K L, Radice P, Stoppa-Lyonnet D, Tavtigian S, Wappenschmidt B, Couch F J, Goldgar D E. ENIGMA-Evidence-based network for the interpretation of germline mutant alleles: an international initiative to evaluate risk and clinical significance associated with sequence variation in BRCA1 and BRCA2 genes. Human Mutation. 2011; doi:10.1002/humu.21628.
11. Tung N, Battelli C, Allen D, Kaldate R, Bhatnagar S, Bowles K, Timms K, Garber J E, Herold C, Ellisen L, Krejdovsky J, DeLeonardis K, Sedgwick K, Soltis K, Roa B, Wenstrup R J, Hartman A R. Frequency of mutations in individuals with breast cancer referred for BRCA 1 and BRCA 2 testing using next-generation sequencing with a 25-gene panel. Cancer. 2014; doi:10.1002/cncr.29010.
12. Bragg L M, Stone G, Butler M K, Hugenholtz P, Tyson G W. Shining a light on dark sequencing: characterising errors in Ion Torrent PGM data. Plos Comput Biol. 2013; doi:10.1371/journal.pcbi.1003031.
13. Quail M, Smith M, Coupland P, Otto T D, Harris S R, Connor T R, Bertoni A, Swerdlow H P, Gu Y. A tale of three next generation sequencing platforms: comparison of Ion torrent, Pacific Biosciences and Illumina MiSeq sequencers. Bmc Genomics. 2012; doi:10.1186/1471-2164-13-341.
14. Yeo Z, Wong J C L, Rozen S G, Lee A S G. Evaluation and optimization of indel detection workflows for ion torrent sequencing of the BRCA1 and BRCA2 genes. Bmc Genomics. 2014; doi:10.1186/1471-2164-15-516.
15. Naslavsky MS, Yamamoto GL, de Almeida TF, Ezquina SAM, Sunaga DY, Pho N, Bozoklian D, Sandberg TOM, Brito LA, Lazar M, Bernardo DV, Amaro E Jr, Duarte YAO, Lebrão ML, Passos-Bueno MR, Zatz M. Exomic variants of an elderly cohort of Brazilians in the ABraOM database. Hum Mutat. 2017 Mar 23. doi:10.1002/humu.23220.

12

Long non-coding RNAs as novel players in β cell function and type 1 diabetes

Aashiq H. Mirza[1,2,3], Simranjeet Kaur[1] and Flemming Pociot[1,2,3*]

Abstract

Background: Long non-coding RNAs (lncRNAs) are a sub-class within non-coding RNA repertoire that have emerged as crucial regulators of the gene expression in various pathophysiological conditions. lncRNAs display remarkable versatility and wield their functions through interactions with RNA, DNA, or proteins. Accumulating body of evidence based on multitude studies has highlighted the role of lncRNAs in many autoimmune and inflammatory diseases, including type 1 diabetes (T1D).

Main body of abstract: This review highlights emerging roles of lncRNAs in immune and islet β cell function as well as some of the challenges and opportunities in understanding the pathogenesis of T1D and its complications.

Conclusion: We accentuate that the lncRNAs within T1D-loci regions in consort with regulatory variants and enhancer clusters orchestrate the chromatin remodeling in β cells and thereby act as cis/trans-regulatory determinants of islet cell transcriptional programs.

Keywords: Long non-coding RNAs, Type 1 diabetes, Enhancers, Regulatory elements, 3D genome architecture

Background

Type 1 diabetes (T1D) is a chronic immune-mediated disease resulting from selective destruction of insulin-producing pancreatic islet β cells. A complex interplay between several environmental and genetic risk factors contribute to the onset of T1D [1, 2]. Defects in both immune system and β cells play an active role in T1D pathogenesis [3]. In recent years, efforts have been accelerated to gain insights into the molecular mechanisms of pathogenesis of T1D and to determine how genetic loci contribute to the T1D risk [1, 4]. Based on genome-wide association studies (GWAS), currently more than 50 genomic risk loci have been identified for T1D [2, 5–7]. Approximately, 50% of the genetic risk for T1D is known to reside within the human leukocyte antigen (HLA) region; however, other non-HLA disease susceptibility loci have been identified based on their direct influence on the risk. Some of the well-established candidate genes in the non-HLA risk loci including *INS* (11p15), *CTLA4* (2q33), *PTPN22* (1p13), *PTPN2* (18p11), *ERBB3* (12q13), *IL2RA* (10p15), and *IFIH1* (2q24) have been associated with immune response, insulin expression, and β cell function [1, 4, 8]. The risk alleles for several T1D susceptibility genes are not exclusively confined to T1D but have been shown to confer risk in other prevalent autoimmune disorders, including multiple sclerosis (MS), systemic lupus erythematosus (SLE), and rheumatoid arthritis (RA) [7]. Furthermore, most of these risk variants are located in non-coding genomic regions including long non-coding RNAs (lncRNAs) and are enriched in distal regulatory elements such as enhancers and promoters. Non-coding variants affecting regulatory elements have the potential to perturb chromatin folding leading to mis-expression of the target gene. These facts suggest that the regulatory landscape of human genome plays an important role in pathology of a disease and newer approaches are needed to identify putative regulatory risk variants affecting gene regulation and immune function.

Recent advances in our understanding of lncRNA biology has offered new perspectives on gene regulation and has allowed us to unveil the regulatory potential of these versatile molecules in a spectrum of biological processes and pathologies, including autoimmune and inflammatory disorders. High-throughput technologies such as ChIP-

* Correspondence: flemming.pociot.01@regionh.dk
[1]CPH-DIRECT, Department of Pediatrics, Herlev University Hospital, Herlev Ringvej 75, DK-2730 Herlev, Denmark
[2]Faculty of Health and Medical Sciences, University of Copenhagen, Copenhagen, Denmark
Full list of author information is available at the end of the article

seq and chromosome conformation capture techniques have also opened new possibilities to investigate in detail potential regulatory roles of non-coding genome in gene regulation and 3D chromatin folding. In this review, we discuss the recent discoveries in the field of lncRNAs, regulatory elements, 3D genome architecture, and their implications for T1D and β cell function. We further highlight the role of active enhancers associated with T1D–loci lncRNAs and protein-coding genes in regulating β cell gene expression programs through both *cis*- and *trans*-regulatory mechanisms involving structural remodeling of chromatin in human islets.

Main text

lncRNAs in T1D and other immune-mediated diseases

lncRNAs are non-coding RNAs that are more than 200 nucleotides in length, and are capped, polyadenylated, and spliced like their well-characterized "cousins," protein-coding transcripts, with one exception; lncRNAs do not code for proteins [9]. Most of the lncRNAs are expressed in a cell-specific manner and are usually expressed in lower abundance than the protein-coding transcripts. In terms of genomic location, lncRNAs have been often categorized as long intergenic non-coding RNAs (lincRNAs), intronic lncRNAs, antisense lncRNAs, divergent lncRNAs and enhancer-derived lncRNAs (lncRNAs arising from enhancer-like regions) [10–12] (Fig. 1). lncRNAs have emerged as important players of gene regulation and have been implicated in various human pathologies [13]. lncRNAs regulate various cellular and biological processes including heterochromatin formation, histone modifications, DNA methylation targeting, and gene silencing [14, 15]. The lncRNA-recruited regulatory complexes orchestrate development and differentiation of various immune cell lineages and actively regulate expression programs within these cells.

Multiple studies have highlighted the potential roles of lncRNAs in pancreatic islets and T1D pathogenesis [10, 16, 17]. Based on transcriptome profiling studies of islets and β cells, more than 1000 islet-specific lncRNAs have been identified in both human and mouse islets [18, 19]. The ability of lncRNAs to regulate gene expression and cell-specific identity provides an exciting opportunity to advance our understanding of T1D pathogenesis. Table 1 lists examples of lncRNAs that have been implicated in β cell function and T1D. lncRNA *MALAT1* has been associated with diabetes-induced microvascular dysfunction in STZ-induced diabetic rats and db/db mice [20]. Knockdown of *MALAT1* prevents the hyper-proliferation of retinal endothelial cells through p38 MAPK signaling and might serve as a potential target for anti-angiogenic therapy for diabetic retinopathy. lncRNA *MEG3* has been associated with paternally inherited risk of T1D [21] and its downregulation affects

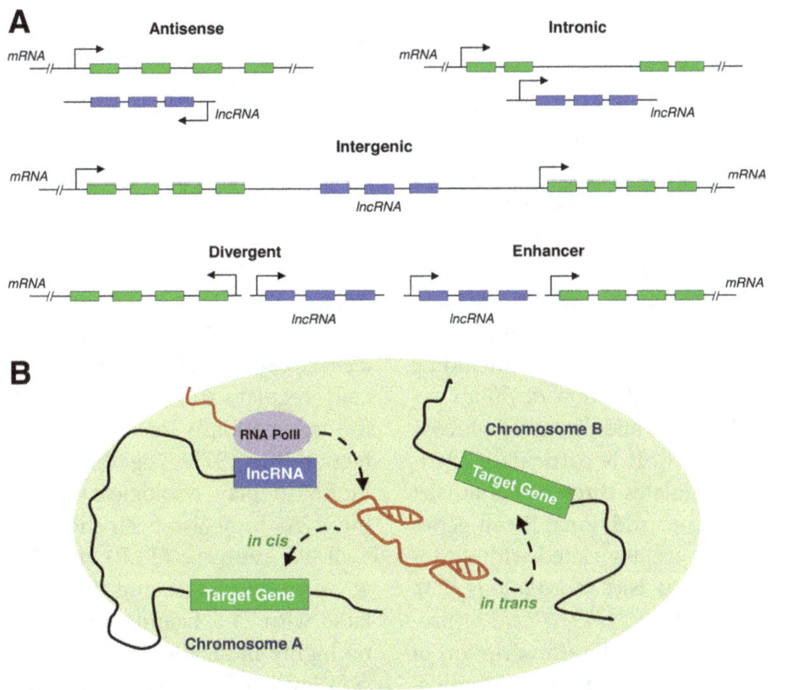

Fig. 1 Bio-types of lncRNAs and enhancer-derived lncRNA function. **a** Different bio-types of lncRNAs based on their genomic location include antisense, intergenic, intronic, divergent and enhancer-derived lncRNAs. lncRNAs are depicted in *blue*, while protein-coding genes are shown in *green*. **b** The postulated role of enhancer-derived lncRNAs for both *cis*- and *trans*-mediated regulation of target genes is shown via chromatin loop formation. Figure modified from Ref. [10, 11]

Table 1 lncRNAs associated with β cell function and type 1 diabetes

lncRNAs	Function	Reference
MEG3	Regulates β cell identity and function via insulin production and apoptosis in mouse MIN6 cells and isolated mouse islets	You et al. 2016 [22]
HI-LNC25	Positively regulates *GLIS3* (which contains both T1D and T2D risk variants) in EndoC-βH1 human β cell line	Moran et al. 2012 [18]
βlinc1 (HI-LNC15)	Regulates β cell identity and function in mouse MIN6 cells and EndoC-βH1 human β cell line; also regulates its neighboring gene NKX2.2 (an islet transcription factor).	Arnes et al. 2016 [23]
TUNAR (HI-LNC78)	Knockdown of *TUNAR* leads to impaired glucose-stimulated insulin secretion in human islets	Akerman et al. 2017 [24]
PLUT (HI-LNC71)	Regulates transcription of *PDX1*, a key pancreatic β cell transcriptional regulator, in EndoC-βH1 cells, primary islet cells, mouse β cell line MIN6	Akerman et al. 2017 [24]
MALAT1	Upregulation of *MALAT1* is associated with microvascular dysfunction (diabetic retinopathy) in STZ-induced diabetic rats and db/db mice	Liu et al. 2014 [20]
TUG1	Downregulation of lncRNA TUG1 expression increased apoptosis and reduced insulin secretion in mouse β cells	Yin et al. 2015 [25]

insulin synthesis and secretion in mouse β cells [22]. The knockdown of *trans*-acting islet-specific lncRNA *HI-LNC25* (*LINC01370*) in mature β cells resulted in down-regulation of *GLIS3* gene [18]. *GLIS3* encodes an islet transcription factor (TF) and is a candidate gene for both type 1 and type 2 diabetes. Another islet-specific lncRNA *βlinc1* (previously known as *HI-LNC15*) has been shown to be essential for proper specification and function of β cells [23]. Knockdown of *βlinc1* in mouse MIN6 cells and human insulin-producing EndoC-βH1 cells resulted in downregulation of several islet-specific TFs, including Nkx2.2, Pax6, and Mafb [23]. Also, deletion of *βlinc1* resulted in defective islet development and disrupted glucose homeostasis in the adult mice [23]. It is particularly intriguing that *βlinc1* specifically regulates three essential islet TFs (Nkx2.2, Pax6, and MafB) and additional β cell genes on chromosome 2, all of which are associated with endocrine development and maintaining islet morphology [23]. Nuclear-enriched β cell lncRNA *PLUTO (PLUT)* (previously known as *HI-LNC71*) regulates the transcription of *PDX1* gene which is a key pancreatic β cell transcriptional regulator [24]. *PLUT* encompasses a cluster of enhancers that make 3D contacts with the *PDX1* promoter in human islets and in human β cell line EndoC-βH1. Loss of *PLUT* was associated with downregulation of *PDX1* at both mRNA and protein levels in EndoC-βH1 cells, primary islet cells, and a similar effect was observed for the mouse lncRNA ortholog in mouse β cell line MIN6 [24]. Knockdown of lncRNA *TUNAR* (*HI-LNC78*) resulted in reduced insulin content and impaired glucose-stimulated insulin secretion in T antigen-excised EndoC-βH3 cells [24]. lncRNA *TUG1* is a highly conserved lncRNA in mammals and is highly expressed in mouse pancreatic tissues [25]. In mouse β cells, downregulation of *TUG1* as a consequence of hyperglycemia resulted in increased apoptosis and reduced insulin synthesis and secretion [25]. These findings suggest that *TUG1* may partially contribute to the impairment of β cell function and could therefore be implicated in diabetes pathogenesis.

In recent years, growing body of evidence has linked dysregulation of lncRNA expression to a spectrum of autoimmune disease [26, 27]. Hrdlickova and colleagues found enrichment of lincRNAs in autoimmune disease-associated loci in a subset of immune cells [28]. A number of studies describe the emerging role of lncRNAs in transcriptional regulation of inflammatory gene expression [29, 30]. For example, in human monocytes, lncRNA *THRIL* has been shown to interact with hnRNP-L and regulate the expression of *TNFα* [31]. Correspondingly, additional examples of lncRNAs involvement in inflammatory signaling cascades and regulation of innate immune responses includes (1) lncRNA *PACER* (*PACERR*) which has been shown to bind p50 subunit of *NFκB* and control the basal expression levels of *Cox2 (PTGS2)* [32]; (2) in primary human monocytes, knockdown of *NFκB* regulated, enhancer-RNA (eRNA) *IL1β-eRNA* and region of bi-directional transcription (RBT) IL1β-RBT46, mitigated bacterial lipopolysaccharide (LPS) pro-inflammatory cytokine IL1β induction and release [33]; (3) overexpression of natural antisense transcript anti-IL1β alters the chromatin structure around the IL1β promoter and consequently inhibits the IL1β expression [34, 35]. In a murine model, lncRNA *NeST* (Nettoie Salmonella pas Theiler's; *cleanup Salmonella not Theiler's*) was shown to epigenetically regulate the interferon-γ (IFN-γ) locus and control the susceptibility to Theiler's virus and Salmonella infection [36, 37]. Together, these findings indicate that lncRNAs play etiological role in autoimmune diseases. lncRNAs have also been shown to play pivotal roles in the Toll-like receptor (TLR) signaling pathway. For example, when macrophages and dendritic cells (DCs) were stimulated with TLR ligands, the *lincRNA-Cox2A* was found to be highly inducible and also controlled the basal expression levels of interferon-stimulated genes (ISGs) and pro-inflammatory cytokines [29]. Intriguingly, pseudogenes lncRNAs have been identified to act as functional regulators of inflammatory signaling with their expression being actively regulated. Stimulation of mouse embryonic fibroblast cells by *TNFα* has been found to induce expression of lncRNAs. *Lethe*, a pseudogene lncRNA, has been shown to function as a novel negative regulator of *NF-κB*. *Lethe*, wields its regulatory function by binding directly RelA, a subunit of *NF-κB* heterodimeric complex, preclude *NF-κB* binding to the promoter regions of target genes [38]. Another pseudogene lncRNA Lnc-dendritic cell (*DC*) (*WFDC21P*) has been shown to be involved in monocyte to DC differentiation [39].

Systemic cell-mediated immunity is known to play a central role in the apoptotic β cell destruction that culminates in T1D. The T helper 17 (Th17) cells are known to protect mucosal barriers from opportunistic infections and are also associated with number of autoimmune inflammatory diseases. Like many other autoimmune diseases, T1D is also a T cell-mediated malady, and imbalance between the Th17 cells and T regulatory (Treg) has been implicated in development of the T1D [40, 41]. Recently, Huang et al. [42] demonstrated role of DEAD-box protein 5 (DDX5) as a binding partner of RORγt, a well-known ligand-regulated nuclear receptor that controls the differentiation of Th17 cells. Interestingly, DDX5 coordinates the transcription of selective Th17 genes through its interaction with RORγt, and it is also required for Th17 cell-mediated inflammatory diseases. The interaction between DDX5 and RORγt is dependent on the inherent RNA helicase activity of DDX5 and the binding of Rmrp, an evolutionarily conserved nuclear lncRNA. Furthermore, Rmrp was found mutated in patients with cartilage-hair hypoplasia, and corresponding mutation in Rmrp in mice resulted in altered chromatin interaction, and diminished interaction between the DDX5 and RORγt, and also downregulated expression of selective Th-17 genes [42].

These examples highlight the importance of lncRNAs in regulating gene expression in immune cells and underscore yet another layer of complexity in gene regulation. Future studies should be focused towards elucidating their molecular functions which in turn could provide crucial insights into novel mechanisms of gene regulation, autoimmune and inflammation-mediated disorders, including T1D.

Genome-wide interactions between T1D SNPs, lncRNAs, enhancers, and other distal regulatory elements

More than 90% of disease-associated single-nucleotide polymorphisms (SNPs) are located within the non-coding regions of the genome such as promoters, enhancers, intergenic regions, and ncRNA genes [43]. The disease-associated SNPs have the potential to be regulatory in nature, particularly if they are significantly enriched in functional regulatory elements such as transcription factor binding sites (TFBSs), histone modification marks, DNase-I hypersensitive sites, and expression quantitative trait loci (eQTLs) [44, 45]. These disease-associated regulatory SNPs are also referred to as "functional SNPs" [44]. Approximately, 10% of the autoimmune disease-associated SNPs are present within lncRNAs and some of these SNPs are also known to act as *cis*-eQTLs [46]. It has been shown that 75% of the lincRNA *cis*-eQTLs specifically alter the expression of lincRNAs in a tissue-dependent fashion but does not affect the nearby protein-coding genes, and many of these *cis*-eQTLs SNPs are known to be associated with complex genetic diseases [47]. Since the expression of protein-coding genes can be regulated by lincRNAs either in *cis* [48] or *trans* [49] manner, this suggests a link between disease-associated SNPs within the non-coding regions with the regulation of protein-coding gene expression.

Distal regulatory elements such as enhancers, locus control regions (LCRs), and insulators are highly abundant in the human genome and play an important role in transcriptional control. These elements represent the primary mechanism by which cell and developmental specific gene expression is accomplished. Enhancers are regulatory sequences that can activate gene expression independent of their proximity to their target genes in a tissue-specific manner [50]. Multiple enhancer elements arrayed over large regions can synergistically regulate the expression of individual genes or gene clusters by altering the TF binding and chromatin states [51, 52]. Additionally, multiple polymorphisms in linkage disequilibrium (LD) impact clusters of enhancer elements active in the same cell type and cooperatively contribute to altered expression of their gene targets [53]. The multiple enhancer variants within a given locus typically target the same gene which results in either gain- or loss-of-function [53]. Additionally, the genes associated with multiple enhancer variants encode proteins that are often functionally related and enriched in common pathways. Recently, several methods have been developed for genome-wide prediction of enhancers primarily based on chromatin marks such as H3K4 monomethyl (H3K4me1) and H3K27 acetyl (H3K27ac) modifications, bi-directional transcription, and binding of p300 [54–57]. The underlying mechanism for enhancer function has been suggested to involve formation of long-range chromatin loops, bringing enhancers and promoters into proximity and allowing interaction of the necessary co-transcriptional factors [58, 59]. Formation of chromatin loops occurs between two distant genomic sequences that are brought in close vicinity by protein complexes and are assumed to be chemically cross-linked. Various chromosomal conformation capture techniques such as 3C (chromosome conformation capture) [60], 4C (circular chromosome conformation capture) [61], 5C (chromosome conformation capture carbon copy) [62], ChIA-PET (Chromatin Interaction Analysis with Paired-End-Tag sequencing)

[63], and Hi-C [64] have been used to detect genome-wide chromosome interactions. Examples of long-range interactions within mammalian gene loci include the locus control region (LCR) and β-globin promoter [65, 66]; the α-globin gene cluster in erythroid cells [67]; the TH2 and MHC loci in T cells [68, 69]; and the imprinted gene clusters Dlx5, Dlx6 [70], and H19-Igf2 [71–73]. Additional example of long-range chromatin loop mediated interaction among regulatory elements on different chromosomes has been observed at the IFNγ and TH2 cytokine loci [74]. The transcriptional regulation of IL-21 gene at the chromatin level was recently uncovered to be mediated through long-range chromatin interaction in CD4+ T cells. IL-21, a pro-inflammatory cytokine with pleiotropic effects, is strongly associated with autoimmunity and inflammation and regulates various immune responses. A study by Park et al. showed that a distal enhancer element within an evolutionary conserved non-coding sequence 49 kb upstream of the IL-21 can upregulate IL-21 gene expression in a STAT3- and NFAT-dependent manner [75]. Stimulation of CD4+ T cells with IL-6 leads to the recruitment of STAT3 to the IL-21 promoter and the distal enhancer region, bringing them in close spatial proximity. As a consequence, this long-range interaction between the promoter and distal enhancer region dependent on IL-6/STAT3 signaling pathway alters the chromatin configuration dynamically, and controls the expression of IL-21 in CD4+ T cells [75].

Based on published genome-wide chromosome conformational capture datasets from various cell-lines and T1D associated SNPs we identified physical interactions between distant regulatory regions in T1D loci. Figure 2 shows an interactive map of T1D loci highlighting the physical interactions between distal regulatory elements and potential functional T1D SNP at each locus. T1D risk SNPs and SNPs in LD (r2 > 0.8, CEU HapMap3 population) were selected and scored based on the original GWAS signal, long range chromosome interactions, overlap with chromatin marks, epigenetic modifications and sequence motifs from various ENCODE cell lines [2, 76–78]. The top most scoring SNP for each region was inferred as the most significant functional SNP and selected for plotting along with the most significant distal chromosomal interaction signal. As an example, in *ERBB3* locus, SNP rs4759229 qualified as the most significant variant. rs4759229 is in perfect LD with T1D risk SNP rs2292239, overlaps a known enhancer region and has a long range interaction signal with an antisense lncRNA *AC008079.1* (Ensembl ID: ENSG00000187979) located at USP18 locus on chromosome 22. In a recent study, we proposed that the *ERBB3* SNP rs2292239 and its proxy SNPs in perfect LD rs3741499 and rs4759229 are putatively functional based on the overlapping open chromatin marks, TFBs and DNase I hypersensitivity peaks [79]. We further showed that SNP rs4759229 overlaps a known enhancer element and is in the vicinity of several lncRNA transcripts overlapping *ERBB3* locus. The potential functional T1D SNPs within known T1D candidate genes such as *GLIS3, ERBB3, CTRB1, CTSH, FUT2, IL27, SKAP2, TNFAIP3* and *PTPN2* had highly significant distal chromosomal interactions including enhancers and lncRNAs that are worthy of specific laboratory investigations (Fig. 2). Intriguingly, the impact of interactions between T1D SNPs and enhancer associated lncRNAs on transcription and ultimately on T1D risk remains to be seen. Based on the above evidence we postulate that the T1D SNPs mapping to enhancer associated lncRNAs could potentially alter the expression of their gene targets through enhancer mediated interactions and thereby significantly impact β cell gene expression.

Many lncRNAs have been reported to be expressed from the enhancer regions that are produced by activity-dependent RNA polymerase II binding of specific enhancers [80]. The expression levels of these enhancer associated lncRNAs positively correlate with the expression of neighboring protein-coding genes, i.e., depletion of enhancer associated lncRNAs led to decreased expression of their neighboring protein-coding genes [48, 80]. In addition, enhancers overlapping lncRNAs have higher H3K4me3/H3K4me1 ratios as compared to enhancers that do not overlap lncRNAs [81]. The enrichment of H3K4me3 marks (which are also associated with active promoters) points towards strong transcriptional capabilities of overlapping lncRNAs. lncRNAs transcribed from active enhancers have been identified as important players in mediating enhancer function [82]. Enhancers associated lncRNA play roles in important physiological processes and influence the activation of protein coding and non-coding genes in both *cis* and *trans* mediated mechanism. For example, lncRNA *NEST* is involved in *cis*-activation of the neighboring interferon γ locus, whereas lncRNA *Jpx* regulates *trans*-activation of another lncRNA, *XIST*, (which is critical for X inactivation) [36, 83]. While acting in *trans*, enhancer associated lncRNAs act over long distances by long range chromatin loop mediated interactions and activate transcription at distal promotors. It has also been suggested that bridging factors such as Mediator/Cohesin complex and enhancer associated lncRNAs are involved in establishment of chromatin looping between the lncRNAs and their regulated distal promotors [84]. Knockdown of either lncRNA or mediator subunits has been shown to abolish the chromosomal interactions [84].

It has been shown that islet-specific lncRNAs and TFs co-regulate genes associated with enhancer clusters [24, 85]. lncRNAs regulating enhancer cluster-associated genes bound by multiple islet-specific TFs include *HI-LNC12, HI-LNC15, HI-LNC30, HI-LNC78, HI-LNC80, HI-LNC85*, and *PLUT* (*HI-LNC71*) [24]. However, further studies are warranted that employ

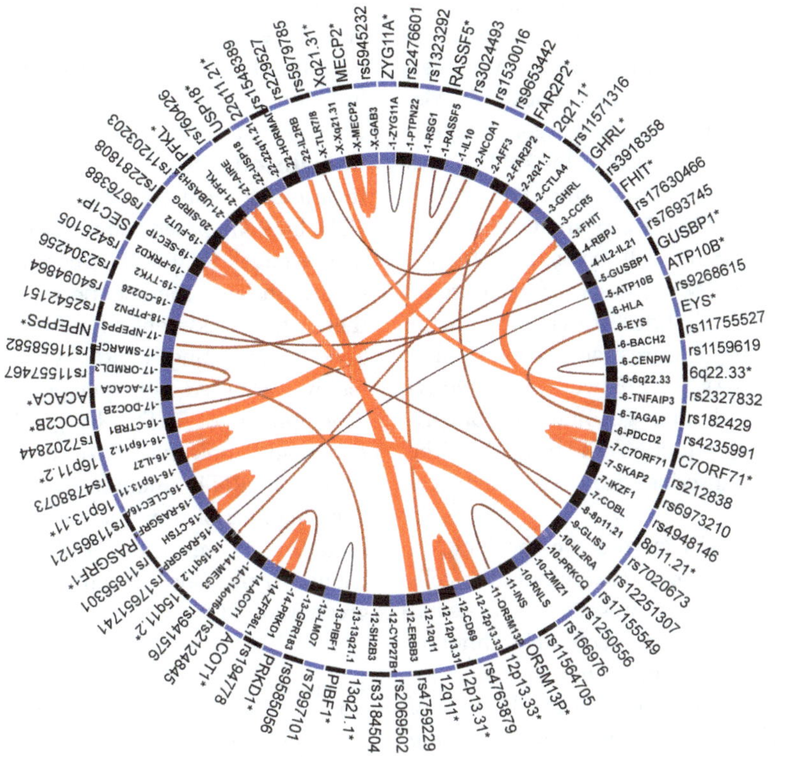

Fig. 2 Distal regulatory elements and potential functional T1D SNPs in T1D susceptibility loci. The *inner circle* represents T1D susceptibility genes and genomic loci and the *outer circle* lists the regulatory variants and distal interaction regions. The distal interactive elements are denoted by an *asterisk* which includes enhancer elements and lncRNAs. The *red lines* indicate long-range chromosome interaction signals to another locus and the intensity of interaction is represented by the width of the *red lines*

chromosomal conformation techniques to identify potential targets of enhancer associated lncRNAs in human islets.

Future challenges and opportunities

Although lncRNAs have achieved formable recognition as key players in gene regulation and disease, there is still a huge gap in our overall understanding of lncRNA regulatory functions and underlying molecular mechanisms, particularly in context of β cell function and development of T1D. The rise of lncRNAs as key regulators of gene expression during normal development and diseases has positioned these pervasive transcripts in the crosshairs of novel disease-specific biomarker discovery. The dysregulation of lncRNA expression not only represents a newfangled layer of intricacy in the molecular architecture of human malady, but it also unveils the potential to use lncRNAs as disease biomarkers. In contrast to their "cousins" mRNA transcripts, the lncRNAs themselves are functional molecules and their expression levels might serve as a better disease indicator. Moreover, expression of lncRNAs is highly tissue-specific and disease-specific which indicates that lncRNA-based expression signatures could effectively be used to accurately diagnose and classify disease. Although, the field of lncRNA-based diagnostics is still in its infancy, the use of distinct lncRNAs in a clinical diagnostics setting has already taken off. Indeed, lncRNAs have already been suggested as potential biomarkers for a number of diseases, including cancer. For example, *PCA3*, a prostate-specific lncRNA notably overexpressed in prostate cancer, has been developed into diagnostic assay to detect prostate cancer [86]. Nevertheless, there are still many challenges ahead of us that need to be addressed in order to fully appreciate the function of lncRNAs in islet biology and T1D contexts.

Most of the functionally characterized lncRNAs exhibit modular-domain architecture that arises from their well-conserved secondary and tertiary structures and is crucial for their biological functions. This assumes importance as it illustrates the importance of the conservation at secondary and tertiary structure level rather than at primary sequence level [87–89]. Therefore, future studies are needed to identify homologous lncRNAs taking a structure-based evolutionary conservation criterion into consideration rather than relying only on the primary sequence-based conservation in cellular and subclinical models of T1D.

Although, a handful of lncRNAs have been functionally characterized, they have certainly emerged as bona fide players in regulating the gene expression at various levels during all the stages of development and disease. With the advent of next-generation sequencing technologies, thousands of lncRNA genes have already been identified and annotated in human and mouse. According to the recent GENCODE v26 (www.gencodegenes.org), more than 15,000 and 11,000 lncRNA genes have already identified in the human and mouse, respectively. In addition, FANTOM5 cap analysis of gene expression (CAGE) in primary cell types and tissues identified 27,919 human lncRNA genes with accurate 5′ termini [90]. Based on multiple lines of evidence, including genomic, epigenomic features and evolutionary conservation of the lncRNAs, 19,175 were reported as potentially functional in the human genome [90]. Surprisingly, most of the intergenic lncRNAs identified in the FANTOM5 project were transcribed from the enhancers and not from the promoters.

One of the major bottlenecks in studying the lncRNA functions has been their low steady-state levels in the cells [91]. Majority of lncRNAs are expressed at low-levels which makes it more challenging to accurately annotate their gene boundaries. The problem of incomplete annotation of lncRNAs is further compounded by the lack of typical genomic hallmarks of transcription initiation and termination that are often used as primary flag posts for defining the gene boundaries [91]. But, recently many methods have been developed and implemented to improve the annotation of lncRNAs, including RNA Capture Sequencing (CaptureSeq) [92], coupling of rapid amplification of cDNA ends (RACE) technique to long-read sequencing (RACE-Seq) [93], RNA Capture Long Seq (CLS) [94], and genome-scale CRISPR-mediated interference (CRISPRi) [95]. So far, these methods have been used for exploring the transcriptomic structure of lncRNA loci using cell or tissue types that are not relevant to diabetes. Nevertheless, these methods provide an excellent experimental framework for future studies to address the lingering questions regarding the roles and molecular mechanisms of lncRNAs in β cell function and T1D pathogenesis. Therefore, employing methods like CLS, RACE-Seq, CAGE and CRISPRi under the proinflammatory cytokines stimulation and control settings will enable to disentangle the transcriptomic landscape of β cells.

It is known that active β cells exhibit extensive allelic imbalance in gene expression [96]. However, the impact of allelic imbalance on the lncRNA expression has been not studied. A robust reassessment of the regulation of allele-specific gene expression in lncRNA loci overlapping or lying in close proximity of T1D GWAS SNPs in islets and β cells derived from cadaveric pancreas with known genotypes would be highly desirable. This could provide important clues linking disease-associated SNPs with the lncRNA expression. Furthermore, these studies have the potential to unravel the diversity of lncRNA repertoire, including the enhancer RNAs (eRNAs) [97] and novel rare transcripts and many of which might have important functional roles in modulating the β cell function.

Conclusions

In immune-mediated and inflammatory diseases such as T1D, lncRNA-based transcriptional signatures might open new avenues for lncRNA-based diagnostics, classification or personalized therapeutic regimens in near future. Furthermore, assessment of functional implications of T1D SNPs overlapping lncRNAs and enhancers regions is highly warranted from perspective of β cell function and development of T1D. The precise biochemical characteristics and molecular basis of β- and immune cells expressed lncRNA functions are necessary to elucidate how deregulations of immune cell-specific T1D loci-associated lncRNAs, as well islet-specific lncRNAs, potentially contribute to the development of islet autoimmunity to progression of T1D.

Abbreviations

eQTL: Expression quantitative trait loci; GWAS: Genome-wide association studies; LD: Linkage disequilibrium; lncRNA: Long non-coding RNA; SNP: Single-nucleotide polymorphism; TF: Transcription factor; TFBS: Transcription factor binding site; T1D: Type 1 diabetes

Funding

Not applicable

Authors' contributions

AHM and SK researched the data and drafted and reviewed the manuscript before submission. FP made substantial contribution to discussion of the content and reviewed the manuscript before submission. All authors read and approved the final manuscript.

Authors' information

AHM is a postdoctoral fellow and received predoctoral and postdoctoral training in the laboratories of Professor Flemming Pociot (Copenhagen Diabetes Research Center, Copenhagen, Denmark), Professor Jan Gorodkin (Center for non-coding RNA in Technology and Health, Copenhagen, Denmark), and Professor Francis Barany (Sandra and Edward Meyer Cancer Center, Weill Cornell Medicine, NY, USA). AHM obtained his PhD degree in Cellular and Genetic Medicine from the University of Copenhagen, Denmark, under the supervision of Professor Jan Gorodkin and Professor Flemming Pociot. AHM's research revolves broadly around understanding the role of non-coding RNAs in autoimmune and inflammatory diseases. AHM is currently involved in development of assays and technologies for early detection of tumors using circulating cell-free nucleic acid based genetic and epigenetic biomarkers in collaboration with Professor Francis Barany and Professor Steven Soper (Department of Chemistry, University of Kansas, KS, USA).
SK is a postdoctoral fellow training in the laboratory of Professor Flemming Pociot. SK obtained her PhD degree in Biostatistics and Bioinformatics from University of Copenhagen, Denmark, under the supervision of Professor Flemming Pociot (Copenhagen Diabetes Research Center, Herlev and Gentofte Hospital, Denmark) and Professor Henrik B. Mortensen (Department of Clinical Medicine, University of Copenhagen, Denmark). SK's research revolves broadly around understanding the role of non-coding RNAs and regulatory elements in β cell function and type 1 diabetes.
FP is a professor of Pediatrics and Clinical Medicine at Herlev and Gentofte Hospital, Denmark and University of Copenhagen, Denmark. FP received his

MD from University of Copenhagen and performed his doctoral research at Steno Diabetes Center, Denmark. FP has a strong focus on clinical markers for residual β cell function and to identify early markers for type 1 diabetes risk. FP has been part of the Type 1 Diabetes Genetics Consortium (T1DGC) Steering Group, which published the largest GWAS (genome-wide association study) in T1D. FP has published more than 300 papers in peer reviewed journals accruing >14,000 citations. FP has been ranked no. 21, worldwide by cited papers within the field of Diabetes 1991–2001 and his H-index is 51.

Consent for publication
Not applicable.

Competing interests
The authors declare that they have no competing interests.

Author details
[1]CPH-DIRECT, Department of Pediatrics, Herlev University Hospital, Herlev Ringvej 75, DK-2730 Herlev, Denmark. [2]Faculty of Health and Medical Sciences, University of Copenhagen, Copenhagen, Denmark. [3]Center for non-coding RNA in Technology and Health, University of Copenhagen, Copenhagen, Denmark.

References
1. Pociot F, Akolkar B, Concannon P, Erlich HA, Julier C, Morahan G, et al. Genetics of type 1 diabetes: what's next? Diabetes. 2010;59:1561–71.
2. Groop L, Pociot F. Genetics of diabetes—are we missing the genes or the disease? Mol Cell Endocrinol. 2014;382:726–39.
3. Soleimanpour SA, Stoffers DA. The pancreatic β cell and type 1 diabetes: innocent bystander or active participant? Trends Endocrinol Metab. 2013;24:324–31.
4. Noble JA, Erlich HA. Genetics of type 1 diabetes. Cold Spring Harb Perspect Med. 2012;2:a007732.
5. Rich SS, Concannon P, Erlich H, Julier C, Morahan G, Nerup J, et al. The type 1 diabetes genetics consortium. Ann N Y Acad Sci. 2006;1079:1–8.
6. Barrett JC, Clayton DG, Concannon P, Akolkar B, Cooper JD, Erlich HA, et al. Genome-wide association study and meta-analysis find that over 40 loci affect risk of type 1 diabetes. Nat Genet. 2009;41:703–7.
7. Onengut-Gumuscu S, Chen W-M, Burren O, Cooper NJ, Quinlan AR, Mychaleckyj JC, et al. Fine mapping of type 1 diabetes susceptibility loci and evidence for colocalization of causal variants with lymphoid gene enhancers. Nat Genet. 2015;47:381–6.
8. Santin I, Eizirik DL. Candidate genes for type 1 diabetes modulate pancreatic islet inflammation and β-cell apoptosis. Diabetes Obes Metab. 2013;15(Suppl 3):71–81.
9. Rinn JL, Chang HY. Genome regulation by long noncoding RNAs. Annu Rev Biochem. 2012;81:145–66.
10. Knoll M, Lodish HF, Sun L. Long non-coding RNAs as regulators of the endocrine system. Nat Rev Endocrinol. 2015;11:151–60.
11. Lam MTY, Li W, Rosenfeld MG, Glass CK. Enhancer RNAs and regulated transcriptional programs. Trends Biochem Sci. 2014;39:170–82.
12. Ulitsky I, Bartel DP. lincRNAs: genomics, evolution, and mechanisms. Cell. 2013;154:26–46.
13. Fitzgerald KA, Caffrey DR. Long noncoding RNAs in innate and adaptive immunity. Curr Opin Immunol. 2014;26:140–6.
14. Khalil AM, Guttman M, Huarte M, Garber M, Raj A, Rivea Morales D, et al. Many human large intergenic noncoding RNAs associate with chromatin-modifying complexes and affect gene expression. Proc Natl Acad Sci U S A. 2009;106:11667–72.
15. Guttman M, Amit I, Garber M, French C, Lin MF, Feldser D, et al. Chromatin signature reveals over a thousand highly conserved large non-coding RNAs in mammals. Nature. 2009;458:223–7.
16. Eliasson L, Esguerra JLS. Role of non-coding RNAs in pancreatic beta-cell development and physiology. Acta Physiol (Oxf). 2014;211:273–84.
17. Motterle A, Gattesco S, Caille D, Meda P, Regazzi R. Involvement of long non-coding RNAs in beta cell failure at the onset of type 1 diabetes in NOD mice. Diabetologia. 2015;58:1827–35.
18. Morán I, Akerman I, van de Bunt M, Xie R, Benazra M, Nammo T, et al. Human β cell transcriptome analysis uncovers lncRNAs that are tissue-specific, dynamically regulated, and abnormally expressed in type 2 diabetes. Cell Metab. 2012;16:435–48.
19. Ku GM, Kim H, Vaughn IW, Hangauer MJ, Myung Oh C, German MS, et al. Research resource: RNA-Seq reveals unique features of the pancreatic β-cell transcriptome. Mol Endocrinol. 2012;26:1783–92.
20. Liu J-Y, Yao J, Li X-M, Song Y-C, Wang X-Q, Li Y-J, et al. Pathogenic role of lncRNA-MALAT1 in endothelial cell dysfunction in diabetes mellitus. Cell Death Dis. 2014;5:e1506.
21. Wallace C, Smyth DJ, Maisuria-Armer M, Walker NM, Todd JA, Clayton DG. The imprinted DLK1-MEG3 gene region on chromosome 14q32.2 alters susceptibility to type 1 diabetes. Nat Genet. 2010;42:68–71.
22. You L, Wang N, Yin D, Wang L, Jin F, Zhu Y, et al. Downregulation of long noncoding RNA Meg3 affects insulin synthesis and secretion in mouse pancreatic beta cells. J Cell Physiol. 2016;231:852–62.
23. Arnes L, Akerman I, Balderes DA, Ferrer J, Sussel L. βlinc1 encodes a long noncoding RNA that regulates islet β-cell formation and function. Genes Dev. 2016;30:502–7.
24. Akerman I, Tu Z, Beucher A, Rolando DMY, Sauty-Colace C, Benazra M, et al. Human pancreatic β cell lncRNAs control cell-specific regulatory networks. Cell Metab. 2017;25:400–11.
25. Yin D, Zhang E, You L, Wang N, Wang L, Jin F, et al. Downregulation of lncRNA TUG1 affects apoptosis and insulin secretion in mouse pancreatic β cells. Cell Physiol Biochem. 2015;35:1892–904.
26. Li J, Xuan Z, Liu C. Long non-coding RNAs and complex human diseases. Int J Mol Sci. 2013;14:18790–808.
27. Hrdlickova B, de Almeida RC, Borek Z, Withoff S. Genetic variation in the non-coding genome: involvement of micro-RNAs and long non-coding RNAs in disease. Biochim Biophys Acta. 1842;2014:1910–22.
28. Hrdlickova B, Kumar V, Kanduri K, Zhernakova DV, Tripathi S, Karjalainen J, et al. Expression profiles of long non-coding RNAs located in autoimmune disease-associated regions reveal immune cell-type specificity. Genome Med. 2014;6:88.
29. Carpenter S, Aiello D, Atianand MK, Ricci EP, Gandhi P, Hall LL, et al. A long noncoding RNA mediates both activation and repression of immune response genes. Science. 2013;341:789–92.
30. Atianand MK, Fitzgerald KA. Long non-coding RNAs and control of gene expression in the immune system. Trends Mol Med. 2014;20:623–31.
31. Li Z, Chao T-C, Chang K-Y, Lin N, Patil VS, Shimizu C, et al. The long noncoding RNA THRIL regulates TNFα expression through its interaction with hnRNPL. Proc Natl Acad Sci U S A. 2014;111:1002–7.
32. Krawczyk M, Emerson BM. p50-associated COX-2 extragenic RNA (PACER) activates COX-2 gene expression by occluding repressive NF-κB complexes. elife. 2014;3:e01776.
33. Ilott NE, Heward JA, Roux B, Tsitsiou E, Fenwick PS, Lenzi L, et al. Long non-coding RNAs and enhancer RNAs regulate the lipopolysaccharide-induced inflammatory response in human monocytes. Nat Commun. 2014;5:3979.
34. Lu J, Wu X, Hong M, Tobias P, Han J. A potential suppressive effect of natural antisense IL-1β RNA on lipopolysaccharide-induced IL-1β expression. J Immunol. 2013;190:6570–8.
35. Carpenter S, Fitzgerald KA. Transcription of inflammatory genes: long noncoding RNA and beyond. J Interf Cytokine Res. 2015;35:79–88.
36. Gomez JA, Wapinski OL, Yang YW, Bureau J-F, Gopinath S, Monack DM, et al. The NeST long ncRNA controls microbial susceptibility and epigenetic activation of the interferon-γ locus. Cell. 2013;152:743–54.
37. Collier SP, Collins PL, Williams CL, Boothby MR, Aune TM. Cutting edge: influence of Tmevpg1, a long intergenic noncoding RNA, on the expression of Ifng by Th1 cells. J Immunol. 2012;189:2084–8.
38. Rapicavoli NA, Qu K, Zhang J, Mikhail M, Laberge R-M, Chang HY. A mammalian pseudogene lncRNA at the interface of inflammation and anti-inflammatory therapeutics. elife. 2013;2:e00762.

39. Wang P, Xue Y, Han Y, Lin L, Wu C, Xu S, et al. The STAT3-binding long noncoding RNA lnc-DC controls human dendritic cell differentiation. Science. 2014;344:310–3.
40. Ryba-Stanisławowska M, Skrzypkowska M, Myśliwiec M, Myśliwska J. Loss of the balance between CD4(+)Foxp3(+) regulatory T cells and CD4(+)IL17A(+) Th17 cells in patients with type 1 diabetes. Hum Immunol. 2013;74:701–7.
41. Ferraro A, Socci C, Stabilini A, Valle A, Monti P, Piemonti L, et al. Expansion of Th17 cells and functional defects in T regulatory cells are key features of the pancreatic lymph nodes in patients with type 1 diabetes. Diabetes. 2011;60:2903–13.
42. Huang W, Thomas B, Flynn RA, Gavzy SJ, Wu L, Kim SV, et al. DDX5 and its associated lncRNA Rmrp modulate TH17 cell effector functions. Nature. 2015;528:517–22.
43. Ricaño-Ponce I, Wijmenga C. Mapping of immune-mediated disease genes. Annu Rev Genomics Hum Genet. 2013;14:325–53.
44. Schaub MA, Boyle AP, Kundaje A, Batzoglou S, Snyder M. Linking disease associations with regulatory information in the human genome. Genome Res. 2012;22:1748–59.
45. Hoffman MM, Ernst J, Wilder SP, Kundaje A, Harris RS, Libbrecht M, et al. Integrative annotation of chromatin elements from ENCODE data. Nucleic Acids Res. 2013;41:827–41.
46. Gong J, Liu W, Zhang J, Miao X, Guo A-Y. lncRNASNP: a database of SNPs in lncRNAs and their potential functions in human and mouse. Nucleic Acids Res. 2015; 43(Database issue):D181–D186.
47. Kumar V, Westra H-J, Karjalainen J, Zhernakova DV, Esko T, Hrdlickova B, et al. Human disease-associated genetic variation impacts large intergenic non-coding RNA expression. PLoS Genet. 2013;9:e1003201.
48. Ørom UA, Derrien T, Beringer M, Gumireddy K, Gardini A, Bussotti G, et al. Long noncoding RNAs with enhancer-like function in human cells. Cell. 2010;143:46–58.
49. Guttman M, Donaghey J, Carey BW, Garber M, Grenier JK, Munson G, et al. lincRNAs act in the circuitry controlling pluripotency and differentiation. Nature. 2011;477:295–300.
50. Visel A, Rubin EM, Pennacchio LA. Genomic views of distant-acting enhancers. Nature. 2009;461:199–205.
51. Sakabe NJ, Savic D, Nobrega MA. Transcriptional enhancers in development and disease. Genome Biol. 2012;13:238.
52. Sanyal A, Lajoie BR, Jain G, Dekker J. The long-range interaction landscape of gene promoters. Nature. 2012;489:109–13.
53. Corradin O, Saiakhova A, Akhtar-Zaidi B, Myeroff L, Willis J, Cowper-Sal lari R, et al. Combinatorial effects of multiple enhancer variants in linkage disequilibrium dictate levels of gene expression to confer susceptibility to common traits. Genome Res. 2014;24:1–13.
54. Visel A, Blow MJ, Li Z, Zhang T, Akiyama JA, Holt A, et al. ChIP-seq accurately predicts tissue-specific activity of enhancers. Nature. 2009;457:854–8.
55. Heintzman ND, Hon GC, Hawkins RD, Kheradpour P, Stark A, Harp LF, et al. Histone modifications at human enhancers reflect global cell-type-specific gene expression. Nature. 2009;459:108–12.
56. Rada-Iglesias A, Bajpai R, Swigut T, Brugmann SA, Flynn RA, Wysocka J. A unique chromatin signature uncovers early developmental enhancers in humans. Nature. 2011;470:279–83.
57. Andersson R, Gebhard C, Miguel-Escalada I, Hoof I, Bornholdt J, Boyd M, et al. An atlas of active enhancers across human cell types and tissues. Nature. 2014;507:455–61.
58. Kadauke S, Blobel GA. Chromatin loops in gene regulation. Biochim Biophys Acta. 1789;2009:17–25.
59. Deng W, Lee J, Wang H, Miller J, Reik A, Gregory PD, et al. Controlling long-range genomic interactions at a native locus by targeted tethering of a looping factor. Cell. 2012;149:1233–44.
60. Dekker J, Rippe K, Dekker M, Kleckner N. Capturing chromosome conformation. Science. 2002;295:1306–11.
61. Zhao Z, Tavoosidana G, Sjölinder M, Göndör A, Mariano P, Wang S, et al. Circular chromosome conformation capture (4C) uncovers extensive networks of epigenetically regulated intra- and interchromosomal interactions. Nat Genet. 2006;38:1341–7.
62. Dostie J, Richmond TA, Arnaout RA, Selzer RR, Lee WL, Honan TA, et al. Chromosome conformation capture carbon copy (5C): a massively parallel solution for mapping interactions between genomic elements. Genome Res. 2006;16:1299–309.
63. Fullwood MJ, Liu MH, Pan YF, Liu J, Xu H, Mohamed YB, et al. An oestrogen-receptor-alpha-bound human chromatin interactome. Nature. 2009;462:58–64.
64. Lieberman-Aiden E, van Berkum NL, Williams L, Imakaev M, Ragoczy T, Telling A, et al. Comprehensive mapping of long-range interactions reveals folding principles of the human genome. Science. 2009;326:289–93.
65. Carter D, Chakalova L, Osborne CS, Dai Y, Fraser P. Long-range chromatin regulatory interactions in vivo. Nat Genet. 2002;32:623–6.
66. Tolhuis B, Palstra RJ, Splinter E, Grosveld F, de Laat W. Looping and interaction between hypersensitive sites in the active beta-globin locus. Mol Cell. 2002;10:1453–65.
67. Vernimmen D, De Gobbi M, Sloane-Stanley JA, Wood WG, Higgs DR. Long-range chromosomal interactions regulate the timing of the transition between poised and active gene expression. EMBO J. 2007;26:2041–51.
68. Spilianakis CG, Flavell RA. Long-range intrachromosomal interactions in the T helper type 2 cytokine locus. Nat Immunol. 2004;5:1017–27.
69. Kumar PP, Bischof O, Purbey PK, Notani D, Urlaub H, Dejean A, et al. Functional interaction between PML and SATB1 regulates chromatin-loop architecture and transcription of the MHC class I locus. Nat Cell Biol. 2007;9:45–56.
70. Horike S, Cai S, Miyano M, Cheng J-F, Kohwi-Shigematsu T. Loss of silent-chromatin looping and impaired imprinting of DLX5 in Rett syndrome. Nat Genet. 2005;37:31–40.
71. Murrell A, Heeson S, Reik W. Interaction between differentially methylated regions partitions the imprinted genes Igf2 and H19 into parent-specific chromatin loops. Nat Genet. 2004;36:889–93.
72. Kurukuti S, Tiwari VK, Tavoosidana G, Pugacheva E, Murrell A, Zhao Z, et al. CTCF binding at the H19 imprinting control region mediates maternally inherited higher-order chromatin conformation to restrict enhancer access to Igf2. Proc Natl Acad Sci U S A. 2006;103:10684–9.
73. Yoon YS, Jeong S, Rong Q, Park K-Y, Chung JH, Pfeifer K. Analysis of the H19ICR insulator. Mol Cell Biol. 2007;27:3499–510.
74. Spilianakis CG, Lalioti MD, Town T, Lee GR, Flavell RA. Interchromosomal associations between alternatively expressed loci. Nature. 2005;435:637–45.
75. Park J-H, Choi Y, Song M-J, Park K, Lee J-J, Kim H-P. Dynamic long-range chromatin interaction controls expression of IL-21 in CD4+ T cells. J Immunol. 2016;196:4378–89.
76. ENCODE Project Consortium, Birney E, Stamatoyannopoulos JA, Dutta A, Guigó R, Gingeras TR, et al. Identification and analysis of functional elements in 1% of the human genome by the ENCODE pilot project. Nature. 2007;447:799–816.
77. Li MJ, Sham PC, Wang J. Genetic variant representation, annotation and prioritization in the post-GWAS era. Cell Res. 2012;22:1505–8.
78. Raychaudhuri S. VIZ-GRAIL: visualizing functional connections across disease loci. Bioinformatics. 2011;27:1589–90.
79. Kaur S, Mirza AH, Brorsson CA, Fløyel T, Størling J, Mortensen HB, et al. The genetic and regulatory architecture of ERBB3-type 1 diabetes susceptibility locus. Mol Cell Endocrinol. 2016;419:83–91.
80. Kim T-K, Hemberg M, Gray JM. Enhancer RNAs: a class of long noncoding RNAs synthesized at enhancers. Cold Spring Harb Perspect Biol. 2015;7:a018622.
81. Murakami S, Gadad SS, Kraus WL. A PreSTIGEous use of LncRNAs to predict enhancers. Cell Cycle. 2015;14:1619–20.
82. Ørom UA, Shiekhattar R. Long noncoding RNAs usher in a new era in the biology of enhancers. Cell. 2013;154:1190–3.
83. Tian D, Sun S, Lee JT. The long noncoding RNA, Jpx, is a molecular switch for X chromosome inactivation. Cell. 2010;143:390–403.
84. Lai F, Orom UA, Cesaroni M, Beringer M, Taatjes DJ, Blobel GA, et al. Activating RNAs associate with mediator to enhance chromatin architecture and transcription. Nature. 2013;494:497–501.
85. Pasquali L, Gaulton KJ, Rodríguez-Seguí SA, Mularoni L, Miguel-Escalada I, Akerman I, et al. Pancreatic islet enhancer clusters enriched in type 2 diabetes risk-associated variants. Nat Genet. 2014;46:136–43.
86. Lee GL, Dobi A, Srivastava S. Prostate cancer: diagnostic performance of the PCA3 urine test. Nat Rev Urol. 2011;8:123–4.
87. Diederichs S. The four dimensions of noncoding RNA conservation. Trends Genet. 2014;30:121–3.
88. Cabili MN, Trapnell C, Goff L, Koziol M, Tazon-Vega B, Regev A, et al. Integrative annotation of human large intergenic noncoding RNAs reveals global properties and specific subclasses. Genes Dev. 2011;25:1915–27.
89. Mercer TR, Mattick JS. Structure and function of long noncoding RNAs in epigenetic regulation. Nat Struct Mol Biol. 2013;20:300–7.
90. Hon CC, Ramilowski JA, Harshbarger J, Bertin N, Rackham OJ, Gough J, et al. An atlas of human long non-coding RNAs with accurate 5′ ends. Nature. 2017;543:199–204.

91. Derrien T, Johnson R, Bussotti G, Tanzer A, Djebali S, Tilgner H, et al. The GENCODE v7 catalog of human long noncoding RNAs: analysis of their gene structure, evolution, and expression. Genome Res. 2012;22:1775–89.
92. Mercer TR, Gerhardt DJ, Dinger ME, Crawford J, Trapnell C, Jeddeloh JA, et al. Targeted RNA sequencing reveals the deep complexity of the human transcriptome. Nat Biotechnol. 2011;30:99–104.
93. Lagarde J, Uszczynska-Ratajczak B, Santoyo-Lopez J, Gonzalez JM, Tapanari E, Mudge JM, et al. Extension of human lncRNA transcripts by RACE coupled with long-read high-throughput sequencing (RACE-Seq). Nat Commun. 2016;7:12339.
94. Lagarde J, Uszczynska-Ratajczak B, Carbonell S, Davis C, Gingeras TR, Frankish A. High-throughput annotation of full-length long noncoding RNAs with capture long-read sequencing (CLS). bioRxiv. 2017;105064. doi: https://doi.org/10.1101/105064.
95. Liu SJ, Horlbeck MA, Cho SW, Birk HS, Malatesta M, He D, et al. CRISPRi-based genome-scale identification of functional long noncoding RNA loci in human cells. Science. 2017;355. doi: 10.1126/science.aah7111.
96. Nica AC, Ongen H, Irminger JC, Bosco D, Berney T, Antonarakis SE, et al. Cell-type, allelic, and genetic signatures in the human pancreatic beta cell transcriptome. Genome Res. 2013;23:1554–62.
97. Li W, Notani D, Rosenfeld MG. Enhancers as non-coding RNA transcription units: recent insights and future perspectives. Nat Rev Genet. 2016;17:207–23.

13

Precision medicine at the crossroads

Maynard V. Olson[1,2]

Abstract: There are bioethical, institutional, economic, legal, and cultural obstacles to creating the robust-precompetitive-data resource that will be required to advance the vision of "precision medicine," the ability to use molecular data to target therapies to patients for whom they offer the most benefit at the least risk. Creation of such an "information commons" was the central recommendation of the 2011 report *Toward Precision Medicine* issued by a committee of the National Research Council of the USA (Committee on a Framework for Development of a New Taxonomy of Disease; National Research Council. Toward precision medicine: building a knowledge network for biomedical research and a new taxonomy of disease. 2011). In this commentary, I review the rationale for creating an information commons and the obstacles to doing so; then, I endorse a path forward based on the dynamic consent of research subjects interacting with researchers through trusted mediators. I assert that the advantages of the proposed system overwhelm alternative ways of handling data on the phenotypes, genotypes, and environmental exposures of individual humans; hence, I argue that its creation should be the central policy objective of early efforts to make precision medicine a reality.

Introduction

In human genomics today, one question looms above all others. How are we going to handle data on the phenotypes, genotypes, and environmental exposures of individual humans [1]? These data are already the lifeblood of our field and will play an increasingly dominant role in human-genomic research for decades, if not centuries, to come. We already collect these data in quantities that were unthinkable a few years ago, and a tsunami of new data will soon be upon us. Indeed, this metaphor is inadequate. Tsunamis are discrete, rare events that do a lot of damage and then recede. Survivors bury the dead, pick up the debris, beef up seawalls, and get on with their lives. In contrast, we are not dealing with a one-time event: the flux of data about human phenotypes, genotypes, and environmental influences will just keep growing, exponentially or super-exponentially, for the foreseeable future. Furthermore, the basic character of these data will differ greatly from those that human genomicists have gathered in the past. We need a strategic plan for managing these data, and it is increasingly obvious we lack one.

Geneticists and genomicists like change and have a good record of adapting to it. Consider the rapidity with which recombinant-DNA and genomic techniques allowed human geneticists to solve longstanding problems in the 1980s and 1990s. In that era, much of the energy of human geneticists went into exploring local features of the human genome in cottage-industry fashion. Once the whole genome had been sequenced, the energy once expended mapping out megabase-pair-sized regions, no easy task in the 1980s, was freed up for more scientifically rewarding endeavors. An optimist might imagine a similarly smooth transition from the current era, in which human genomicists and their collaborators expend enormous energy enrolling patients in one-off research studies, to an era in which huge data sets containing genomic, phenotypic, and environmental data on millions of recontactable people become widely available. In this essay, I argue this will not happen unless we make a big push now to create a true information commons. Inaction or misdirected actions pose an existential threat to the open-science traditions of human genomics. In what follows, I elaborate on this alarmist view and sketch a path forward that offers a more promising future for all stakeholders than the path we are now on.

Correspondence: mvo@u.washington.edu
[1]Department of Medicine, University of Washington, Seattle, Washington 98195, USA
[2]Department of Genome Sciences, University of Washington, Seattle, Washington 98195, USA

Lessons of history

From its inception, genomics has had a split personality. In one guise, genomics is an interdisciplinary field that brings a distinctive point of view and set of increasingly powerful techniques to the analysis of diverse problems in basic biology. From this perspective, although some genomic data have utilitarian value, pursuit of practical applications is not the field's *raison d'être*. In another guise, genomics is on a fast track to providing humans with long, healthy lives and making a few venturesome genomicists rich. During the dot-com bubble of the late 1990s, which was accompanied by a biotech bubble, a company developing gene-analysis platforms ran an advertisement showing a double helix rising up through brightly colored mist, accompanied by the slogan "At the top of this ladder is a world without disease" [2]. This slogan is just plain stupid. Not only do we, like all other mortal agents, lack the ability to banish disease from the human condition, we risk creating new niches for disease at a faster pace than we attenuate or eradicate old ones. There is a reason why pneumonia was once called "the old man's friend." Advances in medicine have always involved a delicate balance, easily gotten wrong, between increasing health and increasing disease, the latter effect arising when heavily medicalized lives are extended beyond reasonable limits. The more effective genomic medicine becomes, the more vulnerable it will be to the latter trap.

This risk notwithstanding, human genomics has managed its dual personality tolerably well. There has been some embarrassment when mostly friendly critics ask "Where are the goods?" but these queries have been little more than polite requests that some of our noisier colleagues lower their voices. We have retained public support because many people recognize that genomics has already delivered a lot of goods, both directly and indirectly. Direct benefits have been realized in areas such as genetic testing and DNA forensics, while indirect ones have accrued on a much broader front. The indirection of most of genomics' contributions to biology is a natural consequence of what genomics is. Genomicists solve few problems on their own, but they empower all biological research at the molecular level and even much research at higher levels of biological organization. A plausible analogy can be made with computer science, most of whose contributions to scientific knowledge and societal wellbeing are also indirect.

Of course, from time to time, tension between genomics' two personae has flared up. Controversies about the wholesale patenting of gene sequences are one example [3]. The conflict between public and private sector participation in the Human Genome Project (HGP) is another [4]. The mantra of the major private sector participant in the HGP was "Discovery can't wait!" Evidently, what discovery could not wait for were the processes that communities of scientists rely on to accumulate broadly accessible knowledge, insure high-quality standards, and keep tabs on each other's behavior. Scientists such as myself, who argued for balancing the desirability of moving quickly in the HGP with that of preserving the Mertonian virtues of communalism, universalism, disinterestedness, and organized skepticism, were attacked for being indifferent to the suffering of patients whose treatment might benefit, in some unspecified way, from turning the HGP into a crash program [2, 5].

Those were yesterday's battles, which were largely won by proponents of open science. In the USA, we now have a unanimous Supreme Court decision that prevents the use of patent law to restrict free use of bulk genome sequences [6]. We have a high-quality reference sequence of the human genome that is accessible to all, large public repositories of human genetic variation data, and a robust research community that continually adds value to these resources through peer-reviewed publications in the open literature.

The present dilemma

Threats to the open-science tradition in human genomics now come from several directions, particularly with regard to research on human phenotype-genotype correlations. Since research in this area is likely to dominate human genomics for the foreseeable future, these threats demand our closest attention. Here is a brief outline of the reasons the open-science traditions of our field are under threat:

- *Exaggerated concerns about patient privacy.* Privacy concerns are the main obstacle to an open-science approach to the study of human phenotype-genotype correlations. An elaborate web of laws, regulations, cultural practices, and entrenched beliefs walls off rich data sets about individual humans from the research community. Given the long history of genetic exceptionalism in attitudes toward privacy [7–9], there is no way to undo or redo past decisions. The only path forward is to empower patients to choose the level of privacy they are comfortable with and then attempt to persuade them, one at a time, to make choices that will allow research to go forward. I outline below how such a system might work and argue that there are reasons to hope that patients and their families will prove more willing to contribute their data to an information commons than many believe they will be. The potential for abusive efforts to identify research participants through their genetic profiles or information in their medical records will only grow in the future. It cannot be eliminated. We simply need to bring genetic privacy into the same tent that houses the escalating privacy concerns that permeate modern life, not treat them as something unique unto themselves. People will always vary greatly in the level and nature of their privacy concerns. Our current impulse to impose paternalistically one-size-fits-all ways of addressing them are both futile and, arguably, unethical.

- Increasing reliance of the biomedical research community on large health care delivery systems. The only feasible way of acquiring phenotypic data on millions of individuals is by capturing information collected in the ordinary course of clinical care. With patient consent and supplementary funding, these data could be augmented with genotypic and phenotypic assessments that are safe and easily carried out, even when not medically indicated. Large health care delivery systems are the only organizations that can house and conduct this activity. No other approach will be affordable, sustainable, or logistically feasible. It is one thing to gather supplementary molecular data on tissue samples collected in the ordinary course of clinical care but quite another to imagine that millions of people are going to participate regularly in a parallel system of phenotypic assessment for much of their lives. A three-way marriage between patients, researchers, and health care delivery systems will be awkward, but it offers the only path forward. The rule in building relationships that make sense for all parties—even if there is little mutual attraction or even natural compatibility among them—is "one step at a time." I outline below an incremental approach that would observe this rule and be a better use of public resources than hurried efforts to enroll a lot of patients in inadequately designed, underfunded, long-term studies.
- *Increasing reliance of everyone on the information technology (IT) industry.* The days are gone when human genomicists should be building and maintaining their own information technology infrastructure. Major resources are presently wasted supporting legacy systems that made sense in the 1990s but should now be retired. At a time when large corporations are downsizing IT departments and outsourcing computing needs to companies that actually know how to deal with the twenty-first century data, most research centers cling to do-it-yourself operations. The good news is that computing, like sequencing, is getting cheap. The bad news is that the growing gap between the computing capabilities of typical research centers and those of the IT industry risks driving population-scale genomics into the arms of this industry without any strategic plan to maintain public control over the data. Health care delivery systems already have the relationships with patients that are the sine qua non of population genomics and have reasons of their own to want to increase their involvement in research on medically relevant phenotypes, genotypes, and environmental influences. IT companies are the only entities capable of managing the data. Hence, for advocates of open science, the obvious risk is that players in these two sectors will join forces, relegating both academic researchers and the public interest to the sidelines. Of course, academic researchers will still be consulted when it suits the needs of private sector genomic companies, but the consultations will occur on their terms, not ours.
- *Self-interest.* So far, I have emphasized the external forces favoring privatization of population-scale genomics. Now, I turn to internal practices within human genomics that contribute to this threat. Communities that aspire to make the world a better place should always start by looking in the mirror. Human genomics has a mixed record on data sharing, and my proposals will be no more welcome to some of my academic colleagues than to many entrepreneurs seeking commercial opportunity in the marriage of genomics and medicine. Human genomics is a fusion discipline forged from two fields with different data-sharing practices. Genomics largely grew out of model-organism biology, in which sharing of strains, protocols, and data have long been the norm. In contrast, human genetics has never had a strong data-sharing tradition: human geneticists "own" their patients and guard access to them zealously. The reasons for these divergent traditions are easy enough to understand. Researchers develop relationships of mutual trust with human research subjects but not with yeast strains and mouse lines. Furthermore, access to patients and patient data is now restricted by a tangle of bureaucratic, regulatory, and legal constraints. Nonetheless, self-interest is a more formidable obstacle to data sharing than laws like the Health Insurance Portability and Accountability Act in the USA [10]. Careers are often built by enrolling valuable patient populations in research studies and then permanently sequestering them from competitors. As the sizes of these populations increase, it is not just individual careers but whole research bureaucracies that sometimes appear more focused on controlling access to their valuable patient resources than solving scientific problems. If we are to create an information commons containing comprehensive data about individual research subjects, this system must be reformed.

These bullet points frame the present dilemma. The task of addressing any one of them would be daunting enough, but, given the way they reinforce each another, advocates of maintaining and enhancing an open-science tradition in human genomics will need to address all at once. Perhaps the impulse to do so is simply Quixotic. What motivates me is a dystopian vision of the way research in our field is likely to evolve if we let current momentum carry us where it will. For starters, a business-as-usual scenario will increasingly marginalize academic researchers in human genomics, a community already under stress. Academic researchers will find that the legal and regulatory systems that once protected their proprietary access to particular patient populations can be deployed to far greater effect by privatized entities formed through alliances between health care delivery systems and the IT industry. These organizations will hire the legal staffs and lobbyists they need to lock down everything they control that has commercial value. Federal agencies such as the National Institutes of Health (NIH) in the USA, created to represent and promote the public interest in biomedical research, are also at risk. The regulatory power of the NIH depends on the ability of its Institutes to make grant funding contingent on agreement by researchers and their institutions to do things the NIH way. The NIH's Institutes are not true regulatory agencies: they lack the experience, staff, and standing to oversee a sprawling, privatized research enterprise that is deeply embedded in a multi-trillion-dollar-per-year industry. Agencies that do regulate that industry will acquire de facto control over most research as an indirect consequence of their responsibilities in regulating patient care. Programs such as the Precision Medicine Initiative (recently rebranded the *All of Us* Research Program), which was launched with great fanfare by an administration no longer in office [11], are likely to end up under-funded, under-powered, over-regulated, and unable to deliver on their promise. Legislators who would welcome increasing privatization of biomedical research and attendant tightening of the link between research and commercial opportunities will see the NIH's mission as increasingly irrelevant to their priorities. The situation in the USA will differ less from that in countries with government-sponsored national health care systems than one might imagine. Federal and state governments already pay for two thirds of health care in the USA with most of the money coming from Washington, D.C. [12].

Not everyone, even within academia, will consider the future scenarios I have sketched as undesirable. Hence, before proposing an alternative future for population-scale genomics, I will briefly defend my view that science, industry, and society would all benefit if key players take bold action now to design a more open future for population-scale genomics. My argument rests on the societal value of defending a line, or perhaps zone is a better descriptor, separating precompetitive and proprietary knowledge. I think all players—science, industry, and the larger society—win if we give careful consideration to the types of data and knowledge that belong on one side of the line or the other. Science wins when researchers have unencumbered access to as much data and knowledge as possible since, at least on a time scale of decades, the messy processes associated with open science overwhelm the transient advantages that sometimes accrue to closed organizations. As private sector partisans like to point out, academia cannot match the ability of closed organizations to raise capital, build infrastructure, manage skilled workforces, and act decisively. However, one cannot manage one's way to identifying and exploring the "unknown unknowns" that stand in the way of our ability to achieve better health. Industry wins because commercial organizations can focus on what they do best: determining whether or not seemingly good ideas are market-ready and, if so, shepherding them through the research and development pipeline that actually delivers drugs, diagnostic tests, and medical devices from bench to bedside. Society wins for the simple reason that practical advances in the modern world are tightly linked to expanding knowledge, and open science has a large edge over other systems as a way of learning new things. For these reasons, I am confident that bold action to create a precompetitive information commons would be a win-win-win proposition for science, industry, and society.

What should be done

Questions about what should be done are ultimately about power: in whose hands should it reside and how should it be deployed? I will borrow my answer to this question from the title of a paper by Sharon and Patrick Terry [13], two tireless advocates of increased data sharing in biomedical research: "Power to the People!" Empowering the people on whose cooperation population-scale genomics will depend, and for whose benefit it should be carried out, would solve a whole nexus of problems. I have been referring to these volunteers as "patients" and "research subjects," but, first and foremost, they are just us. The volunteers who will have to contribute DNA, images of their internal organs, samples of their body fluids, and access to their electronic medical records to the commons are just us, all of us.

We need to promote a new social contract between patients and the health care systems on which they depend. Susan Desmond-Hellmann, who co-chaired the committee of the United States National Research Council that issued the report *Toward Precision Medicine*, a committee on which I served, articulated the need for this new contract in an editorial in *Science Translational Medicine* [14]:

I believe that the most important requirement for the new knowledge network envisaged by the *Precision Medicine* report is that it be driven by patients. Indeed, it is patients who particularly understand the potential value of a social contract in which patients both contribute personal clinical data and benefit from the knowledge gained through the collaboration... Patient advocacy can best ensure that policy-makers in the U.S. Congress and elsewhere understand that well-intended efforts to guard patient privacy could impede the kind of data sharing required to accelerate the cures all are awaiting.

I see no alternative to a patient-centered approach. We must dismantle the paternalistic system administered by self-interested and self-appointed protectors of research subjects. Increasingly, what these parties actually protect patients from are the potential benefits of a system in which precompetitive information flows freely from bedside to lab bench (or computer terminal!) and then, largely via commercial enterprises, back to the bedside again. I am not advocating relieving institutions of the responsibility to guarantee that research subjects are fully informed and that the studies they enroll in are safely and expertly carried out. However, institutions should focus on protecting patients from procedural harm and careless handling of their medical records, not from hypothetical informational risks: if blood is to be drawn, the quantity should be reasonable and the draw conducted professionally; if images are to be acquired, associated risks should be clearly explained and the images competently acquired and interpreted; electronic medical records should be maintained in standard formats and stored on secure computer systems. However, if I, as an independent researcher with no ties to the initial study in which a patient enrolled, want access to raw data about the patient, my request should go directly to the patient, or to his or her designated agent, not to the researchers who carried out the original study or the institutions that employ them.

Fortunately, there is already significant experience designing systems that work this way [13, 15–17]. What we need is the will to use them and the vision to understand the central role they could play in coupling basic science to medicine. To make a patient-centered system work on the scale required, we would need to foster the development of a new type of organization, which Erlich et al. have dubbed the "trusted mediator" [17]. The trust in question is between the research participant and the mediator; the mediation is between the research participant and researchers who want access to the participant's data. In many cases, existing patient-advocacy organizations could expand their missions to play this role. Over the long haul, a variety of trusted-mediation models would undoubtedly emerge since the needs of different classes of research participants would vary greatly; for example, patients suffering from a rare genetic disease that manifests itself at or soon after birth would require different protections than healthy adults who simply want to contribute their data to the general good. Competition between trusted-mediator organizations should be encouraged, and patients should be free to transfer their loyalties from one to another at any time. The key point is to eliminate the conflicts of interest that corrupt the current system. The fiduciary duty of an idealized trusted mediator should be to a single individual, the research participant whose data are at issue.

Of course, as databases grow to include information about millions of individuals, grouping of individuals into classes is inevitable. Most research participants would be willing to select one of a modest number of standard protocols, ranging from unrestricted sharing to case-by-case consideration of data access requests. For large studies, this system could evolve into a far more efficient system for assembling research subjects than current methods since subject acquisition would largely be a matter of computers talking to other computers. The sensitive steps involved in informing subjects of the risks and benefits of participation and allowing them time to consider their personal preferences would have already occurred before any particular study entered the picture.

Through social media, research participants could discuss their experiences with other individuals who are considering adopting particular sharing protocols. Given the scarcity of documented instances of informational harm to research participants, a reasonable expectation is that these discussions would often reassure newcomers that even the most permissive protocols pose minimal risk. Peer counseling would be particularly important in shaping the willingness of research participants to be recontacted by researchers for specific purposes. We have inflated recontact of research subjects into an unnecessarily vexing issue. It should become a routine option in all research studies. The key to making it one would be to channel recontact requests through trusted mediators. These mediators would know which option patients have chosen from a menu of choices. For example:

- "Allow researchers to do anything they want with the data they already have but leave me alone."
- "Screen recontact requests and pass along the ones my physician thinks might be relevant to my health or that of my family."
- "Subject recontact requests to peer review and approve the ones judged to have high scientific merit; and, by the way, do not recontact me more often than once a year!"

As population-genomic studies come to encompass millions of individuals, all of whom have had full genome sequences, recontact could become the standard method of recruiting subjects for specialized studies, including clinical trials. In populations of this size, it would become possible to acquire subjects by genotype, even for studies of rare genetic diseases. We know that the current system of acquiring subjects by phenotype is distorting our view of phenotype-genotype correlations, and it is time to act on this knowledge [18].

Importantly, the system I describe would be self-correcting since there is strength in numbers. If research participants become unhappy with the way their data are being managed, they would be able to demand and obtain changes in data-sharing protocols. As just one example, some groups of patients may want proposals for access to their data to be reviewed in particular ways. For instance, they might believe that review committees should have stronger participation by patients, ethicists, health economists, or other stakeholders and sources of expertise. There is every reason to think that trusted-mediator organizations would be more responsive to these requests than the institutional bureaucracies that now assess both the scientific merits and ethical acceptability of research studies. If different legal protections than those now in place prove necessary, legislators would hear from groups of patients who are well organized and in communication with one another through social media. None of this happens effectively now since, in a paternalistic model, protections are designed by researchers and institutions, not by the people who need and deserve protection.

Who should pay for this system? This vexing question is best approached by elimination. Obviously, we are not going to charge research participants for sharing their data. Public subsidies would be welcome, and perhaps essential, but it would be politically unrealistic and ethically problematic to socialize this system. Among other difficulties, over-reliance on public support would guarantee sequestration of data into geopolitically demarcated silos and bureaucratization of their administration. Privatization schemes in which data are provided to researchers for free should be viewed with suspicion: most such schemes are thinly veiled bait-and-switch inducements to use a company's products. If we eliminate research participants, public agencies, and private companies as payers, we are left with user fees. Data about the genotypes, phenotypes, environmental exposures, and health of enormous numbers of individuals are becoming an essential research resource. Just as laboratories, libraries, and accounting systems are accepted costs of doing research, access to these data should be viewed similarly. Within a few decades, access to the information commons will overshadow the importance of all other research resources. The approach to managing these data proposed here would allow recapture of costs by patient-centered organizations, while leaving in place the sacrosanct principle that individuals should not be paid to participate in research studies except under exceptional circumstances. In contrast, the privatized alternative I sketched out above would almost certainly lead to bidding wars for enrollment of particularly valuable research subjects and routine payments to millions of others to insure their ongoing loyalty to particular data aggregators.

Conclusion Human genomics is at a crossroads. It may even be a bit past the crossroads, but I see little likelihood that any of the routes we are presently following will take us where we want to go. Fortunately, these are still early days in the mammoth undertaking of attempting to understand the interplay between human phenotypes, genotypes, and environmental exposures and to use what we learn to improve health. Humans are an outbred species with a complex population structure that is in the process of breaking down. We can, for the most part, only study ourselves observationally. Despite these obstacles, we are seeking to address a whole nexus of issues that have perplexed biologists since Darwin, Mendel, and the architects of the New Synthesis framed questions that have now moved to center stage in biomedical research. We should envision this undertaking as trans-generational. On this point, I quote from the NRC's *Precision Medicine* report (full disclosure—I wrote this passage myself):

In a sense, this challenge has parallels with the building of Europe's great cathedrals–studies started by one generation will be completed by another, and plans will change over time as new techniques are developed and knowledge evolves. As costs in the health care system are increasingly dominated by the health problems of a long-lived, aging population, one can imagine that [only] studies that last 5, 10, or even 50 years can answer many of the key questions on which clinicians will look to researchers for guidance. Many patients are already put on powerful drugs in their 40s, 50s, and 60s that they will take for the rest of their lives. The very success of some cancer treatments is shifting attention from short-term survival to the long-term sequelae of treatment. For all these reasons, the era during which a genetic researcher simply needed a blood sample and a reliable diagnosis is passing [19].

We must avoid cathedral-building initiatives that lead to bureaucratic science or premature commercialization. I have attempted to sketch an alternative future that preserves the ability of individual investigators and small laboratories to tap directly into a truly communal resource. Anyone who thinks we can do better by turning this project over to large, tightly managed teams analyzing their own siloed data sources, ignores the lessons of history. The policies I advocate will take time to put in place. At present, priority should go to medium-scale pilot projects, not to building large cohorts under hastily constructed rules of engagement. We need to hunker down for the long haul. The future of health care does lie with increasingly precise targeting of therapies to the right patients. Progress toward this future will require the best basic and applied science we can muster. The place to start in mobilizing this effort is by paying close attention to how we handle the data.

Abbreviations
HGP: Human Genome Project; IT: Information technology; NIH: National Institutes of Health

Acknowledgements
I initially approached the challenges of merging genomic and clinical data on individuals from the vantage point of a genome scientist primarily involved in technology development and basic research. I provide an informal account of my avocational involvement in policy issues in Ref. [5]. On the specific issue of how we ought to handle population-scale genomic data, I have benefited from discussions with many stakeholders in the debate. A conference on Protecting Genomic Data Privacy, held at the Banbury Center of the Cold Spring Harbor Laboratory on December 11–12, 2013, had a strong influence on my thinking. Ref. [16] summarizes ideas discussed at this conference and identifies many of the participants. Robert Shelton, the author of Ref. [14], was at the Banbury conference and played a particularly direct role in persuading me that a patient-centered system based on dynamic consent would be practicable. Stephen Friend, a co-founder of SAGE Bionetworks and a co-author of Ref. [15], has also encouraged my interest in data sharing during the many years he has promoted new data-sharing models. Amy McGuire and Robert Cook-Deegan organized a conference, held at Baylor University on March 2–3, 2016, that examined the proposal to build an information commons in detail; I am indebted to participants in this stimulating meeting for helping me refine my ideas.

Funding
None.

Consent for publication
Not applicable.

Competing interests
The author declares that he has no competing interests.

References
1. Committee on a Framework for Development of a New Taxonomy of Disease; National Research Council. Toward precision medicine: building a knowledge network for biomedical research and a new taxonomy of disease. Washington: National Academies Press; 2011. Available for download at https://www.nap.edu/catalog/13284/toward-precision-medicine-building-a-knowledge-network-for-biomedical-research. Accessed 11 Apr 2017.
2. Olson MV. The Human Genome Project: a player's perspective. J Mol Biol. 2002;319:931–42.
3. Caplan AL, Merz J. Patenting gene sequences. BMJ. 1996;312:926.
4. Cook-Deegan RM. The gene wars: science, politics, and the human genome. New York: W.W. Norton & Co; 1994.
5. Olson MV. A behind-the-scenes story of precision medicine. Genomics Proteomics Bioinformatics. 2017. https://doi.org/10.1016/j.gpb.2017.01.002.
6. Kesselheim AS, Cook-Deegan RM, Winickoff DE, Mello MM. Gene patenting—the supreme court finally speaks. N Engl J Med. 2013;369:869–75.
7. Murray TH. Genetic exceptionalism and 'future diaries': is genetic information different from other medical information? In: Rothstein MA, editor. Genetic secrets: protecting privacy and confidentiality in the genetic era. New Haven: Yale University Press; 1997. p. 60–73.
8. McGee G. Foreward: genetic exceptionalism. Harv J Law Technol. 1998;11: 565–70.
9. Ilkilic I. Coming to grips with genetic exceptionalism: roots and reach of an explanatory model. Medicine Studies. 2009;1:131–42.
10. Lane J, Schur C. Balancing access to health data and privacy: a review of the issues and approaches for the future. Health Serv Res. 2010;45:1456–67.
11. Precision Medicine Initiative (PMI) Working Group Report to the Advisory Committee to the Director, NIH. The Precision Medicine Initiative cohort program—building a research foundation for 21st century medicine. 2015. Available for download at https://www.nih.gov/sites/default/files/research-training/initiatives/pmi/pmi-working-group-report-20150917-2.pdf. Accessed 17 Apr 2017.
12. Himmelstein DU, Woolhandler S. The current and projected taxpayer shares of US health costs. Am J Public Health. 2016;106:449–52.
13. Terry SF, Terry PF. Power to the people: participant ownership of clinical trial data. Sci Trans Med. 2011. https://doi.org/10.1126/scitranslmed.3001857.
14. Desmond-Hellmann S. Toward precision medicine: a new social contract? Sci Trans Med. 2012. https://doi.org/10.1126/scitranslmed.3003473
15. Shelton RH. Electronic consent channels: preserving patient privacy without handcuffing researchers. Sci Trans Med. 2011. https://doi.org/10.1126/scitranslmed.3002037.
16. Wilbanks J, Friend SH. First, design for data sharing. Nature Biotech. 2016;34: 377–9.
17. Erlich Y, Williams JB, Glazer D, Yocum K, Farahany N, Olson M, et al. Redefining genomic privacy: trust and empowerment. PLoS Biol. 2014. https://doi.org/10.1371/journal.pbio.1001983.
18. McGuire SE, McGuire AL. Don't throw the baby out with the bathwater: enabling a bottom-up approach in genome-wide association studies. Genome Res. 2008;18:1683–5.
19. Committee on a Framework for Development of a New Taxonomy of Disease; National Research Council. Toward precision medicine: building a knowledge network for biomedical research and a new taxonomy of disease. Washington: National Academies Press; 2011. p. 36. Available for download at https://www.nap.edu/catalog/13284/toward-precision-medicine-building-a-knowledge-network-for-biomedical-research.

14

Ethical frameworks for obtaining informed consent in tumour profiling: an evidence-based case for Singapore

Yasmin Bylstra[1,2,3*], Tamra Lysaght[4], Jyothi Thrivikraman[1], Sangeetha Watson[4] and Patrick Tan[2,5,6]

Abstract

Background: Genomic profiling of malignant tumours has assisted clinicians in providing targeted therapies for many serious cancer-related illnesses. Although the characterisation of somatic mutations is the primary aim of tumour profiling for treatment, germline mutations may also be detected given the heterogenous origin of mutations observed in tumours. Guidance documents address the return of germline findings that have health implications for patients and their genetic relations. However, the implications of discovering a potential but unconfirmed germline finding from tumour profiling are yet to be fully explored. Moreover, as tumour profiling is increasingly applied in oncology, robust ethical frameworks are required to encourage large-scale data sharing and data aggregation linking molecular data to clinical outcomes, to further understand the role of genetics in oncogenesis and to develop improved cancer therapies.

Results: This paper reports on the results of empirical research that is broadly aimed at developing an ethical framework for obtaining informed consent to return results from tumour profiling tests and to share the biomolecular data sourced from tumour tissues of cancer patients. Specifically, qualitative data were gathered from 36 semi-structured interviews with cancer patients and oncology clinicians at a cancer treatment centre in Singapore. The interview data indicated that patients had a limited comprehension of cancer genetics and implications of tumour testing. Furthermore, oncology clinicians stated that they lacked the time to provide in depth explanations of the tumour profile tests. However, it was accepted from both patients and oncologist that the return potential germline variants and the sharing of de-identified tumour profiling data nationally and internationally should be discussed and provided as an option during the consent process.

Conclusions: Findings provide support for the return of tumour profiling results provided that they are accompanied with an adequate explanation from qualified personnel. They also support the use of broad consent regiments within an ethical framework that promotes trust and benefit sharing with stakeholders and provides accountability and transparency in the storage and sharing of biomolecular data for research.

Keywords: Tumour profiling, Informed consent, Genomic data sharing, Germline mutations

Background

Advances in genomic technologies and declining costs of sequencing have expanded opportunities to conduct genetic profiling of diseased cells routinely. In oncology, molecular testing of tumours, such as breast cancer, has been practiced for over 20 years. These tests can define the tumour subtype, which has important implications for the selection of therapeutic options. However, testing has since evolved to differentiate both heritable (germline) and tumour-specific (somatic) mutations in tumours. These developments have revolutionised cancer care and bridged a new era of chemotherapy and targeted treatments.

The value in delineating somatic and germline genomics for therapeutic purposes has already been demonstrated with the efficacy of ADP-ribose polymerase (PARP) inhibitors for patients with a germline BRCA

* Correspondence: yasmin.bylstra@singhealth.com.sg
[1]POLARIS, Genome Institute of Singapore, Agency for Science, Technology and Research, Singapore, Singapore
[2]SingHealth Duke-NUS Institute of Precision Medicine, Singapore, Singapore
Full list of author information is available at the end of the article

mutation [1]. In parallel, next generation sequencing (NGS) platforms are also integral to translational cancer research in identifying and validating promising new biomarkers for the development of cancer treatment. Worldwide collaborative efforts, such as The Cancer Genome Atlas (TCGA) and the International Cancer Genome Consortium (ICGC), have catalogued the genomic landscapes of thousands of tumours. In such settings, germline DNA has been routinely collected for comparative analysis with tumour DNA from the same patient to distinguish unambiguously true somatic mutations from rare germline polymorphisms. However, clinical practice is currently shifting towards a preference of routinely sequencing a patient's tumour tissue alone, to characterise its molecular profile: reasons for this preference include cost reduction and simplifying the logistics of sample collection [2, 3]. Sequencing a patient's tumour tissue alone, in the absence of a matched germline sample, challenges accurate delineation of somatic versus germline mutations due to the heterogeneous nature of mutations observed in tumours.

Until recently, there was no clear guidance on whether or how findings that only imply germline variations from genomic tumour profiling should be returned to patients. International governance bodies, such as the World Health Organization (WHO) and the Organisation for Economic Co-Operation Development (OECD), as well as national regulatory authorities around the world, have issued guidelines on the management of genetic databases; although few have developed explicit guidance on the return of incidental findings [4]. These guidance documents address the return of germline findings known to have health implications for individual participants as well as their genetic relations. However, none address the situation where tumour profiles results in a potential, but unconfirmed germline finding. In response to the increasing utility of tumour-only testing in clinical practice, the American Society of Clinical Oncology (ASCO) updated their policy statement to include recommendations that the patients should be made aware of the possible detection of germline mutations [5]. However, the implications of these recommendations in day-to-day clinical practice have not yet been fully explored, particularly in Asia.

In addition to the uncertainty around managing incidental findings, the need for sharing biomolecular data internationally is increasingly being recognised as critical to understanding the role of genetics in oncogenesis and delivering more effective target therapies for cancer [6]. However, researchers require common guidelines to ensure accountability and ethical oversight for the protection of patient data that is shared between institutions and across international borders [6, 7]. In 2014, the Global Alliance for Genomics and Health (GA4GH) published the *Framework for Responsible Sharing of Genomic and Health-Related Data* that establishes a set of foundational principles for sharing genomic and health-related data [8]. According to this framework, best practices for sharing genomic and health-related data should 'promote and protect respect for the commitment to informed consent' as the foundational principle that underlies the ethical conduct of all research involving human subjects [9]. However, while intended to facilitate compliance with international norms, this framework should also be interpreted in a manner that recognises local cultural practices and the different contexts for storing and sharing data.

In developing an ethical framework that is culturally appropriate and sensitive to local norms, systems and preferences, we initiated a qualitative study in Singapore to explore the understandings, attitudes and preferences that cancer patients and clinicians have towards the return of results of tumour profiling tests as well as the usage and sharing of the data for research purposes. Singapore is an ethnically diverse and multi-cultured country of 5 million situated in South East Asia. As most published studies on patient understandings of genetic testing have focused predominantly on Caucasian populations, there is value in gaining further insights from a diverse Asian perspective. Currently, there are no laws in Singapore to protect patients against employment and insurance discrimination due to their genetic status. Any framework for obtaining informed consent in this context should also take into account local concerns about genetic discrimination and trust in governance mechanisms that oversee the storage and sharing of genome data.

Methods

The study was designed with the aims of exploring and describing the attitudes, understandings and preferences that clinicians and cancer patients have towards participation in tumour profiling research, storage and sharing of tumour genetic data, and the return of tumour profiling results. To achieve these aims, the study design employed qualitative research methods, which are useful for documenting and explaining variation in a wide range of views, needs, values, practices and beliefs [10]. These methods are not designed to estimate proportions in a wider population, quantify relationships between pre-determined variables or provide a single representative or average view or opinion [11]. However, they are particularly useful for policy development and for the design and delivery of health care and are especially well-suited to exploring the understandings and attitudes towards highly complex concepts and subjects that cannot be fully captured with quantitative methodologies.

Evidence for this study was collected from semi-structured qualitative interviews with patients and clinicians at the National Cancer Centre Singapore (NCCS). This method was chosen to provide a contextualised dataset that focused on the specified issues and could generate themes from clearly defined, homogeneous populations within an already known context [10, 12]. Ethics approval for this protocol was obtained from the Domain Specific Research Board (DSRB) of SingHealth on 9 July 2015 to conduct up to 40 semi-structured interviews with SingHealth staff and cancer patients: (2015/2522).

Recruitment

Participants were selected using purposive sampling techniques to allow for greater flexibility in targeting informants and capture a broad range of perspectives [13] until thematic saturation was reached (i.e. no new themes were emerging from the data analysis to justify continued recruitment) [14]. To identify relevant clinicians, clinical members of the research team provided a list of 25 key oncologists at the NCCS. Three emails were sent to these individuals over 3 weeks starting at the end of July 2015. From these emails, six clinicians agreed to be interviewed, resulting in a response rate of 24%. To increase the sample size, a second email invitation was sent to an additional 59 SingHealth oncology staff in early August. Of these, 15 responded and five agreed to participate. This process resulted in a total of 11 participants being recruited from a pool of 74 contacts (a response rate of 14.8%). No further attempts were made to increase the sample size after the data were thematically saturated at 11 interviews. These interviews were conducted between July and September 2015 on the phone and face-to-face based on the preferences of participants.

For the patient group, eligible participants were recruited from the waiting room at the NCCS with the assistance of staff at the registration desk in the public clinic as well as the nurses in the private clinic. Participants were offered a $50 supermarket voucher as fair compensation for their time. Of the 28 patients approached, only three declined to be interviewed resulting in a sample of 25 informants. The much higher response rate of 89.3% in this group was likely due to the support of their treating physician, being present onsite, face-to-face recruitment and compensation. The patient interviews were conducted in October 2015.

Interview protocol

An interview protocol for both groups was developed from the issues identified in a literature review (see Additional file 1). The clinician interviews were structured around three key issues to describe their attitudes and preferences towards (1) how information on the cancer diagnosis and the role of genetics (if any) is delivered to the patient; (2) delivery of the tumour profiling test results; and (3) the type of informed consent document needed to explain storing, sharing and withdrawal of tumour profile data. The interview protocol for the patient group was designed to explore participant attitudes, understandings and preferences of key issues including the purpose of the test; preferred linguistic labels and options of delivering the informed consent; the test procedures (sharing, storing and re-contact for additional research); perceived benefits and risks; ideas of altruism and solidarity; attitudes towards withdrawal options; and role of family and medical professionals in decision-making. The interview guide was piloted with one patient in the colon cancer clinic before full data collection proceeded.

Data analysis

All interviews were digitally recorded, transcribed verbatim and analysed using qualitative content analysis to identify, categorise and interpret key themes in relation to the consent process for storing and sharing of biomolecular data. Transcripts were read multiple times by the interviewer along with two study team members (YB and TL) to identify major themes and sub-themes. These themes and sub-themes were discussed together by the three study team members to corroborate categories and placement of relevant quotes. A coding frame was developed using these themes, which a fourth research applied to the data using NVivo© software (QSR International). Reliability was checked with two of the team members (YB and TL) independently coding pages of randomly selected interview transcripts. Agreement was measured using Cohen's kappa coefficient [15]. Demographics (age, ethnicity, gender and type of cancer diagnosis) were also collected for each patient and analysed using summative descriptive statistics (averages, median and frequencies).

Results

From August to October 2015, 11 clinicians (7 oncologists, 2 cancer genetic specialists and 3 palliative care doctors) were interviewed at the NCCS. Patients in both the private and public breast cancer clinics were recruited. In total, 25 patients were interviewed (see Table 1 for demographic descriptions of patients).

The average age of those interviewed was 52, with a median age of 54 years (ranging from 27 to 69). The majority were ethnic Chinese (10), with Indian (6) being the next largest group. The process of obtaining informed consent for the tumour profiling tests was discussed to explore patient understandings of consent and their attitudes towards the return of results and sharing of biomolecular data for research. From these discussions,

Table 1 Demographics of breast cancer patients interviewed

Patient ID	Age	Ethnicity	No. of patients
1	43	Bangladeshi	2 (8%)
2	59	Bangladeshi	
3	39	Chinese	10 (40%)
4	46	Chinese	
5	49	Chinese	
6	52	Chinese	
7	52	Chinese	
8	54	Chinese	
9	55	Chinese	
10	59	Chinese	
11	60	Chinese	
12	60	Chinese	
13	58	Filipino	1 (4%)
14	40	Indian	6 (24%)
15	40	Indian	
16	53	Indian	
17	58	Indian	
18	64	Indian	
19	69	Indian	
20	35	Malay	3 (12%)
21	63	Malay	
22	68	Malay	
23	27	Malay-Chinese	1 (4%)
24	50	Pakistani	1 (4%)
25	46	Vietnamese	1 (4%)
Total no. of patients			25

broad themes emerged that described several issues concerning participant understandings of cancer genetics and tumour testing results, therapeutic misconceptions, privacy and confidentiality. Results were supportive of a broad consent model in these contexts.

Current practice for discussing tumour profiling tests

To frame the clinical context of discussions around tumour profiling tests, the communication of this information was explored with both clinicians and patients. Clinicians indicated that their conversations about tumour testing with their patients were heavily simplified and that cancer genetics terms, such as somatic and germline mutations, were not distinguished. Instead, information regarding the test was briefly summarised by explaining that results would clarify treatment options. Clinicians explained that family history was raised if appropriate, or if patients had any concerns, referrals would be made to the cancer genetic clinics for further review.

> 'And if you tell them that they have this mutation, it means you can receive this drug. It will work on you or not work on you. I think about, that is how we explain it.' (Clinician 1)

Likewise, patients also indicated that discussions around genetics were limited, although some recalled being asked about their family history of cancer. When explored further about the information needs the patients desired, the response ranged widely. Some preferred brief information whereas others wanted to be well-informed. In discussions with patients about cancer genetics and tumour profiling, it became apparent that they had very limited understandings of these concepts and many appeared confused about somatic and germline genetics when raised. Cancer was generally perceived as being primarily hereditary, even by one highly educated patient who had a background in health communications:

> 'Generally as a lay person we are more inclined to look at family genetics. We would not think about, what you told me. When I say mutations, I was referring to the family genes you mention to me...I know every cancer cell is a mutation... normally when we talk about mutations, we talk about family history.' (Patient 9)

Clinicians interviewed also agreed that patients had limited understandings of genetics, mutations and cancer development. Some suggested that these limitations would even apply to clinicians who did not specialise in cancer genetics:

> 'It is does not stop at patients. Even physicians. I've had so many...mis...even from physicians referring to me you can understand that their grasp of it is very low between driver and passenger mutations, between actionable and not actionable. So you can't blame patients for not knowing this.' (Clinician 11)

It emerged from both clinicians and patients that the concepts around tumour profiling were complex and would require in depth explanations for an appropriate level of comprehension to be achieved.

Return of tumour profiling results

Current practices were explored regarding the return tumour test results. Some clinicians gave their patients the option of receiving the results as standard practice and others believed that the results should be returned to both the participant and their treating oncologist without any opportunities for either party to opt out. However, not all clinicians agreed with this approach, as with many clinical tests, there can be uncertainty around the results and their implications for treatment. For example, the pathogenicity of a variant may be unclear (known as 'variant of unknown significance') or a variant may be reported for research opportunities, such as clinical trials, rather than for immediate clinical benefit.

> '...if you just give consent and say, "Here are the clinical one and these are research ones", and you just say that, nothing else, no support about possible uncertainty. And the patient comes back and says "What does this mean?", and the doctor says this means "uncertainty". And the patient says "Oh, this is something you never told me, we [didn't] know and I don't really want this.' (Clinician 2)

As the tumour test panels can contain genes that are associated with hereditary conditions, there is the possibility that mutations in these genes derive from germline origin and have familial implications. The prospect of identifying germline incidental findings generated conflicting ideas amongst clinicians. Some clinicians discussed the possibility of discrimination that could follow from germline analyses and suggested that more legal protections, such as the Genetic Information Nondisclosure Act (2008) in the USA, should be in place before these types of tests are introduced widely into precision oncology. Hence, there were stated preferences for tumour profiling tests to exclude analysis of genes that could imply germline mutations until measures were in place. Others felt that patients should know, but should be referred to another healthcare professional trained in discussing germline implications:

> 'I don't think I can hide this from the patient. You have to tell the patient. Patient's interest for me to tell them to get tested. This has implications for you. I will send you to a trained cancer genetics oncologist or counsellor or whatever to sort this out. It should not be done in my clinic. It has to be someone trained.' (Clinician 10)

Most of the clinicians interviewed were clear about their professional boundaries and limitations. They understood that further evidence would be required to support the origin of a germline finding and that this was usually beyond their role as an oncologist. They also agreed that they did not have sufficient training to counsel and educate patients about germline implications.

Patients, on the other hand, were clearer in their preferences to receive their tumour profiling results. They were informed that this information could include a risk to hereditary conditions, such as breast cancer or cardiac conditions, or new treatments currently under research. Yet they were clear that they wanted to know about these findings even if they had implications outside their own cancer diagnosis. They indicated that they were open to receiving any information that may help them understand why they were diagnosed with cancer or advance their treatment:

> 'I'm completely okay with that. So if there is a way that we can receive then why not. We would like to have the information.' (Patient 21)

Many patients interviewed indicated a strong preference to receive results with the provision that their oncologist or another trusted healthcare professional explain the implications of the results. They agreed that receiving such information independent of any explanation could create unnecessary confusion or worry. Therefore, if the option of returning tumour tests is available to patients, the inclusion and management of such incidental findings must also be considered.

Data sharing

Significant to the advancements in research for new therapies is the generation and accessibility of large and diverse genomic data sets. The possibility of sharing the genomic data obtained from the tumour tests with external researchers, both locally and internationally, was discussed with clinicians and patients. Both groups expressed the view that personal information had to be delinked from the stored data before being shared with third parties. Some clinicians also felt that the sociopolitical culture in Singapore would mean that few patients would be overly concerned about the storage and sharing of their results, and that they would likely consent on the basis of assurances that their personal data would be kept confidential in compliance with local laws and regulations:

> 'We in Singapore are not so worried about big brother or privacy like you in the West. We are used to big brother. We are a democracy, but have an overlay of authoritarianism...we are used to having government know about us and having access to our information. Singaporeans will not be bothered about the storing and sharing of data.' (Clinician 6)

These cultural views were shared amongst some of the patients interviewed who felt that there were sufficient safeguards in Singapore to protect privacy and prevent the data from being disclosed inappropriately and misused, such as the Personal Data Protection Act (2012). However, some patients were concerned about possible misuses, particularly with respect to the potential for discrimination:

> 'If it is only for the purpose of research it is okay. There is no problem. But if for whatever reason my name will be shown and published in a publically available media, okay then basically I need to see it and basically I need to have a positive consent for myself before it is published.' (Patient 6)

Some of the clinicians interviewed expressed concerns about sharing patient data with research institutions in other countries that lacked the accountability of publicly funded institutions like in Singapore. It was also expressed that sharing participant data for profit-orientated research might create mistrust between oncologists and their patients if such information were revealed at a later point. Such perceptions of 'profit-orientated' institutions being driven towards the commercial development of products for private benefit conflicted with views of genome research as a 'public good'.

On the other hand, the patients interviewed did not draw strong distinctions between public and private goods, although the possibility of commercial products being developed from shared tumour profile data was not raised with these informants either. All patients interviewed appeared to understand that they would not benefit directly from the sharing of tumour profile data. However, their willingness to allow their data to be stored and shared with other institutions was sometimes premised on an understanding that the research was aimed at benefiting future cancer patients:

> 'I feel very excited that someone can look at this and figure it out. And if they can figure it out here or in Argentina, I don't really care. It is going to be helpful to other people with a similar tumor profile I would actually be very interested in donating my tumor to science.' (Patient 14)

There were also indications amongst clinicians that patients would agree to participate in research altruistically if they believe it had the potential to benefit patients in future as a societal good:

> 'I think a lot of patients will do it for altruistic reasons.. most patients will do it. But I think they don't want to be made to feel as if they are guinea pigs. And so I think that's the balance you want to strike. I think you might want to say "Look whatever profits we get from these cell lines, we will donate it back to cancer". They don't feel as if they are being taken for granted and they are helping the future.' (Clinician 9)

The reciprocation of indirect benefits back to the cancer community would likely be a strong moral justification for sharing tumour profile data. Most patients interviewed in this study did not have a family history, many wanted to understand why they had developed cancer, and were trying to make sense of their diagnosis. The possibility of having those questions answered through increased knowledge of the causes and pathology of cancer was highly valued, and patients could view themselves as contributing to that cause as a benefit. Trust in the potential to generate further knowledge around cancer causation may provide the strongest moral justification for consenting to sharing data under a broad consent regiment.

Broad consent as a model

Ensuring that patients understand test outcomes and documenting preferences in both research and clinical settings is conditional for informed consent. The process of obtaining informed consent from patients to take part in the tumour profiling tests was discussed with patients and clinicians. These discussions centred on the length and complexity of the consent form, the management of test results and incidental findings, participation in research and sharing of biomolecular data, the type of preferred consent and withdrawal options. In general, both patients and clinicians preferred that information be provided within a broad or blanket consent regiment with an option to withdraw from the research.

Clinicians were generally familiar with the various types of consent regiments (Table 2), and all but one clinician felt that a blanket or broad consent would be most appropriate in this setting. With respect the usage of tumour profiling data for research, one clinician preferred a categorical consent out of concerns for sharing genetic data outside cancer-related research. However, most of the clinicians felt that documentation with multiple consent tiers would be confusing to patients and cumbersome to manage:

> "It would be more easier for scientists or researchers to get the one that the patient already say "Okay, I agree you can use it freely for research" and cover all the parameters with the patient. It is easier for the researcher. For the patient, they will feel "Why I have to consent for so many things?" (Clinician 2)

Patients on the other hand were, at times, confused about the concept of informed consent and the different types of consent needed careful explaining. As discussed above, although most patients preferred to receive any potential incidental findings, this preference still needs to be documented during the consent process.

As patients displayed a limited comprehension of tumour testing and the clinicians expressed they had limited time, additional support such as a dedicated

Table 2 Glossary of terms for informed consent

Types of consent	
Implied consent	Whereby consent is not explicitly sought from participants to use their samples in research.
Blanket consent	Consent that is sought from the participant once, either at or prior to sample collection, for use in any and all future research without the need obtain any further consent.
Broad consent	Consent that is sought from the participant once, either at or prior to sample collection, for use in any and all research without the need obtain further consent from the participant, who then delegates their decision making authority to an IRB (or another institution) for specific research projects.
Categorical consent	Consent that is sought from the participant to use samples in particular categories of research, and may include an option that allows researchers to recontact participants for consent to use samples outside of nominated areas of research.
Specific consent	Consent that is sought from the participant to use samples in specific research projects only, and may include an option that allows researchers to recontact participants for consent to use samples in other projects.
Tiered consent	Provision of multiple options for participants to choose the type of consent they wish to provide.
Types of consent methods	
Opt out	Whereby consent is not explicitly sought for a given action, but participants are informed about the option to withdraw.
Opt in	Whereby verbal or written consent is explicitly sought from the participant to use samples in research.
Types of withdrawal options	
Tiered withdrawal	Whereby participants are given numerous options to withdraw in varying degrees. I.e. to withdraw from further contact while leaving samples and data in the study, or withdraw samples while leaving data, or withdraw all samples, personal information and discontinued use of data
Single withdrawal	Whereby participants are given the option to either continue participation or withdraw completely.

coordinator or counsellor to explain the test in detail and facilitate informed consent was suggested:

> 'It may be better if someone else that is trained can do it... you just need a trained counsellor or a trained coordinator, research coordinator who is trained to explain it. And then obviously, we have to take the consent, we sort of don't have to go through the details of explaining. We just wrap up and answer any specific questions or concerns.' (Clinician 1)

While some clinicians agreed that a facilitator would be helpful, in contrast others felt that the responsibility to explain the results to participants should lie with the oncologist who has professional obligations to stay updated on current evidence of best practice:

> 'They can provide additional information to assist the oncologists, but I think it is incumbent on the individual oncologist to know the information. Because at the end of the day they are physicians; it is their responsibility to keep up to date. Genomics is so much a part of oncology that you have to know.' (Clinician 7)

While patients supported the assistance of a dedicated coordinator or counsellor, there were some concerns about a nurse being able to adequately answer questions, given the perceived complexity of content in the consent form:

> 'Definitely it's not the nurse; doctor should be fine, if they have the time, looking at the patients. So I think a neutral person before this test carried out. I think it would be much better, so that they can understand. But the words are pretty tough here for people to understand.' (Patient 16)

There was recognition from patients and clinicians that support from an additional healthcare professional would allow more time for questions, which may not currently be possible in busy clinical settings. The costs of appointing such a professional in a clinical context were not explored with the informants, although the findings suggest that the existing infrastructure would not be well-equipped to absorb those costs.

Discussion

This paper reports on qualitative research with cancer patients and oncology clinicians in Singapore to explore current practices with tumour profiling tests and consent preferences for the return of results and sharing of their tumour profiling data. The results should be interpreted within the limitations of the study; notably, the small sample size, low response rates from clinicians, and restriction to breast cancer patients interviewed at a single site in Singapore limits the generalisability of results to facilities outside of this context. However, the aim of this study was not to produce generalizable findings about patients and clinicians everywhere, but to explore and describe the perspectives, understandings and attitudes of stakeholders who will likely engage and contribute to the expansion of tumour profiling tests from within the healthcare settings of Singapore. Thus, findings are informative for obtaining consent in these contexts and may be relevant to other types of genome-related research in Singapore and beyond. From the analysis, three major themes emerged: limited comprehension of cancer genetics and the consent process indicating that decision support is required; the consent preferences regarding the return of test results and usage of tumour profiling data for research; and the issues of trust and accountability in relation to research involvement. These findings are discussed in further detail below.

Decision support for obtaining consent

One significant finding that emerged from the data was the limited comprehension that patients may have of cancer genetics and implications of the tumour profiling results. It was also evident confusion arose around the concept of consent and preferences to obtaining consent. These findings are not limited to Singapore, as previously reported evidence is suggestive of limited comprehension amongst participants in genome research of genomics and cancer genetics [16–19]. In addition, comprehension limits can also be complicated by the multi-lingual context and cultural beliefs within local healthcare settings that may contribute to the varied understandings of genes and inheritance in cancer development [20]. Although cancer healthcare professionals interviewed were aware of the possibility tumour testing panels contained genes associated with hereditary conditions, there was no indication that this was discussed with their patients. In fact, if there were any indications of hereditary implications, clinicians made referrals to inherited cancer services.

Recently, recommendations from both ASCO and National Comprehensive Cancer Network (NCCN) support the view that patients should be informed about the potential of tumour profiling results inferring hereditary conditions, as well as the potential benefits, limitations and risks prior to the test taking place [5, 21]. Clinicians stated that they often lacked the time to explain medical protocols and outcomes in detail with their patients, and indicated that would they would not have time to provide lengthy explanations of the tumour profile tests. This reality of the local healthcare setting suggests that additional resources would be required to support the consent process. In research settings, dedicated co-ordinators are frequently appointed to support the recruitment and consent process. In the context of genomic research, some scholars have recommended the appointment of trained genetic counsellors to deliver the consent documentation and explain to participants the implications of consenting as they are trained to discuss issues related to germline genetic tests [17, 22].

With the significance of tumour profiling panels containing genes associated with hereditary risk, it has been proposed that the role of a genetic counsellor to deliver counselling around such tests should become more predominant in oncology as consultations parallel germline testing [21]. In countries where genetic counselling services are limited, such as Singapore, the involvement of a trained co-ordinator was proposed. With a few exceptions, the clinicians were generally supportive of a dedicated clinical co-ordinator or researcher being available to explain the consent documentation in detail and take the written consent from participants. The additional support to assist with consent will require funding to compensate for the cost of this service. This responsibility may extend to the role of existing hospital employees to assist with the consent or this service could be included in the cost of the tumour profiling test. Institutions will need to consider how the cost of such support can be absorbed.

Consent preferences for returning results and data sharing

Recommendations provided by the ASCO and NCCN also emphasise that patients should be given the opportunity to opt out of receiving possible incidental germline findings. In addition, for those patients interested learning more about germline origin should be further investigated for their pathogenicity [5, 21]. The obligation to return research results and incidental findings to patients in genetics research is contested and currently lacks consensus [4]. In Singapore, there are currently no laws that create legal duties for clinicians or researchers to return results or incidental findings to participants; nor are there any explicit rights 'not to know'. As recommended, results from this study also suggest that participants should be given the option to receive the results of their tumour profiling test, and be made aware of the potential for incidental findings during the consent process.

However, discussions became more complex regarding how incidental findings should be highlighted if patients opted to receive a copy of their tumour profiling results. While one clinician interviewed suggested the removal of those genes with germline implications from the tumour test report, most clinicians and patients were generally comfortable with the inclusion of these genes providing that they were accompanied with an adequate explanation. In recommendations for the delivery of tumour profiling results, it has been suggested that oncologists draw on the expertise of genetics specialists to assist with the interpretation and discussions of those findings with participants [21, 23]. The possibility of incidental germline findings and genetic discrimination also emerged from interview data. As there are currently no laws in Singapore to protect patients against employment and insurance discrimination due to their genetic status this approach also justifies a role for genetics specialists having a role to raise awareness of such issues. Therefore, the possibility of incidental findings being revealed with the return of tumour profiling results should be acknowledged along with ensuring that participants are referred to relevant specialists to validate the findings and take action where appropriate.

There are currently no guidelines or recommendations on how these preferences towards the return of results should be captured. It is also apparent from literature that the consent framework and clinical processes to inform patients and document preferences about the hereditary implications of tumour profiling tests remain uncertain. Results from the present study suggest that clinicians and cancer patients would prefer a simple model where consent is given just once. This model was preferred by clinicians because they lacked the time needed to explain adequately the implications of multiple consent options. Some also felt that participants would not fully comprehend different categories of research and would be happy to provide a one-off consent. They also specified that if testing revealed information beyond somatic implications that this should be captured separately, by including a tick box, to consenting for tumour profiling to be performed.

This view also extended to preferences around the usage of tumour profiling data for research applications. Patients were generally unconcerned about the provision of their data providing it was shared with external researchers in a de-identified format, and in compliance with Singapore laws and regulations. Similar to the many other studies published previously, the findings indicated support for a broad consent model that delegates decision-making authority to an independent oversight body, such as an ethics review committee or institutional review board [24, 25].

Trust and governance

From the results of this study, it is clear that the storage and sharing of tumour profiling data cannot be ethically justified as merely an exercise of personal autonomy when the informed consent of participants is inherently limited. Even with the support of dedicated research staff and a simplified consent process, the degree to which cancer patients can be truly informed of the implications for consenting to the storage and sharing of these data with researchers in Singapore and abroad is uncertain. Thus, it is important to ensure that other measures are in place to protect participants from unnecessary harms and that their data is shared within the morally accepted parameters of the consent. In short, participants must be able to trust that their data will be protected and used for the purposes they consented to.

A lack of trust with clinicians and patients would have significant implications for the value of biomolecular databanks specific to the health needs of the Singaporean population. Storage and sharing these data with external researchers will be key to fostering research and ensuring the widest public health benefits [6]. The potential for these benefits justifies the enormous public resources that are invested in genomic databanks and their purpose as a public good. Maintaining trust in this public good not only requires security measures to protect the data of participants, but will also require transparency in how the data are accessed and how social and economic benefits are distributed [26]. Any intention to privatise these benefits should be disclosed to participants prior to consenting and policies should be in place to restrict access to the data for purposes participants have consented to.

The results of this study support the adoption of a broad consent model where participants would not consent to specific projects or types of research. However, they also suggest that participants would consent altruistically on the condition that their data is used for research that has the potential to benefit other cancer patients in the future. This finding is supported in the literature with other evidence that solidarity with future patients incentivises participation in research that is unlikely to have direct benefits for participants [27]. The solidarity principle forms the basis of ethical arguments that justify the use of broad consent regiments for genomic research [28] and is strongly advocated by the HUGO Committee on Ethics, Law and Society [29]. Yet, the acceptability of this approach is also attached with provisions for governance mechanisms that ensure transparency and accountability in how data are stored and shared with other researchers and institutions. Such mechanisms may include approval from an ethics review committee for specific projects, or a separate independent body comprised of members with relevant expertise to provide oversight for the release of data to external institutions and the distribution of benefits [7].

While the results of this study indicate that participants would consent to tumour profiling data being shared for the purposes of cancer research, this might not be limited to cancer research only as other types of biomedical research were not discussed in the interviews. However, the consent might not extend to non-medical related research, such as military research or forensic investigations. Concerns over the use of genetic data for these purposes has been raised in the literature [30, 31], and while they are most relevant to germline research rather than somatic tumour profiling, participants are unlikely to understand these differences well enough to assume that they appreciate the risks of sharing these data. In these circumstances, institutions must assume a guardianship role to ensure that the data entrusted to them is not misused or perceived as such.

Finally, the concept of benefit sharing is another principle that has emerged to justify the use of broad consent regiments for genomic research [28] and is also endorsed by HUGO [32] Committee on Ethics, Law and Society. This principle does not imply that participants should benefit directly, as it is important not to promote therapeutic misconception. Rather, the principle prioritises benefits to be shared with *communities*. In the context of this study, the principle implies that mechanisms should be in place for the expedient dissemination of published research results as new discoveries in cancer treatments emerge and the reclassification of variants becomes clinically significant.

Conclusions

As the integration of NGS to inform patient care is continually evolving in oncology practice, this is experience is novel to clinicians, researchers and especially to patients. Therefore, developing a framework for obtaining consent from participants for this type of testing becomes challenging when recommendations specific to tumour profiling worldwide are only emerging and there are no best practice principles explicit to genomic testing in a Singaporean context.

This study has highlighted that there is limited public awareness around cancer causation and genetics as well as an understanding of what informed consent entails. As genomics advances, communication of these concepts will become increasingly complicated, yet highly relevant to ensure realistic expectations of the test outcomes. It has become evident that support is required when tumour profiling tests are offered, from either a clinic co-ordinator or genetic counsellor, so that information and test outcomes are explained, ultimately ensuring that informed consent can be obtained in precision oncology settings.

Abbreviations

ASCO: American Society of Clinical Oncology; DSRB: Domain Specific Research Board; GA4GH: Global Alliance for Genomics and Health; ICGC: International Cancer Genome Consortium; NCCN: National Comprehensive Cancer Network; NCCS: National Cancer Centre Singapore; NGS: Next generation sequencing; OECD: Organisation for Economic Co-Operation Development; PARP: ADP-ribose polymerase; TCGA: The Cancer Genome Atlas; WHO: World Health Organization

Acknowledgements

We would like to acknowledge Dr. Rebecca Dent, Dr. Joanne Ngeow, Dr. Iain Beehuat Tan, Dr. Daniel Tan and their team for their assistance in recruiting our research participants and Professor Alastair Campbell for his support with conceiving this study. We would also like to acknowledge the oncology clinicians and patients for their contributions to our research findings and the POLARIS team members for their support and input.

Funding

This research was funded by the POLARIS program under the Agency for Science, Technology, and Research (A*STAR) Strategic Positioning Fund (SPF) scheme and supported with a Start-Up Grant from the National University of Singapore (WBS: R-171-000-058-133).

Authors' contributions

PT conceived the study. YB, TL and JT contributed to study design, results analysis and manuscript preparation. SJ contributed to results analysis and manuscript preparation. All authors read and approved the final manuscript.

Consent for publication

Not applicable.

Competing interests

The authors declare that they have no competing interests.

Author details

[1]POLARIS, Genome Institute of Singapore, Agency for Science, Technology and Research, Singapore, Singapore. [2]SingHealth Duke-NUS Institute of Precision Medicine, Singapore, Singapore. [3]Inherited Cardiac Clinic, National University Hospital, Singapore, Singapore. [4]Centre for Biomedical Ethics, Yong Loo Lin School of Medicine, National University of Singapore, Singapore, Singapore. [5]Cancer and Stem Biology, Duke-NUS Medical School, Singapore, Singapore. [6]Biomedical Research Council, Agency for Science, Technology and Research, Singapore, Singapore.

References

1. Farmer H, McCabe N, Lord CJ, Tutt AN, Johnson DA, Richardson TB, Santarosa M, Dillon KJ, Hickson I, Knights C, et al. Targeting the DNA repair defect in BRCA mutant cells as a therapeutic strategy. Nature. 2005;434:917–21.
2. Jones S, Anagnostou V, Lytle K, Parpart-Li S, Nesselbush M, Riley DR, Shukla M, Chesnick B, Kadan M, Papp E, et al. Personalized genomic analyses for cancer mutation discovery and interpretation. Sci Transl Med. 2015;7:283ra253.
3. Catenacci DV, Amico AL, Nielsen SM, Geynisman DM, Rambo B, Carey GB, Gulden C, Fackenthal J, Marsh RD, Kindler HL, Olopade OI. Tumor genome analysis includes germline genome: are we ready for surprises? Int J Cancer. 2015;136:1559–67.
4. Zawati MH, Knoppers BM. International normative perspectives on the return of individual research results and incidental findings in genomic biobanks. Genet Med. 2012;14:484–9.
5. Robson ME, Bradbury AR, Arun B, Domchek SM, Ford JM, Hampel HL, Lipkin SM, Syngal S, Wollins DS, Lindor NM. American Society of Clinical Oncology policy statement update: genetic and genomic testing for cancer susceptibility. J Clin Oncol. 2015;33:3660–7.
6. Knoppers BM, Harris JR, Tasse AM, Budin-Ljosne I, Kaye J, Deschenes M. Zawati MnH: towards a data sharing code of conduct for international genomic research. Genome Med. 2011;3(7):46.
7. Caulfield T, McGruire AL, Cho M, Buchanan JA, Burgess MM, DAnilcyk U, Diaz CM, Fryer-Edwards K, Green SK, Hodosh MA, et al. Research ethics recommendations for whole-genome research: consensus statement. PLoS Biol. 2008;6(3):e73.
8. Knoppers BM. Framework for responsible sharing of genomic and health-related data. HUGO J. 2014;8:1–6.
9. Global Alliance for Genomics and Health: Framework for responsible sharing of genomic and health-related data: development of policies. In 3rd plenary meeting of the global alliance for genomics and health; Leiden, The Netherlands. 2015.
10. Denzin NK, Lincoln YS (Eds.): The SAGE handbook of qualitative research. Thousand Oaks, CA: Sage Publications; 2005.
11. Kuper A, Reeves S, Levinson W. An introduction to reading and appraising qualitative research. BMJ. 2008;337(7666):404–7.
12. Miller WL, Crabtree BF. In: Hesse-Biber SN, Leavy P, editors. Depth interviewing. In approaches to qualitative research: a reader on theory and practice. New York: Oxford University Press; 2004. p. 185–202.
13. Merriam SB: Case study research in education: a qualitative approach. San Francisco, CA: Jossey-Bass Publishers; 1988.
14. Saunders B, Sim J, Kingstone T, Baker S, Waterfield J, Bartlam B, Burroughs H, Jinks C. Saturation in qualitative research: exploring its conceptualization and operationalization. Quality & Quantity. 2017;14:1–15.
15. Berelson B: Content analysis in communication research. Glencose, IL: The Free Press; 1952.
16. Gray SW, Hicks-Courant K, Lathan CS, Garraway L, Park ER, Weeks JC. Attitudes of patients with cancer about personalised medicine and somatic genetic testing. J Oncol Pract. 2012;8(6):329–35.

17. Kaphingst KA, Facio FM, Cheng MR, Brooks S, Eidem H, Linn A, Biesecker BB, Biesecker LG. Effects of informed consent for individual genome sequencing on relevant knowledge. Clin Genet. 2012;82:408–15.
18. McGowan ML, Settersten RA Jr, Juengst ET, Fishman JR. Integrating genomics into clinical oncology: ethical and social challenges from proponents of personalized medicine. Urol Oncol. 2014;32:187–92.
19. Lea DH, Kaphingst KA, Bowen D, Lipkus I, Hadley DW. Communicating genetic and genomic information: health literacy and numeracy considerations. Public Health Genom. 2011;14:279–89.
20. Lim MK. Transforming Singapore health care: public-private partnership. Annals-Academy Med Singapore. 2005;34(7):461–7.
21. Jain R, Savage MJ, Forman AD, Mukherji R, Hall MJ. The relevance of hereditary cancer risks to precision oncology: what should providers consider when conducting tumor genomic profiling? J Natl Compr Cancer Netw. 2016;14:795–806.
22. Levenseller BL, Soucier DJ, Miller VA, Harris D, Conway L, Bernhardt BA. Stakeholders' opinions on the implementation of pediatric whole exome sequencing: implications for informed consent. J Genet Couns. 2014;23:552–65.
23. Raymond VM, Gray SW, Roychowdhury S, Joffe S, Chinnaiyan AM, Parsons DW, Plon SE. Germline findings in tumor-only sequencing: points to consider for clinicians and laboratories. J Natl Cancer Inst. 2016;108(4)
24. Hansson MG. Building on relationships of trust in biobank research. J Med Ethics. 2005;31:415–8.
25. Hansson MG, Dillner J, Bartram CR, Carlson JA, Helgesson G. Should donors be allowed to give broad consent to future biobank research? Lancet Oncol. 2006;7:266–9.
26. Caulfield T, McGuire AL, Cho M, Buchanan JA, Burgess MM, Danilczyk U, Diaz CM, Fryer-Edwards K, Green SK, Hodosh MA, et al. Research ethics recommendations for whole-genome research: consensus statement. PLoS Biol. 2008;6:e73.
27. Felt U, Bister MD, Strassnig M, Wagner U. Refusing the information paradigm: informed consent, medical research, and patient participation. Health (London). 2009;13:87–106.
28. Knoppers BM, Chadwick R. Human genetic research: emerging trends in ethics. Nature Rev Genetics. 2005;6:75–9.
29. Mulvihill JJ, Capps B, Joly Y, Lysaght T, Zwart HAE, Chadwick R. Ethical issues of CRISPR technology and gene editing through the lens of solidarity. Br Med Bull. 2017;122:17–29.
30. Hofmann B. Broadening consent—and diluting ethics? J Med Ethics. 2009; 35:125–9.
31. O'Neill O. Autonomy and Trust in Bioethics. Cambridge: Cambridge University Press; 2002.
32. Statement on Benefit Sharing. [http://www.hugo-international.org/Resources/Documents/CELS_Statement-BenefitSharing_2000.pdf].

15

Yale school of public health symposium on lifetime exposures and human health: the exposome; summary and future reflections

Caroline H. Johnson[1*], Toby J. Athersuch[2,3], Gwen W. Collman[4], Suraj Dhungana[5], David F. Grant[6], Dean P. Jones[7], Chirag J. Patel[8] and Vasilis Vasiliou[1*]

Abstract

The exposome is defined as "the totality of environmental exposures encountered from birth to death" and was developed to address the need for comprehensive environmental exposure assessment to better understand disease etiology. Due to the complexity of the exposome, significant efforts have been made to develop technologies for longitudinal, internal and external exposure monitoring, and bioinformatics to integrate and analyze datasets generated. Our objectives were to bring together leaders in the field of exposomics, at a recent Symposium on "Lifetime Exposures and Human Health: The Exposome," held at Yale School of Public Health. Our aim was to highlight the most recent technological advancements for measurement of the exposome, bioinformatics development, current limitations, and future needs in environmental health. In the discussions, an emphasis was placed on moving away from a one-chemical one-health outcome model toward a new paradigm of monitoring the totality of exposures that individuals may experience over their lifetime. This is critical to better understand the underlying biological impact on human health, particularly during windows of susceptibility. Recent advancements in metabolomics and bioinformatics are driving the field forward in biomonitoring and understanding the biological impact, and the technological and logistical challenges involved in the analyses were highlighted. In conclusion, further developments and support are needed for large-scale biomonitoring and management of big data, standardization for exposure and data analyses, bioinformatics tools for co-exposure or mixture analyses, and methods for data sharing.

Background

Since the completion of the Human Genome Project in 2003, it has become apparent that most chronic diseases are attributable to both genetic and environmental influences; the environment is, however, the major contributor to the global disease burden [1–3]. In 2005, Christopher Wild put forth the concept of the exposome, which highlighted the need for comprehensive environmental exposure assessment tools to better delineate causality and disease [4]. The exposome, originally defined as "the totality of environmental exposures encountered from birth to death" [4], has moved from a concept to a reality and was recently redefined as the "cumulative measure of environmental influences and associated biological responses throughout the lifespan, including exposures from the environment, behavior, diet, and endogenous processes" [5]. To begin the epic task of attempting to analyze all exposures that an individual may encounter over their lifespan and connect those to biological impact, there have been significant technological advancements to enable the study of the exposome. Herein, the Department of Environmental Health Sciences at Yale School of Public Health (YSPH) brought together leaders in exposome technology advancements to discuss recent developments, limitations, and future needs, also with the intention to bring increased awareness to this growing and important field.

* Correspondence: caroline.johnson@yale.edu; vasilis.vasiliou@yale.edu
[1]Department of Environmental Health Sciences, Yale School of Public Health, New Haven, CT, USA
Full list of author information is available at the end of the article

Findings

The Symposium was initially opened by YSPH Dean Dr. Sten Vermund and National Institute of Environmental Health Sciences (NIEHS) Director Dr. Linda Birnbaum (by prerecorded video), who expressed the importance and value of the exposome in environmental health and epidemiology. The exposome is a highly interdisciplinary holistic approach that intersects environmental exposure monitoring with modern technologies such as genomics and metabolomics. It is a valuable science particularly important for understanding how environmental factors affect children's health and later-life outcomes.

The Symposium discussed some current important considerations, developments, and future perspectives for exposome research which are discussed below.

Moving away from a single exposure-disease approach

Environmental health research has traditionally focused on how a specific chemical, or class of chemicals, influences a specific health outcome. This single exposure-disease approach does not, however, represent the complexity of exposures encountered throughout life. Environmental exposures are complex, widespread, and play a role in human health and the development of disease. Researchers are now beginning to consider the totality of external and internal exposures across the life course, a concept called the exposome. Since the concept was developed, most efforts have focused on defining the exposome and challenges to its application into scientific research. Three studies in Europe—the Health and Environment-wide Associations based on Large population Surveys (HEALS), Human Early-Life Exposome (HELIX), and EXPoSOMICS projects—represent early coordinated efforts to advance exposome research [6, 7]. To further advance and promote implementation of the exposome in environmental health research, NIEHS convened a workshop in 2015 to review the state of the science and develop recommendations in key domains. Takeaways from each group included:

- Biomonitoring: Exploring cumulative exposure history requires a hybrid of traditional (targeted) and exposomic (untargeted) biomonitoring approaches and utilizing advantages of both methods [8].
- Biological response and impact: External and internal exposures interact to alter biological processes and trigger production of new chemical intermediates. Exposomic technologies can link exposures to these downstream effects [9].
- Epidemiology: The exposome is a complement to environmental epidemiology. Untargeted analyses can generate findings that need to be investigated using hypothesis-driven approaches central to epidemiology. Merging data across cohorts with different life stages enables characterization of the exposome across the life course [10].
- Data science: Exposomic approaches generate extensive data to be stored, managed, analyzed, integrated, and shared. Development of community-based data standards and ontologies is critical [3].

While specific challenges exist in each domain, there are cross-cutting themes and needs, central to implementing the exposome into scientific research. Infrastructure support is needed for large-scale untargeted biomonitoring and managing big data. Advancement and standardization of technologies and methods for exposomic analyses as well as data analyses, integration, and sharing are another area requiring considerable support. Training environmental health scientists in big data and use of exposomic approaches in human health research is also critical. Promotion of the concept in research areas that can benefit from the exposome approach, such as epidemiology, can accelerate its implementation.

The NIEHS Children's Health Exposure Analysis Resource (CHEAR) Program addresses many of these challenges. CHEAR laboratory services span the breadth of the exposome and offer targeted and untargeted analyses. The CHEAR Data Center serves as a data repository, providing statistical analyses, data integration, and interpretation services. This data center is also developing community-based data standards and ontologies. NIEHS supports a hybrid approach to investigating the exposome, which depends upon interactive workshops, established resources (e.g., CHEAR), and new research initiatives. In these efforts, NIEHS interacts with other institutes within the National Institutes of Health, as well as with other federal agencies and international consortia as mentioned above. By taking this comprehensive approach, the exposome can be implemented into environmental health research.

Inter- and intraindividual variability and analytical advancements

Many burdensome diseases are complex and result from a combination of hereditary and environmental factors. For example, the heritability, or the phenotypic variation in the population attributable to inherited factors is on average 50%, leaving the other 50% of phenotypic variation to specific influences of the environment [11]. Additional analytic tools and data are needed to discover exposures to explain missing phenotypic variation in the population. In contrast, genomic investigations have accelerated the pace for discovery of inherited factors in disease, and the same advances should be applied to discover the influences of exposures in disease [3]. For exposome studies to deliver the promised benefits and causal understanding we seek, and to inform public health policy and chemical risk assessment, it is important to understand metabolic (and other) networks in a holistic manner to link toxic exposures, responses, and disease endpoints. However, modeling such networks may be confounded by uncertainty in both the interactions that occur and the variability of network components; some components of urinary and blood metabolomes (pool of low molecular weight compounds in the sample) exhibit high variability, whereas, others appear to be tightly regulated. Contributions of genetic and environmental factors to metabolic phenotypes have been identified, alongside differences in stability and resilience of components of the metabolomes over long periods in individuals [12, 13].

In addition, inter- and intraindividual variability in specific subpopulations or strata that are of importance to exposome studies should be characterized, including those in critical periods of life (including in utero, early life, and old age) where susceptibility to adverse consequences of exposure may be increased. Such subpopulations exist in the European Union FP7-funded HELIX project. This project is focused on studying the early life exposome by combining six mother-child cohorts in Europe: BiB (Born in Bradford, UK), EDEN (Étude des Déterminants pré-et postnatals du développement et de la santé de l'Enfant, France), INMA (INfancia y Medio Ambiente, Spain), KANC (Kaunus Cohort, Lithuania), MoBa (Norwegian Mother and Child Cohort Study, Norway), and the Rhea Mother-Child Cohort Study (Rhea, Greece) [6]. Within these cohorts, a total of 1200 mother-child pairs were selected for exposome characterization using a multitude of analytical approaches, including both internal and external measures. To assess variability in one of the measured parameters, the metabolome, a panel study within the INMA component of the subcohort was conducted to investigate the temporal variability of metabolite concentrations in children's urine over a week, relative to the interindividual variation. Variations attributable to experimental and biological factors (analytics, cohort, etc.) were assessed, giving a better understanding of the sources of variability in these metabolic phenotyping data [14]. The study showed that one of the sources of variation was diurnal and resulted in the recommendation that a pooled sample should be used made from urine samples collected at different times of the day, or a 24-h urine collection for exposome analysis. There was also interindividual variability in metabolites between males and females (citric acid) and in dietary metabolites such as *N*-methylnicotinic acid, which is derived from coffee, soda drinks, and chocolate.

An approach called "exposome-wide association studies" or equivalently "environment-wide association studies" (EWAS) is another methodology to drive discovery of new exposures in disease and the missing phenotypic variation in the population (e.g., [15–18]). EWAS offers a few advantages, including explicitly mitigating false positive findings and assessing the entire database of potential environmental correlates systematically to avoid a fragmented literature of associations [19–21]. While far from causal (and observational), the associations that emerge are those that can be prioritized to investigate in biological experiments. For example, Patel and colleagues, after using an EWAS-like approach to find exposure factors putatively correlated with telomere length, investigated how the exposure factors potentially influence changes in gene expression using publicly available data from the *Gene Expression Omnibus* [22]. Exposures must influence changes in biological function if causal, and gene expression investigations are among the important approaches to decipher causal routes to disease.

Recent technological advancements in metabolomics for exposomics

Exposome studies ultimately promise to help identify causal pathways that link environmental exposures to disease endpoints, by combining a range of state-of-the-art technologies that probe external and internal exposures, and concomitant responses. Central to the task of implementing human exposome studies is to characterize the metabolome, a phenotypic measure that encodes a wealth of information relating to genes, environmental exposures, and their various interactions [23–25]. Accordingly, high-resolution platforms such as ultraperformance liquid chromatography-mass spectrometry (UPLC-MS) and ^{1}H nuclear magnetic resonance (NMR) spectroscopy for generating metabolic phenotypic data are now commonly included in molecular epidemiological studies of chronic disease [26, 27]. For exposomics, it is essential that these platforms can (1) capture the diversity of the chemical space, (2) assign chemical identify to the associated mass spectral features, and (3) accurately quantify them. Both mass spectrometry (MS) and NMR spectroscopy have been used for analyses of the exposome; however, MS was a predominant focus of this Symposium which highlighted advancements in hardware and software for large-scale exposome analysis.

High-resolution metabolomics (HRM) of plasma has the potential to be a central platform for affordable, high-throughput, biomonitoring of environmental chemical exposures [28, 29]. The platform takes advantage of the ultra-high mass resolution, mass accuracy, sensitivity, and improved scan speed of modern Fourier-transform (FT) mass spectrometers. Improved data extraction methods support routine measurement of more than 20,000 mass spectral features in microliter volumes of plasma and other human samples, and advanced software packages support both knowledge-driven and data-driven approaches for interpretation of these data. These developments, listed below in more detail, create exciting new opportunities for large-scale, systematic exposome research.

Fourier-transform mass spectrometry

Comisarow and Marshall [30] showed that FT of signals from the free induction decay (FID) of ions responding to an oscillating electric field that is orthogonal to a fixed ion cyclotron resonance (ICR) magnetic field could be used to measure the mass-to-charge ratio (m/z) of an ionized metabolite. Application of FT-ICR MS to crude oil showed that 17,000 ions could be detected [31]. These instruments showed linear response characteristics for quantification over at least five orders of magnitude [32], but were limited for high-throughput analyses because of the slow scan speed required, and thus run times needed of 10 minutes or longer. Introduction of a new FT instrument, termed an Orbitrap [33], supported faster scan speeds, and scan speed has been further improved with a high-field version. Importantly, unlike time-of-flight instruments, the mass resolution and mass accuracy are preserved at low ion intensities, and this allows quantification of chemicals over nearly eight orders of magnitude [34]. This extensive dynamic range is an important capability for high-throughput exposome research because environmental chemicals are frequently encountered three-to-five orders of magnitude lower abundance than endogenous metabolites [35]. Early results from gas chromatography (GC)-Orbitrap analyses provide optimism for expansion of high-throughput biomonitoring to include more non-polar, hydrophobic environmental chemicals. Hundreds of environmental chemicals in different pesticide groups have been detected in single analyses of human samples (D.I. Walker, unpublished). Thus, a combination of liquid chromatography (LC) and GC analyses could provide a standardized central platform for longitudinal studies to initiate a human exposome project. Results are already available to show that analyses can be performed on samples stored for decades [36]. Therefore, rapid progress can be made by analysis of existing samples for which health outcome data are available. These high-throughput methods could provide a central resource on which to build a more extensive exposome research capability [28, 29].

Large-scale, systematic exposome research

Humans are thought to experience more than a million exposures in a lifetime [37], so detailed understanding of life-stage-specific effects represent an enormous challenge. Using the Human Genome Project as a reference, one can focus on several criteria needed for exposome research explained below. These criteria have already been established for HRM, which further supports the use of HRM for exposome research.

First, assays need to be simple enough that they can be easily performed in multiple facilities; samples can now be processed using just a single extraction and centrifugation prior to analysis [38]. Second, assays need to be high-throughput and automated with extensive coverage; the extraction and injection workflow for LC-MS can be fully automated, and run-times can be as short as 2.5 min (to detect more than 20,000 mass spectral features in batches of samples) [29]. Third, the assays need to be reproducible; analyzing each sample in triplicate, one can verify the reproducibility of an individual signal in an individual sample; however, a second biological sample set is always necessary when available. Fourth, standards are required; reference standardization [34] has been developed to support creation of cumulative data libraries; a pooled reference sample is calibrated against a National Institute of Standards and Technology (NIST) Standard Reference Material (e.g., SRM1950 containing approximately 100 metabolites) and concurrently analyzed with each batch of 20 samples. This analytic structure allows estimation of the absolute concentration of any known compound that is measured in the NIST standard. There are numerous standards available for different environmental chemical classes such as pesticides, organic contaminants from cigarettes, chemicals in drinking water, drugs, and their online spectral library are for approximately 267,376 chemical compounds. However, we know from a recent expansion to the METLIN metabolite database that the number of endogenous and environmental chemical compounds is at least 1 million, so some standards are still needed for complete coverage [39]. Finally, fifth, assays need to be affordable; the use of a dual chromatography [40], and dual ionization approach [41], provides a very broad spectrum of chemicals that can be analyzed in triplicate for about $100/sample [28], with possibilities to lower this to below $10/sample [36].

Tools for data extraction and analysis

Extraction of ultra-high resolution mass spectral data can be effectively obtained with software language tools such as apLCMS [42] and XCMS [43]. A wrapper function in xMSanalyzer [44] allows re-extraction of the same data with different parameter settings to improve capture of signals with different characteristics, and also provides quality control, batch normalization, and other capabilities. xMSannotator [45] provides an automated computational framework using existing databases (ChemSpider, KEGG, HMDB, T3DB, LipidMaps) and a multistage clustering algorithm to assign confidence scores for chemical identity by evaluating intensity profiles, retention time characteristics, mass defect, isotope patterns, adduct patterns, and correlations with matches to other metabolites in known metabolic pathways. The resulting annotated data are compatible with any of the many pathway analysis tools, e.g., KEGG [46], MetaboAnalyst [47] and MetaCore [Thomson Reuters (https://portal.genego.com/)]. To complement these knowledge-based tools, which require knowledge of chemical identities prior to pathway analysis, *mummichog* is a set of computational algorithms to predict metabolic pathway effects directly from spectral feature tables without prior identification of metabolites [48].

Chemical identification

One of the major issues for metabolomics in studies of the exposome has been chemical/structural identification. Less than half of the ions detected by mass spectrometry are associated with known chemicals and essentially the rest are the "dark matter of the exposome." Of critical importance for exposome research, about half of the mass spectral features associated with disease are currently unidentified [37]. It was recognized early on that the structural identification of detected metabolites might be problematic [49]. However, this was considered a temporary problem, easily solved by constructing databases containing all known mammalian metabolites. At the time, the mammalian metabolome was estimated to contain ≤ 5000 compounds, so the assertion that a complete metabolite database would be readily available seemed reasonable. Thanks to the diligent work of many individuals, there are now several excellent and freely available metabolite databases (METLIN, HMDB, KEGG, HumanCyc, and others) that contain these 5000 compounds, and many more [50–53]. Unfortunately, despite the availability of databases, high-throughput instrumentation, ophisticated statistical, and cheminformatics tools, the "structure identification" problem has not been solved. What has replaced the initial expectation of identifying the structures of hundreds or thousands of metabolites is the disappointing realization that most discovery metabolomics studies report the chemical structure of fewer than 100 compounds, and very often less than 50 [54]. Thus, the most significant barrier to progress and a seemingly intractable limitation of the field of metabolomics is the inability to identify the structures of most detected compounds.

A novel approach to help overcome this problem is the development of algorithms that predict physical/chemical properties of compounds contained in chemical databases. The properties chosen are those that can be experimentally measured for any unknown compound by LC-MS. These include retention indices, precursor ion survival curves, collision-induced dissociation fragmentation spectra, biological relevance, and collisional cross-sectional area. Compounds in databases (for example PubChem) whose predicted properties most closely match experimentally measured properties are returned as the most likely candidates for the unknown peak. This system is currently being validated in an in vivo model of acute trauma and could be of value for exposome studies. In addition, a multilevel framework to include unidentified signals in cumulative databases has been proposed in which ion characteristics are defined in multivector space, which will aid in overcoming this problem [37].

Orthogonal technologies in MS can also separate and capture the chemical complexity of the samples, aiding structural identification. LC is a proven technology that is orthogonal to MS, and it can be adequately optimized to target the chemical space of interest, for example, hydrophilic interaction liquid chromatography is appropriate for hydrophilic molecules while a reversed-phase method provides optimal separation for lipophilic molecules. The correct chromatography allows separation of isomers and removes isobaric interference in a mass spectrometer and makes identification of unknowns easier. Similar to LC, ion mobility, a gas phase separation of ions based on their mobility, has been shown to be very useful in separating and capturing the components of a complex sample and providing with clean mass spectra needed for identification [55]. It has been recognized that appropriate fractionation of samples at the sample preparation step as well as on-line separations (chromatography and ion mobility) all assist in capturing the chemical complexity of a matrix, such as blood, by decoupling the overlapping interferences. Accurate quantification is the next logical step following detection and identification of exposure-associated molecular species. Molecular species originating from food and drugs fall in the same concentration regime as endogenous metabolites, while the blood concentration levels of environmental pollutants are 1000 times lower. Modern mass spectrometers have a dynamic range of six orders of magnitude, therefore assessment and validation of the dynamic range of the analytical assay used to measure these molecular species are critical [56]. Dynamic range of an analytical method is defined as the concentration range over which a signal response is linear to the concentration. It is important that the dynamic range in exposure analysis be defined in the context of a molecule, especially in MS-based analysis where the ionization of molecular ions can be vastly different. Furthermore, interference in the samples can easily result in ion suppression or enhancement, which can result in inaccurate quantification. Use of hyphenated technologies such as LC-MS is even more important in quantification since chromatography can separate out the interfering ions and alleviate ion suppression or enhancement challenges.

Integrated omics methodologies

An important need is to link external exposures to internal body burden, and internal body burden to biologic responses and disease outcomes. A recent example of this analysis continuum was presented in an HRM study of occupational exposure to trichloroethylene (TCE) [57]. This study showed that TCE exposure was associated with known TCE metabolites in the blood and urine and that other halogenated compounds were correlated both with TCE metabolites and disease biomarkers. Thus, the results showed the use of HRM to connect external exposures, internal body burden, biologic response, and biomarkers of disease outcome. These analyses used a new R script, xMWAS [https://sourceforge.net/projects/xmwas/] [58], which advances capabilities to integrate HRM data with any other omics data, as already shown for transcriptome x metabolome [59], microbiome x metabolome [60], cytokine x metabolome [61], and suitable for genome, epigenome, proteome, and other integrated omics analyses that will be essential for mechanistic understanding of the exposome.

Current limitations in exposomics

Mixtures of exposure profiles

One major limitation of approaching exposure-disease associations is the number, diversity, and mixture of environmental exposure profiles at the individual level; such an array of exposures is a challenge for both measurement science and in efforts to identify components or combinations that are associated with adverse outcomes. Several publications have shown how perturbations in metabolic networks (and others such as those of gene regulation and protein-protein interactions) can help describe complex phenomena such as multimorbidity; nodes in the underlying biochemical networks connect disease phenotypes [62, 63]. It may, therefore, be useful to consider a set of these network perturbations as endpoint proxies when identifying the effects of exposure. Similarly, the conceptual framework for defining adverse outcome pathways (AOPs), i.e., making causal links from molecular initiating events (MIEs) to subsequent key events (KEs), may help reduce the complexity through identifying common MIEs for multiple environmental stressors [64].

False-positives

With big data come big analytical challenges. EWASs are observational studies and prone to biases such as confounding and reverse causality (e.g., disease coming before the exposure) [65]. While there are analytic and epidemiological study designs that attempt to mitigate these biases, they have yet to be harnessed in high-throughput exposure investigations. Yet another issue includes multiple significant associations (low *p* values) with small effect sizes. A recent "prescription-wide association study" on time-to-cancer in a large and comprehensive Swedish database [66] found that when examining > 500 drugs prescribed, almost a quarter of them were associated with cancer with small effect. Furthermore, these effects changed as a function of analytic method chosen (e.g., case-crossover vs. Cox proportional hazard), leaving an investigator with many potential false positives to sift through. This may be the norm in exposome-wide analytics, where correlations may be small but seemingly correlated with everything else and it will be a challenge to ascertain causality [67, 68].

Future perspectives

With respect to the future, the thirst for metabolic phenotype data, to complement other available omics, personal monitoring, and activity data, is only likely to increase, as the concept of the human exposome is developed and deployed around the world. As mentioned previously, methods that can integrate metabolomic data with other system-level data can provide valuable insight for exposomics and provide a way to link these datasets together in a meaningful way. It is therefore timely that several national and international initiatives have been started to provide high-throughput, multiplatform analyses with the capacity to serve the wider scientific community. These initiatives will benefit from a renewed commitment to analytical and data standards harmonization, and opportunities for wider access through open data agreements. If the recent efforts to make large, well-curated, EWAS datasets available alongside tools for their interrogation (e.g., Patel et al. [69]) can be mirrored for MWAS, then progress in exposome studies is likely to move forward at pace.

While recent advances in MS have been enabling, we still need to take advantage of the orthogonally complementing technologies to separate and capture the chemical complexity of the samples. In addition, standardization needs to be addressed, as more exposome studies are developed, reproducibility across sample cohorts will inevitably become an issue. As biobanks are being amassed, there is no current standardization for sample collection, thus data generated will be biased to collection procedure and quality of sample during long-term storage. Currently, data repositories exist for metabolomics and genomics but are missing important additional detailed information such as the type of sample collection tube, time between collection and freezing, number of freeze-thaw cycles, and analytical platform used (vendor/model). Thus, these important points need to be considered for widespread integration of the exposome.

Conclusions

In a new era of high-throughput environmental exposure assessment, there is an urgent need for new analytic approaches to drive discovery of new exposures associated with disease and phenotype [70]. Herein, the Symposium provided increased awareness of the utility of the exposome in environmental health research, as well as recent updates on technological innovation and challenges that still need to be overcome to enable the study of the exposome, particularly in metabolomics. Despite these challenges, the exposome paradigm may bear fruit in enhancing discoveries to identify exogenous factors that have up to now been elusive in disease risk. Moving forward, new technologies to measure environmental exposures in large populations in a cost-effective manner are needed, along with harnessing sound epidemiological designs to extract potential signals from noise, with data deposited in the public domain for investigators of all ilk to analyze results.

Acknowledgments
We would like to thank the Waters Corporation for their support and sponsorship for the Symposium Drs. Dustin Yaworksy and Ray Chen. We would also like to thank Ms. Donna Cropley and Ms. Damaris Faustine for their invaluable help in organizing the Symposium.

Funding
The authors would like to acknowledge the following funding sources: NIH R01 EY017963 (VV), NIH U01 AA021724 (VV), NIH R24 AA022057 (VV), NIH R00 ES023504 (CP), R21 ES025052 (CP), R01 ES023485 (DJ), R21 ES025632 (DJ), P30 ES019776 (DJ), NIH S10 OD018006 (DJ), U2C ES026560 (DJ), Women's Health Research at Yale (CJ), and Yale Comprehensive Cancer Center (CJ),

Authors' contributions
All authors were involved in writing and contributing to the manuscript. All authors read and approved the final manuscript.

Consent for publication
Not applicable.

Competing interests
The authors declare that they have no competing interests.

Author details
[1]Department of Environmental Health Sciences, Yale School of Public Health, New Haven, CT, USA. [2]Department of Surgery and Cancer, Faculty of Medicine, Imperial College London, London, UK. [3]MRC-PHE Centre for Environment and Health, School of Public Health, Imperial College Norfolk Place, London, UK. [4]Division of Extramural Research and Training, National Institute of Environmental Health Sciences, National Institutes of Health, Morrisville, NC, USA. [5]Waters Corporation, Metabolomics and Translational Research, Milford, MA, USA. [6]Department of Pharmaceutical Sciences, University of Connecticut, Storrs, CT, USA. [7]Department of Medicine, Emory University School of Medicine, Atlanta, GA, USA. [8]Department of Biomedical Informatics, Harvard Medical School, Boston, MA, USA.

References

1. Willett WC. Balancing life-style and genomics research for disease prevention. Science. 2002;296:695–8.
2. Rappaport SM, Smith MT. Epidemiology. Environment and disease risks. Science. 2010;330:460–1.
3. Manrai AK, Cui Y, Bushel PR, Hall M, Karakitsios S, Mattingly CJ, Ritchie M, Schmitt C, Sarigiannis DA, Thomas DC, et al. Informatics and data analytics to support exposome-based discovery for public health. Annu Rev Public Health. 2017;38:279–94.
4. Wild CP. Complementing the genome with an "exposome": the outstanding challenge of environmental exposure measurement in molecular epidemiology. Cancer Epidemiol Biomark Prev. 2005;14:1847–50.
5. Miller GW, Jones DP. The nature of nurture: refining the definition of the exposome. Toxicol Sci. 2014;137:1–2.
6. Vrijheid M, Slama R, Robinson O, Chatzi L, Coen M, van den Hazel P, Thomsen C, Wright J, Athersuch TJ, Avellana N, et al. The human early-life exposome (HELIX): project rationale and design. Environ Health Perspect. 2014;122:535–44.
7. Vineis P, Chadeau-Hyam M, Gmuender H, Gulliver J, Herceg Z, Kleinjans J, Kogevinas M, Kyrtopoulos S, Nieuwenhuijsen M, Phillips DH, et al. The exposome in practice: design of the EXPOsOMICS project. Int J Hyg Environ Health. 2017;220:142–51.
8. Dennis KK, Marder E, Balshaw DM, Cui Y, Lynes MA, Patti GJ, Rappaport SM, Shaughnessy DT, Vrijheid M, Barr DB. Biomonitoring in the era of the exposome. Environ Health Perspect. 2016;125:502–10.
9. Dennis KK, Auerbach SS, Balshaw DM, Cui Y, Fallin MD, Smith MT, Spira A, Sumner S, Miller GW. The importance of the biological impact of exposure to the concept of the exposome. Environ Health Perspect. 2016;124:1504–10.
10. Stingone JA, Buck Louis GM, Nakayama SF, Vermeulen RC, Kwok RK, Cui Y, Balshaw DM, Teitelbaum SL. Toward greater implementation of the exposome research paradigm within environmental epidemiology. Annu Rev Public Health. 2017;38:315–27.
11. Polderman TJ, Benyamin B, de Leeuw CA, Sullivan PF, van Bochoven A, Visscher PM, Posthuma D. Meta-analysis of the heritability of human traits based on fifty years of twin studies. Nat Genet. 2015;47:702–9.
12. Nicholson G, Rantalainen M, Maher AD, Li JV, Malmodin D, Ahmadi KR, Faber JH, Hallgrimsdottir IB, Barrett A, Toft H, et al. Human metabolic profiles are stably controlled by genetic and environmental variation. Mol Syst Biol. 2011;7:525.
13. Ghini V, Saccenti E, Tenori L, Assfalg M, Luchinat C. Allostasis and resilience of the human individual metabolic phenotype. J Proteome Res. 2015;14: 2951–62.
14. Maitre L, Lau CE, Vizcaino E, Robinson O, Casas M, Siskos AP, Want EJ, Athersuch T, Slama R, Vrijheid M, et al. Assessment of metabolic phenotypic variability in children's urine using 1H NMR spectroscopy. Sci Rep. 2017;7: 46082.
15. Patel CJ, Rehkopf DH, Leppert JT, Bortz WM, Cullen MR, Chertow GM, Ioannidis JP. Systematic evaluation of environmental and behavioural factors associated with all-cause mortality in the United States national health and nutrition examination survey. Int J Epidemiol. 2013;42:1795–810.
16. Patel CJ, Cullen MR, Ioannidis JP, Butte AJ. Systematic evaluation of environmental factors: persistent pollutants and nutrients correlated with serum lipid levels. Int J Epidemiol. 2012;41:828–43.
17. Patel CJ, Bhattacharya J, Butte AJ. An environment-wide association study (EWAS) on type 2 diabetes mellitus. PLoS One. 2010;5:e10746.
18. McGinnis DP, Brownstein JS, Patel CJ. Environment-wide association study of blood pressure in the National Health and Nutrition Examination Survey (1999–2012). Sci Rep. 2016;6:30373.
19. Ioannidis JP. Exposure-wide epidemiology: revisiting Bradford Hill. Stat Med. 2016;35:1749–62.
20. Ioannidis JP, Tarone R, McLaughlin JK. The false-positive to false-negative ratio in epidemiologic studies. Epidemiology. 2011;22:450–6.
21. Patel CJ, Burford B, Ioannidis JP. Assessment of vibration of effects due to model specification can demonstrate the instability of observational associations. J Clin Epidemiol. 2015;68:1046–58.
22. Patel CJ, Manrai AK, Corona E, Kohane IS. Systematic correlation of environmental exposure and physiological and self-reported behaviour factors with leukocyte telomere length. Int J Epidemiol. 2017;46:44–56.
23. Athersuch TJ. The role of metabolomics in characterizing the human exposome. Bioanalysis. 2012;4:2207–12.
24. Athersuch T. Metabolome analyses in exposome studies: profiling methods for a vast chemical space. Arch Biochem Biophys. 2016;589:177–86.
25. Athersuch TJ, Keun HC. Metabolic profiling in human exposome studies. Mutagenesis. 2015;30:755–62.
26. Dona AC, Jimenez B, Schafer H, Humpfer E, Spraul M, Lewis MR, Pearce JT, Holmes E, Lindon JC, Nicholson JK. Precision high-throughput proton NMR spectroscopy of human urine, serum, and plasma for large-scale metabolic phenotyping. Anal Chem. 2014;86:9887–94.
27. Lewis MR, Pearce JT, Spagou K, Green M, Dona AC, Yuen AH, David M, Berry DJ, Chappell K, Horneffer-van der Sluis V, et al. Development and

application of ultra-performance liquid chromatography-TOF MS for precision large scale urinary metabolic phenotyping. Anal Chem. 2016;88: 9004–13.
28. Jones DP. Sequencing the exposome: a call to action. Tox Rep. 2016;3:29–45.
29. Walker DI, Go YM, Liu K, Pennell KD, Jones DP. Population screening for biological and environmental properties of the human metabolic phenotype: implications for personalized medicine. In: Holmes E, Nicholson JK, Darzi AW, Lindon JC, editors. Metabolic Phenotyping in personalized and public healthcare. London: Elsevier; 2016. p. 167–211.
30. Comisarow MB, Marshall AG. Fourier-transform ion-cyclotron resonance spectroscopy. Chem Phys Lett. 1974;25:282–3.
31. Rodgers RP, Schaub TM, Marshall AG. Petroleomics: MS returns to its roots. Anal Chem. 2005;77:20. **A-27 A**
32. Johnson JM, Strobel FH, Reed M, Pohl J, Jones DP. A rapid LC-FTMS method for the analysis of cysteine, cystine and cysteine/cystine steady-state redox potential in human plasma. Clin Chim Acta. 2008;396:43–8.
33. Hu Q, Noll RJ, Li H, Makarov A, Hardman M, Graham Cooks R. The Orbitrap: a new mass spectrometer. J Mass Spectrom. 2005;40:430–43.
34. Go YM, Walker DI, Liang Y, Uppal K, Soltow QA, Tran V, Strobel F, Quyyumi AA, Ziegler TR, Pennell KD, et al. Reference standardization for mass spectrometry and high-resolution metabolomics applications to exposome research. Toxicol Sci. 2015;148:531–43.
35. Rappaport SM, Barupal DK, Wishart D, Vineis P, Scalbert A. The blood exposome and its role in discovering causes of disease. Environ Health Perspect. 2014;122:769–74.
36. Walker DI, Mallon CT, Hopke PK, Uppal K, Go YM, Rohrbeck P, Pennell KD, Jones DP. Deployment-associated exposure surveillance with high-resolution metabolomics. J Occup Environ Med. 2016;58:S12–21.
37. Uppal K, Walker DI, Liu K, Li S, Go YM, Jones DP. Computational metabolomics: a framework for the million metabolome. Chem Res Toxicol. 2016;29:1956–75.
38. Johnson JM, Yu T, Strobel FH, Jones DP. A practical approach to detect unique metabolic patterns for personalized medicine. Analyst. 2010;135:2864–70.
39. Warth B, Spangler S, Fang M, Johnson CH, Forsberg EM, Granados A, Martin RL, Domingo-Almenara X, Huan T, Rinehart D, et al. Exposome-scale investigations guided by global metabolomics, pathway analysis, and cognitive computing. Anal Chem. 2017;89:11505–13.
40. Soltow QA, Strobel FH, Mansfield KG, Wachtman L, Park Y, Jones DP. High-performance metabolic profiling with dual chromatography-Fourier-transform mass spectrometry (DC-FTMS) for study of the exposome. Metabolomics. 2013;9:S132–43.
41. Liu KH, Walker DI, Uppal K, Tran V, Rohrbeck P, Mallon TM, Jones DP. High-resolution metabolomics assessment of military personnel: evaluating analytical strategies for chemical detection. J Occup Environ Med. 2016;58:S53–61.
42. Yu T, Park Y, Johnson JM, Jones DP. apLCMS—adaptive processing of high-resolution LC/MS data. Bioinformatics. 2009;25:1930–6.
43. Libiseller G, Dvorzak M, Kleb U, Gander E, Eisenberg T, Madeo F, Neumann S, Trausinger G, Sinner F, Pieber T, Magnes C. IPO: a tool for automated optimization of XCMS parameters. BMC Bioinform. 2015;16:118.
44. Uppal K, Soltow QA, Strobel FH, Pittard WS, Gernert KM, Yu T, Jones DP. xMSanalyzer: automated pipeline for improved feature detection and downstream analysis of large-scale, non-targeted metabolomics data. BMC Bioinform. 2013;14:15.
45. Uppal K, Walker DI, Jones DP. xMSannotator: an R package for network-based annotation of high-resolution metabolomics data. Anal Chem. 2017;89:1063–7.
46. Kanehisa M, Goto S, Sato Y, Kawashima M, Furumichi M, Tanabe M. Data, information, knowledge and principle: back to metabolism in KEGG. Nucleic Acids Res. 2014;42:D199–205.
47. Xia J, Mandal R, Sinelnikov IV, Broadhurst D, Wishart DS. MetaboAnalyst 2. 0—a comprehensive server for metabolomic data analysis. Nucleic Acids Res. 2012;40:W127–33.
48. Li S, Park Y, Duraisingham S, Strobel FH, Khan N, Soltow QA, Jones DP, Pulendran B. Predicting network activity from high throughput metabolomics. PLoS Comput Biol. 2013;9:e1003123.
49. Walker DI, Uppal K, Zhang L, Vermeulen R, Smith M, Hu W, Purdue MP, Tang X, Reiss B, Kim S, et al. High-resolution metabolomics of occupational exposure to trichloroethylene. Int J Epidemiol. 2016;45:1517–27.
50. Smith CA, O'Maille G, Want EJ, Qin C, Trauger SA, Brandon TR, Custodio DE, Abagyan R, Siuzdak G. METLIN—a metabolite mass spectral database. Ther Drug Monit. 2005;27:747–51.
51. Wishart DS, Jewison T, Guo AC, Wilson M, Knox C, Liu YF, Djoumbou Y, Mandal R, Aziat F, Dong E, et al. HMDB 3.0—The Human Metabolome Database in 2013. Nucleic Acids Res. 2013;41:D801–7.
52. Kanehisa M, Goto S, Sato Y, Furumichi M, Tanabe M. KEGG for integration and interpretation of large-scale molecular data sets. Nucleic Acids Res. 2012;40:10.
53. Trupp M, Altman T, Fulcher CA, Caspi R, Krummenacker M, Paley S, Karp PD. Beyond the genome (BTG) is a (PGDB) pathway genome database: HumanCyc. Genome Biol. 2010;11:O12.
54. Zamboni N, Saghatelian A, Patti GJ. Defining the metabolome: size, flux, and regulation. Mol Cell. 2015;58:699–706.
55. Paglia G, Astarita G. Metabolomics and lipidomics using traveling-wave ion mobility mass spectrometry. Nat Protoc. 2017;12:797–813.
56. Metz TO, Baker ES, Schymanski EL, Renslow RS, Thomas DG, Causon TJ, Webb IK, Hann S, Smith RD, Teeguarden JG. Integrating ion mobility spectrometry into mass spectrometry-based exposome measurements: what can it add and how far can it go? Bioanalysis. 2017;9:81–98.
57. Castle AL, Fiehn O, Kaddurah-Daouk R, Lindon JC. Metabolomics standards workshop and the development of international standards for reporting metabolomics experimental results. Brief Bioinform. 2006;7:159–65.
58. Uppal K, Ma C, Go YM, Jones DP. xMWAS: a data-driven integration and differential network analysis tool. Bioinformatics. 2017:btx656.
59. Roede JR, Uppal K, Park Y, Tran V, Jones DP. Transcriptome-metabolome wide association study (TMWAS) of maneb and paraquat neurotoxicity reveals network level interactions in toxicologic mechanism. Toxicol Rep. 2014;1:435–44.
60. Cribbs SK, Uppal K, Li S, Jones DP, Huang L, Tipton L, Fitch A, Greenblatt RM, Kingsley L, Guidot DM, et al. Correlation of the lung microbiota with metabolic profiles in bronchoalveolar lavage fluid in HIV infection. Microbiome. 2016;4:3.
61. Chandler JD, Hu X, Ko EJ, Park S, Lee YT, Orr M, Fernandes J, Uppal K, Kang SM, Jones DP, Go YM. Metabolic pathways of lung inflammation revealed by high-resolution metabolomics (HRM) of H1N1 influenza virus infection in mice. Am J Physiol Regul Integr Comp Physiol. 2016;311:R906–16.
62. Lee DS, Park J, Kay KA, Christakis NA, Oltvai ZN, Barabasi AL. The implications of human metabolic network topology for disease comorbidity. Proc Natl Acad Sci U S A. 2008;105:9880–5.
63. Sturmberg JP, Bennett JM, Martin CM, Picard M. 'Multimorbidity' as the manifestation of network disturbances. J Eval Clin Pract. 2017;23:199–208.
64. Sturla SJ, Boobis AR, FitzGerald RE, Hoeng J, Kavlock RJ, Schirmer K, Whelan M, Wilks MF, Peitsch MC. Systems toxicology: from basic research to risk assessment. Chem Res Toxicol. 2014;27:314–29.
65. Ioannidis JP, Loy EY, Poulton R, Chia KS. Researching genetic versus nongenetic determinants of disease: a comparison and proposed unification. Sci Transl Med. 2009;1:7ps8.
66. Patel CJ, Ji J, Sundquist J, Ioannidis JP, Sundquist K. Systematic assessment of pharmaceutical prescriptions in association with cancer risk: a method to conduct a population-wide medication-wide longitudinal study. Sci Rep. 2016;6:31308.
67. Patel CJ, Ioannidis JP. Placing epidemiological results in the context of multiplicity and typical correlations of exposures. J Epidemiol Community Health. 2014;68:1096–100.
68. Patel CJ, Manrai AK. Development of exposome correlation globes to map out environment-wide associations. In: Altman RB, Dunker AK, Hunter L, Ritchie MD, Murray TA, Klein TE, editors. Biocomputing 2015 Proceedings of the Pacific Symposium: Kohala Coast, Hawaii, USA: 4-8 January 2015. New Jersey: World Scientific Pub Co Inc.; 2015. p. 231-42.
69. Patel CJ, Pho N, McDuffie M, Easton-Marks J, Kothan C, Kohane IS, Avillach P. A database of human exposomes and phenomes from the US National Health and Nutrition Examination Survey. Sci Data. 2017;3.
70. Patel CJ, Ioannidis JP. Studying the elusive environment in large scale. JAMA. 2014;311:2173–4.

Ensemble genomic analysis in human lung tissue identifies novel genes for chronic obstructive pulmonary disease

Jarrett D. Morrow[1*], Michael H. Cho[1,2], John Platig[3], Xiaobo Zhou[1], Dawn L. DeMeo[1,2], Weiliang Qiu[1], Bartholome Celli[2], Nathaniel Marchetti[4], Gerard J. Criner[4], Raphael Bueno[5], George R. Washko[2], Kimberly Glass[1], John Quackenbush[3], Edwin K. Silverman[1,2] and Craig P. Hersh[1,2]

Abstract

Background: Genome-wide association studies (GWAS) have identified single nucleotide polymorphisms (SNPs) significantly associated with chronic obstructive pulmonary disease (COPD). However, many genetic variants show suggestive evidence for association but do not meet the strict threshold for genome-wide significance. Integrative analysis of multiple omics datasets has the potential to identify novel genes involved in disease pathogenesis by leveraging these variants in a functional, regulatory context.

Results: We performed expression quantitative trait locus (eQTL) analysis using genome-wide SNP genotyping and gene expression profiling of lung tissue samples from 86 COPD cases and 31 controls, testing for SNPs associated with gene expression levels. These results were integrated with a prior COPD GWAS using an ensemble statistical and network methods approach to identify relevant genes and observe them in the context of overall genetic control of gene expression to highlight co-regulated genes and disease pathways. We identified 250,312 unique SNPs and 4997 genes in the cis(local)-eQTL analysis (5% false discovery rate). The top gene from the integrative analysis was *MAPT*, a gene recently identified in an independent GWAS of lung function. The genes *HNRNPAB* and *PCBP2* with RNA binding activity and the gene *ACVR1B* were identified in network communities with validated disease relevance.

Conclusions: The integration of lung tissue gene expression with genome-wide SNP genotyping and subsequent intersection with prior GWAS and omics studies highlighted candidate genes within COPD loci and in communities harboring known COPD genes. This integration also identified novel disease genes in sub-threshold regions that would otherwise have been missed through GWAS.

Keywords: eQTL, Expression QTL, Integrative genomics, Network medicine, Ensemble methods, Bayesian methods

Background

Chronic obstructive pulmonary disease (COPD) is characterized by progressive airflow obstruction accompanied by chronic inflammation. It is a major cause of morbidity and mortality worldwide [1]. Although environmental exposures such as cigarette smoking are risk factors, a genetic component to susceptibility has been observed [2–5]. Multiple genome-wide association studies (GWAS) have identified loci associated with COPD susceptibility across various populations [6–9]. However, most of these associations have small effect sizes, so there are likely additional COPD genes to be discovered. Understanding the gene regulatory implications of the significant and sub-genome-wide significant (sub-threshold) GWAS variants in lung tissue may identify genes and loci relevant to COPD for future validation experiments.

Prioritization of previously identified genomic loci enhances the molecular understanding of complex disease [10, 11]. Additionally, sub-threshold genetic loci may play a role in complex diseases [12] such as COPD, as

* Correspondence: jarrett.morrow@channing.harvard.edu
[1]Channing Division of Network Medicine, Brigham and Women's Hospital, 181 Longwood Avenue, Boston, MA 02115, USA
Full list of author information is available at the end of the article

they likely carry a significant biological signal and may reach significance in later higher powered studies. Increasing the power to identify additional associations often requires a much larger sample size [13], which greatly increases study expense. Integration with omics data can provide insight into the regulatory effects of these variants [12, 14, 15], without increasing sample size. Expression quantitative trait locus (eQTL) analysis tests the association between genetic variants and gene expression and can point to relevant single nucleotide polymorphisms (SNPs) and genes within GWAS loci [15–17] using the observation that trait-associated SNPs are likely to be eQTLs/eSNPs [17] and/or have gene regulatory implications [18].

In this study of genetic control of gene expression, we performed eQTL analysis in lung tissue samples from severe COPD cases and ex-smoker controls and integrated the findings with results from a prior GWAS [8]. We used the Bayesian method Sherlock [19] to identify genes having collective associations within the significant and sub-threshold GWAS SNPs. To observe these genes in the overall context of genetic control of gene expression, we constructed a bipartite network and identified communities [20] harboring the Sherlock-derived genes. We observed that some of these communities contained differentially expressed genes and genes with CpG sites differentially methylated by COPD status. This integration of previous omics studies hones in on the communities demonstrating greater relevance to COPD.

The central hypothesis of this study is that sub-threshold GWAS SNPs, in addition to genome-wide significant SNPs, both influence gene expression and confer disease susceptibility through effects better observed using network and integrative statistical methods. The foundation of this study is the aggregation of the gene expression signals from SNPs identified in prior GWAS, both significant and sub-threshold, using regulatory evidence via an ensemble Bayesian and network approach. This integrative method extracts the additional genetic and genomic signals contained in the sub-threshold SNPs by combining evidence across genotyping, gene expression and DNA methylation datasets and highlights novel genes and loci within regions that may not have been identified through GWAS. This motivates hypotheses regarding the biological role of these findings in disease and informs selection of targets for further functional investigations.

Results

Gene expression data were available for lung tissue samples from 86 severe COPD cases (mean FEV_1 26.4% predicted) and 31 controls with normal spirometry, all Caucasians (Additional file 1: Table S1). There were no significant differences between cases and controls by sex or age. The cases had higher lifetime smoking intensity in pack-years and quit smoking on average 8.7 fewer years in the past ($p = 0.0006$). We identified eQTLs using the gene expression and imputed genotyping data and integrated them with prior GWAS and omics studies using an ensemble approach of statistical and network methods (Fig. 1).

Using the lung tissue gene expression profiling and imputed genotyping data from the cases and controls, we performed cis- and trans-eQTL analysis (see the "Methods" section). We identified 347,251 significant cis-eQTL results (FDR < 5%) out of 55,550,191 total tests. Within these results, there were 250,312 unique cis-eQTL SNPs (eSNPs) and 5878 unique eQTL genes (eGenes, 4997 gene symbols) (Additional file 1: Table S2). This represents 4.2% of the SNPs and 24% of the expression probes tested. The trans results contain 8519 significant results (FDR < 5%), out of 146,665,850,054 total tests, with 6930 unique eSNPs and 451 unique eGenes (434 gene symbols) (Additional file 1: Table S3).

We intersected the significant cis-eQTL results with the GWAS at a suggestive level of significance ($p < 10^{-4}$) [8] and observed that 292 of these 1847 significant and sub-threshold GWAS SNPs were eSNPs (4.3 fold enrichment, hypergeometric p value < 0.00001). The top intersection results are shown in (Additional file 1: Table S4). Regional genomic plots of significant cis-eQTLs (FDR < 5%) for 5 of these 13 loci highlight the regulatory information for the top eSNPs and SNPs in linkage disequilibrium (LD) (Additional file 1: Figures S1–S5). Two of the eSNPs from (Additional file 1: Table S4) are located within the

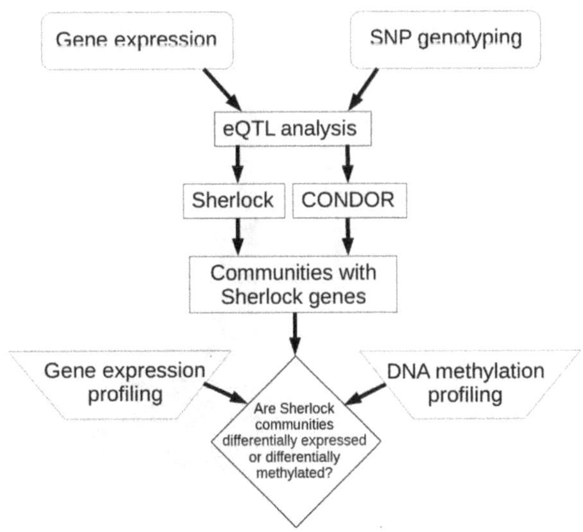

Fig. 1 Graphical overview of the study methods and process. The cis- and trans-eQTLs identified in lung tissue were integrated with prior GWAS using Bayesian and network methods. The network communities identified were interrogated for evidence of differential gene expression and differential DNA methylation by COPD status

associated eGene (rs1504550-*IREB2* and rs2252518-*ACVR1B*; Additional file 1: Figures S1 and S2). Two others (rs12461383-*C19orf54* and rs11852372-*CHRNA5*; Additional file 1: Figures S3 and S4) are in promoter flanking and transcription factor binding regions within DNase hypersensitivity (DHS) sites. The last eSNP (rs151321-*SULT1A2*; Additional file 1: Figure S5) is in LD (shaded in red) with several SNPs located in regulatory regions. To observe overall genetic control of gene expression in a disease context, we intersected all cis-eQTL results with the nominally significant GWAS SNPs ($p < 0.05$) [8] and plotted the p values from the two sets (Fig. 2). Each point in the plot represents an eQTL result (eSNP-eGene pair); prior COPD gene expression profiling results [21] are overlaid in color. We observed that eQTLs with COPD GWAS associations are generally not enriched for differentially expressed genes; regions with sub-threshold GWAS p values ($p < 10^{-4}$) and significant eQTL p values lack differentially expressed genes (FDR < 5%). Therefore, we used additional statistical and network methods to extract the signal in these results, given this complex relationship between the disease and the genetic control of gene expression.

We integrated the nominally significant cis-eQTLs ($p < 10^{-3}$) and trans-eQTLs ($p < 10^{-6}$) with prior GWAS using the Bayesian method Sherlock [19], seeking genes with collective associations across the significant and sub-threshold GWAS results. The 438,536 SNPs common to the eQTL, GWAS, and GWAS permutation data were the basis for this integrative analysis. A total of 50 Sherlock results had p values $< 10^{-3}$ (Table 1, Additional file 2: Table S5). This p value threshold corresponds to a LBF (logarithm of Bayes factor) sum of 1.94. Of the 50 genes identified, 13 were previously found in the intersection between cis-eQTLs and GWAS ($p < 10^{-4}$) results. Several genes have been identified in previous COPD GWAS studies. We repeated the Sherlock analysis using the eQTL results from GTEx V7 (using the same p value thresholds) and observed the results for these top 50 genes (Table 1). We further sought to place our 50 Sherlock-derived genes in the context of overall genetic control of gene expression using network methods, since co-regulated genes may have shared function. This process has the potential to reveal additional COPD genes of interest.

We constructed a bipartite network using the cis- and trans-eQTLs with p value thresholds identical to those for Sherlock (cis: $p < 10^{-3}$ and trans: $p < 10^{-6}$). After all filtering steps (see the "Methods" section), 171,490 eSNPs and 11,348 eGenes were used in the construction of the network. The power-law nature of the degree distribution for this network is heavy-tailed (Additional file 1: Figure. S6) and similar to that seen in other bipartite eQTL networks [20], suggesting a scale-free structure characterized by the presence of hubs. We identified 250 communities within this network and focused on the 14 that contain Sherlock-derived genes (Table 2, Additional file 1: Table S6). We also examined two communities that contained putative interactors (*HMGB1* and *CD79A*) of genes near GWAS loci from our previous study [21]. These differentially expressed interactors were identified using gene expression profiling in lung tissue and in vitro, in vivo, and in silico datasets that identified genes with evidence of

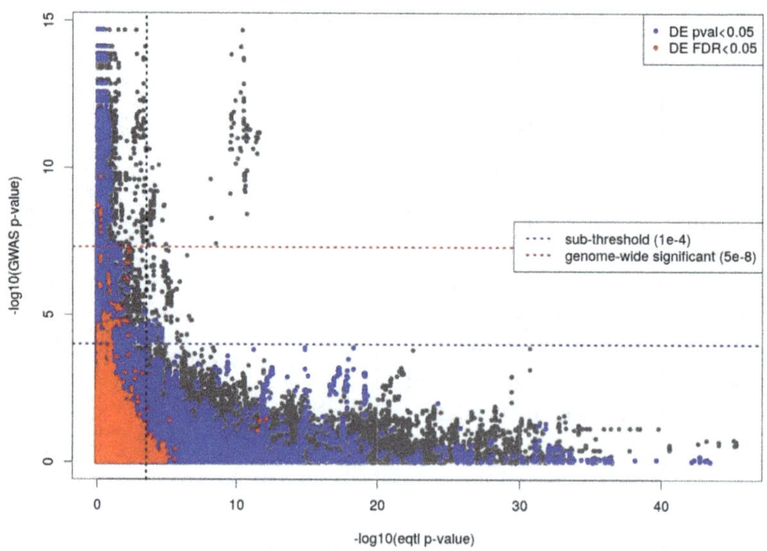

Fig. 2 Plot of COPD GWAS p values vs. the cis-eQTL p values. Each point in the plot represents a cis-eQTL result with an rsID found in the prior GWAS. GWAS p values (y axis) are plotted against the expression QTL p values (x axis). A vertical dotted line indicates the threshold of significance (FDR < 5%) for the eQTL. Horizontal lines delineate genome-wide significant (red) and sub-threshold (blue) GWAS p values. The significant (red; FDR < 5%) and nominally significant (blue; $p < 0.05$) eGenes from gene expression profiling in COPD lung tissue are highlighted

Table 1 COPD genes identified in the Sherlock analysis

Gene symbol	Total LBF score	Sherlock *p* value	Differentially expressed probe ($p < 0.05$)	Differentially methylated site ($p < 0.05$, effect > 5%)	GTEx V7 (cis-only, LBF score)	GTEx V7 (cis-only, *p* value)
MAPT	7.65	6.91E-07	Yes	No	7.31	6.41E-07
LRRC37A4	7.46	6.91E-07	No	No	2.13	1.8E-3
C17orf69	7.38	6.91E-07	Yes	No	2.39	1.3E-3
IREB2 *	6.40	6.91E-07	No	No	4.37	5.89E-05
C19orf54 *	5.45	5.53E-06	No	No	5.01	1.79E-05
ACVR1B *	5.40	5.53E-06	No	Yes	4.77	2.82E-05
EIF3CL *	4.45	1.94E-05	No	No	N/A	N/A
TUFM *	4.29	2.49E-05	Yes	No	5.31	8.97E-06
FAM13A	4.09	3.60E-05	No	No	5.69	3.84E-06
PCBP2	3.97	4.43E-05	No	No	N/A	N/A
CYP2B7 *	3.87	5.67E-05	No	No	N/A	N/A
SULT1A1 *	3.81	6.08E-05	Yes	No	5.38	8.97E-06
SULT1A2 *	3.80	6.08E-05	Yes	Yes	5.01	1.79E-05
TIGD2	3.58	7.88E-05	No	No	2.48	1.10E-03
CHRNA5 *	3.37	1.05E-04	No	No	5.27	1.15E-05
BZRAP1	3.27	1.20E-04	No	Yes	−0.20	7.28E-01
GPX8 *	3.25	1.20E-04	No	No	N/A	N/A
TEKT3	3.19	1.31E-04	No	No	0.00	1.59E-01
SNRPB	3.06	1.63E-04	No	No	0.00	1.61E-01
ZNF652	3.03	1.69E-04	No	No	−0.02	2.69E-01
AHSA2 *	2.86	2.14E-04	No	No	2.22	1.63E-03
CDH23	2.82	2.21E-04	No	Yes	0.01	1.38E-01
NOP2	2.69	2.99E-04	No	No	N/A	N/A
AASDH	2.68	3.06E-04	No	No	2.45	1.14E-03
DAGLA	2.68	3.06E-04	No	No	N/A	N/A
IFI27L2 *	2.65	3.24E-04	No	No	2.90	5.98E-04
APIP	2.60	3.48E-04	No	No	2.52	1.03E-03
AXIN2	2.59	3.55E-04	No	No	−0.04	4.10E-01
WDR47	2.49	4.20E-04	Yes	No	N/A	N/A
C4orf33	2.41	4.74E-04	No	No	1.68	3.71E-03
HNRNPAB	2.34	5.23E-04	No	No	N/A	N/A
GFPT1	2.33	5.24E-04	Yes	No	−0.02	2.04E-01
LOC644172	2.32	5.30E-04	No	No	N/A	N/A
SNORD25	2.25	5.86E-04	No	No	N/A	N/A
PPAT	2.23	6.06E-04	Yes	No	−0.03	3.22E-01
FBRSL1	2.23	6.08E-04	No	No	−0.09	5.90E-01
FSTL5	2.22	6.14E-04	No	No	N/A	N/A
SMG6	2.18	6.44E-04	No	Yes	−0.01	1.85E-01
CHIAP2	2.09	7.58E-04	No	No	N/A	N/A
RPL23A	2.07	7.77E-04	Yes	No	N/A	N/A
C2orf74 *	2.06	7.85E-04	No	No	N/A	N/A
CTSH	2.04	8.17E-04	No	No	1.40	5.59E-03
UBE2J1	2.03	8.27E-04	Yes	No	N/A	N/A

Table 1 COPD genes identified in the Sherlock analysis *(Continued)*

Gene symbol	Total LBF score	Sherlock *p* value	Differentially expressed probe ($p < 0.05$)	Differentially methylated site ($p < 0.05$, effect > 5%)	GTEx V7 (cis-only, LBF score)	GTEx V7 (cis-only, *p* value)
AEN	2.01	8.50E-04	No	No	0.36	3.61E-02
CUL1	2.00	8.88E-04	No	No	−0.02	3.02E-01
DSP	2.00	8.91E-04	No	No	1.51	4.77E-03
MYCN	1.97	9.32E-04	No	No	−0.04	4.13E-01
TRIM4	1.96	9.43E-04	Yes	No	1.57	4.37E-03
ZNF57	1.94	9.64E-04	No	No	−0.02	2.16E-01
NARS2	1.94	9.74E-04	No	No	2.89	6.10E-04

LBF logarithm of Bayes factor
*Gene identified in the cis-eQTL-GWAS intersection in (Additional file 1: Table S4)

interaction with one of the three genes (*HHIP, FAM13A*, and *IREB2*) implicated by in-depth functional studies at COPD GWAS loci.

To validate the disease relevance of the communities, we calculated the differential expression and differential DNA methylation meta-analysis *p* values (see the "Methods" section) for these 16 communities. Seven communities were validated based on nominally significant (meta-$p < 0.05$) differential expression and differential methylation results (Table 2). These communities contain the Sherlock-derived genes *CDH23, CHRNA5, HNRNPAB, IREB2, PCBP2, ZNF652, ACVR1B*, and *RPL23A* (Figs. 3, 4, and 5 and Additional file 1: Figures S7–S8) or the interactors *HMGB1* and *CD79A* (Additional file 1: Figures S9–S10). There was significant pathway enrichment (FDR *q* value < 0.05) using ConsensusPathDB [22] for two validated communities (ID = 222:*ACVR1B* and ID = 135:*CD79A*) in Table 2 (Additional file 1: Table S7), highlighting cGMP-PKG signaling, focal adhesion, and actin and immune system-related pathways. Six of the nine remaining communities, which were lacking joint evidence, had either nominally significant differential expression or differential methylation.

Discussion

Although many genome-wide significant loci from COPD GWAS were not eSNPs in lung tissue, we found

Table 2 CONDOR communities that contain Sherlock-derived genes or putative COPD GWAS gene interactors

Community ID	Sherlock or interactor gene(s)	Total SNPs	Sub-threshold SNPs	Total genes	Number of differentially expressed genes	Number of differentially methylated genes	Expression meta-*p* value	Methylation meta-*p* value
98**	*HMGB1*	143	0	4	3	1	2.26E-19	0.0028
113**	*CDH23*	489	0	12	2	1	0.0184	4.95E-05
135**	*CD79A*	1959	0	162	29	13	9.27E-11	4.27E-33
202**	*CHRNA5, HNRNPAB, IREB2, PCBP2*	293	57	17	4	1	0.0032	0.0026
218**	*ZNF652*	410	0	47	8	3	0.0017	4.85E-06
222**	*ACVR1B*	790	0	67	12	9	0.0003	8.23E-16
223**	*RPL23A*	509	4	32	10	6	3.26E-06	8.82E-18
20*	*WDR47*	476	0	6	3	0	0.0021	–
78*	*CHIAP2*	631	0	18	3	1	0.0907	0.0019
131	*AHSA2 C2orf74*	599	8	4	1	0	0.0634	–
161*	*SMG6*	633	0	18	1	2	0.3723	3.38E-09
179*	*DSP*	68	0	7	3	0	0.0060	–
181*	*FSTL5*	475	0	23	4	1	0.0503	0.0069
187*	*SNRPB*	178	0	14	1	2	0.5669	0.0001
210	*CTSH*	439	5	12	0	0	0.5741	–
249	*TRIM4*	555	0	11	3	0	0.0957	–

*Communities with either significant differential expression or differential methylation ($p < 0.05$)
**Communities with both significant differential expression and differential methylation ($p < 0.05$)

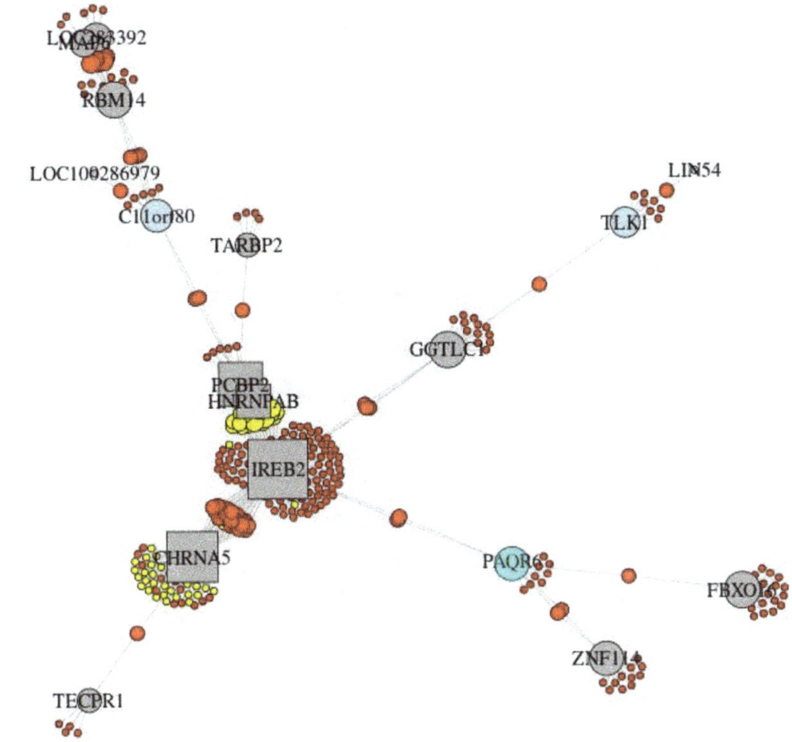

Fig. 3 Community 202 from CONDOR analysis that contains the Sherlock-derived genes *CHRNA5*, *HNRNPAB*, *IREB2*, and *PCBP2*. Community genes are listed in (Additional file 1**:** Table S6). (Red = SNP, yellow = SNP with GWAS $p < 10^{-4}$, square = Sherlock gene, gray = gene, green = gene with differentially methylated site ($p < 0.05$ and effect > 5%), light blue = gene with differentially expressed probe ($p < 0.05$), and cyan = gene with differentially methylated site and differentially expressed probe)

that the sub-threshold GWAS findings are enriched in eSNPs. We also observed that eQTLs with GWAS associations did not have eGenes significantly differentially expressed in severe COPD cases vs controls, demonstrating the complex nature of genetic control of gene expression. We employed an ensemble approach involving Bayesian and network methods to investigate these eQTL results, which yielded 16 relevant bipartite communities. Based on the differential gene expression and/or differential DNA methylation of all of the genes or CpG sites within each community, we validated the disease relevance for 13 of these communities, highlighting potential COPD genes within the significant and sub-threshold GWAS results.

One of the seven communities (community 202) which was validated by both differential expression and DNA methylation contains two previously identified COPD GWAS genes located in a genome-wide significant region: *IREB2* (iron responsive element binding protein 2) and *CHRNA5* (cholinergic receptor nicotinic alpha 5 subunit) [23–25]. The product of *IREB2* is known to interact with mRNA to influence translation or degradation. Two other Sherlock-derived genes in community 202 also have putative RNA binding activity, *PCBP2* (poly(rC) binding protein 2) and *HNRNPAB* (heterogeneous nuclear ribonucleoprotein A/B). *PCBP2* plays a role in mRNA stability, and it has been suggested that deregulation of this stability may contribute to COPD pathogenesis [26]. A recent study of breast cancer highlighted the regulatory role of RNA binding by *PCBP3* (paralog of *PCBP1* along with *PCBP2*) on mRNA stability and induction of epithelial-mesenchymal transition (EMT) [27]. Additionally, *HNRNPAB* has been shown to induce EMT [28], a potential contributor to airway disease [29, 30]. Together, this suggests a role for this community in COPD pathogenesis. Community 222 contains the Sherlock-derived gene *ACVR1B* (activin A receptor type 1B), a gene identified in a previous eQTL study in blood and sputum in COPD [31]. *ACVR1B* was a sub-threshold finding in a GWAS of lung function in COPD [32] and was identified in our intersection of eQTLs with the sub-threshold GWAS of case-control status. The genes in community 222 were enriched for cGMP-PKG signaling, bacterial invasion of epithelial cells, and focal adhesion pathways [33], with possible relevance to COPD pathogenesis and exacerbations. Community 113 includes the Sherlock-derived gene *CDH23* (cadherin-related 23), involved in cell-cell adhesion and perhaps EMT as a calcium-dependent cell adhesion molecule [34]. This gene was contained within sub-threshold loci in GWAS of lung

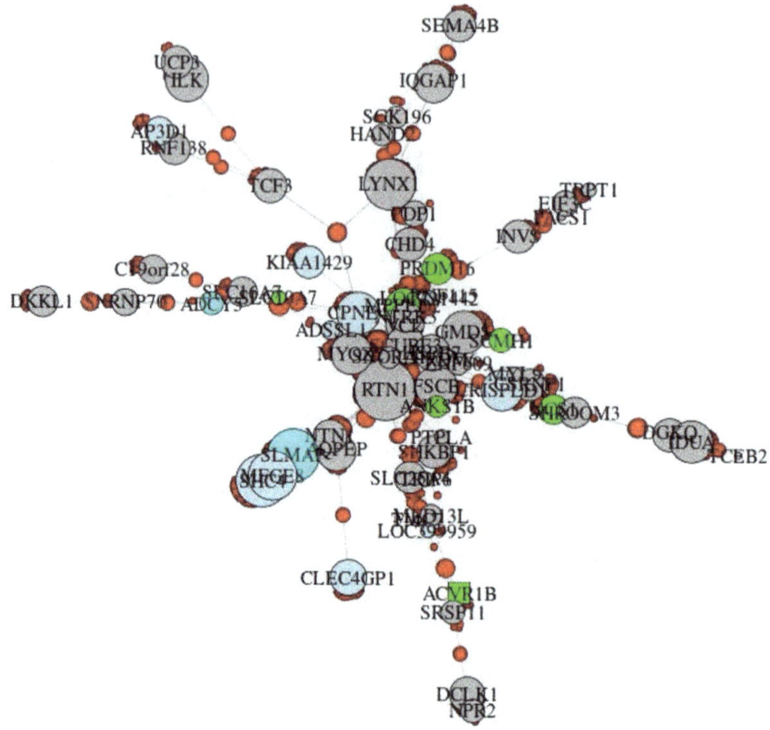

Fig. 4 Community 222 from CONDOR analysis that contains the Sherlock-derived gene *ACVR1B*. Community genes are listed in (Additional file 1: Table S6). (Red = SNP, yellow = SNP with GWAS $p < 10^{-4}$, square = Sherlock gene, gray = gene, green = gene with differentially methylated site ($p < 0.05$ and effect > 5%), light blue = gene with differentially expressed probe ($p < 0.05$), and cyan = gene with differentially methylated site and differentially expressed probe)

function decline [35], occupational asthma [36], and age at smoking initiation [37]. *DSP* (desmoplakin) was in a community (ID = 179) validated by differential expression but not differential methylation. *DSP* has been identified in a recent COPD GWAS meta-analysis [9] and in a study of interstitial lung disease [38]. Identifying this gene, which has only been highlighted in recent higher powered studies, supports our hypothesis that sub-threshold SNPs have the potential to confer disease susceptibility; genes in communities 222 and 113 may also be found significant in future GWAS.

The Sherlock analysis itself, prior to network integration, identified genes of interest that were not found through the simple intersection of eQTL and GWAS results. One of these genes, *MAPT* (microtubule associated protein tau), was previously found in a locus associated with extremes of lung function [39] and was suggestive in a recent COPD GWAS meta-analysis ($p = 4.5 \times 10^{-3}$) [9]. Genome-wide significant loci near *MAPT* were found to be associated with pulmonary fibrosis [38, 40]. In our previous gene expression profiling study, we observed a *MAPT* expression probe nominally differentially expressed ($p < 0.05$) in lung tissue of COPD cases vs. controls [21]. In the Sherlock analysis of the GTEx V7 results, we observed robust replication, with high scores from GTEx (LBF > 2.1) for eight of our top ten findings. Overall, 17 of the 35 genes that overlap our top 50 Sherlock genes attained a LBF of 1.94 or higher in the GTEx data. Trans-eQTL results are not available in GTEx (see the "Methods" section), preventing a complete replication of our findings, as the trans-eQTLs contributed important information to the COPD lung tissue Sherlock analysis. In addition, seven of the COPD lung tissue Sherlock genes were not included in the GTEx Sherlock input and eight other genes were not available in GTEx V7 eQTL data.

Four genes in a complex region on chromosome 16 associated with COPD in an exome array study [41] were identified in the Sherlock analysis and in the eQTL-GWAS intersection: *TUFM* (Tu translation elongation factor, mitochondrial), *EIF3CL* (eukaryotic translation initiation factor 3 subunit C like), *SULT1A1* (sulfotransferase family 1A member 1), and *SULT1A2* (sulfotransferase family 1A member 2). Nominal associations ($p < 0.05$) for *SULT1A2* were found in both previous gene expression profiling [21] and DNA methylation profiling [42] studies; nominal results for only gene expression were observed for *SULT1A1* and *TUFM*. Two genes in the Sherlock results, *CYP2B7* (cytochrome P450 family 2 subfamily B member 7, pseudogene) and *C19orf54* (chromosome 19 open reading frame 54), are located in another complex COPD locus on chromosome 19

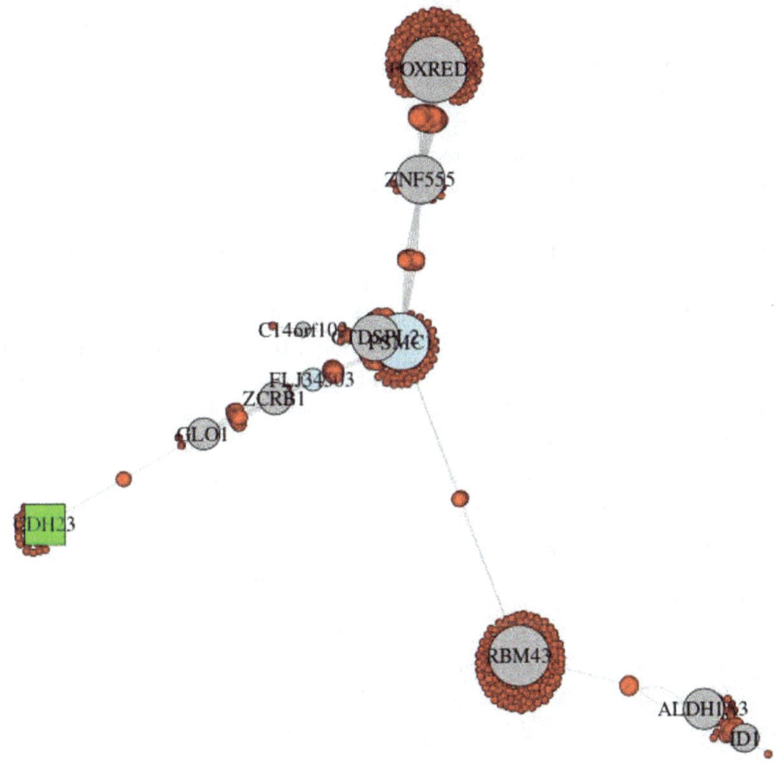

Fig. 5 Community 113 from CONDOR analysis that contains the Sherlock-derived gene *CDH23*. The central genes *PSMC1* and *CTDSPL2* partially overlap and are obstructed in the figure. Community genes are listed in (Additional file 1: Table S6). (Red = SNP, yellow = SNP with GWAS $p < 10^{-4}$, square = Sherlock gene, gray = gene, green = gene with differentially methylated site ($p < 0.05$ and effect > 5%), light blue = gene with differentially expressed probe ($p < 0.05$), cyan = gene with differentially methylated site and differentially expressed probe)

[7]. Further efforts will be required to determine which of these genes is relevant for COPD pathogenesis.

In a previous gene expression profiling study [21], we identified several putative interactors of three known COPD GWAS genes (*HHIP, FAM13A*, and *IREB2)*. Communities harboring two of these interactors were identified in the current study. Both community 98 with *HMGB1* (high-mobility group box 1) and community 135 with *CD79A* (CD79a molecule) had evidence of differential expression and differential methylation. Additionally, there may also be a role for *HMGB1* in the development of EMT in airway epithelial cells [43].

Our study has several limitations. The omics datasets in this study were generated using homogenized lung tissue, so we could not determine the cellular specificity of the eQTLs, differential expression, and differential methylation. Studies in single lung cell types will address this cellular heterogeneity and provide validation of the findings. Our study focused on severe COPD and was enriched for subjects with emphysema and therefore may miss genes relevant for milder disease or other COPD phenotypes such as airway disease. Lastly, future integrative studies using these datasets will explore in more detail the gene regulatory impact of DNA methylation in lung tissue.

This study of the genetic control of gene expression in human lung has revealed potential genes of interest co-regulated with known COPD genes. The ensemble approach using statistical and network methods also pointed to specific genes in complex genomic regions found through prior GWAS, and genes within loci that would not meet strict thresholds for genome-wide significance, thereby extracting additional information from these results and supporting our hypothesis regarding the relevance of sub-threshold SNPs. We integrated three omics datasets, providing regulatory characterization of significant and sub-threshold GWAS variants, and highlighted genes for further functional investigation that may be involved in COPD pathogenesis. These genes would otherwise not have been identified through GWAS and could potentially meet the strict threshold for statistical significance in larger GWAS in COPD.

Methods

Study subjects

We collected lung tissue samples from former smokers undergoing thoracic surgery for lung transplantation, lung volume reduction surgery, or lung nodule resection at three medical centers; all subjects quit smoking at least 1 month prior to surgery [21, 42]. Distant normal tissue was sourced from lung nodule resection samples. The COPD subjects had severe airflow obstruction, with GOLD grade 3–4 spirometry (FEV1% predicted < 50% and FEV1/FVC < 0.7) and the controls had normal spirometry (FEV1% predicted ≥ 80% and FEV1/FVC ≥ 0.7). IRB approval was obtained at the three centers (Brigham and Women's Hospital, Boston, MA; St. Elizabeth's Hospital; Boston, MA; and Temple University Hospital, Philadelphia, PA), and subjects provided written informed consent.

eQTL analysis

Microarray expression profiling was available for 111 cases and 40 controls [21] (GEO Series GSE76925). Of the 32,831 expression probes, 24,495 had genomic location information and were retained for integration with genotyping data. Genome-wide SNP genotyping data was obtained from lung tissue DNA using the HumanOmni2.5Exome-8 V1.0 BeadChip (Illumina, Inc., San Diego, CA) as previously described [21]. After quality control, genotypes were phased using SHAPEIT2 [44] and imputed using IMPUTE2 [45, 46] with the 1000 Genomes Phase3 V5 reference. The analyses were performed using only data from the Caucasian subjects. Data for markers with an imputation info metric > 0.5 and minor allele frequency > 5% were retained for the 117 Caucasian subjects that had both high-quality genotyping and gene expression data (86 cases and 31 controls; Additional file 1: Table S8). To account for population stratification, two principal components (PC) based on the Tracy-Widom statistic for the Caucasian population were retained [47]. Both cis- and trans-eQTL analyses were performed using the R/Bioconductor package Matrix eQTL (version 2.1.1) [48]. A total window size of 1 million bases was used for the cis analysis (500 kb upstream and downstream from the gene); trans analysis was performed genome-wide. This analysis identifies associations between genotype dosage and gene expression levels, adjusting for age, sex, pack-years of smoking, and the two ancestry PCs. An iterative method was used to determine the number of PCs for the matrix of expression values to add as covariates to mitigate batch effects [21]; 13 PCs were included in the eQTL analyses. An eQTL association result consists of an eGene (microarray expression probe) and eSNP pair.

Integration using Sherlock

The Sherlock method performs genetic signature matching using a Bayesian statistical framework [19]. The hypothesis is that SNPs associated with expression of disease-relevant genes are also likely to influence disease risk and be identified through GWAS. Using Sherlock, we integrated the cis- and trans-eQTLs with all results from a published COPD GWAS [8]. Sherlock provides a total score for each gene, along with the score for each of the individual eQTL contributions. This total score is the sum of the LBFs (logarithm of Bayes factor) for each of these contributions. For interpretation of individual results, a value of 4.0 is typically required for significance. To output a p value, we created permuted GWAS results with similar linkage disequilibrium structure to the GWAS using the set of 379 EUR genotypes available in 1000 Genomes Phase1 V3 [49]. Specifically, we randomly permuted the case-control phenotypes 50 times as recommended in the Sherlock method (190 cases and 189 controls) and applied Plink2 [50] to calculate association p values for each iteration and used these results as inputs for Sherlock. Only overlapping SNPs (loci with rsIDs) present across the eQTL, GWAS, and permutation results were included in the analysis; minor allele frequencies for these markers were obtained from 1000 Genomes data. In the ensemble analysis, we applied a p value threshold of 10^{-3} to select a more significant set of Sherlock-derived genes for downstream analysis. We performed a replication of the Sherlock analysis using the GTEx V7 lung tissue eQTL results [51]. Only the GTEx markers found across the COPD GWAS [8] and our permutation results were included in the analysis. The GTEx project produced cis-eQTL results using a window of 1 million bases upstream and downstream. To align this Sherlock input with our study, we labeled eSNPs located 500 kb to 1 million bases from the gene transcription start site as trans-eQTLs.

Network construction

A bipartite network was constructed using the cis- and trans-eQTLs. Network nodes are eGenes represented by their gene symbol annotation and eSNPs represented by their rsIDs. Edges only connect eSNPs to eGenes; no edges are present between pairs of eSNPs or pairs of eGenes. Only eSNPs represented in the GWAS were included in the network. Cis- or trans-eQTLs with only a single edge between an eSNP and eGene were excluded, since they did not create additional connections in the network. We identified communities within this bipartite network using the R package CONDOR [20] and visualized them using the R package igraph [52], with the Fruchterman-Reingold algorithm. A differential expression meta-analysis p value was computed for each community of interest. Specifically, the differential expression p values from prior expression profiling [21] for each expression probe annotated to genes in the community were combined using Fisher's method via the R package metap. For differential DNA methylation, we used a similar approach based on prior methylation profiling results [42] for CpG sites annotated to genes in the community. In order to focus on CpG sites more likely to be biologically relevant, we required that the mean difference in methylation between cases and controls be greater than 5%.

Regulatory annotation

The R package Sushi [53] was used with gene annotation and regulatory information from Ensemble BioMart [54] (CTCF Binding Site, TF binding site, Open chromatin, Promoter and Enhancer information produced from ENCODE, Roadmap Epigenomics, and Blueprint projects [55] for GRCh37) and DNaseI Hypersensitivity Clusters in 125 cell types from ENCODE (V3) from the UCSC database [56] (GRCh37). Linkage disequilibrium information in these regional plots was produced using correlation r^2 values for SNP pairs from PLINK, using genotyping data from 1000 Genomes Phase3 V5.

Acknowledgements

Funding: NIH grants K25 HL136846, P01 HL105339, R01 HL111759, R01 HL125583, R01 HL130512, P01 HL132825, R01 HL089856, R01 HL089897, and K25 HL133599 funded this study.

We thank Drs. Amund Gulsvik, Per Bakke, Augusto Litonjua, Pantel Vokonas, Ruth Tal-Singer, and the GenKOLS, NETT/NAS, ECLIPSE, and COPDGene studies for use of the GWAS meta-analysis data.

R01 HL089856 and R01 HL089897 are from the COPDGene study. NCT00608764 was funded by the National Institutes of Health is also supported by the COPD Foundation through contributions made to an Industry Advisory Board comprised of AstraZeneca, Boehringer Ingelheim, Novartis, Pfizer, Siemens, GSK, and Sunovion. The National Emphysema Treatment Trial was supported by the NHLBI N01HR76101, N01HR76102, N01HR76103, N01HR76104, N01HR76105, N01HR76106, N01HR76107, N01HR76108, N01HR76109, N01HR76110, N01HR76111, N01HR76112, N01HR76113, N01HR76114, N01HR76115, N01HR76116, N01HR76118, and N01HR76119; the Centers for Medicare and Medicaid Services; and the Agency for Healthcare Research and Quality. The Normative Aging Study is supported by the Cooperative Studies Program/ERIC of the US Department of Veterans Affairs and is a component of the Massachusetts Veterans Epidemiology Research and Information Center (MAVERIC). The Norway GenKOLS study (Genetics of Chronic Obstructive Lung Disease, GSK code RES11080), the ECLIPSE study (NCT00292552; GSK code SCO104960), and the ICGN study were funded by GlaxoSmithKline.

Authors' contributions

JM was responsible for the concept and design, analysis and interpretation of the data, manuscript preparation, and approval of final manuscript. MC contributed to the acquisition of the data, analysis and interpretation of the data, manuscript preparation, and approval of the final manuscript. JP contributed to the analysis and interpretation of data, statistical support, and approval of the final manuscript. XZ took part in the analysis and interpretation of the data, manuscript preparation, and approval of final manuscript. DD contributed to the acquisition of data, manuscript preparation, and approval of the final manuscript. WQ contributed to the analysis and interpretation of data, statistical support, and approval of the final manuscript. BC, NM, GC, and RB contributed to the acquisition of data, approval of final manuscript. GW took part in the acquisition of the data, analysis and interpretation of the data, and approval of the final manuscript. KG contributed to the analysis and interpretation of the data, statistical support, manuscript preparation, and approval of the final manuscript. JQ provided statistical support and approval of the final manuscript. ES contributed to the concept and design, acquisition of the data, manuscript preparation, and approval of the final manuscript. CH was responsible for the concept and design, acquisition of the data, analysis and interpretation of data, manuscript preparation, and approval of the final manuscript.

Competing interests

Drs. Morrow, Platig, Zhou, Qiu, Marchetti, Criner, Celli, Glass, Quackenbush report no competing interests related to this manuscript.

Dr. Cho has received compensation from GSK.

Dr. DeMeo has received compensation from Novartis.

Dr. Bueno has received compensation from Myriad Genetics, Inc., Siemens, Verastem, Inc., Genentech, Inc., Gritstone Oncology, Inc., HTG Molecular Diagnostics, Inc., Neil Leifer, Esq, Morrison Mahoney, David Weiss, LLC, Balick & Balick, LLC, Hartford Hospital, Cleveland Clinic/Conference, Aspen Lung Conference, Case Western Reserve, North Shore University, Castle Bioscience, Novartis Institutes for Biomedical Research, AstraZebeca, imCORE/Roche, Arthur Tuverson, LLC, Ferraro Law Firm, Rice Dolan & Kershaw, Satterly & Kelly, LLC, Exosome, Inc.

Dr. Washko has received compensation from Boehringer Ingelheim, GlaxoSmithKline, Janssen Pharmaceuticals, BTG Interventional Medicine, Regeneron, Quantitative Imaging Solutions and ModoSpira, and his Spouse works for Biogen.

Dr. Silverman has received compensation from COPD Foundation, GlaxoSmithKline, Merck and Novartis,

Dr. Hersh has received consulting fees from AstraZeneca, Concert Pharmaceuticals, Mylan, and grant support from Boehrinher Ingelheim.

Author details

[1]Channing Division of Network Medicine, Brigham and Women's Hospital, 181 Longwood Avenue, Boston, MA 02115, USA. [2]Division of Pulmonary and Critical Care Medicine, Brigham and Women's Hospital, Boston, MA 02115, USA. [3]Department of Biostatistics and Computational Biology, Dana-Farber Cancer Institute, Boston, MA 02115, USA. [4]Division of Pulmonary and Critical Care Medicine, Temple University, Philadelphia, PA 19140, USA. [5]Division of Thoracic Surgery, Brigham and Women's Hospital, Boston, MA 02115, USA.

References

1. Vestbo J, Hurd SS, Agustí AG, Jones PW, Vogelmeier C, Anzueto A, et al. Global strategy for the diagnosis, management, and prevention of chronic obstructive pulmonary disease: GOLD executive summary. Am J Respir Crit Care Med. 2013;187:347–65.
2. Hersh CP, Hokanson JE, Lynch DA, Washko GR, Make BJ, Crapo JD, et al. Family history is a risk factor for copd. Chest. 2011;140:343–50.
3. McCloskey S, Patel B, Hinchliffe S, Reid E, Wareham N, Lomas D. Siblings of patients with severe chronic obstructive pulmonary disease have a significant risk of airflow obstruction. Am J Respir Crit Care Med. 2001;164: 1419–24.
4. Silverman EK. Genetics of chronic obstructive pulmonary disease. In: Organizer DC, Goode JA, editors. Chronic Obstr. Pulm. Dis. Pathog. Treat. John Wiley & Sons, Ltd; 2000. p. 45–64.
5. Silverman EK, Chapman HA, Drazen JM, Weiss ST, Rosner B, Campbell EJ, et al. Genetic epidemiology of severe, early-onset chronic obstructive pulmonary disease. Risk to relatives for airflow obstruction and chronic bronchitis. Am J Respir Crit Care Med. 1998;157:1770–8.
6. Cho MH, Boutaoui N, Klanderman BJ, Sylvia JS, Ziniti JP, Hersh CP, et al. Variants in FAM13A are associated with chronic obstructive pulmonary disease. Nat Genet. 2010;42:200–2.
7. Cho MH, Castaldi PJ, Wan ES, Siedlinski M, Hersh CP, Demeo DL, et al. A genome-wide association study of COPD identifies a susceptibility locus on chromosome 19q13. Hum Mol Genet. 2012;21:947–57.

8. Cho MH, McDonald M-LN, Zhou X, Mattheisen M, Castaldi PJ, Hersh CP, et al. Risk loci for chronic obstructive pulmonary disease: a genome-wide association study and meta-analysis. Lancet Respir Med. 2014;2:214–25.
9. Hobbs BD, de Jong K, Lamontagne M, Bossé Y, Shrine N, Artigas MS, et al. Genetic loci associated with chronic obstructive pulmonary disease overlap with loci for lung function and pulmonary fibrosis. Nat Genet. 2017;49:426–32.
10. Bjornsson H. An integrated epigenetic and genetic approach to common human disease. Trends Genet. 2004;20:350–8.
11. Feinberg AP. Epigenomics reveals a functional genome anatomy and a new approach to common disease. Nat Biotechnol. 2010;28:1049–52.
12. Wang X, Tucker NR, Rizki G, Mills R, Krijger PH, de Wit E, et al. Discovery and validation of sub-threshold genome-wide association study loci using epigenomic signatures. elife. 2016;5:e10557.
13. Bush WS, Moore JH. Chapter 11: genome-wide association studies. Lewitter F, Kann M, editors. PLoS Comput Biol. 2012;8:e1002822.
14. Civelek M, Lusis AJ. Systems genetics approaches to understand complex traits. Nat Rev Genet. 2013;15:34–48.
15. Li L, Kabesch M, Bouzigon E, Demenais F, Farrall M, Moffatt MF, et al. Using eQTL weights to improve power for genome-wide association studies: a genetic study of childhood asthma. Front Genet. 2013;4:103. doi:10.3389/fgene.2013.00103.
16. Nica AC, Montgomery SB, Dimas AS, Stranger BE, Beazley C, Barroso I, et al. Candidate causal regulatory effects by integration of expression QTLs with complex trait genetic associations. Gibson G, editor. PLoS Genet. 2010;6:e1000895.
17. Nicolae DL, Gamazon E, Zhang W, Duan S, Dolan ME, Cox NJ. Trait-associated SNPs are more likely to be eQTLs: annotation to enhance discovery from GWAS. PLoS Genet. 2010;6:e1000888.
18. Maurano MT, Humbert R, Rynes E, Thurman RE, Haugen E, Wang H, et al. Systematic localization of common disease-associated variation in regulatory DNA. Science. 2012;337:1190–5.
19. He X, Fuller CK, Song Y, Meng Q, Zhang B, Yang X, et al. Sherlock: detecting gene-disease associations by matching patterns of expression QTL and GWAS. Am J Hum Genet. 2013;92:667–80.
20. Platig J, Castaldi PJ, DeMeo D, Quackenbush J. Bipartite community structure of eQTLs. Markowetz F, editor. PLoS Comput Biol. 2016;12:e1005033.
21. Morrow JD, Zhou X, Lao T, Jiang Z, DeMeo DL, Cho MH, et al. Functional interactors of three genome-wide association study genes are differentially expressed in severe chronic obstructive pulmonary disease lung tissue. Sci Rep. 2017;7:44232.
22. Kamburov A, Stelzl U, Lehrach H, Herwig R. The ConsensusPathDB interaction database: 2013 update. Nucleic Acids Res. 2013;41:D793–800.
23. DeMeo DL, Mariani T, Bhattacharya S, Srisuma S, Lange C, Litonjua A, et al. Integration of genomic and genetic approaches implicates IREB2 as a COPD susceptibility gene. Am J Hum Genet. 2009;85:493–502.
24. Hardin M, Zielinski J, Wan ES, Hersh CP, Castaldi PJ, Schwinder E, et al. CHRNA3/5, IREB2, and ADCY2 are associated with severe chronic obstructive pulmonary disease in Poland. Am J Respir Cell Mol Biol. 2012;47:203–8.
25. Pillai SG, Ge D, Zhu G, Kong X, Shianna KV, Need AC, et al. A genome-wide association study in chronic obstructive pulmonary disease (COPD): identification of two major susceptibility loci. PLoS Genet. 2009;5:e1000421.
26. Navratilova Z, Krsjakova T, Novosadova E, Zatloukal J, Kolek V, Petrek M. Genes affecting mRNA stability and metalloproteinase inhibitor RECK are down-regulated in patients with COPD. Eur Respir J. 2013; 42(Suppl 57):3512.
27. Hou P, Li L, Chen F, Chen Y, Liu H, Li J, et al. PTBP3-mediated regulation of ZEB1 mRNA stability promotes epithelial-mesenchymal transition in breast cancer. Cancer Res. 2017;canres.0883.2017.
28. Zhou Z-J, Dai Z, Zhou S-L, Hu Z-Q, Chen Q, Zhao Y-M, et al. HNRNPAB induces epithelial-mesenchymal transition and promotes metastasis of hepatocellular carcinoma by transcriptionally activating SNAIL. Cancer Res. 2014;74:2750–62.
29. Nowrin K, Sohal SS, Peterson G, Patel R, Walters EH. Epithelial-mesenchymal transition as a fundamental underlying pathogenic process in COPD airways: fibrosis, remodeling and cancer. Expert Rev Respir Med. 2014;8:547–59.
30. Sohal SS, Mahmood MQ, Walters EH. Clinical significance of epithelial mesenchymal transition (EMT) in chronic obstructive pulmonary disease (COPD): potential target for prevention of airway fibrosis and lung cancer. Clin Transl Med. 2014;3:33.
31. Castaldi PJ, Cho MH, Zhou X, Qiu W, Mcgeachie M, Celli B, et al. Genetic control of gene expression at novel and established chronic obstructive pulmonary disease loci. Hum Mol Genet. 2015;24:1200–10.
32. Lutz SM, Cho MH, Young K, Hersh CP, Castaldi PJ, McDonald M-L, et al. A genome-wide association study identifies risk loci for spirometric measures among smokers of European and African ancestry. BMC Genet. 2015;16(1):138.
33. Ezzie ME, Crawford M, Cho J-H, Orellana R, Zhang S, Gelinas R, et al. Gene expression networks in COPD: microRNA and mRNA regulation. Thorax. 2012;67:122–31.
34. Gheldof A, Berx G. Cadherins and epithelial-to-mesenchymal transition. Prog Mol Biol Transl Sci. 2013;116:317–36.
35. Imboden M, Bouzigon E, Curjuric I, Ramasamy A, Kumar A, Hancock DB, et al. Genome-wide association study of lung function decline in adults with and without asthma. J Allergy Clin Immunol. 2012;129:1218–28.
36. Yucesoy B, Kaufman KM, Lummus ZL, Weirauch MT, Zhang G, Cartier A, et al. Genome-wide association study identifies novel loci associated with diisocyanate-induced occupational asthma. Toxicol Sci. 2015;146:192–201.
37. Siedlinski M, Cho MH, Bakke P, Gulsvik A, Lomas DA, Anderson W, et al. Genome-wide association study of smoking behaviours in patients with COPD. Thorax. 2011;66:894–902.
38. Fingerlin TE, Murphy E, Zhang W, Peljto AL, Brown KK, Steele MP, et al. Genome-wide association study identifies multiple susceptibility loci for pulmonary fibrosis. Nat Genet. 2013;45:613–20.
39. Wain LV, Shrine N, Miller S, Jackson VE, Ntalla I, Artigas MS, et al. Novel insights into the genetics of smoking behaviour, lung function, and chronic obstructive pulmonary disease (UK BiLEVE): a genetic association study in UK Biobank. Lancet Respir Med. 2015;3:769–81.
40. Noth I, Zhang Y, Ma S-F, Flores C, Barber M, Huang Y, et al. Genetic variants associated with idiopathic pulmonary fibrosis susceptibility and mortality: a genome-wide association study. Lancet Respir Med. 2013;1:309–17.
41. Hobbs BD, Parker MM, Chen H, Lao T, Hardin M, Qiao D, et al. Exome array analysis identifies a common variant in *IL27* associated with chronic obstructive pulmonary disease. Am J Respir Crit Care Med. 2016;194:48–57.
42. Morrow JD, Cho MH, Hersh CP, Pinto-Plata V, Celli B, Marchetti N, et al. DNA methylation profiling in human lung tissue identifies genes associated with COPD. Epigenetics. 2016;11:730–9.
43. Chen Y-C, Statt S, Wu R, Chang H-T, Liao J-W, Wang C-N, et al. High mobility group box 1-induced epithelial mesenchymal transition in human airway epithelial cells. Sci Rep. 2016;6:18815. doi:10.1038/srep18815.
44. Delaneau O, Marchini J, Zagury J-F. A linear complexity phasing method for thousands of genomes. Nat Methods. 2011;9:179–81.
45. Howie B, Marchini J, Stephens M. Genotype imputation with thousands of genomes. Chakravarti a, editor. G3amp58 GenesGenomesGenetics. 2011;1: 457–470.
46. Howie BN, Donnelly P, Marchini J. A flexible and accurate genotype imputation method for the next generation of genome-wide association studies. Schork NJ, editor. PLoS Genet. 2009;5:e1000529.
47. Price AL, Patterson NJ, Plenge RM, Weinblatt ME, Shadick NA, Reich D. Principal components analysis corrects for stratification in genome-wide association studies. Nat Genet. 2006;38:904–9.
48. Shabalin AA. Matrix eQTL: ultra fast eQTL analysis via large matrix operations. Bioinformatics. 2012;28:1353–8.
49. Auton A, Abecasis GR, Altshuler DM, Durbin RM, Abecasis GR, Bentley DR, et al. A global reference for human genetic variation. Nature. 2015;526:68–74.
50. Chang CC, Chow CC, Tellier LC, Vattikuti S, Purcell SM, Lee JJ. Second-generation PLINK: rising to the challenge of larger and richer datasets. GigaScience. 2015;4:7.
51. Aguet F, Ardlie KG, Cummings BB, Gelfand ET, Getz G, Hadley K, et al. Genetic effects on gene expression across human tissues. Nature. 2017; 550:204–13.
52. Csardi G, Nepusz T. The igraph software package for complex network research. InterJournal 2006;Complex Systems:1695.

53. Phanstiel DH, Boyle AP, Araya CL, Snyder MP. Sushi.R: flexible, quantitative and integrative genomic visualizations for publication-quality multi-panel figures. Bioinformatics. 2014;30:2808–10.
54. Durinck S, Moreau Y, Kasprzyk A, Davis S, De Moor B, Brazma A, et al. BioMart and bioconductor: a powerful link between biological databases and microarray data analysis. Bioinformatics. 2005;21:3439–40.
55. Zerbino DR, Wilder SP, Johnson N, Juettemann T, Flicek PR. The Ensembl Regulatory Build. Genome Biol. 2015;16:56.
56. Rosenbloom KR, Sloan CA, Malladi VS, Dreszer TR, Learned K, Kirkup VM, et al. ENCODE Data in the UCSC Genome Browser: year 5 update. Nucleic Acids Res. 2013;41:D56–63.

2-deoxy-2-[18]fluoro-D-glucose PET/CT (18FDG PET/CT) may not be a viable biomarker in Pompe disease

U. Plöckinger[1*], V. Prasad[2,3], A. Ziagaki[1], N. Tiling[1] and A. Poellinger[4]

Abstract

Background: Pompe disease (PD) is an autosomal recessive, lysosomal storage disease due to a mutation of the acid α-glucosidase (*GAA*) gene. In adult patients, PD is characterized by slowly progressive limb-girdle and trunk myopathy and restrictive respiratory insufficiency. Enzyme replacement therapy (ERT) is available, improving or stabilizing muscle-function in some and slowing deterioration in other patients. Unfortunately, there is no biomarker available to indicate therapeutic efficacy and/or disease activity. Whole body MRI depicts all skeletal muscles demonstrating foci of atrophic muscles, i.e., late and irreversible pathological changes. Any method indicating the localizations of increased muscle glycogen storage, muscle inflammation and/or degradation could possibly help identifying newly afflicted tissue and may be of prognostic value. We therefore investigated 2-deoxy-2-[18]fluoro-D-glucose (FDG) PET, a biomarker for glucose-metabolism, as a tool to evaluate disease activity and prognosis in PD.

Methods: In a pilot study, we investigated four patients by FDG dynamic PET/CT while on ERT. One patient had FDG-PET/CT twice, before and after 12 months on ERT. Dynamic FDG-PET/CT quantifies the metabolic rate of glucose utilisation in mg/ml/min. MRI was performed in parallel with pelvic and thigh muscles semi-quantitatively scored for atrophy and disease-activity.

Results: None of the muscles analysed showed a focally increased FDG-uptake. Thus, quantification of muscle glucose metabolism could not be calculated. However, increased FDG-uptake, i.e., increased glucose utilisation, was observed in the respiratory muscles of one patient with severe, restrictive respiratory failure. In contrast, specific MRI sequences showed oedematous as well as atrophic muscle areas in PD.

Conclusions: Our pilot study demonstrates that FDG-uptake does not correlate with glycogen storage in vivo. In contrast, MRI is an excellent tool to demonstrate the extent of muscle involvement. Specific MRI sequences may even demonstrate early changes possibly allowing prognostic predictions or localization of early stages of PD.

Keywords: Pompe disease, 2-deoxy-2-[18]fluoro-D-glucose PET/CT, Biomarker, MRI

Background

Pompe disease (OMIM 232300) or glycogenosis type 2 is a lysosomal storage disease characterized by a mutation of the acid α-glucosidase (*GAA*) gene. Pompe disease (PD) is inherited in an autosomal recessive mode. Manifestations of PD in adult patients are a myopathy of limb-girdle and trunk muscles, with restrictive respiratory insufficiency as a possible complication. The disease is chronic and slowly progressive with some patients becoming wheel-chair-bound and respirator-dependent. The available enzyme replacement therapy effectively improves or stabilizes muscle function in some and slows deterioration of the disease in other patients [1, 2].

The phenotype/genotype correlation is poor and many patients harbour private mutations. Thus, genotyping is unable to predict the clinical course of an individual patient [3]. Clinical monitoring, i.e., follow-up of the individual patient, relies mainly either on semi-quantitative analysis of muscle function, like 6-min walk test, quick

* Correspondence: Ursula.Ploeckinger@charite.de
[1]Kompetenzzentrum Seltene Stoffwechselkrankheiten, Interdisziplinäres Stoffwechsel-Centrum: Endokrinologie, Diabetes und Stoffwechsel, Charité Universitätsmedizin Berlin, Augustenburger Platz 1, Campus Virchow-Klinikum, 13352 Berlin, Germany
Full list of author information is available at the end of the article

motor function test [4] or magnetic resonance tomographic imaging (MRI) of limb-girdle, paravertebral and thighs musculature and sometimes proximal arm musculature, or in rare cases, repeated muscle biopsies. Respiratory function is evaluated by lung function testing [forced expiratory vital capacity (FVC) and vital capacity (VC)], both while seated and supine. However, these clinical evaluations are flawed by a high intra- and inter-observer variation, as is the case for functional testing [6-min walk test [5, 6] and quick motor function test [4]. In addition, the test-results vary depending on the patient's sex, age and day-to-day state of health. A reliable positive predictive result is therefore difficult to achieve and intra-individual variability is high. Due to the lack of more sensitive and accurate measurements, the 6-min walk test is defined as the gold-standard and has been used in clinical studies for the evaluation of motor function in adult patients with PD [3, 7].

Biochemical parameters, i.e., muscle enzymes like aspartate aminotransferase/glutamat-pyruvat-transaminase (AST/GOT), alanine aminotransferase/glutamat-oxalacetat-transaminase (ALT/GPT), creatinine-kinase (CK) or lactate dehydrogenase (LDH) are non-specifically increased in PD and fail to correlate with disease severity or activity. The glucose tetra-saccharide, Glcalpha1-6Glcalpha1-4glcalpha1-4Glc (Glc(4)), is a glycogen-derived limit dextrin that correlates with the extent of glycogen accumulation in skeletal muscle. A retrospective analysis of clinical records of 208 patients evaluated for PD by this approach showed Glc(4) having 94% sensitivity and 84% specificity for the diagnosis of PD. However, while indicating the overall disease burden, Glc(4) provided no information on the location and distribution of excess glycogen accumulation [8]. In addition Glc(4) excretion in adult-onset PD is low and ERT-induced declines may be very small [8].

MRI imaging demonstrates the distribution pattern of muscular atrophy, compensatory muscular hypertrophy and vacuolised muscle fibres. A study with 34 adult-onset PD patients compared whole body muscle MRI using T1w and 3-point Dixon imaging of thighs and the lower trunk region to a wide range of functional scales. This comparison demonstrated a strong correlation between muscle strength, muscle functional scales and the degree of muscle fatty replacement in muscle MRI. In addition, muscle MRI detected mild degree of fatty replacement in para-spinal muscles in pre-symptomatic patients [9]. Others used either quantitative proton-density fat-fraction (PDFF) whole-body MRI or quantitative MRI in late-onset PD and compared the results with manual muscle testing. According to their results, MRI was more sensitive than physical examination for detection of abnormalities in multiple muscle groups [10, 11]. Yet, the rather slow disease progression in PD is one difficulty for MRI monitoring of muscles changes. A retrospective study by Carlier et al. using quantitative MRI demonstrated muscle fatty infiltration increase on average by 0.9%/year, with the hamstring and adductor muscles showing the fastest degradation. Muscle water T2 mapping revealed that 32% of all muscles had abnormally high T2 in at least one of two successive examinations. When muscle water T2 was abnormal, fatty degenerative changes increased by 0.61%/year. Enzyme replacement therapy resulted in 0.68%/year slow-down of the muscle fatty infiltration, in both muscles with normal and high T2s [12]. Unfortunately, most MRI findings all indicate a rather late event in the course of the disease, i.e., muscle atrophy. Furthermore, an overall slow-down of muscle fatty infiltration of 0.68%/year may not allow an individual prognosis, neither on the natural course of the disease nor on the effectiveness of enzyme replacement therapy. In addition, MRI imaging poses a burden on patients with claustrophobia, is difficult to perform in patients with respiratory insufficiency in the supine position and can be painful due to the long duration of laying still on a hard bench.

Muscle biopsies using ultrastructural examination of the tissue demonstrated reduced lysosomal glycogen after 6 months of ERT, consistent with stabilization of the disease that was not represented in the MRI images acquired parallel to the biopsies [13]. However, muscle biopsies are fraught due to (i) changing tissue localization at repeated biopsies and (ii) the invasiveness of the procedure.

Thus, to date, none of the aforementioned methods allow for a simple, reproducible measurement of disease activity, localization of active disease and monitoring of therapeutic efficacy.

Glucose and/or FDG uptake by the cell is a receptor-mediated process. Glucose binds to the membrane bound glucose-transporter (GLUT), as does FDG. The receptor-ligand complex is taken up into the cell by endocytosis. There the receptor separates from its substrate in early endosomes and is passed on to recycling endosomes and, subsequently, stored in the GLUT-containing vesicular compartment. Once inside the cell, FDG is phosphorylated to FDG-6P, which cannot enter the glycolytic pathways and is therefore trapped within the cell (Fig. 1).

The mutation of acid α-glucosidase (*GAA*) gene leads to reduced concentration/activity of the enzyme. This results in a defective metabolism of lysosomal glycogen with tissue-specific glycogen accumulation. We hypothesized that the uptake of 2-deoxy-2-[18]fluoro-D-glucose should lead to an accumulation of the labelled glucose molecule in cells with pathological glycogen storage. The extent of accumulation would indicate the extent of glycogen storage, correlating with disease activity and possible therapeutic efficacy. The method would therefore allow for early detection of active foci of glycogen deposits, well before fat accumulation or muscle atrophy occurs.

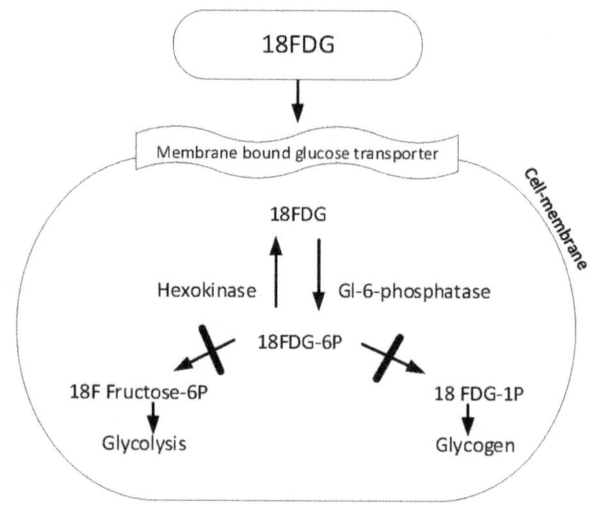

Fig. 1 Scheme delineating cellular uptake of FDG

We therefore undertook an explorative study investigating the usefulness of dynamic FDG-PET as an indicator of disease activity in late-onset PD and compared these results to routinely performed quantitative whole-body muscle MRI.

Methods

We performed five FDG dynamic PET/CTs in four patients with late onset PD. In one patient, FDG-PET/CT was performed twice, before and 1 year after the initiation of ERT, while in all other patients FDG-PET/CT took place during ongoing ERT. Patient characteristics are given in Table 1.

FDG-PET Acquisition Dynamic FDG-PET allows to quantify the metabolic rate of utilisation of glucose in mg/ml/min. Patients were kept fasting for more than 6 h, and serum glucose was measured prior to the injection of FDG. Patients were given 350 MBq of FDG as slow bolus over 20 s, and scanning was performed with the patients supine. Dynamic images were acquired over 60 min in list-mode immediately after the injection of the tracer. Images were reconstructed as follows: 3 × 20 s, 8 × 30 s, 5 × 1 min, 5 × 2 min, 4 × 5 min and 2 × 10 min. After the dynamic images, whole body images were acquired from base of skull to mid-thigh with 1.5 min/bed position. Lean body mass maximum standardized uptake value (SUVmax) was calculated for involved muscles; region of interest was drawn on the muscles showing hyperintensity on MRI. In addition, background activity was measured on the subcutaneous fat at the level of gluteus muscle as well as over the left ventricular cavity. For correction of the PET images, we used a CT attenuation correction map.

MRI: standard T1w spin echo (SE) of the pelvis and thigh muscles was performed (TR = 472 ms, TE = 18 ms) and muscle fatty degenerative changes were scored according to a 5-grade modified Mercuri score (grade 0: normal, grade1: < 25%; grade 2: > 25% and < 50%; grade 3: > 50% and < 75%; grade 4: > 75%). Short TI inversion recovery (STIR) sequences of the same body regions were acquired with TR = 3240 ms, TE = 42 ms. Finally, after administration of 0.1 mmol/kg of a gadolinium-based contrast agent (Gadovist; Bayer Healthcare), a T1w fat-sat sequence was acquired (TR = 709 ms, TE = 18 ms). All MR scans were acquired axially. For STIR and T1w fat-sat contrast-enhanced (CE) images hyperintensities were again scored according to a 5-grade modified Mercuri score (grade 0: no hyperintensities, grade 1: mild; grade 2: moderate; grade 3: intermediate; grade 4: severe amount of hyperintensities). All MRIs were performed within 6 months of the FDG-PET. An experienced radiologist (AP) analysed the MRI scans. Fatty infiltration as a marker for muscular atrophy was scored based on T1w scans. Hyperintensities in T1w FS CE and STIR scans show hypervascularisation or leakage of contrast material and oedema, respectively. The following pelvic and thigh muscles were scored: autochthonous back muscle, iliopsoas, gluteus maximus, medius and minimus (lateral, mid, medial) quadriceps femoris, sartorius, obturator and pectineus. Activity and atrophy on MRI were scored as follows: from 0 to 4 (0 = no atrophy; 1 = minimal, 2 = moderate, 4 =

Table 1 Patients characteristics

Patient number	1	2	3	4
Age (years)	51	59	27	45
Years of ERT	1.5	6.5	7	0
Sex	M	M	M	M
Age at diagnosis (years)	50	45	20	44
Mutation	c.(336-13 T > G); (1927G > A)	IVC-45 T > G; 536bpDel (IVS16 + 102_IVS17 + 31)	c.32-13 T > G; c.1128_1129delinsC	c-32-13 T > G; c.2214G > A
6-min walk test (m)	484	204	201	510
Wheelchair bound	No	No	No	No
Respiratory failure	Yes	Yes	Yes	No

[a]*SD* standard deviation

severe). The FDG-uptake in the abovementioned muscles was visually analysed. An example for the analysis of MRI images is given in Fig. 2.

Statistics

Statistical analysis was performed using STATISTICA 6.0 and IBM SPSS Statistics (IBM, Armonk, NY), Version 21. Data were calculated as median and interquartile range, for correlation Spearman's coefficient of correlation was used. A p value < 0.05 was considered significant.

Results

Four male patients (median age 48, interquartile range 36–55 years) participated in this explorative study. All patients were on ERT. One patient was investigated twice, before and after 1 year on ERT. All the patients demonstrated clinical improvement compared to before ERT and had either a stable (patients AB, FR) or slowly progressive (patients GH, SK) course of their disease. Details of the mutation and further clinical characteristics are indicated in Table 1. Classification [14] of disease severity of was moderate (one patient) and severe (three patients).

MRI fatty infiltration in T1w images as a sign for muscular atrophy was found in all patients to varying degrees and localizations (Table 2) and correlated well with the clinical status of the patients. For all four patients, the most atrophic muscles were the intrinsic back muscles (autochthonous back muscles) and the gluteus muscles, especially the gluteus minimus. Muscles with a high degree of atrophy (score = 4) showed only low signal-intensity in STIR and T1w FS CE images (score = 0–1; score = 2 only in one case and muscle). When there was no evidence of muscular atrophy (T1w score = 0), the STIR and T1w FS CE images mostly also scored 0 in these locations. However, in two patients there were muscles without atrophic changes but with elevated STIR and T1w FS CE values. Highest score for both STIR and T1w FS CE were observed when muscular atrophy scores were between 1 and 3 (Fig. 3). Atrophy scores 0–2 positively correlated with T1w and STIR (Spearman's R: 0.693, $p < 0.05$) and T1w and T1w FS CE values (Spearman's R: 0.644, $p < 0.05$). In contrast, atrophy scores 2-4 demonstrated a negative correlation for T1w and STIR (Spearman's R: – 0.426, $p < 0.05$) and for T1w and T1w FS CE, respectively (Spearman's R: – 0.334, $p < 0.05$). There was a strong positive correlation between STIR and T1w FS CE values (Spearman's R: 0.854, $p < 0.05$).

For all sequences, measured alterations were rather symmetrically distributed (Spearman's R for atrophy = 0.875, $p < 0.05$; activity = 0.829 $p < 0.05$; T1w FS CE = 0.92 $p < 0.05$).

Assuming an alpha error of 0.05, we receive an a posteriori power of 1.000, 0.987 and 0.958 for T1, STIR and T1FSCE, respectively.

Repeated MRI in one patient demonstrated a reduction of the MRI scores at the tensor fasciae latae muscle after 1 year (Fig. 4). No other muscle group showed similar improvements.

FDG-PET/CT. None of the muscles and/or regions of muscles demonstrating hyperintensity on MRI showed a quantifiable focally increased FDG metabolism. Nor did we detect increased FDG-metabolism in trunk or thigh muscles. Thus, dynamic PET quantification of glucose metabolism in muscles could not be calculated. Figure 5 gives an example of the results of FDG-PET.

FDG-PET was positive in one patient with respiratory failure. We observed a high uptake of FDG in the respiratory muscles. This clearly demonstrates the increased glucose metabolism due to the high muscle workload in a patient with restrictive respiratory insufficiency (Fig. 5).

Discussion

Our pilot study confirms the usefulness of MRI to delineate affected muscles in PD [9, 12, 14–16]. The pattern of involvement was similar in patients with and without ERT [14] and disease severity and duration were correlated to quantitative MRI findings.

We analysed 26 different muscle regions of the pelvis and thighs in four different patients with late onset PD. Within individual patients, there were considerable differences in

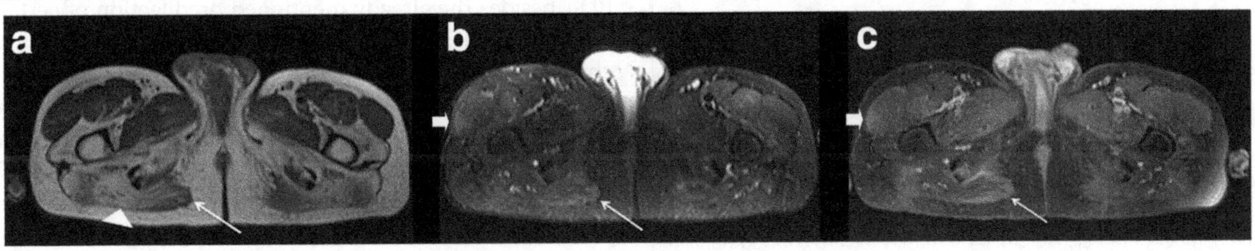

Fig. 2 MR scans of a Pompe patient at the level just below the pelvic floor. There are different stages of muscular inflammation, or atrophy respectively, visible: T1w images show fatty atrophy in various muscles, pronounced in the middle part of the gluteus maximus (**a**, arrow head). The medial part of the gluteus maximus shows only beginning atrophy at T1w (**a**, arrow) together with high signal in the STIR images (**b**). T1w FS scans also display high signal after gadolinium administration (**c**). While the tensor fasciae latae muscle (wide arrow) seems to be unaffected in the T1w images, there is high signal on STIR and T1w FS scans suggesting early changes

Table 2 Semi-quantitative results of MRI evaluation for each muscle group in Pompe disease

Muscle	T1w (Median)	T1w (IQR[a])	STIR (Median)	STIR (IQR[a])	T1 FS CE (Median)	T1 FS CE (IQR[a])
Intrinsic back muscles (lower back)	3.0	3.0–3.0	0.0	0.0–3.0	0.0	0.0–3.0
Iliopsoas	2.0	0.5–3.5	1.0	0.0–2.5	1.5	0.0–2.5
Gluteus maximus (lateral)	2.0	0.5–4.0	1.0	0.0–2.0	1.5	0.5–2.0
Gluteus maximus (center)	0.0	0.0–1.5	0.0	0.0–1.5	0.0	0.0–1.5
Gluteus maximus (medial)	1.5	0.0–3.0	1.0	0.0–2.0	1.0	0.0–2.5
Gluteus medius (ventral)	2.0	1.0–3.5	1.5	1.0–2.0	2.0	1.0–3.5
Gluteus medius (dorsal)	3.5	1.5–4.0	1.0	0.0–1.5	0.5	0.0–1.5
Gluteus minimus (ventral)	4.0	3.5–4.0	0.5	0.0–1.5	0.5	0.0–1.5
Gluteus minimus (dorsal)	4.0	3.5–4.0	0.5	0.0–1.5	0.5	0.0–1.5
Rectus femoris	0.0	0.0–0.0	0.0	0.0–0.0	0.0	0.0–0.0
Sartorius	0.0	0.0–0.0	0.0	0.0–0.0	0.0	0.0–0.0
Obturator ext.	1.0	0.5–2.0	0.0	0.0–0.5	0.0	0.0–0.5
Pectineus	0.0	0.0–2.5	0.0	0.0–0.0	0.0	0.0–0.0

[a]Interquartile range

T1 images were scored according to a 5-grade score (grade 0: normal, grade 1: < 25%; grade 2: > 25% and < 50%; grade 3: > 50% and < 75%; grade 4: > 75%). STIR and T1w fat-sat contrast-enhanced (CE) images were scored according to a 5-grade score (grade 0: no hyperintensities, grade1: mild; grade 2: moderate; grade 3: intermediate; grade 4: severe amount of hyperintensities)

muscular atrophy of different muscles ranging from no visible atrophy (score = 0) to severe atrophy (score = 4) with the intrinsic back muscles and the gluteus minimus muscle displaying the highest scores of atrophy. We found no observable atrophy in the quadriceps femoris (rectus femoris) and sartorius muscle. Why these muscles display minor damage while others are heavily involved is a matter of debate and was also observed in earlier studies [13, 15]. Van der Ploeg et al. [13] suggests that muscle groups, like the gluteus muscles and intrinsic back muscles, performing continuous or repetitive contraction are more prone to earlier damage than muscles that are subject to relatively intermittent contraction.

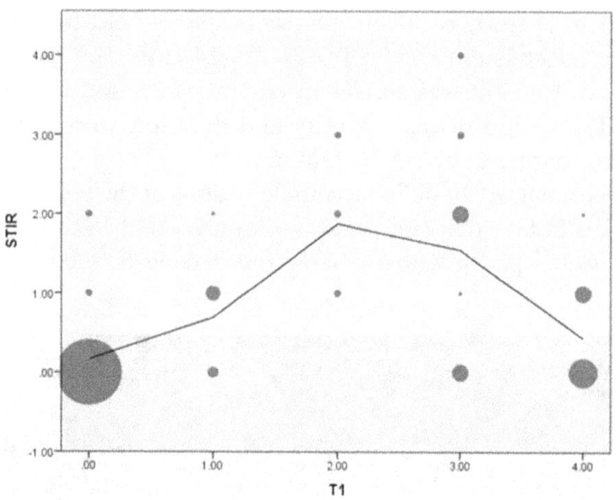

Fig. 3 Scatterplot between the semi-quantitative assessment of T1 (atrophy) and STIR (muscle oedema): the size of the circle displays the number of muscle regions. Most muscle regions showed no atrophy (T1 = 0) and no oedema (STIR = 0). As atrophy increases so does muscular oedema, but only up to a score of T1 = 2. From there, further atrophy is associated with less oedema. Of note, some muscles showing no atrophy (T1 = 0) already exhibited oedema, possibly an early sign of affected muscle

STIR images revealing muscular oedema were only partly in line with the results of the T1w images showing atrophy: when muscular atrophy was not visible (score = 0) in most of the muscles analysed there was also no oedema. Oedematous changes increased with increasing atrophy, but only up to an atrophy score of 2–3 (correlation of Spearman's *R*: 0.693). When atrophy was more prevalent (score 4) oedematous changes decreased (Spearman's *R*: – 0.426). None of the T1w changes with a score of 4 showed an oedema score higher than 2. As a rule, similar changes as for the STIR images were noted for the T1w FS CE images in most of the muscles analysed.

The varying degree of atrophy and oedema/inflammation in different muscles in a given individual with PD—besides the already mentioned predilection of certain muscles—indicates a temporal heterogeneity of muscular changes. We hypothesize that disease manifestation in a muscle initially demonstrates only little atrophy but an increasing amount of oedema and inflammatory changes as reflected by increased STIR and T1w FS CE values. Of note, in some muscles, oedematous and inflammatory changes were visible in muscles showing no atrophy at all, consistent with results by van der Ploeg et al. [13].

After this initial stage, atrophic, oedematous and inflammatory changes seem to develop rather synchronously up to the point when inflammation and oedema are less visible, but atrophy further increases. Finally, at

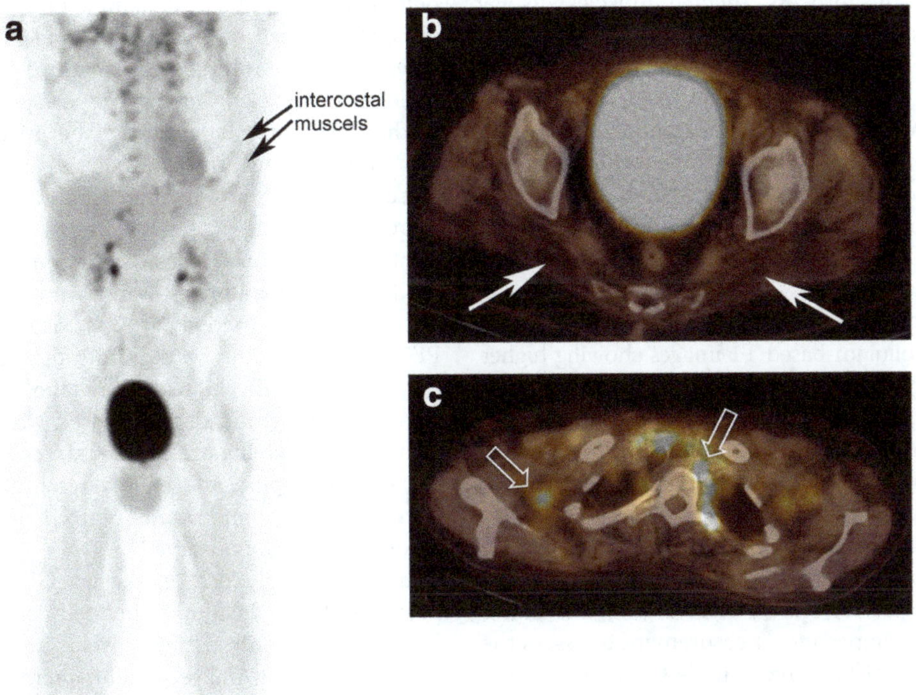

Fig. 4 a Maximum intensity projection image showing the paravertebral brown fat as well as intercostal muscle. **b** Upper panel showing fused FDG PET/CT image with gluteus muscle atrophy and almost no FDG-uptake (white arrows). **c** Lower panel showing paravertebral and axillary brown fat (open arrows)

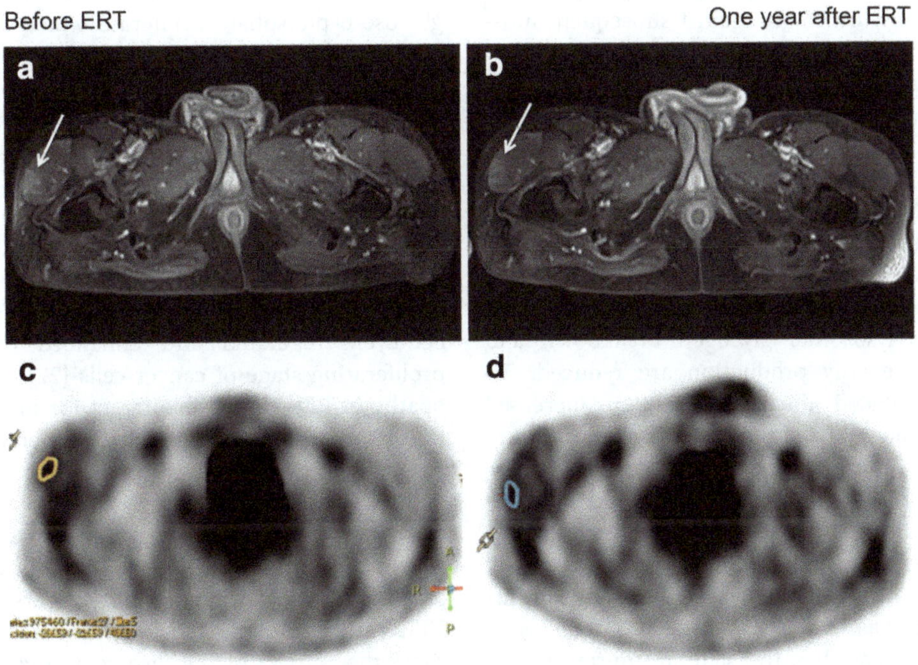

Fig. 5 MRI (**a**, **b**) and FDG PET (**c**, **d**) before and after 1 year of ERT. MRI shows slight improvement, i.e., less hyperintensity of the tensor fasciae latae muscle (arrow) in the T1w sequence after gadolinium administration 1 year after ERT. FDG-PET show no significantly different tracer uptake in the region of interest (orange and blue lines) pre- and post-therapy

the end-stage of this process affected muscles display fatty infiltration as a result of atrophy but no more inflammation or oedema.

This study is the first study that used gadolinium-enhanced MR imaging for the evaluation of non-cardiac muscle involvement in late-onset PD patients. Gadolinium-based studies have shown benefits in other forms of myositis for differentiation and staging [17]. In the present study, we found a strong positive correlation between STIR and T1 FS CE images ($R = 0.854$). However, there was one significant difference between the STIR and T1 FS CE images, with the gadolinium-based T1 images showing higher values on the modified Mercuri scale. This may indicate that T1 FS CE might be more sensitive to early muscle changes in late-onset PD patients. If gadolinium studies are really necessary for early detection needs to be evaluated in further studies, especially in light of the problem of gadolinium deposition that was first described in 2014 [18].

Due to MRI limitations (claustrophobia, non-MRI compatible devices, severe respiratory disease) [10], alternative approaches like bio-impedance measurement to assess the relative proportions of fatty and muscle tissue may give a correlation between the degree of replacement of the muscle tissue with fatty tissue and the severity of the disease evaluated clinically [19], diagnosing the late phase of the disease.

In conclusion, MRI is an excellent tool to demonstrate the extent of muscle involvement in late-onset PD. MRI may even pick up early, i.e., oedematous stages of the disease. Focusing on these early signs may allow more specific training early on to set against subsequent muscular atrophy. Whether these early changes may allow prognostic predictions has yet to be demonstrated.

In well-prepared (after 6-h fast, serum glucose < 150 mg/dl and adequate rest prior to image acquisition) non-PD patients no or only faint muscular FDG uptake can be observed. We hypothesized that in PD FDG-PET/CT would delineate increased accumulation of glucose into glycogen-enriched depots and thus diagnose the early phases of the disease. In α-glucosidase-deficient muscles lysosomal glycogen breakdown and thus glucose and energy production are reduced. To compensate for reduced glucose production, increased glucose and in analogy FDG uptake may be an option in these cells. In α-glucosidase-deficient muscles intracytoplasmatic GLUT4 expression is increased in damaged and normal in unafflicted muscle fibres [20]. We hypothesized that this increased GLUT4 expression may correlate with an increased glucose and thus an increased FDG uptake as well.

This information may then translate in improved local physiotherapy and/or anti-inflammatory treatment. Unfortunately, no focally increased FDG accumulation in relation or unrelated to MRI-signal changes could be demonstrated. Thus, dynamic PET quantification of glycogen deposition in muscles could not be calculated. There might be multiple explanations for this result. Nutritional status, i.e., fasting or post-prandial application of the tracer may be an issue. We injected FDG in fasting patients and thus glycolysis may have prevailed glycogenesis. This is in line with our observation of an increased uptake in the respiratory muscles in the patient with severe restrictive respiratory failure. Due to the high workload of respiratory muscles glucose metabolism was increased as it was visualized in the FDG PET/CT. Again, this would indicate a rather late state of the disease, as the increased metabolic needs are correlated with a significantly increased workload on the few remaining/surviving muscles. On the other hand, with the patient supine, the energy requirement of all other muscles was low and therefore no increased glucose metabolism could be observed.

In addition, glucose uptake via GLUT4 occurs either post-prandially insulin-stimulated or during exercise [21]. However, all patients were investigated after an overnight resting phase without increased muscular energy needs. Whether post-exercise FDG may have given different results, remains to be investigated.

Alternatively, deposition of the tracer into glycogen may not have taken place at all. Glycogen is synthesized from the activated glucose-donor, uridine diphosphate glucose (UDP-glucose), catalysed by glycogen synthase, the key regulatory enzyme in glycogenesis. To be incorporated into glycogen, FDG has to be modified by glucose-6-phosphate isomerase which catalyses the second step during glycolysis. It has been suggested that the substitution of the C-2 hydroxyl moiety by ^{18}F prevents this process [22]. Subsequently, FDG could possibly not be integrated into glycogen. A new tracer, 18F-N-(methyl-(2-fluoroethyl)-1H-[1,2,3]triazole-4-yl) glucosamine (^{18}F-NFTG), recently developed, may be a more effective biomarker in PD. So far, 18F-NFTG PET has been used in animal tumour models to visualize tumours of the upper thorax where the rate of glycogen synthesis is cell-cycle regulated and enhanced during the non-proliferating stage of cancer cells [22]. Whether the myopathy of PD is a feasible target for integrating this new tracer for demonstrating early glycogen accumulation remains to be demonstrated.

Conclusions

In conclusion, MRI delineated the localisation and extent of muscle atrophy in all patients. Changes in the STIR and gadolinium-based T1w sequences probably show the activity of the disease and can serve as earlier markers in the disease process than late changes revealed by fatty infiltration of atrophic muscles as measured by T1-weighted sequences.

FDG PET/CT did not demonstrate increased uptake in glycogen, neither in the early nor late phase of the tracer accumulation. A positive signal was detected by FDG PET/CT in the patient with respiratory failure. Due to the increased respiratory muscle workload, glucose utilisation and thus FDG-uptake was increased as well.

Author details
[1]Kompetenzzentrum Seltene Stoffwechselkrankheiten, Interdisziplinäres Stoffwechsel-Centrum: Endokrinologie, Diabetes und Stoffwechsel, Charité Universitätsmedizin Berlin, Augustenburger Platz 1, Campus Virchow-Klinikum, 13352 Berlin, Germany. [2]Department of Nuclear Medicine, Charité Universitätsmedizin Berlin, Berlin, Germany. [3]Department of Nuclear Medicine Universitätsklinik Ulm, Ulm, Germany. [4]Department of Diagnostic, Interventional and Pediatric Radiology, Inselspital Bern University Hospital, University of Bern, Bern, Switzerland.

Abbreviations
^{18}F: ^{18}Fluoro; ^{18}F-NFTG: 18F-N-(methyl-(2-fluoroethyl)-1H-[1,2,3]triazole-4-yl) glucosamine; CE: Contrast enhanced; CK: Creatinine kinase; CT: Computer tomography; ERT: Enzyme replacement therapy; FDG: 2-deoxy-2-[18]fluoro-D-glucose; FVC: Forced expiratory vital capacity; *GAA*: Acid α-glucosidase gene; Glc(4): Glcalpha1-6Glcalpha1-4glcalpha1-4Glc; GOT: Glutamat-Oxalacetet-Transaminase; GPT: Glutamat-Pyruvat-Transaminase; GS: Glycogen synthase; LDH: Lactate dehydrogenase; MBq: Megabecquerel; MRI: Magnetic resonance imaging; OMIM: Online Mendelian Inheritance in Man; PD: Pompe disease; PDFF: Proton-density fat-fraction; PET: Positron emission tomography; SD: Standard deviation; SE: Spin echo; STIR: Short TI inversion recovery; T1: T1-weighted image; TE: Echo time; TI: Inversion time; TR: Repetition time; VC: Vital capacity; Years: Years

Acknowledgements
Not applicable.

Funding
The investigation was funded by an unrestricted grant from Sanofi Genzyme to Ursula Plöckinger. Sanofi Genzyme was not involved in the design of the study, collection, analysis and interpretation of data or in writing the manuscript.

Authors' contributions
UP conceived the study in cooperation with VP and AP. UP cared for the patients and drafted the manuscript with the technical details concerning FDG-PET/CT and MRI written by VP and AP, respectively. VP was responsible for the implementation and interpretation of the FDG-PET/CT, AP was responsible for the implementation and interpretation of the MRIs. NT collected the clinical details from the patients' files. AZ was responsible for the legal aspects of the study, critically read the manuscript and helped with the revised version. All authors read and approved the final manuscript.

Ethics approval and consent to participate
All procedures were in accordance with the ethical standards of the responsible committee on human experimentation (institutional and national) and with the Helsinki Declaration of 1964, as revised in 2000 [23]. Informed written consent was obtained from all patients. All patients consented to the publication of their data. The institutional Ethic Committee of the Charité consented to the procedures and the publication of the data (EA2/089/15).

Competing interests
Ursula Plöckinger was the recipient of an unrestricted grant by Genzyme, Germany, received speaker honorarium from Sanofi Genzyme, Germany; BioMarin Germany, and a research grant from Pfizer, Germany. Nikolaus Tiling has received a speaker honorarium from Shire, Germany and Sanofi Genzyme, Germany. V. Prasad, A. Poellinger and A. Ziagaki have nothing to declare.

References

1. Schuller A, Kornblum C, Deschauer M, Vorgerd M, Schrank B, Mengel E, et al. Diagnosis and therapy of late onset Pompe disease. Nervenarzt. 2013;84:1467–72.
2. Teener JW. Late-onset Pompe's disease. Semin Neurol. 2012;32:506–11.
3. Regnery C, Kornblum C, Hanisch F, Vielhaber S, Strigl-Pill N, Grunert B, et al. 36 months observational clinical study of 38 adult Pompe disease patients under alglucosidase alfa enzyme replacement therapy. J Inherit Metab Dis. 2012;35:837–45.
4. van Capelle CI, van der Beek NA, de Vries JM, van Doorn PA, Duivenvoorden HJ, Leshner RT, et al. The quick motor function test: a new tool to rate clinical severity and motor function in Pompe patients. J Inherit Metab Dis. 2012;35:317–23.
5. Casanova C, Celli BR, Barria P, Casas A, Cote C, de Torres JP, et al. The 6-min walk distance in healthy subjects: reference standards from seven countries. Eur Respir J. 2011;37:150–6.
6. Laboratories ATSCoPSfCPF. ATS statement: guidelines for the six-minute walk test. Am J Respir Crit Care Med. 2002;166:111–7.
7. Andreassen CS, Schlutter JM, Vissing J, Andersen H. Effect of enzyme replacement therapy on isokinetic strength for all major muscle groups in four patients with Pompe disease-a long-term follow-up. Mol Genet Metab. 2014;112:40–3.
8. Young SP, Piraud M, Goldstein JL, Zhang H, Rehder C, Laforet P, et al. Assessing disease severity in Pompe disease: the roles of a urinary glucose tetrasaccharide biomarker and imaging techniques. Am J Med Genet Part C Sem Med Genet. 2012;160c:50–8.
9. Figueroa-Bonaparte S, Segovia S, Llauger J, Belmonte I, Pedrosa I, Alejaldre A, et al. Muscle MRI findings in childhood/adult onset Pompe disease correlate with muscle function. PLoS One. 2016;11:e0163493. https://doi.org/10.1371/journal.pone.0163493.
10. Horvath JJ, Austin SL, Case LE, Greene KB, Jones HN, Soher BJ, et al. Correlation between quantitative whole-body muscle magnetic resonance imaging and clinical muscle weakness in Pompe disease. Muscle Nerve. 2015;51:722–30.
11. Pichiecchio A, Berardinelli A, Moggio M, Rossi M, Balottin U, Comi GP, et al. Asymptomatic Pompe disease: can muscle magnetic resonance imaging facilitate diagnosis? Muscle Nerve. 2016;53:326–7.
12. Carlier PG, Azzabou N, de Sousa PL, Hicks A, Boisserie JM, Amadon A, et al. Skeletal muscle quantitative nuclear magnetic resonance imaging follow-up of adult Pompe patients. J Inherit Metab Dis. 2015;38:565–72.
13. van der Ploeg A, Carlier PG, Carlier RY, Kissel JT, Schoser B, Wenninger S, et al. Prospective exploratory muscle biopsy, imaging, and functional assessment in patients with late-onset Pompe disease treated with alglucosidase alfa: the EMBASSY study. Mol Genet Metab. 2016;119:115–23.
14. Alejaldre A, Diaz-Manera J, Ravaglia S, Tibaldi EC, D'Amore F, Moris G, et al. Trunk muscle involvement in late-onset Pompe disease: study of thirty patients. Neuromuscul Disord. 2012;22(Suppl 2):S148–54.
15. Carlier RY, Laforet P, Wary C, Mompoint D, Laloui K, Pellegrini N, et al. Whole-body muscle MRI in 20 patients suffering from late onset Pompe disease: involvement patterns. Neuromuscul Disord. 2011;21:791–9.
16. Gruhn KM, Heyer CM, Guttsches AK, Rehmann R, Nicolas V, Schmidt-Wilcke T, et al. Muscle imaging data in late-onset Pompe disease reveal a correlation between the pre-existing degree of lipomatous muscle alterations and the efficacy of long-term enzyme replacement therapy. MGM Rep. 2015;3:58–64.
17. Schulze M, Kotter I, Ernemann U, Fenchel M, Tzaribatchev N, Claussen CD, et al. MRI findings in inflammatory muscle diseases and their noninflammatory mimics. AJR. 2009;192:1708–16.

18. Kanda T, Ishii K, Kawaguchi H, Kitajima K, Takenaka D. High signal intensity in the dentate nucleus and globus pallidus on unenhanced T1-weighted MR images: relationship with increasing cumulative dose of a gadolinium-based contrast material. Radiology. 2014;270:834–41.
19. Rozdzynska-Swiatkowska A, Jurkiewicz E, Tylki-Szymanska A. Bioimpedance analysis as a method to evaluate the proportion of fatty and muscle tissues in progressive myopathy in Pompe disease. JIMD Rep. 2016;26:45–51.
20. Orth M, Mundegar RR. Effect of acid maltase deficiency on the endosomal/lysosomal system and glucose transporter 4. NMD. 2003;13:49–54.
21. Lauritzen HP, Schertzer JD. Measuring GLUT4 translocation in mature muscle fibers. Am J Physiol Endocrinol Metab. 2010;299:E169–79.
22. Witney TH, Carroll L, Alam IS, Chandrashekran A, Nguyen QD, Sala R, et al. A novel radiotracer to image glycogen metabolism in tumors by positron emission tomography. Cancer Res. 2014;74:1319–28.
23. Association WM. World medical association declaration of Helsinki ethical principles for medical research involving human subjects. JAMA. 2013;310:2191–4.

18

The development of large-scale de-identified biomedical databases in the age of genomics—principles and challenges

Fida K. Dankar[1*], Andrey Ptitsyn[2] and Samar K. Dankar[3]

Abstract

Contemporary biomedical databases include a wide range of information types from various observational and instrumental sources. Among the most important features that unite biomedical databases across the field are high volume of information and high potential to cause damage through data corruption, loss of performance, and loss of patient privacy. Thus, issues of data governance and privacy protection are essential for the construction of data depositories for biomedical research and healthcare. In this paper, we discuss various challenges of data governance in the context of population genome projects. The various challenges along with best practices and current research efforts are discussed through the steps of data collection, storage, sharing, analysis, and knowledge dissemination.

Keywords: Biomedical database, Data privacy, Data governance, Whole genome sequencing

Background

Overview

Databases are both the result and the instrument of research. From the earliest times, assembling collections of samples and stories was essential for any research project. The results of research feeding back into the libraries and collections create a positive feedback in the accumulation of knowledge limited only by the technological platform for storage and retrieval of information. The modern times did not change the principle but further emphasized it with the advent of computers, mass information storage, and high-throughput research instrumentation. Modern biomedical databases may vary in size, specialization, and type of access but with a few exceptions are voluminous and include complex data from multiple sources. Arguably, the first integrated database of the population scale was initiated in Iceland when Decode Genetics started in 1996 [1]. This new generation of integrated biomedical databases incorporates both phenotype (medical records, clinical studies, etc.) and genotype (variation screening at first, now increasingly shifting to whole exome and whole genome sequencing [2, 3]). The project started by Decode has generated one of the best resources for discovery in biomedical sciences and inspired development of multiple populational and national genomics projects, also feeding into integrated databases. Genomics England [4], Human Longevity [5], All of US (formerly known as Precision Medicine Initiative) [6], China's Precision Medicine Initiative [7], Korean Reference Genome Project [8], Saudi Human Genome Program [9], and Qatar Genome [10] programs are just a few recent examples of active large-scale projects generating enormous databases of complex biomedical information. Large-scale population genomics projects proliferating in the second decade of the twenty-first century show enormous diversity in goals and strategies. The Icelandic genome program has evolved from the largest population genetics study of the time and has primary objectives in advancing biomedical research. China's Precision Medicine Initiative is one of the most ambitious programs with an aim to sequence 100 million whole human genomes by 2030. The objective is to improve disease diagnosis, develop targeted treatments, and provide better wellness regimes. Genomics

* Correspondence: fida.dankar@uaeu.ac.ae
[1]College of IT, UAEU, Al Ain, UAE
Full list of author information is available at the end of the article

England is an augmented (100,000) research cohort study that implies sampling of the most common diseases and reflecting the genetic diversity of the population in Great Britain. The All of Us project has similar objectives and aims to collect a sufficiently large cohort (1,000,000). The numbers alone have a great ameliorating effect on statistical power of association studies. Deep phenotyping and follow-up sampling in All of Us are aiming to develop the new level of precision in diagnostic and treatment of multiple diseases. The declared aims of the Human Longevity project are even more focused on a specific range of age-associated diseases. To achieve its goals, Human Longevity plans to recruit about 1,000,000 donors. The Saudi Human Genome Program has a very different focus; it aims to develop effective methods and facilities for early diagnostics and treatment of heritable diseases. Such goal does not require the genome sequencing effort on the same scale as All of Us or Genomics England. The program implements only a small number of whole genome sequencing and up to 100,000 whole exome sequencing to collect the data reflecting local genetic variation and design a microarray chip for cost-effective mass neonatal screening. In contrast, the national genome program in Kuwait requires complete sampling of the entire population including nationals and non-citizen residents because the principal goal, according to the recently adopted DNA Law [11], is to counteract terrorist activity by precise unequivocal identification of every human being. The Qatar Genome Programme (QGP) aims to integrate genome sequencing information of all Qatari nationals with electronic medical records (EMRs) and results of clinical studies to provide quick and precise personalized diagnostic and treatment of diseases. The goal is to provide a solid basis for the biomedical research in the country.

These biomedical databases are often viewed as a platform for regional and worldwide collaborative research projects. Both the construction of these resources and serving them to a growing research community (national and international) present a significant challenge toward preserving the privacy of the participants.

Particularities of genomic data

In 2008, James Watson, a co-discoverer of the double-helix DNA model, opted to release his sequenced genome in a public database with the exception of his APOE gene (which has been associated with Alzheimer's disease). However, a statistical model was later developed that inferred the missing gene with a high degree of confidence [12]. This incident conveys one of many new privacy concerns that genomic data raises and that are difficult to deal with:

- First, genomic data is highly distinguishable. There is confirmation that a sequence of 30 to 80 SNPs could uniquely identify an individual [13]. Genomic data is also very stable [14]. It undergoes little changes over the lifetime of an individual and thus has a long-lived value (as opposed to other biomedical data such as blood tests which have expiry dates).
- Second, genetic data provides sensitive information about genetic conditions and predispositions to certain diseases such as cancer, Alzheimer, and schizophrenia. If breached, such information can be stigmatizing to participants and can be used against them in employment and insurance opportunities, even if these pre-dispositions never materialize.
- Third, genetic data does not only provide information about the sequenced individuals but also about their ancestors and off springs. Whole genome data increases our ability to predict information related to relatives' present and future health risks, which raises the question as to the obligation of a consented participant towards their family members (the authors in [15] describe privacy risks to family members of individuals who shared their genetic data for medical research).
- Finally, and most concerning, there is great fear from the potential information hidden within genomic data [16]. As our knowledge in genomics evolves, so will our view on the sensitivity of genomic data (in other words, it is not possible to quantify the amount and sensitivity of personal information that can be derived from it).

Paper outline

In this paper, we discuss various privacy and governance challenges encountered during the construction and deployment of population-scale sequencing projects. The various challenges are discussed through the stages of:

1. Initial data collection,
2. Data storage,
3. Data sharing (utilization), and
4. Dissemination of research findings to the community.

At each stage, we discuss current practices and challenges, as well as contemporary research efforts, with a particular interest in *data sharing for research purposes* [17]. We provide examples from a diversity of large-scale population sequencing projects and reflect on their scope and data governance models.

Note that the above division is simplistic as the different stages are not mutually exclusive; however, it makes for a simpler and more organized presentation of the different ideas.

Data collection

The data for the different genome projects is sought from the community and results from the efforts on part of the community. Thus, it is important to consult with the concerned population to establish the basic principles for data collection and research oversight. To achieve that, *a community engagement model* should be defined. The model should establish the basic principles for data collection and research oversight such as:

(i) *An advocating technique* for advertising the project to the community and raising the number of individuals who are aware of the project. Such technique should strive to reach different elements within the society, provide clear dissemination of risks and benefits, and establish methods for recurrent evaluation of the community attitudes and understanding of the project.
(ii) *Enrollment criteria* to define the basis for enrollment (should it be disease-based or volunteer-based) as well as the acceptable age for volunteers.
(iii) *An enrollment process* to define the scope of subjects' consent (a general opt in/out or an informed consent) and to set a clear boundary between research and clinical practice, and
(iv) *An institutional and community-based oversight process* to discuss and establish oversight for the program by the community and by independent ethics committees. The scope of these committees should include oversight on data repositories, oversight on research studies and oversight on any changes to the protocol (data use agreements, communications, etc.).

In many cases, regulations require the organization to establish an independent institutional review board, (IRB). The IRB's mandate (at the data collection and storage phases) is to review and approve all proposals related to the data collection protocol and to approve/manage the participant's consent process for the data collection activity.

One of the most comprehensive community engagement models is that of the Electronic Medical Records and Genomics (eMERGE) network [18]. eMERGE, a National Institute of Health Initiative, is a consortium of nine US medical research institutes (including Vanderbilt Genome-Electronic Records (VGER) project and North Western University biorepository (NUgene)) that combine DNA repositories and EMR systems for advancing genetic research. In the case of VGER [19], the community engagement model was established in consultation with the community through surveys, focus groups (from different ethnic, racial, and socioeconomic backgrounds), posters, and in-person interviews. These activities helped in shaping the principles of data collection, data sharing, and community oversight. The established oversight bodies include The Vanderbilt IRB, the medical center's ethics committee, and several newly established ethics, scientific, and community advisory boards. The community advisory board's role is to evaluate the projects' adherence to the established security and privacy measures, to voice the concerns/issues of the community with regards to the use of their genetic information for research, and to monitor any social/ethical issues arising in the process and help in providing the necessary measures to resolve them [19].

In the case of the NUgene project (North Western University biorepository, another eMERGE network member), the NUMC (Northwestern Medical Center) scientific, medical, and ethics community; the North Western University IRB; community researchers; external advisors; and public health experts were all involved early in establishing issues of consent for genome-wide association studies (GWASs), means to inform participants about data sharing, means to keep participants informed about research activities, and means to engage participants and learn their concern regarding data sharing.

For the case of the Qatar Genome Programme, oversight is provided mainly by an IRB and an access committee (involving prominent members of the community). Although some effort was exercised to publicize the long-term goals and benefits of the project and to get the community involved, the major recruitment incentive is the comprehensive health check provided as part of the sample collection visits by the Qatar Biobank [10]. The appointment takes two 2 days and includes an extensive set of studies and measurement. The measurements include height, weight, blood pressure, grip strength, waist and hip measurements, and body fat composition. The study proceeds to lung function, ultrasound carotid artery scan, 12-lead electrocardiogram, full body iDXA scan, artery stiffness measurement, and treadmill walking test. Finally, samples of blood, saliva, and urine are collected and analyzed.

Most large-scale population genomics programs collect some phenotypic data; the type and volume adjusted to the goals of the study. For instance, the Estonian Genome Project data collection is performed by the Estonian Biobank. The emphasis is on collection of personal data by computer-assisted personal interview (CAPI) within hours of appointment at a doctor's office. The CAPI includes personal and genealogical data (place of birth, ethnicity, family history of medical conditions, etc.), educational and occupational history, and lifestyle data (physical activity, dietary habits, smoking, alcohol consumption, etc.). During the appointment, additional anthropometric, blood pressure, and heart rate data are collected along with the blood sample. The particular feature of the Estonian Genome Project is its strong association with electronic health records providing access to the past and current health status of each sample donor. However, the phenotype study is by far less intensive than that of the Qatar Genome Programme. Saudi Human Genome Program [20] collects virtually no individual phenotype data since this information is not essential to the goals of the program. In the most extreme example, the Kuwait DNA Law [11] showed no interest in phenotype data; mandatory DNA sampling from all residents and visitors also implied no need for consent on the part of the sample donor. Remarkably, after the international outcries pointing out potential abuse of such law, local protests, and challenge from the lawyers, the law has been amended in its most controversial parts.

Protecting participants' data from privacy breaches is a key issue to the success of any genome project. Prospective participants in research studies ranked privacy as one of their top worries and as a major determinant toward their participation in a study [21–23]. Privacy is a socially bound concept; it is deeply affected by language, religion, traditions, and cultural expectations. A simple question such as "how much rent do you pay?" is considered inappropriate in some societies while perfectly normal in others. In the Arab world, for example, personal reputation and family ties are among the highest moral values. As explained by Abokhodair and Vieweg [24], "membership in a family or tribe are of the utmost importance; there is no individual separate from a family ... asserting one's individuality is viewed in a negative light"; in fact, individuals often rely on their family members and communities for significant decisions, while in western societies, asserting one's individuality is celebrated. For these reasons, privacy breaches from genetic testing may differ in their impact on individuals from different backgrounds. Thus, it is important to investigate and understand the cultural values of concerned communities and to tailor the specifics of data collection and data sharing accordingly. Unfortunately, privacy is still treated as a universal notion, and little research has been done to understand the cultural impact.

In the next two sections, we discuss current practice and challenges in protecting participants' sensitive data while in storage (data storage) and while in use (data sharing).

Data storage

EMR and Biobank data are highly sensitive and require significant storage space (the total length of an individual genome is over 3 billion base pairs). As such, one of the biggest challenges for a data warehouse is to decide *where* and *how* to store this data.

Where to store the data?

Data storage presents a significant technological challenge for many large-scale genome projects. The total volume of deep whole genome sequencing (WGS) with raw read, aligned, and variant calling data can reach 0. 5 TB per genome. Phenotyping, imaging, and omics data add additional volume. The specific number may vary widely depending on the types of data collected. Questionnaires and physiological tests, even as comprehensive as those conducted by Qatar Biobank, when collecting samples for the Genome Sequencing Program, add only a small percent to the total volume. Digital images can potentially add large volumes on the same scale as genome sequencing (i.e., on TB scale). However, the real imaging data associated with a particular sample donor in current projects is relatively small and does not exceed gigabyte (GB) scale. Omics data (such as gene expression, methylation, or metabolomics) can also be as large as genome sequencing data. Some of such data is produced using similar next-generation sequencing techniques that result in the same volumes of raw data, which can be stored to reproduce the downstream analysis. Multiple tissue samples can be taken for omics analysis from different organs of the same donor, at different times or in different disease states. This potentially can multiply the volume of data by as many times as more samples are taken. However, at this time, this kind of data is rarely added in significant amounts due to the high costs of high-throughput methods. WGS data remains the most voluminous part of genomic databases. With reserve copy and redundancy, the overall data volume requires petabytes of storage space even for relatively small population studies with tens of thousands of samples. Data compression and selective saving of key data files (while other types of data can be reproduced from initial and intermediate data) can reduce the requirements. Nevertheless, the overall data storage demand in population sequencing is enormous. In the QGP example, it has been originally estimated as 300 PB. The challenge is further compounded by requirement of fast access to individual data files, high-throughput access to multiple genomes in research cohort studies, and long-term storage keeping the data safe and actively used for decades ahead. On the other hand, the price of storage has a hard ceiling dictated by the progress in sequencing technology: the price for data storage per gigabyte should not exceed (and better be significantly lower than) the price of sequencing of the same data from a stored sample. Such demands and limitations make engineering the data storage facility extremely challenging.

In general, the data can be outsourced to a cloud provider or stored on a private—locally managed—cloud. The former approach obscures the complexity of technology but demands highly developed broadband network infrastructure and limits the control over data security and access performance. The overall performance of a cloud-based data storage solution in a large-scale project is gated by the availability of broadband infrastructure. Nevertheless, when local conditions offer adequate answers to security and broadband infrastructure challenges, cloud solution can be very attractive. Genomics England with a goal of 100,000 WGS and full complement of phenotype data is the most brilliant example [25]. The latter approach can be more expensive in terms of engineering, capital expenses, and running costs. In the QGP example, the storage is engineered as a complex solution that involves multiple redundancy and multi-tier storage on different information carriers ranging from flash drives to tape libraries. However, the storage service is provided in a form of a single name space private cloud (see overview in Fig. 1).

In other examples of local storage solution for large-scale genomic and biomedical data, the technical details of storage architecture are rarely detailed and rely on the local policies of the data center for data integrity, security, and safety. Examples of such projects include the Estonian Genome Project and Saudi Human Genome Program [26, 27].

It is increasingly advocated that individuals should be the guardians of their own biomedical data. As such, they should have the ability to access, modify, and grant access (to family, health authorities, or research facilities) as they see fit. However, numerous challenges (in terms of data storage) have to be solved before such model can be adopted, such as:

1. Where should individual data be stored (individual's private PC or on a private access-controlled cloud?), and how to ensure the security of the data in either case?
2. How to grant access to different authorities and how to manage such access?
3. Should the data be backed up, where and how?
4. Does the individual have the right to withdraw authorized access or to delete their data, and how can either be done [28]?

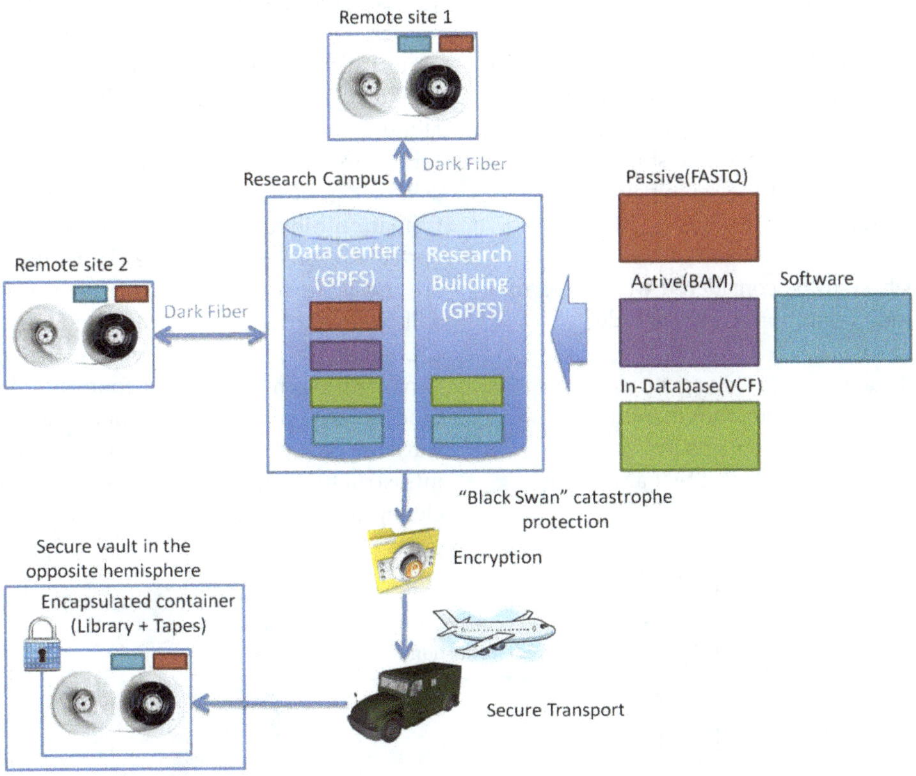

Fig. 1 Secure storage strategy for a large-scale population sequencing project. All data is stored in a secure data center with partial mirroring for research on site, partial archival mirroring for backup at geographically distant remote sites within the country, and additional mirror copy for protection against unforeseeable rare catastrophic (aka "Black Swan") events.

How to store the data?

To minimize the risk of harm, most research platforms store de-identified clinical and biobank data while retaining the link between both data sources (the de-identified EMR data and the biobank data). This can be achieved by applying the following two operations:

1. The first operation (known as pseudonymization) identifies a stable and unique identifier(s) (such as Social Security numbers and national IDs) that is included in both data sources and replaces it with a unique random ID or pseudonym (refer to Fig. 2). The pseudonym can be obtained by encrypting or hashing one or several identifiers. Decode genetics uses a symmetric encryption algorithm (TwoFish) to convert the Social Security number (SSN) to an alphabet-derived string. VGER hashes the medical record number using the public hashing algorithm SHA-512.
2. The second operation removes all uniquely identifying information (such as names, record number, and emails) from the structured data and masks all unique identifiers from the unstructured data (such as doctors' notes), (refer to Table 1 for examples of unique identifiers). Additional fields can be also removed from the data for added privacy; the VGER project, as an example, removes all geographic information smaller than a state and all elements of dates (except year) directly related to the individual (such as date of birth and date of death) and shifts all hospital visit dates by a random value between 1 and 364 days (the shift being the same across the record of the same patient to preserve temporal analysis).

Multiple aspects have to be considered when designing the pseudonymization operation; these include:

1. Ensuring that each subject is assigned the same random ID (pseudonym) across different data sources. This consistency will ensure that data belonging to a particular subject will always be mapped to one record.
2. Deciding whether the pseudonymization process should be reversible or not. Reversible systems allow reverting back to the identity of the subjects through a process called de-pseudonymization. For the case of Decode Genetics and QGP, reversibility was chosen because communication with patients was deemed to be a foreseen possibility (to communicate novel treatments and/or possible preventative measures). While for the VGER case, reversibility is not possible as the link between the pseudonym and the medical record number was not maintained.
3. When communication is forecasted, a secure de-pseudonymization mechanism should be specified; the mechanism should define (i) the cases for which de-identification can occur, (ii) the bodies that can initiate re-identification requests, (iii) those that rule and regulate these requests, and (iv) the actual re-identification mechanism.

Privacy breaches can occur if the data is leaked to an unauthorized party. Such leakage can happen if (i) the *stored data is hacked/handled recklessly* or if it is (ii) *shared with a pretentious/irresponsible third party*. After applying the pseudonymization process, the data remains vulnerable to de-identification attacks (in other words, although de-identification makes re-identification harder, it does not eliminate the risk). Thus, a strong security layer is needed to ensure that unauthorized individuals cannot access/modify the data. Encryption alone is not an adequate security solution, particularly for genomic data. As explained in [28], encryption schemes gradually weaken in the long run, while the information hidden inside a genome remains stable and is better interpreted with time. Thus, if encrypted genomes are available to an unauthorized third party, the party will be able to decrypt it with time (40–50 years).

Commercial cloud providers (such as IBM and Amazon) claim to employ foolproof security, but their models are not shared publicly and thus cannot be learned and evaluated. Security of the privately held infrastructure and private clouds depends on the proficiency of system administrators and security specialists

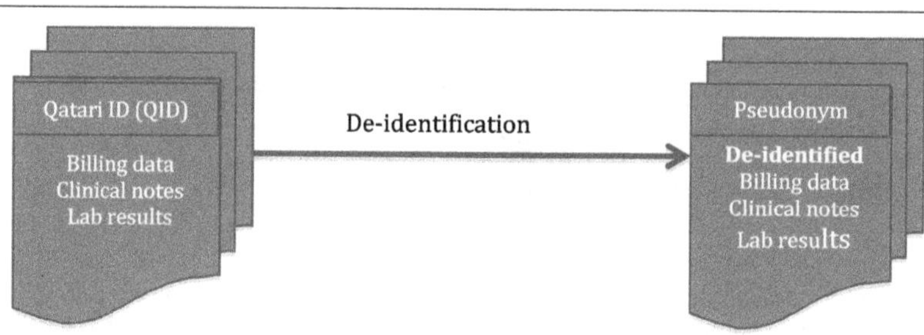

Fig. 2 De-identification of clinical data

Table 1 Examples of unique identifiers

Uniquely identifying fields	Remarks
National ID (or SSN)	
Name	Names of patients and caregivers
Email	
Source ID	Hospital/Biobank-assigned IDs
Passport number	
Exact address	

employed by the custodian organization. In some cases, like the Qatar Genome Programme, geographic location and state-regulated data access may provide additional protective layer against sporadic attacks and "social engineering" hacks. However, the ability of genomic data storage to withstand a determined and competent invasion is yet to be tested.

Data sharing

Electronic medical records (EMRs) hold diverse clinical information about large populations. When this information is coupled with genetic data, it has the potential to make unprecedented associations between genes and diseases. The incorporation of these discoveries into healthcare practice offers the hope to improve healthcare through personalized treatments. However, the availability of such data for widespread research activities is dependent *on the protection of a subject's privacy.* Current technological methods for privacy preservation are outdated and cannot provide protection for genomic and longitudinal data (EMR).

Access mechanisms and privacy

Data sharing mechanisms can be categorized into two broad categories: open-access and controlled-access. While both were widely used for regulating genomic data sharing, open-access datasets have been used in many more studies per year [29]. Open-access models either operate under a mandate from participants (who want to publish their genomic data in public platforms) or under the assumption that the shared data is de-identified and possibly aggregated [30]. However, as demonstrated by multiple recent studies, the risk of re-identification is strongly present. It was shown, in multiple independent studies, that it is possible to learn the identities of people who participate in research studies by matching their data with publicly available data [31]. In a recent study [32], the authors showed that they can infer the identity of 50 anonymous male subjects whose Y-chromosome has been sequenced as part of the 1000 Genomes Project. The researchers were not only able to discover the identities of these anonymized research participants but also their family members using available/public pedigrees. In response to this study, the NIH removed the age information from the project's database. In another recent study, [33, 34], the authors reported that they can confirm whether a person participated in a genome-wide association study, by using information from the person's DNA sample, "even if the study reported only summary statistics on hundreds or thousands of participants" [31]. In response, the NIH shifted to a controlled access mechanism. In fact, currently, most human genome projects use controlled-access mechanisms.

The personal information derived from genomic data (and EMR data) can be very damaging to the participants. It can be used against them to limit insurance coverage, to guide employment decisions, or to apply social stigma. In [35], the authors report on a case of genetic discrimination by a railroad company. The case occurred in 2002 when the company forced its employees to undergo a genetic test; employees who refused to participate in the test were threatened with disciplinary actions. The company was later forced (in an out-of-court settlement) to compensate 36 of its employees. That is hardly a consolation because if such genetic data was obtained from online sources or breached through illegal means, the company may have been able to get away with its discrimination practices.

Regulations

In many countries, the use of sensitive human-subject data for research purposes has been studied extensively from the legal aspect. Resulting legislations aimed to ensure that private information is properly used and adequately protected when disclosed for research purposes [36, 37]. The legislations (such as the Common Rule [36], Health Information Portability and Accountability Act (HIPAA) [38], and EU data protection directive [39]) generally permit data sharing under one of the following guidelines:

G1. For the use of identifiable data, an approval from an Institutional Review Board (IRB) is required. To approve data requests, IRBs require:
   a. Informed consents from the participants for the specific data use, or
   b. When consents are deemed impractical, IRBs can grant data access if the study accrues more benefit than risk. Such decision requires a thorough and lengthy evaluation of each data access request from the IRB part.

G2. For adequately de-identified data, researchers can be exempt from IRB approval. The adequacy of the de-identification is generally established by the IRB or by pre-approved policies such as the United States HIPAA privacy rule [37].

Guideline G2 depends on the availability of robust de-identification techniques, but as current techniques are outdated, and unable to deal with genetic and EMR data (as evident from the privacy breaches cited earlier), G2 cannot be adopted. The Vanderbilt genome project is the only project we are aware of that was ruled by Vanderbilt IRB to be a "non-human subject data" as it was deemed to be properly de-identified. However, given the potential impact of the project on the community, guidelines adhering to G1.b were enforced.

Guideline G1.a requires informed consent from participants. The problem with such requirement is that data collectors have to forecast all possible uses of the data and create a comprehensive consent detailing the benefits and risks related to all different data uses. Something that is not easily achievable. In fact, most biobanks collect consents in the form of opt in/opt out [19]. The issues/challenges in implementing proper informed consent will be discussed in depth later in this section.

Almost all existing biomedical data warehouses that house (non-aggregate) genetic data coupled with EMR data follow guideline *G1.b*. These warehouses lightly de-identify their data and regulate investigators' access to the data through an IRB [18, 19, 40]. Only researchers with studies that involve less risk than benefit are allowed access to requested data and only after they pass a thorough identity check. However, IRB procedures are extensive and can obstruct timely research and discoveries [41–43]. Studies on platforms that rely on IRB for all data accesses reveal unsatisfied users. The application process is strenuous and approvals take a long time often delaying project initiation significantly [43, 44].

In Qatar, as an example, access to the biomedical data collected in Qatar is governed by the QSCH "guidelines, regulations and policies for research involving human subjects", which adheres to guideline *G1.b*. A recently formed IRB will regulate all accesses to the research data and services by all research institutes within Qatar and outside.

With such massive mandates, a principal feature for IRBs is to have the capacity to foster timely research and discoveries. Data application processes and approvals should be smooth and should not delay project initiation significantly. Thus, the traditional "IRB-based" data sharing will produce unsatisfied users.

Methods under investigation

The inadequacy of current de-identification methods and the delays in IRB processes prompted privacy experts to seek new solutions. Rapid progress is taking place in privacy research in the biomedical area, driven by the need to protect and benefit from the large biomedical data warehouses being built worldwide. The novel methods can be divided into two main categories, legislative and technical:

(i) *Legislative:* Legislative methods define privacy rights and responsibilities. Research in this area aims to understand and define individuals' privacy perspectives and expectations and to update policies and laws that govern data sharing. Genetic data introduces a difficult and unique regulatory situation (with respect to data collection laws and data sharing laws) that is not found with other types of health data [16]. So, until effective privacy protection solutions are made into law, scientists and civil right advocates are calling for the adoption of anti-genetic discrimination laws to mitigate the effect of genetic data breaches. An example is the Genetic Information Non-discrimination Act (GINA) adopted by the US government in 2008. GINA forbids discrimination by insurers or employers on the basis of genetic information. The problem with such regulations is that they are enforced only when discrimination on the basis of genetic information is proven, which necessitates the difficult task of proving malicious intentions.

(ii) *Technical:* Technical controls aim to create data sharing systems/methods that fulfill the requirements specified in privacy legislation. Current technical approaches to privacy, such as de-identification, are not effective in the genomic context (in fact, the genome is itself an identifier and as such cannot be de-identified (yet) while retaining its utility), thus the need for innovative methods to deal with our new data realities. We classify current research in privacy-preserving mechanisms into three categories: process-driven mechanisms, risk-aware systems, and consent-based systems. In process-driven mechanisms, such as differential privacy and cryptographic techniques, the dataset is held by a trusted server, users query the data through the server, and privacy is built into the algorithms that access the data. Risk-aware systems aim at speeding the IRB processes through partial/full automation, and consent-based systems aim to empower participants by allowing them to control how and by whom their data can be used. This is being done through the introduction of novel dynamic consent mechanisms.

In what follows, we briefly describe recent efforts within each of the three technical categories.

Dynamic consent

Consent-based mechanisms provide data subjects with control over who can access their stored data/specimens, for what purposes, and for how long. Thus, a researcher requesting access to data will receive the data records for which the consent is fulfilled.

The current (mostly paper-based) consent process is static and locks consent information to a single time point (typically during sample collection) [45], requiring all future data usages to be specified at the time of initial consent. This is not feasible with current (multi-purpose and evolving) biomedical data warehouses. The current process also requires limiting the amount of information conveyed to participants to ensure that their consent is informed (i.e., the educational program), since individuals can only absorb limited information at any one time. Re-contacting participants to obtain additional consents and/or to provide additional education materials is arduous, time-consuming, and expensive. Moreover, it can have a negative impact on the participants and on the enterprise.

Active research is underway to overcome this problem. It attempts to provide consent dynamicity to make it easier on the participants and data holders to continuously provide/update consent information. The authors of [46] are working on ways to represent and manage consent information. They focus on defining the different dimensions of a consent. Such dimensions include (i) the characteristics of the institutions that can access the patient's data, (ii) the level of details that each institution can access, and (ii) the type of research allowed on the data (all possible uses of the data). The authors' approach is to codify the different consent dimensions. The benefit of the codification "is to provide a common language to capture consented uses of data and specimens" and to "select those data for the investigator's study that are compliant with the subjects' consented uses and the investigator's permissions." Thus, given a particular study, the characteristics of the study could be matched against the subjects' codified consent to determine the data subset that conforms. In [47, 48], the authors discuss several challenges in designing dynamic consents, particularly, participant's consent withdrawal and its implications. It is worth noting that some commercial sequencing companies, such as 23andme [49], already provide a limited form of dynamic consent models through secure online portal systems. Such systems allow users to fill/change their consent information at their own will.

Additional aspects that need to be resolved are consent withdrawal, continuous participant education, and the cultural aspect of the consent:

- *Consent withdrawal:* Withdrawal is an essential motivator for research participation; thus, research participants must be allowed to withdraw their participation at any time without any penalties. However, withdrawal is complicated by the fact that participants' samples/data may already have been shared by other research organizations. Current best practices recommend that any leftover specimens be discarded and that medical data no longer be updated or used but that shared samples and data do not necessarily need to be revoked [50]. It is important for the consent process to highlight these issues and to make sure that participants understand the limitations of consent withdrawal. Additionally, more investigation should be done around different forms of withdrawals to understand their impact on the willingness to participate and to update best practices accordingly.
- *Continuous participants' education:* Biomedical sciences are complex and are evolving very fast, which warrants the need for continuous participant education.
- *Cultural aspect:* The purpose of informed consent is to give the right of self-determination to individuals based on complete understanding of risks and benefits of research participation and without any interference or control by others. However, the right of self-determination is deeply affected by culture (some communities value the relationship with family members and turn to them for support when making critical decisions), and thus, consent should be adapted to the specifics of the underlying culture in terms of information sharing and disclosure [51].

Risk-aware access control

The risk of granting data access to a user depends on the characteristics of the request. For example, as stated in [52], "access to highly sensitive data at the data-holder's location by a trusted user is inherently less risky than providing the same user with a copy of the dataset. Similarly, access to de-identified clinical data from a secure remote system is inherently less risky than access to identifiable data from an unknown location." Risk-aware access control tries to quantify the risk posed by a data request and to apply mitigation measures on the data to counter the posed risk.

Risk aware access control received growing attention in the past few years. Several of the studies attempted to quantify/model privacy risk, both from the participants' perspective and the data holder's perspective. In [53], Adams attempts to model users' perceptions of privacy in multimedia environments. He identified three factors that determine users' perceptions of privacy: information sensitivity (user's perception of the sensitivity of the released information), information receiver (the level of trust the user has in the information recipient(s)), and information usage (costs and benefits of the perceived usages). Lederer [54] uses Adams' model as a framework for conceptualizing privacy in ubiquitous computing environments in addition to the Lessig model [55] for conceptualizing the influence of societal forces on the understanding of privacy. These efforts concentrate on privacy quantification from the participant perspective rather than the data holder.

Barker at al. [56] introduce a four-dimensional model for privacy: purpose (data uses), visibility (who will access the data), granularity (data specificity), and retention (time data is kept in storage). Barker et al.'s model was later used by Banerjee et al. [57] to quantify privacy violations. Along the same lines, and in multiple consecutive studies [58, 59], El Emam et al. defined three criteria that contribute to privacy risk; these are users' motives, the sensitivity of the requested data, and the security controls employed by the data requestor. The authors state that, according to their long experience in private data sharing [58, 60–62], these are the main criteria used (informally) by data holders.

Recently, in [52, 63], the authors defined a conceptual risk-based access model for a biomedical data warehouse; the model defines the risk posed by data requests using four dimensions:

1. Data sensitivity, or the extent of privacy invasion that would result from inappropriate disclosure of the requested data,
2. Access purpose, or the usages for which the data was requested,
3. Location of the investigator's institution, which is critical for checking the privacy legislation (if any) that applies at the data requester's end and whether the same laws are enforceable, and
4. User risk, which measures:
   a. The user's institution ability to secure the data (the research institution to which the user is affiliated). This is evaluated by looking at the privacy practices followed/enforced within their headquarters and
   b. The risk associated with the particular user/requestor; it is measured by tracking whether the user caused any past inconveniences.

Once calculated, the risk is fed into an access control decision module. The decision module imposes mitigation measures to counter the posed risk. The defined data-sharing mechanism would impose more mitigation measures on requests of higher sensitivity. The mitigations could manifest as reductions in the granularity of the data (de-identification) and/or as restrictions on when and how a user can access the data. The implementation of this model still requires significant efforts toward (i) assigning sensitivities to the different data attributes, (ii) assigning a score to institutions' privacy and security practices (such as certifications), and (iii) creating universal user records for storing data breach information.

The issue of assigning sensitivity to data attributes is gaining more consideration. In [64], the authors define a method to detect privacy-sensitive DNA segments in an input stream. In [65], the authors present a privacy test to distinguish degrees of sensitivity within different attributes recognized as sensitive.

Secure multiparty computation

Secure multiparty computations (SMCs) are an attractive approach that allows a researcher to run a function on data owned by multiple parties (each holding a fraction of the data to be analyzed). The calculation is carried out on the overall dataset without any party having to reveal any of their own raw data. Such scenario can be particularly useful for cross-institutional studies (or even cross-countries studies) particularly when no site has enough data to conduct the study in question (for example, studies on rare diseases).

Figure 3 illustrates the SMC concept. In the figure, a researcher wants to run a computation *f* over the private inputs of three remote databases (data1, data2, data3) while keeping these inputs private. The different parties are allowed to exchange messages with each other and with the researcher. However, such messages are encrypted so as to prevent the different parties from learning any private information through interaction.

SMC is gaining more popularity in the biomedical domain. SMCs are supported by robust mathematical proofs demonstrating their ability to securely protect privacy and thus proving their ability to support data sharing without fear of privacy abuse. In [66, 67], the authors designed a secure linear regression using homomorphic encryption for a multi-hospital quality improvement study. In [68], a secure genome-wide association study (GWAS) was designed using homomorphic

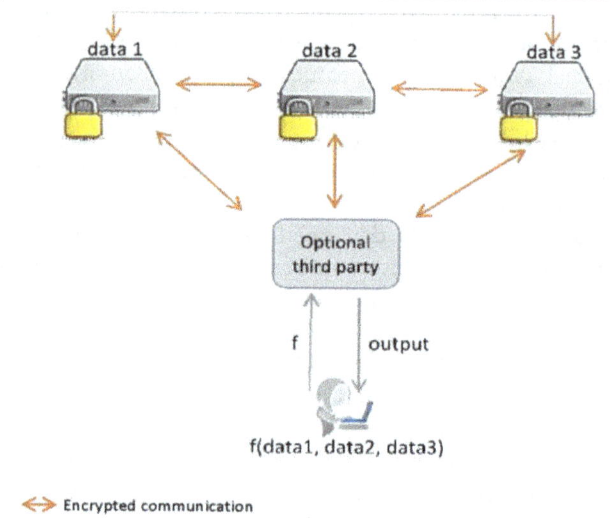

Fig. 3 Framework for the secure multiparty computation

encryption, and in [69], a GWAS protocol was designed using secret sharing. In [70], the authors use garbled circuits to perform metagenomics analysis.

In general, the protocols for secure computation have achieved outstanding results; it has been shown that any function (no matter how complex) can be computed securely. Efficiency however is the major drawback of these computations; they are much more complex than regular protocols (that do not provide any security) [71]. The complexity is driven by the extensive message passing between the involved parties as well as the cryptographic functions employed. Recently, the authors in [72] presented a fast and secure computation for linear regression over distributed data based on secure matrix multiplication. And, the authors in [73] designed another efficient secure multiparty linear regression protocol; their method was based on mathematical results in estimation theory. It remains to be seen whether these methods are generalizable to other estimators.

Dissemination of findings

Prior work demonstrated that in order to affirm the value of research participation and contribute to public education, it is important to have a mechanism for disseminating research findings to the public. This will keep the community aware of how their participation is facilitating research and improving knowledge in the biomedical field.

The mechanism should also tackle the issue of disseminating individual research findings to specific participants. The recommendations governing the return of individual results are usually driven by the psychological harm that could affect the subjects from knowing a result weighted by the benefits in learning it. As such, recommendations are usually aligned with returning "clinically actionable" results, that is, results that are considered *scientifically valid* and that constitute *valuable information* for the recipient, i.e., results associated with some kind of preventive/cautionary strategy.

For example, a finding of deleterious mutations in the BRCA1 or BRCA2 genes associates diagnosed women with high frequency of developing breast or ovarian cancer. Such valid findings help the participants choose to undergo more screening (yearly mammograms, yearly MRI), frequent clinical breast screenings, or bilateral risk-reducing mastectomy which is known to reduce the risk of cancer up to 95% [74–76].

Another example concerns the incidence of mutations in chromosome 12 in the gene coding for phenylalanine hydroxylase (PAH). The mutation may result in the absence of or a defect in PAH enzyme. Phenylketonuria (PKU) can be prevented if PKU is diagnosed soon after birth; children can be placed on diets low in phenylalanine and the detrimental effects of accumulated phenylalanine are avoided. Such highly valuable information for the recipient might prevent severe mental retardation as a result of PKU.

Other findings might not put the participants at risk of developing a disease but could give them the necessary information to guide some of their life choices; an example is whether the participant is a carrier for albinism.

The American College of Medical Genetics and Genomics (ACMG) published a policy statement in 2013 specifying the mutations that should be sought and reported back to the participants (in the context of clinical sequencing). ACMG updates these recommendations annually.

Although the ACMG recommendations were put forth by experts in the field, these underwent a thorough deliberation process and were reviewed (before publication) by external geneticists; they were criticized for excluding the community from the discussion [77]. In fact, there is a growing push to empower members of the public regarding genetic research in general and regarding the return of individual results to research participants in particular. Empirical studies have shown that the majority of participants would like to learn a broader array of genetic results than what is recommended and that they would like to be given the opportunity to decide on that matter [78]. This however necessitates the design of an educational and dynamic consent process to capture the informed (and fluctuating) choices of participants with regards to returning their interpreted data and to continuously educate participants (refer to the "Regulations" section). Such individual consent coupled with educational material could be provided to participants through a secure online portal system for them to complete at their own pace and as the need arises. This allows consent documents to be tied to real events as they occur in the data life cycle, rather than requiring all consent issues to be defined at the beginning of the study. Thus, for example, as new information is generated that changes a variant's status from ambiguous to actionable, additional educational programs and consent documents can be created to allow participants to decide if they want to receive information about the variant and/or to allow that information to be transmitted to their physicians.

Another difficult issue at the core of information dissemination is that of interpretation of the genome sequence information. Interpretation requires the storage of additional information in a form that is easily understood by medical doctors (and other caregivers). It also necessitates the continuous updating of this information with any relevant findings.

A table summarizing several characteristics of select genome projects is presented at the end of the manuscript (Table 2). For every project, it indicates the target number of genomes to be sequenced, the number of genomes sequenced to date, the project's context, the initiation date, the data access model (open versus controlled), the consent process, whether it supports notification (or dissemination) of relevant clinical data, and whether a de-identification mechanism is applied.

Conclusion

Biomedical sciences have been evolving faster than the societies' ability to cope with them. On one hand, current technical approaches to privacy are not adequate for modern biomedical data, and on the other hand, privacy laws have not been updated to deal with the special features of genomic data. As a result, common practice for biomedical data sharing is either rule-based or relies on an IRB for data-sharing decisions. These processes lack a clear and quantitative measurement of privacy risks.

Moreover, calls for participants' empowerment and data ownership are increasing. Data ownership gives the right to individuals to be the guardians of their own data, allowing them to access their data, modify it, set access rules, and modify the rules at will. Informed consent is believed to grant such right of self-determination to the individuals by specifying how they like their data to be accessed (data sharing) and what findings (from their data) they would like to receive back (data dissemination).

However, we cannot talk about participants' empowerment without talking about culture and education. As mentioned earlier in the paper, the right of self-determination is deeply affected by culture. More studies are needed to understand the role of religion, cultures, and traditions in constructing norms around privacy and self-determination.

On the education front, more effort should be made to (continuously and dynamically) educate the public and

Table 2 Characteristics of selected genome projects. In *opt-out* consent process, consent is presumed (for clinical data and left-over hospital samples) with an opportunity to opt out. *Opt-out* is usually coupled with *paper-based consent* for individuals who want to volunteer samples at the biobank. In *local access* model, researchers are not allowed to download the data; they can only access it on the data holder's site. – indicates missing information, *Intra-country* indicates that data is not allowed to leave the country (collaborations should be done through a local researcher)

Projects	Declared target #genomes/ exomes	#Genomes sequenced to date	Context	Start date	Data access model	Consent process	Notification of relevant data	De-identification process
Human Longevity	1000,000 WGS	–	Research	2013	Controlled	paper based	Yes	Yes
All of US	1000,000 WGS	0	Research	2017	Multi-tier (open to controlled), based on risk of request	Dynamic consent	Yes	Yes
Korean Genome Project	1000 WGS for 2016 10,000 WGS for 2018 50,000,000 WGS for 2030	1722	Research	2012	Open	–	–	Yes
QGP	300,000 WGS	4000	Research	2013	Controlled (multi-ethics/ review boards)	Paper-based (11 simple questions)	Yes	Yes
Estonian Genome Project	–	52,000[a] samples	Research	2000	Controlled (multi-ethics/ review boards	broad paper-based consent	Yes	Yes
Saudi Human Genome Program	100,000 WES	–	Research, diagnostic screening	2013	Controlled	Informed Paper based consent	Yes	Yes
Decode Genetics	300,000 WGS (with imputation)	160,000	Research	1996	Controlled (intra-country)	Opt-out/ paper-based consent	Yes	Yes
The Faroe Genome Project	50,000 WGS	–	Research	2011	Controlled (multi-ethics/ review boards)	Informed consent (one for each research project)	No[b]	Yes
Genomics England	100,000	52,065	Research	2015	Controlled (access committee)	Paper-based	Yes	Yes, coupled with local access

[a]The number of biological specimens collected up to date
[b]Upon participation in a research study, subjects may opt to receive notification about different genetic results that may be revealed

inform them about the great benefits arising from sharing their data and the potential risk and damage that could result on the individual and their close relatives should their information be breached.

On another related topic, that of genomic medicine, advancements are needed on many fronts to integrate genetic knowledge into medical practice. On one hand, consent issues regarding dissemination of findings should be resolved, and on the other hand, issues that require development are (i) genetic knowledge representation and the technical limitations of EMR systems, (ii) the lack of genetic training programs for practitioners, and (iii) the difficulty in interpreting genetic results (due to their probabilistic nature and their dependency on phenotypic data).

Abbreviations

ACMG: American College of Medical Genetics and Genomics; APOE: Apolipoprotein E; CAPI: Computer-Assisted Personal Anterview; DNA: DeoxyriboNucleic Acid; DXA: Dual X-ray Absorptiometry; eMERGE: Electronic Medical Records and Genomics; EMR: Electronic Medical Record; EU: European Union; GINA: Genetic Information Non-discrimination Act; GWAS: Genome-Wide Association Study; HIPAA: Health Information Portability and Accountability Act; IRB: Institutional Review Board; NIH: National Institute of Health; NUgene: North Western University biorepository; NUMC: North Western University Medical Center; PAH: PhenylAlanine Hydroxylase; PKU: PhenylKetonUria; PMI: Precision Medicine Initiative; QGP: Qatar Genome Programme; QSCH: Qatar Council for Healthcare Practitioners; SHA-512: Secure Hash Algorithm; SMC: Secure Multiparty Communication; SNP: Single Nucleotide Polymorphism; SSN: Social Security Number; VGER: Vanderbilt Genome-Electronic Records; WGS: Whole Genome Sequencing

Acknowledgements

We are deeply grateful to the late Professor Mahmud Micheal Barmada for the long informative discussions we had during his short time with us. He has shown, by his example, what a good scientist (and person) should be. Also, we would like to thank the two anonymous reviewers for their helpful comments/suggestions on earlier drafts of the manuscript.

Funding

This work is supported by the UAE University research grant #31T084 Research Start-up.

Authors' contributions

FKD designed the paper and contributed to writing and editing the manuscript. AP contributed to writing and editing the manuscript. SKD contributed to writing the manuscript. All authors read and approved the final manuscript.

Consent for publication

Not applicable.

Competing interests

The authors declare that they have no competing interests.

Author details

[1]College of IT, UAEU, Al Ain, UAE. [2]Gloucester Marine Genomics Institute, Gloucester, MA, USA. [3]Faculty of Sciences, University of Balamand, Souk El Ghareb, Lebanon.

References

1. Decode genetics. http://www.decode.com/.
2. Gulcher J, Stefansson K. An Icelandic saga on a centralized healthcare database and democratic decision making. Nat Biotechnol. 1999;17:620.
3. Gudbjartsson DF, Helgason H, Gudjonsson SA, Zink F, Oddson A, Gylfason A, et al. Large-scale whole-genome sequencing of the Icelandic population. Nat Genet. 2015;47:435–44.
4. Genome England. http://genomicsengland.co.uk.
5. Human Longevity. http://www.humanlongevity.com/.
6. Precision Medicine Initiative. http://www.nih.gov/precisionmedicine/.
7. Cyranoski D. China embraces precision medicine on a massive scale. Nat News. 2016;529:9.
8. Korean Reference Genome Project. http://152.99.75.168/KRGDB/menuPages/intro.jsp.
9. Abu-Elmagd M, Assidi M, Schulten H-J, Dallol A, Pushparaj PN, Ahmed F, et al. Individualized medicine enabled by genomics in Saudi Arabia. BMC Merd Genomics. 2015;8(Suppl 1):S3.
10. Qatar BioBank. http://www.qatarbiobank.org.qa/media-center/event-detail?item=33&backArt=29.
11. The DNA law. Kuwait Times. 2016. http://news.kuwaittimes.net/website/the-dna-law/. Accessed 26 Feb 2017.
12. Nyholt DR, Yu C-E, Visscher PM. On Jim Watson's APOE status: genetic information is hard to hide. Eur J Hum Genet. 2009;17:147.
13. El Emam K. Methods for the de-identification of electronic health records for genomic research. Genome Med. 2011;3:25.
14. Gelfand A. Privacy and biomedical research: building a trust infrastructure. 2012. http://biomedicalcomputationreview.org/content/privacy-and-biomedical-research-building-trust-infrastructure.
15. Cassa CA, Schmidt B, Kohane IS, Mandl KD. My sister's keeper?: genomic research and the identifiability of siblings. BMC Med Genomics. 2008;1. https://doi.org/10.1186/1755-8794-1-32.
16. Naveed M, Ayday E, Clayton EW, Fellay J, Gunter CA, Hubaux J-P, et al. Privacy in the genomic era. ACM Comput Surv CSUR. 2015;48:6.
17. Dankar FK, Al-Ali R. Building of a large scale de-identified biomedical database in Qatar—principles and challenges. Qatar Found Annu Res Conf Proc. 2016;2016:HBPP3324.
18. McCarty CA, Chisholm RL, Chute CG, Kullo IJ, Jarvik GP, Larson EB, et al. The eMERGE network: a consortium of biorepositories linked to electronic medical records data for conducting genomic studies. BMC Med Genomics. 2011;4:13.
19. Roden DM, Pulley JM, Basford MA, Bernard GR, Clayton EW, Balser JR, et al. Development of a large-scale de-identified DNA biobank to enable personalized medicine. Clin Pharmacol Ther. 2008;84:362–9.
20. All About The Human Genome Project (HGP). National Human Genome Research Institute (NHGRI). https://www.genome.gov/10001772/All-About-The%2D-Human-Genome-Project-HGP. Accessed 26 Feb 2017.
21. McGuire AL, Oliver JM, Slashinski MJ, Graves JL, Wang T, Kelly PA, et al. To share or not to share: a randomized trial of consent for data sharing in genome research. Genet Med. 2011;13:948–55.
22. McGuire AL, Hamilton JA, Lunstroth R, McCullough LB, Goldman A. DNA data sharing: research participants' perspectives. Genet Med. 2008;10:46–53.
23. Oliver JM, Slashinski MJ, Wang T, Kelly PA, Hilsenbeck SG, McGuire AL. Balancing the risks and benefits of genomic data sharing: genome research participants' perspectives. Public Health Genomics. 2011;15:106–14.
24. Abokhodair N, Vieweg S. Privacy & social media in the context of the Arab Gulf. In: Proceedings of the 2016 ACM Conference on Designing Interactive Systems. New York: ACM; 2016. p. 672–83. https://doi.org/10.1145/2901790.2901873.
25. Hubbard T. HPC infrastructure at King's College London and Genomics England. In: Farr-ADRN-MB eInfrastructure Workshop. 2015.

26. Leitsalu L, Metspalu A. Chapter 8—from biobanking to precision medicine: the Estonian experience. In: Ginsburg GS, Willard HF, editors. Genomic and precision medicine. Third ed. Boston: Academic Press; 2017. p. 119–29. https://doi.org/10.1016/B978-0-12-800681-8.00008-6.
27. Abouelhoda M. The informatics side of the Saudi human genome project. In: GenoME. 2016.
28. Ayday E, Cristofaro ED, Hubaux JP, Tsudik G. The Chills and Thrills of Whole Genome Sequencing. IEEE Computer Magazine; 2013.
29. Wang S, Jiang X, Singh S, Marmor R, Bonomi L, Fox D, et al. Genome privacy: challenges, technical approaches to mitigate risk, and ethical considerations in the United States. Ann N Y Acad Sci. 2017; 1387:73–83.
30. ExAC Browser. http://exac.broadinstitute.org/about. Accessed 6 Mar 2018.
31. Check Hayden E. Privacy protections: the genome hacker. Nature. 2013;497: 172–4.
32. Gymrek M, McGuire AL, Golan D, Halperin E, Erlich Y. Identifying personal genomes by surname inference. Science. 2013;339:321–4.
33. Sweeney L, Abu A, Winn J. Identifying participants in the personal genome project by name. 2013.
34. Homer N, Szelinger S, Redman M, Duggan D, Tembe W, Muehling J, et al. Resolving individuals contributing trace amounts of DNA to highly complex mixtures using high-density SNP genotyping microarrays. PLoS Genet. 2008; 4:e1000167.
35. Malin B, Cassa C, Kantarcioglu M. A survey of challenges and solutions for privacy in clinical genomics data mining. In: Bonchi F, Ferrari E, editors. Privacy-Preserving Knowledge Discovery. New York: Chapman & Hall/CRC Press; 2011.
36. Federal policy for the protection of human subjects ('Common Rule'). http:// www.hhs.gov/ohrp/humansubjects/commonrule/.
37. Sweeney L. Data sharing under HIPAA: 12 years later. In: Workshop on the HIPAA Privacy Rule's de-identification standard. 2010.
38. U.S. Department of Health & Human Services. http://www.hhs.gov/. Accessed 22 Sept 2015.
39. European Data Protection Directive. https://ico.org.uk/media/about-the-ico/ documents/1042349/review-of-eu-dp-directive.pdf.
40. Murphy SN, Weber G, Mendis M, Gainer V, Chueh HC, Churchill S, et al. Serving the enterprise and beyond with informatics for integrating biology and the bedside (i2b2). J Am Med Inform Assoc JAMIA. 2010;17:124–30.
41. Wolf LE, Walden JF, Lo B. Human subjects issues and IRB review in practice-based research. Ann Fam Med. 2005;3(suppl 1):S30–7.
42. Graham DG, Spano MS, Manning B. The IRB challenge for practice-based research: strategies of the American Academy of Family Physicians National Research Network (AAFP NRN). J Am Board Fam Med. 2007;20:181–7.
43. He S, Narus SP, Facelli JC, Lau LM, Botkin JR, Hurdle JF. A domain analysis model for eIRB systems: addressing the weak link in clinical research informatics. J Biomed Inform. 2014;52:121–9.
44. Silberman G, Kahn KL. Burdens on research imposed by institutional review boards: the state of the evidence and its implications for regulatory reform. Milbank Q. 2011;89:599–627.
45. Appelbaum PS, Waldman CR, Fyer A, Klitzman R, Parens E, Martinez J, et al. Informed consent for return of incidental findings in genomic research. Genet Med. 2013;16:367–73.
46. Ohno-Machado L, Bafna V, Boxwala AA, Chapman BE, Chapman WW, Chaudhuri K, et al. iDASH: integrating data for analysis, anonymization, and sharing. J Am Med Inform Assoc. 2011;19(2):196-201.
47. Whitley EA, Kanellopoulou N, Kaye J. Consent and research governance in biobanks: evidence from focus groups with medical researchers. Public Health Genomics. 2012;15:232–42.
48. Steinsbekk KS, Myskja BK are, Solberg B. Broad consent versus dynamic consent in biobank research: is passive participation an ethical problem? Eur J Hum Genet 2013;21:897–902.
49. Goetz T. 23andMe will decode your DNA for $1,000: welcome to the age of genomics. Wired Mag. 2007. http://davehakes.com/weblog/wp-content/ uploads/2007/11/11-17-07_wired_welcome_to_the_age_of_genomics.pdf. Accessed 26 Feb 2017.
50. McGuire AL, Beskow LM. Informed consent in genomics and genetic research. Annu Rev Genomics Hum Genet. 2010;11:361–81.
51. Grady, C. Enduring and emerging challenges of informed consent. New Engl J Med. 2015;372(9):855-62.
52. Dankar FK, Badji R. A risk-based framework for biomedical data sharing. J Biomed Inform. 2017;66:231–40.
53. Adams A. The implications of users' multimedia privacy perceptions on communication and information privacy policies. In: Proceedings of Telecommunications Policy Research Conference. 1999. http://www. researchgate.net/profile/Anne_Adams4/publication/228641284_The_ Implications_of_Users'_Multimedia_Privacy_Perceptions_on_ Communication_and_Information_Privacy_Policies/links/ 0046352a751ad9c417000000.pdf. Accessed 14 Jun 2015.
54. Lederer S, Dey AK, Mankoff J. A conceptual model and a metaphor of everyday privacy in ubiquitous. Berkeley: University of California at Berkeley; 2002.
55. Lessig L. Architecture of privacy. The Vand J Ent Pr. 1999;1:56.
56. Barker K, Askari M, Banerjee M, Ghazinour K, Mackas B, Majedi M, et al. A data privacy taxonomy. In: Dataspace: the final frontier. Springer; 2009. p. 42–54. http://link.springer.com/chapter/10.1007/978-3-642-02843-4_7. Accessed 7 Jul 2015.
57. Banerjee M, Adl RK, Wu L, Barker K. Quantifying privacy violations. In: Secure data management. Springer; 2011. p. 1–17. http://link.springer.com/chapter/ 10.1007/978-3-642-23556-6_1. Accessed 7 Jul 2015.
58. El Emam K, Dankar FK, Vaillancourt R, Roffey T, Lysyk M. Evaluating the risk of re-identification of patients from hospital prescription records. Can J Hosp Pharm. 2009;62:307.
59. El Emam K. Risk-based de-identification of health data. IEEE Secur Priv. 2010; 8:64–7.
60. El Emam K, Jonker E, Fineberg A. The case for de-identifying personal health information. Soc Sci Res Netw. 2011. http://papers.ssrn.com/sol3/papers. cfm?abstract_id=1744038. Accessed 18 Sep 2012.
61. Dankar FK, El Emam K, Neisa A, Roffey T. Estimating the re-identification risk of clinical data sets. BMC Med Inform Decis Mak. 2012;12:66.
62. El Emam K, Dankar FK, Neisa A, Jonker E. Evaluating the risk of patient re-identification from adverse drug event reports. BMC Med Inform Decis Mak. 2013;13:114.
63. Dankar FK, Al-Ali R. A theoretical multi-level privacy protection framework for biomedical data warehouses. Procedia Comput Sci. 2015;63:569–74.
64. Cogo VV, Bessani A, Couto FM, Verissimo P. A high-throughput method to detect privacy-sensitive human genomic data. In: Proceedings of the 14th ACM Workshop on Privacy in the Electronic Society. New York: ACM; 2015. p. 101–10. https://doi.org/10.1145/2808138.2808139.
65. Dyke SO, Dove ES, Knoppers BM. Sharing health-related data: a privacy test? Npj Genomic Med 2016;1:16024.
66. Dankar F, Brien R, Adams C, Matwin S. Secure multi-party linear regression. In: EDBT/ICDT workshops. 2014. p. 406–414. http://ceur-ws.org/Vol-1133/ paper-68.pdf. Accessed 14 Jan 2015.
67. Dankar F. Privacy preserving linear regression on distributed databases. Trans Data Priv. 2015;8:3–28.
68. Ugwuoke C, Erkin Z, Lagendijk I. A Privacy-Preserving GWAS Computation with Homomorphic Encryption. 37th WIC Symposium on Information Theory in the Benelux/6th WIC/IEEE SP Symposium on Information Theory and Signal Processing in the Benelux, Louvain, Belgium. 2016. p. 166-73. https://pure.tudelft.nl/portal/files/11312239/11312198.pdf.
69. Kamm L, Bogdanov D, Laur S, Vilo J. A new way to protect privacy in large-scale genome-wide association studies. Bioinformatics. 2013;29:886–93.
70. Wagner J, Paulson JN, Wang X, Bhattacharjee B, Corrada Bravo H. Privacy-preserving microbiome analysis using secure computation. Bioinformatics. 2016;32(12):1873-9.
71. Lindell Y, Pinkas B. Secure multiparty computation for privacy-preserving data mining. J Priv Confidentiality. 2009;1:5.
72. de CM, Dowsley R, Nascimento ACA, Newman SC. Fast, privacy preserving linear regression over distributed datasets based on pre-distributed data. In: Proceedings of the 8th ACM Workshop on Artificial Intelligence and Security. New York: ACM; 2015. p. 3–14. https://doi.org/10.1145/2808769. 2808774.
73. Dankar FK, Boughorbel S, Badji R. Using robust estimation theory to design efficient secure multiparty linear regression. In: Proceedings of the 2016 Joint EDBT/ICDT Workshops. 2016. http://ceur-ws.org/Vol-1558/paper33.pdf. Accessed 9 Sept 2016.
74. Rebbeck TR, Friebel T, Lynch HT, Neuhausen SL, van't Veer L, Garber JE, et al. Bilateral prophylactic mastectomy reduces breast cancer risk in BRCA1 and BRCA2 mutation carriers: the PROSE study group. J Clin Oncol. 2004;22: 1055–62.
75. Domchek SM, Friebel TM, Singer CF, Evans DG, Lynch HT, Isaacs C, et al. Association of risk-reducing surgery in BRCA1 or BRCA2 mutation carriers with cancer risk and mortality. JAMA. 2010;304:967–75.

19

Tensions in ethics and policy created by National Precision Medicine Programs

Jusaku Minari[1], Kyle B. Brothers[2*] and Michael Morrison[3*]

Abstract

Precision medicine promises to use genomics and other data-intensive approaches to improve diagnosis and develop new treatments for major diseases, but also raises a range of ethical and governance challenges. Implementation of precision medicine in "real world" healthcare systems blurs the boundary between research and care. This has implications for the meaning and validity of consent, and increased potential for discrimination, among other challenges. Increased sharing of personal information raises concerns about privacy, commercialization, and public trust. This paper considers national precision medicine schemes from the USA, the UK, and Japan, comparing how these challenges manifest in each national context and examining the range of approaches deployed to mitigate the potential undesirable social consequences. There is rarely a "one size" fits all solution to these complex problems, but the most viable approaches are those which take account of cultural preferences and attitudes, available resources, and the wider political landscape in which national healthcare systems are embedded.

Keywords: Precision medicine, Genomics, Consent, Insurance, Privacy, Sustainability

Introduction

Across the globe, governments are promoting precision medicine (PM) through national initiatives. High-profile examples include the 100,000 Genomes Project in the UK and the All of Us Research Program (formerly known as the Precision Medicine Initiative Cohort Program) in the USA [1, 2]. These state-supported endeavors aim to realize the potential of genomics and other data-intensive biomedical technologies to improve the accuracy of diagnosis, prevention, and treatment in clinical care. These national programs involve collecting data, building infrastructure, and constructing organizational arrangements to share this data, and to a lesser extent, building capacity among physicians, nurses, and genetic counselors to deliver PM services.

Several important challenges to the implementation of PM have been identified and widely discussed [3–6]. Notable concerns include those related to privacy, data protection, insurance, genetic discrimination, and the management of unanticipated results whose clinical significance is uncertain. However, with the possible exception of the well-publicized divergence on so-called incidental or secondary findings between the American College of Medical Genetics and Genomics and its European counterpart [7–9], many discussions consider these issues at a general or theoretical level rather than at a practical policy level. In particular, relatively little work has been undertaken to compare the approaches taken by different countries. This is an important gap in the literature, since national strategies for the translation of PM necessarily involve a range of trade-offs with respect to ethical and policy matters. Given that the implementation of PM potentially blurs traditional boundaries between research and clinical care in ways that challenge established models for consent, participation, social justice, and sustainability, it is important to consider these issues in real-life contexts.

The aim of this article is to compare the emerging strategies for translating PM, including learning healthcare system approaches, across three countries: the UK, the USA, and Japan. We focus on "precision medicine" as a topic that encompasses personalized, or at least highly stratified [10, 11], approaches to prevention, diagnosis, and treatment of diseases. Although many

* Correspondence: kyle.brothers@louisville.edu; michael.morrison@dph.ox.ac.uk
[2]Kosair Charities Pediatric Clinical Research Unit, University of Louisville School of Medicine, Louisville, KY, USA
[3]Centre for Health, Law and Emerging Technologies (HeLEX), Nuffield Department of Population Health, University of Oxford, Ewert House, Ewert Place, Banbury Road, Oxford OX2 7DD, UK
Full list of author information is available at the end of the article

technologies might be used to inform such approaches, this analysis concentrates on genomic sequencing technologies, since this is a major component of all three national strategies we will examine. The USA and UK are each implementing significant national PM initiatives, but in the context of strikingly different healthcare systems. Japan's PM program is in an earlier stage of implementation but represents an important non-Western example of such an initiative. All three countries have different legal and regulatory frameworks and different cultural backgrounds, although there is some evidence of growing convergence in public attitudes to linking and sharing of health data for research and communication between physicians and patients [12, 13]. It is not feasible within the scope of this paper to review the full scope of differences that could potentially affect the design and implementation of PM initiatives in each country. Instead, this analysis will begin by outlining the current approach taken by each country to promote PM. We then examine a number of major areas where PM presents key ethical, regulatory, and policy challenges and discuss how each national strategy has dealt with these challenges and what this reveals about their strengths and limitations. These challenges naturally involve, and therefore highlight, relevant aspects of each country such as healthcare systems, policy-making apparatus, and public attitudes and opinions that affect the implementation of PM in each territory. Ultimately, by examining these considerations across three distinct countries, we hope to identify key ethical, cultural, and regulatory factors that can inform similar initiatives in other countries and perhaps even support efforts to harmonize policies and ethical norms on an international scale.

National strategies for precision medicine

UK

The UK's flagship PM initiative, the 100,000 Genomes Project, was announced in 2012. In 2013, Genomics England was founded to organize and coordinate the planned work of sequencing 100,000 genomes from around 70,000 patients in the UK's National Health Service (NHS). Genomics England is configured as a company but is wholly owned by the UK Department of Health. The company is managed by a board that includes several prominent UK scientists. Patients are recruited through 13 designated NHS Genomic Medical Centers located across England. Participation from the UK's other constituent regions—Scotland, Wales, and Northern Ireland—is subject to various local arrangements. More than 30,000 participant genomes are reported to have been sequenced. According to the Chief Medical Officer's 2016 annual report, the desired outcome of the government's PM programs is to transform the NHS into a model of a learning healthcare system with "research and care being alloyed together so that each activity is dependent on the other" (Chapter 16 page 9) [14]. However, the same report also observes that reaching this goal will require changes to several elements of the traditional social contract between healthcare professionals and the public including the meaning and function of consent, how uncertainty and contingency are dealt with in medical encounters, and how health data is collected, stored, and used (or not used). The UK government has currently committed to fund the venture through 2021.

Academic and other public sector researchers can access data from the 100,000 Genomes Project by joining one or more consortia known as Genomics England Clinical Interpretation Partnerships (GeCIPs). While the 100,000 Genomes Project focuses on two main disease areas—cancer and rare disease—each GeCIP is dedicated to a specific aspect of one of these disease areas, for example, "ovarian and endometrial cancer" or "pediatric rare disease." Genomics England also coordinates with the UK Genetic Testing Network (UKGTN), which assesses single-gene tests for commissioning on the NHS, to share knowledge about existing variant-disease associations. In addition, Genomics England is set up to facilitate partnerships with private companies. Illumina (San Diego, USA) is the project's official sequencing partner, while several other companies including Congenica (Cambridge, UK) and the multinational WuXi NextCode are also involved in developing tools for analyzing and interpreting the sequence data and associated health records. Genomics England's strategy involves exploring the utility of different bioinformatics platforms through a series of "test phase" contracts where different firms work with a subset of sequence data from the project to demonstrate the capacities (and limitations) of their platforms [1].

Genomics England also operated a 2-year program (2015–2017) known as the Genetics Expert Network for Enterprises (GENE) consortium that brought together academics, NHS Genomic Medicine Centers, and private sector partners from the biotechnology and pharmaceutical sectors. Unlike the bioinformatics partnerships, GENE focused on the development of new diagnostics and treatments based on PM data from the 100,000 Genomes Project. The aim was to facilitate upstream engagement with commercial partners to ensure that the development and eventual outputs of the 100,000 Genomes Project are compatible with industry needs, which explains the relatively short-term nature of the collaboration. Further industry partnerships are reportedly planned.

USA

The Precision Medicine Initiative (PMI), which was announced by then President Barack Obama in 2015, was originally envisioned as a multi-faceted research program focused on PM. The facet of this program that has received the greatest attention, however, is the All of Us Research Program, a biorepository and cohort study that plans to enroll over one million Americans. Coordinated and managed through the NIH Office of the Director, the All of Us Research Program pursues its recruitment, enrollment, data storage, and biosample collection and storage efforts through grants and contractual arrangements with corporations, non-profit organizations, healthcare systems, and universities. The program is currently developing two methods for recruiting and enrolling participants. In the first, eight healthcare provider organizations will recruit participants from their patient populations. In the second, individuals will volunteer to participate online and then visit a retail pharmacy or other contracted location to have their blood or other biosamples collected. The approach to making data and biosamples available to researchers is currently in development, but the PMI has expressed its intention to make these resources widely available to both academic and commercial investigators. Funding for the PMI, including the All of Us Research Program, is determined by the US Congress as a part of its overall budget process. Given the political nature of this process, the potential for long-term funding of the All of Us Research Program remains unknown, although it has received continued support in the transition from the Obama administration to the Trump administration [15].

The All of Us Research Program is just one of a number of federally funded efforts in the USA to develop PM. Another dimension of the PMI focuses on developing precision medicine to treat cancer, as does a related effort termed the "Cancer Moonshot." The Electronic Medical Records and Genomics (eMERGE) Network started out as a federally funded network of biorepositories but has more recently evolved into a program that also focuses on delivering predictive genomic research results into clinical care. The Clinical Sequencing Evidence-Generating Research (CSER2) Consortium, funded by the National Human Genome Research Institute (NHGRI) and the National Cancer Institute (NCI), is designed to integrate genomic sequencing tests into the routine practice of medicine, including in the diagnosis and treatment of rare diseases [16].

In their current iterations, none of these national efforts involves full-fledged implementations of a learning healthcare system. The All of Us Research Program, the eMERGE Network, and the CSER Consortium all involve strategies for returning findings from genomic sequencing to research participants and their healthcare providers, with research aims designed to observe how these results affect clinical care and clinical outcomes. However, these efforts are not yet designed to create the feedback loop between clinical care and research envisioned for the learning healthcare system model.

Japan

In Japan, the government has responded to the advent of an aging population by launching a healthcare innovation initiative to ensure a healthy, long-living society [17]. In 2014, two acts regarding healthcare innovation policy were passed: the Act on Promotion of Healthcare Policy and the Act on the Independent Administrative Agency of Japan Agency for Medical Research and Development. These acts led to the establishment of the Headquarters for Healthcare Policy (HHP), which is located in the Cabinet[1], and the Japan Agency for Medical Research and Development (AMED), as a funding agency attached to three ministries. The Headquarters for Healthcare Policy provides a central organizational hub to strategically promote healthcare innovation, while AMED's goal is to "accelerate the seamless and cooperative translation of basic research to clinical application" through the award of research grants. The mandate for these organizations signals that Japan's nationally driven healthcare initiative incorporates the realization of genomic medicine as one of its key goals. As a part of this initiative, the Council for Realization of Genomic Medicine (CRGM), which is composed of representatives from cabinet secretariat, ministries, agencies, academia, and others, was established in 2015. The purpose of the council is to consider and present a specific national vision and approach to realize genomic medicine. Although an operational learning healthcare system has not been addressed yet, several initiatives to collect genomic data and connect this with electrical health records have been promoted, especially in relation to cancer.

AMED which "has a wide-ranging mandate to smooth the flow of basic discoveries to the clinic and the market" is promoting three research projects [18]: "Platform Program for Promotion of Genome Medicine" (a 5–10-year project for common diseases, in coordination with the Ministry of Education, Culture, Sports, Science and Technology (MEXT)), "Program for an Integrated Database of Clinical and Genomic Information" (a 3–5-year project for rare disease, cancer, and others with the Ministry of Health, Labor and Welfare (MHLW)), and "Program for Promoting Platform of Genomics based Drug Discovery" (a 3-year project for clinical implementation with MHLW). AMED also established a genomic data sharing policy in 2016. As a result, the sharing of genomic data is increasingly required for Japanese databases. For example, the NBDC Human Database is designed with both a managed/controlled system and an open access system. Several large-scale biobanks have been provided with ongoing support, including the Tohoku Medical Megabank Organization (ToMMo). This program has collected samples from more than 150,000 healthy people and analyzed a few thousand whole genome, high-coverage sequences. This resource has been used to estimate the frequencies of actionable pathogenic variants (as specified by the ACMG) in the Japanese population [19], and the active utilization of this and other biobanks for broader stakeholders is being strongly encouraged.

Another relevant activity, the Initiative on Rare and Undiagnosed Disease (IRUD), was launched in 2015 to "maximize the benefit of whole-exome and whole-genome analyses for patients searching a diagnosis [20]." It has already achieved a registry of more than 2000 undiagnosed patients. In these research programs, collaborative efforts to utilize the existing sequencers located in universities, research institutes, and emerging sequencing companies are being strongly encouraged. Several elements of these efforts are starting to reach clinical care. For example, in 2016, significant effort was undertaken by the national healthcare services, expanding the number of rare diseases for which genetic testing is covered from 36 conditions to 72 conditions. In addition, the MHLW released a 2017 report representing a new direction in cancer genomic medicine. This will involve the identification of core centers of cancer genomic medicine in Japan, followed by the translation of genome panel testing into national healthcare services.

Ethics and policy trade-offs

The areas of cancer and rare diseases, which are addressed by national programs in all three countries, are widely regarded as "low-hanging fruit" for this approach. Although the evidence base in these two domains is still developing, early findings indicate that the balance of risks and benefits created by PM may be favorable. In rare diseases in particular, simply improving the chances of providing a diagnosis creates a substantial benefit. However, many scientists, policymakers, and industry leaders in all three countries aspire to the development of PM as an entirely new model for the way medical science addresses a wide array of diseases and conditions, including areas where the risks and benefits of PM remain undefined. Given this aspiration, it is particularly important to consider carefully the opportunities and challenges that PM poses in the domains of ethics and policy. Potential trade-offs between opportunities and challenges in at least three overarching domains will prove particularly important to further efforts to implement PM: (1) genomic sequencing in the context of the learning healthcare system, (2) implications for healthy individuals, and (3) sustainability and private-public coordination. In the sections that follow, we examine the trade-offs in each of these domains.

Genome-wide sequencing and the learning healthcare system

The concept of the learning healthcare system [21–24] envisions that both scientific insights from emerging technologies and the technologies themselves can be applied to clinical care on an ongoing, though flexible and contingent, basis. Although this framework is, in theory, applicable to any technology, PM efforts tend to emphasize the application of genome-wide sequencing (GWS)[2] within learning healthcare systems. Research using GWS has started to generate knowledge in focused areas that can be useful for clinical practice [8], but this technology can also generate a wide array of results whose implications are not yet well understood. The learning healthcare system approach suggests that if GWS is utilized in clinical contexts, despite this incomplete knowledge, both scientific knowledge and clinical care will be improved. For genetic variants that are thought to be clinically actionable, the clinical application of GWS will supply evidence to assess this value. For genetic variants that are not well understood, national PM efforts provide an opportunity to collect genomic data and clinical phenotypes from populations that are more representative than those involved in previous case-control studies, thus improving the understanding of the penetrance and pathogenicity of these poorly understood genetic variants. As more reference genomes from healthy volunteers and patients with milder phenotypes enter databases, the clinical significance of these variants may be revised, leading to additional changes in clinical practice.

Taken as a whole, the learning healthcare system is based on the strategy of integrating information into clinical practice prior to the availability of clinical evidence for its benefit and perhaps even when it is uncertain whether this information is clinically valid or relevant. An inherent dimension of the learning healthcare system, then, is the idea that the evidence base for the utility of genomic sequencing and other technologies can be built by utilizing these technologies in practice and observing what happens. A central debate, both from a medical perspective and from an ethics and policy perspective, is whether this should be thought of as a "feature" of the learning healthcare system or a "bug." On the one hand, much of the scientific value of this strategy lies in the opportunity to observe what happens when results that are currently uncertain are integrated into clinical care. On the other hand, this strategy inevitably involves the application of technologies to clinical care while their risks and benefits remain poorly defined. Learning healthcare system approaches, then, must also account for the potential risks created by feeding uncertain information into the clinical enterprise and must utilize strategies to prevent and reduce potential harms to patients. Moreover, in all three case study countries, the separation between research and clinical care is inscribed in current legal instruments and regulatory systems.

The issue of risk created by returning uncertain information naturally leads to ethical and policy issues, primarily related to informed consent. In a translational research setting, the pitfalls associated with informed consent for GWS are already well-documented [25]. These include difficulty with anticipating and explaining all of the potential findings along with their associated risks and benefits. In the context of the learning healthcare system, these challenges multiply. Research and clinical care are blurred, potentially creating confusion for patients about whether GWS is being recommended to answer a research question or because the provider believes available evidence supports its use in the patient's particular circumstances. In addition, because the learning healthcare system by design involves frequent changes to clinical management, the difficulty with providing a meaningful accounting of the risks and benefits of participation is increased immensely. Therefore, bridging the gap on informed consent between research and clinical care is potentially critical to the application of GWS in the learning healthcare system.

National PM programs, if they are to implement the learning healthcare system framework, will need to carefully consider these concerns. In the short term, many of these programs, such as the eMERGE Network in the USA and the 100,000 Genomes Project in the UK, have simplified this challenge by demarcating return of research results from clinical care. During a recent American Society of Human Genetics workshop, Genomics England chief scientist Mark Caulfield explained that although findings from the project are fed back to patients by their NHS clinician, the results are not regarded as a diagnosis that the clinician is obligated to return as part of the patient's care [26]. 100,000 Genomes Project participants are also offered the choice to opt out of receiving information about "secondary" or additional findings (those not related to the condition that made the participant eligible to take part in the study). In the eMERGE Network in the USA, individual sites develop their own methods for returning results, although in general these approaches make it clear to participants that results are being provided as a result of the research study to which they had consented and not as a part of their routine clinical care. In the longer term, national efforts to implement a learning healthcare system will need to pursue process innovations that adapt informed consent and return of results to this dynamic context [12, 27–29], and further develop appropriate systems of regulations, governance, and oversight adapted to the learning healthcare system framework.

Considerations for healthy individuals

Recruitments of healthy people have several advantages for research. At present, the USA is aiming to incorporate large-scale analysis of genomic and health data from healthy people as part of its national PM initiatives, and Japan is also promoting WGS for a considerable number of healthy people. As noted above, analysis of healthy people provides a reference point for comparing data from patients with various conditions as a means of evaluating the penetrance and pathogenic effect of variants. Sequencing asymptomatic individuals also creates opportunities for the early detection of disease risk, pharmacogenetics-informed prescribing, reproductive decision-making, and counseling on preventive health strategies. Long-term population cohort studies can provide valuable insight into the genetic contribution to the development and progression of diseases. In addition, research on the perspectives of research participants indicates that participation in medical research can be beneficial in a number of ways, including satisfaction from contributing to future public benefits.

Many contemporary PM initiatives, including those pursuing the learning healthcare system model, offer healthy participants the opportunity to obtain individual genomic data, including "incidental findings" with potential clinical significance. Recent research suggests that a small, but significant percent of healthy participants might harbor clinically actionable variants associated with significant conditions [19, 30, 31]. This emerging practice is a significant departure from past research, where it was uncommon to return individual genetic results to healthy research participants.

These changes in research on healthy volunteers will create new tensions between benefits and risks in PM research [31–33]. Although the genetic results returned to healthy participants in the national programs we have highlighted are typically limited to "actionable" genomic variants, the outcomes from reporting these findings remain unknown. Actions taken because of an unexpected result are likely to expose participants to risks they would not have encountered in routine care (such as additional radiation exposure due to imaging). This is critical, since a significant proportion of the individuals who have these variants will in fact never develop the associated conditions. This is especially problematic for variants that are poorly understood, where the likelihood that individuals will develop the associated conditions—the penetrance of the variants—is often overestimated [34]. Reporting genomic results to patients can also create anxiety, fear, or confusion, with patients left wondering when and if they may develop the associated condition. Therefore, returning those results to healthy volunteers should be carefully considered, and when returning following ethical and legal requirements, those results should not be regarded as conclusive data but as supportive or reference data for clinical decision-making at least in the near-to-medium term.

There are also important questions about who else should receive this information including insurance companies, employers, and relatives. The detection of variants of unknown or uncertain significance could carry ramifications for life insurance or other services. For healthy individuals, altered eligibility for insurance based on this information may be perceived as unwelcome and unjust. At the same time, people who discover previously undetected health risks because of PM initiatives may be incentivized to purchase additional insurance if uncertainty over the status of genomic findings means they do not have to disclose that information to insurers [35]. Several nations have already adopted specific legal provisions to address concerns about insurance [36–40]. In the USA, the *Genetic Non-Discrimination Act*, often referred to as GINA, prohibits insurers from utilizing genetic information in health insurance decisions, including the setting of insurance rates, but there is no prohibition against this practice in life insurance or long-term care insurance. For most European countries, basic healthcare coverage is provided by the state, but life insurance and other coverage is not and must still be purchased from private providers. The UK (along with Germany and the Netherlands) has a voluntary moratorium on the use of genetic data in calculating insurance premiums. Most other European countries have opted for formal legal prohibitions. In contrast, most East Asian countries have not implemented these kinds of specific legal regulations [36–38, 41]. In Japan, there is ongoing debate about whether a specific law on genetic discrimination is needed, especially given the existence of other legal instruments regulating the protection of personal information and prohibiting unjust discrimination by the insurance industry.

It is also important to consider effects on family members [29, 42–44]. When a variant with potential clinical implications is detected in one person, it potentially has implications for the provision of care to relatives. This issue also arises with some existing practices, such as when a clinical diagnosis of breast cancer is made, but the prospect of implementing PM in routine care will constitute a massive expansion of tests that require healthcare professionals to consider family health as well as care of individual patients. If sequenced individuals do not wish to share these results with family members, this can create "a conflict of normative duties and values: respecting individual confidentiality and autonomy on one and preventing potential harm to a relative on the other [44]." While the appropriate measures for addressing this challenge may vary from country to country, in the countries selected for our case studies, there are no legal instruments that unequivocally establish a duty for healthcare providers and researchers to disclose genomic information from family members. In the UK, non-binding guidelines advocate that patients voluntarily disclose genomic and other medical data when it has implications for the health of relatives but permit physicians to disclose confidential medical data to a patient's relatives even in the absence of consent if the benefits of disclosure clearly outweigh the risks [45]. Non-binding guidelines in the USA similarly support the sharing of genetic information with family members when this could be helpful. However, the provisions of the Health Information Portability and Accountability Act (HIPAA) arguably prevent the disclosure of a genetic finding to family members if the patient objects [46]. In Japan, non-binding governmental guidelines stipulate that priority be given to ensure consent by research participants, but there are also exemptions to enable healthcare providers to disclose genomic results to family members where consent has not been given for their disclosure [47]. Again, these exemptions exist where disclosing the information is likely to prevent serious damage to the wellbeing of the people affected by the disclosure.

As national efforts to explore the learning healthcare system model expand, the challenges related to disclosing genomic findings to healthy people and their family members will become more common. Providers will more frequently face questions about how to balance the (sometimes conflicting) obligations of participant confidentiality and a "duty to rescue" family members from genetic risk. They will also face questions about privacy and discrimination. Although policies and regulations to provide protections related to privacy and discrimination have been implemented in all three countries, there is substantial evidence that these policies and regulations do not necessarily assuage the concerns of patients and research participants [39, 48–50]. Ultimately, decisions about how to address these challenges will need to be based on a number of contextual factors, including the structure of research and healthcare systems, available resources, cultural preferences and attitudes, and government priorities.

Sustainability and private-public coordination

Implementing PM in routine practice is likely to involve significant costs beyond those associated with single-gene tests. In the USA, access to single-gene testing is determined by insurance coverage, while in the UK and Japan, provision of specific tests is governed by national healthcare systems. In particular, the UK case, where each potential new test is assessed by the UK Genetic Testing Network in terms of potential to reduce mortality/morbidity and the impact of offering testing on existing services, illustrates that cost and resource management is already a factor in this domain. While the cost of a high-quality GWS for an individual has dramatically fallen due to the development of next-generation sequencers, national PM initiatives are likely to incur a range of other costs, not least developing and maintaining the necessary digital and physical infrastructure to manage samples and data [51]. Government funding is often organized around specific projects or missions and is generally for a fixed period. Long-term funding depends on a range of factors, including evaluations of earlier work performed, the perceived importance of the activity being supported, and other strategic and economic concerns. The sustainability of PM efforts, including biobanks, registries, and other types of infrastructure, is a recurring challenge [52–57].

Greater private sector involvement with PM is one way to address the challenge of sustainability for national initiatives. Public-private partnerships offer one mechanism for facilitating commercial access to samples and data on a non-exclusive basis. A commercial firm can access the samples and data held in a public biobank or repository for purposes such as validating existing biomarkers or developing diagnostic, prognostic, or pharmacogenetic tests without inhibiting future access through ownership or intellectual property claims [55]. However, public-private partnerships for PM, which involve the use of samples and data that were obtained through public institutions using public funds, can also create a number of major ethical and social challenges, especially related to participants' trust in research and concerns about privacy.

Although is often assumed that the involvement of biomedical or pharmaceutical companies in research will raise concerns about privacy, there is evidence that it is not simply the presence or absence of industry partners that affects public opinion. Rather, the type of private firm and the nature of their involvement are important. Several recent surveys found that a slight majority of respondents would be in favor of sharing health data with commercial companies if they could envisage a benefit, such as better medicines, while access to data for insurance and marketing was not well-received [13, 58]. Balancing the involvement of private interests is critical. Involving companies in ways that decrease public trust may also lead to reduced rates of participation and reduced willingness for broad data sharing [59, 60].

A range of different models for private involvement has been explored. Genomics England employs a direct contractual approach for its bioinformatics partnerships. In its contracts for sequencing (Illumina) and analytic (WuXi NextCode and others) services, payment is provided on a pre-negotiated fee-for-service basis, and other benefits to the companies are contractually limited. Illumina, for example, does not own any of the sequence data generated, and the company does not get any access to non-genomic patient data. The GENE consortium, in contrast, utilizes a public-private partnership model. Commercial partners are required to pay a fee to join the consortium and in return are granted access to a subset of aggregate sequence data and de-identified patient records. The research, carried out collaboratively by industry, academic, and NHS members, is positioned as a pre-competitive space. Participating partners have certain contractually mandated rights and obligations; for example, all results of the research must be published, but this can be delayed to allow intellectual property claims arising from the research to be secured.

These lessons from the UK demonstrate only a small sample of the numerous funding strategies that can be utilized to move PM forward while laying the groundwork for future sustainability in the private sector. In the USA, for example, Geisinger Health, a regional healthcare system, has established a contractual arrangement with Regeneron, a pharmaceutical company. Through this arrangement, GWS data is combined with electronic healthcare data to create a significant PM resource. As a result, Geisinger is able to pursue academic research, often with federal research funding, while Regeneron is able to pursue the identification and development of new drug targets [61]. While governmental funding approaches have previously been a cornerstone of genome research, public-private partnerships can contribute to achieving sustainable PM. This means, however, that while the privacy of biosamples and data providers will need to be carefully managed, the sharing of benefits among stakeholders will also need to be adequately facilitated through prospective contractual arrangements.

Conclusions

The above discussion has highlighted a number of challenges facing the successful implementation of PM at the national level. This is by no means an exhaustive list. We have focused on ethical and social challenges that arise from the "real world" implementation of national PM programs. Conducting research, even with the most laudable of aims, requires a "social license" in terms of ensuring that both the conduct of the research and its impact are in line with widespread ideas of what is desirable, fair, and appropriate. The scope and scale of implementing PM, especially as part of a learning healthcare system, is such that securing a social license requires attention to multiple dimensions: public trust, financial viability and sustainability, legal and regulatory considerations, organizational factors, and issues of equity and social justice. PM ultimately involves developing new ways of classifying people and groups. In order to reap the benefits of these new classifications, it is therefore important to ensure that appropriate structures are in place to mitigate or prevent any potential negative outcomes of these new taxonomies.

The comparative effort we have undertaken in this paper provides some useful insights, but it is only a first step. A range of significant issues remains in need of analysis including ownership and other legal rights related to genomic data [62], the distribution of benefits among patient communities who contributed data to PM research, and the potential relationship between more "precise," but less homogenous, treatment strategies and pay-for-performance payment models. Furthermore, this variation between nations will likely create challenges for the global harmonization of PM efforts that will need to be explored further in future work. For example, the sharing of biosamples across international boundaries and the use of cloud computing systems to share and analyze genomic data on an international scale both raise ethical and regulatory concerns about privacy and security, which can be also deeply associated with the policy and direction of national data infrastructures [63]. In order to address these issues, the role of local data access committees and the limitations of global regulations and oversight systems will need to be explored further [64, 65]. Our comparison of three countries makes it clear that the global PM community still has a great deal of work to do.

Funding

JM is partially supported by RISTEX, Japan Science and Technology Agency (JST), JSPS Grant-in-Aid for Young Scientists (B) (15K19149), and the Uehiro Foundation on Ethics and Education.

MM is funded by the UK Economic and Social Research Council (ESRC) through grant no ES/P002943/1.

Authors' contributions

JM, KB, and MM each contributed equally to the drafting of the manuscript and shared the final approval of the text.

Competing interests

The authors declare that they have no competing interests.

Author details

[1]Uehiro Research Division for iPS Cell Ethics, Center for iPS Cell Research and Application (CiRA), Kyoto University, Kyoto, Japan. [2]Kosair Charities Pediatric Clinical Research Unit, University of Louisville School of Medicine, Louisville, KY, USA. [3]Centre for Health, Law and Emerging Technologies (HeLEX), Nuffield Department of Population Health, University of Oxford, Ewert House, Ewert Place, Banbury Road, Oxford OX2 7DD, UK.

References

1. Marx V. The DNA of a nation. Nature. 2015;524:503–5. https://doi.org/10.1038/524503a.
2. Collins FS, Varmus H. A new initiative on precision medicine. N Engl J Med. 2015;372:793–5. https://doi.org/10.1056/NEJMp1500523.
3. Wright CF, Middleton A, Burton H, Cunningham F, Humphries SE, Hurst J, et al. Policy challenges of clinical genome sequencing. BMJ. 2013;347:f6845. https://doi.org/10.1136/bmj.f6845.
4. Manolio TA, Chisholm RL, Ozenberger B, Roden DM, Williams MS, Wilson R, et al. Implementing genomic medicine in the clinic: the future is here. Genet Med. 2013;15:258–67. https://doi.org/10.1038/gim.2012.157.
5. Brothers KB, Rothstein MA. Ethical, legal and social implications of incorporating personalized medicine into healthcare. Per Med. 2015;12:43–51.
6. Korngiebel DM, Thummel KE, Burke W. Implementing precision medicine: the ethical challenges. Trends Pharmacol Sci. 2017;38:8–14. https://doi.org/10.1016/j.tips.2016.11.007. Epub 2016 Dec 7
7. Green RC, Berg JS, Grody WW, Kalia SS, Korf BR, Martin CL, et al. ACMG recommendations for reporting of incidental findings in clinical exome and genome sequencing. Genet Med. 2013;15:565–74. https://doi.org/10.1038/gim.2013.73.
8. Kalia SS, Adelman K, Bale SJ, Chung WK, Eng C, Evans JP, et al. Recommendations for reporting of secondary findings in clinical exome and genome sequencing, 2016 update (ACMG SF v2.0): a policy statement of the American College of Medical Genetics and Genomics. Genet Med. 2017;19:249–55. https://doi.org/10.1038/gim.2016.190.
9. Van El CG, Cornel MC, Borry P, Hastings RJ, Fellmann F, Hodgson SV, et al. Whole-genome sequencing in health care: recommendations of the European Society of Human Genetics. Eur J Hum Genet. 2013;21:580–4. https://doi.org/10.1038/ejhg.2013.46.
10. Day S, Coombes RC, McGrath-Lone L, Schoenborn C, Ward H. Stratified, precision or personalised medicine? Cancer services in the 'real world' of a London hospital. Sociol Health Illn. 2017;39:143–58. https://doi.org/10.1111/1467-9566.12457.
11. Trusheim MR, Berndt ER, Douglas FL. Stratified medicine: strategic and economic implications of combining drugs and clinical biomarkers. Nat Rev Drug Discov. 2007;6:287–93. https://doi.org/10.1038/nrd2251.
12. Coathup V, Teare HJA, Minari J, Yoshizawa G, Kaye J, Masanori MP, et al. Using digital technologies to engage with medical research: views of myotonic dystrophy patients in Japan. BMC Med Ethics. 2016;17:51. https://doi.org/10.1186/s12910-016-0132-2.
13. Aitken M, de St Jorre J, Pagliari C, Jepson R, Cunningham-Burley S. Public responses to the sharing and linkage of health data for research purposes: a systematic review and thematic synthesis of qualitative studies. BMC Med Ethics. 2016;17:73. https://doi.org/10.1186/s12910-016-0153-x.
14. Department of Health, Annual report of the Chief Medical Officer 2016. https://www.gov.uk/government/uploads/system/uploads/attachment_data/file/631043/CMO_annual_report_generation_genome.pdf.
15. How science fares in the U.S. budget deal. Science. 2017. http://www.sciencemag.org/news/2017/05/how-science-fares-us-budget-deal.
16. Green RC, Goddard KA, Jarvik GP, Amendola LM, Appelbaum PS, Berg JS, et al. Clinical sequencing exploratory research consortium: accelerating evidence-based practice of genomic medicine. Am J Hum Genet. 2016;99:246. https://doi.org/10.1016/j.ajhg.2016.06.002.
17. Headquarters for Healthcare Policy. The healthcare policy. 2014. http://www.kantei.go.jp/jp/singi/kenkouiryou/en/pdf/policy.pdf
18. Normile D. Biomedical research. Japan's 'NIH' starts with modest funding but high ambitions. Science. 2015;348:616. https://doi.org/10.1126/science.348.6235.616.
19. Yamaguchi-Kabata Y, Yasuda J, Tanabe O, Suzuki Y, Kawame H, Fuse N, et al. Evaluation of reported pathogenic variants and their frequencies in a Japanese population based on a whole-genome reference panel of 2049 individuals. J Hum Genet. 2017 (epub ahead of print); https://doi.org/10.1038/s10038-017-0347-1.
20. Adachi T, Kawamura K, Furusawa Y, Nishizaki Y, Imanishi N, Umehara S, et al. Japan's initiative on rare and undiagnosed diseases (IRUD): towards an end to the diagnostic odyssey. Eur J Hum Genet. 2017;25:1025–8. https://doi.org/10.1038/ejhg.2017.106.
21. Friedman CP, Wong AK, Blumenthal D. Achieving a nationwide learning health system. Sci Transl Med. 2010;2:57cm29. https://doi.org/10.1126/scitranslmed.3001456.

22. Slutsky JR. Moving closer to a rapid-learning health care system. Health Aff. 2007;26:w122–4. https://doi.org/10.1377/hlthaff.26.2.w122.
23. Etheredge LM. A rapid-learning health system. Health Aff. 2007;26:w107–18. https://doi.org/10.1377/hlthaff.26.2.w107.
24. Etheredge LM. Rapid learning: a breakthrough agenda. Health Aff. 2014;33:1155–62. https://doi.org/10.1377/hlthaff.2014.0043.
25. ACMG Board of Directors. Points to consider for informed consent for genome/exome sequencing. Genet Med. 2013;15:748–9. https://doi.org/10.1038/gim.2013.94.
26. Karow, J. (2017) As 100K genomes project returns patient reports, NHS prepares to commission WGS for diagnostics. GenomeWeb 06 November 2017. Available at: https://www.genomeweb.com/molecular-diagnostics/100k-genomes-project-returns-patient-reports-nhs-prepares-commission-wgs (Accessed 12 Aug 2017).
27. Budin-Ljøsne I, Teare HJ, Kaye J, Beck S, Bentzen HB, Caenazzo L, et al. Dynamic consent: a potential solution to some of the challenges of modern biomedical research. BMC Med Ethics. 2017;18:4. https://doi.org/10.1186/s12910-016-0162-9.
28. Tabor HK, Jamal SM, Yu JH, Crouch JM, Shankar AG, Dent KM, et al. My46: a Web-based tool for self-guided management of genomic test results in research and clinical settings. Genet Med. 2017;19:467–75. https://doi.org/10.1038/gim.2016.133.
29. Minari J, Teare H, Mitchell C, Kaye J, Kato K. The emerging need for family-centric initiatives for obtaining consent in personal genome research. Genome Med. 2014;6:118. https://doi.org/10.1186/s13073-014-0118-y.
30. Dorschner MO, Amendola LM, Turner EH, Robertson PD, Shirts BH, Gallego CJ, et al. Actionable, pathogenic incidental findings in 1,000 participants' exomes. Am J Hum Genet. 2013;93:631–40. https://doi.org/10.1016/j.ajhg.2013.08.006.
31. Lindor NM, Thibodeau SN, Burke W. Whole-genome sequencing in healthy people. Mayo Clin Proc. 2017;92:159–72. https://doi.org/10.1016/j.mayocp.2016.10.019.
32. Sanderson SC. Genome sequencing for healthy individuals. Trends Genet. 2013;29:556–8. https://doi.org/10.1016/j.tig.2013.08.005.
33. Sanderson SC, Linderman MD, Suckiel SA, Diaz GA, Zinberg RE, Ferryman K, et al. Motivations, concerns and preferences of personal genome sequencing research participants: baseline findings from the HealthSeq project. Eur J Hum Genet. 2016;24:14–20. https://doi.org/10.1038/ejhg.2015.118.
34. Cassa CA, Tong MY, Jordan DM. Large numbers of genetic variants considered to be pathogenic are common in asymptomatic individuals. Hum Mutat. 2013;34:1216–20. https://doi.org/10.1002/humu.22375.
35. Taylor DH Jr, Cook-Deegan RM, Hiraki S, Roberts JS, Blazer DG, Green RC. Genetic testing for Alzheimer's and long-term care insurance. Health Aff. 2010;29:102–8. https://doi.org/10.1377/hlthaff.2009.0525.
36. Joly Y, Braker M, Le Huynh M. Genetic discrimination in private insurance: global perspectives. New Genet Soc. 2010;29:351–68. https://doi.org/10.1080/14636778.2010.528189.
37. Otlowski M, Taylor S, Bombard Y. Genetic discrimination: international perspectives. Ann Rev Genomics Hum Genet. 2012;13:433–54. https://doi.org/10.1146/annurev-genom-090711-163800.
38. Joly Y, Feze IN, Song L, Knoppers BM. Comparative approaches to genetic discrimination: chasing shadows? Trends Genet. 2017;33:299–302. https://doi.org/10.1016/j.tig.2017.02.002.
39. Green RC, Lautenbach D, McGuire AL. GINA, genetic discrimination, and genomic medicine. N Engl J Med. 2015;372:397–9. https://doi.org/10.1056/NEJMp1404776.
40. Joly Y, Burton H, Knoppers BM, Feze IN, Dent T, Pashayan N, et al. Life insurance: genomic stratification and risk classification. Eur J Hum Genet. 2014;22:575–9. https://doi.org/10.1038/ejhg.2013.228.
41. Yoshizawa G, Sasongko TH, Ho CH, Kato K. Social and communicative functions of informed consent forms in East Asia and beyond. Front Genet. 2017;8:99. https://doi.org/10.3389/fgene.2017.00099.
42. Branum R, Wolf SM. International policies on sharing genomic research results with relatives: approaches to balancing privacy with access. J Law Med Ethics. 2015;43:576–93. https://doi.org/10.1111/jlme.12301.
43. Dheensa S, Crawford G, Salter C, Parker M, Fenwick A, Lucassen A. How do clinical genetics consent forms address the familial approach to confidentiality and incidental findings? A mixed-methods study. Familial Cancer. 2017 (epub ahead of print). https://doi.org/10.1007/s10689-017-9994-9.
44. Dheensa S, Fenwick A, Lucassen A. Approaching confidentiality at a familial level in genomic medicine: a focus group study with healthcare professionals. BMJ Open. 2017;7:e012443. https://doi.org/10.1136/bmjopen-2016-012443.
45. Dheensa S, Fenwick A, Lucassen A. 'Is this knowledge mine and nobody else's? I don't feel that.' Patient views about consent, confidentiality and information sharing in genetic medicine. J Med Ethics. 2016;42:174–9. https://doi.org/10.1136/medethics-2015-102781.
46. Rothstein MA. HIPAA privacy rule 2.0. J Law Med Ethics. 2013;41:525–8.
47. Ministry of Education, Culture, Sports, Science and Technology, Ministry of Health, Labour and Welfare, Ministry of Economy, Trade and Industry. Ethical guidelines for human genome/gene analysis research. 2001 (fully revised in 2004 and 2013, partially revised in 2005, 2008, 2014 and 2017).
48. Parkman AA, Foland J, Anderson B, Duquette D, Sobotka H, Lynn M, et al. Public awareness of genetic nondiscrimination laws in four states and perceived importance of life insurance protections. J Genet Couns. 2015;24:512–21. https://doi.org/10.1007/s10897-014-9771-y.
49. Wauters A, Van Hoyweghen I. Global trends on fears and concerns of genetic discrimination: a systematic literature review. J Hum Genet. 2016;61:275–82. https://doi.org/10.1038/jhg.2015.151.
50. Ikeda W. The public's attitudes towards the use of genetic information for medical purposes and its related factors in Japan. Community Genet. 2008;11:18–25. https://doi.org/10.1159/000111636.
51. Schwarze K, Buchanan J, Taylor JC, Wordsworth S. Are whole-exome and whole-genome sequencing approaches cost-effective? A systematic review of the literature. Genet Med. 2018 (epub ahead of print). https://doi.org/10.1038/gim.2017.247.
52. Chalmers D, Nicol D, Kaye J, Bell J, Campbell AV, Ho CW, et al. Has the biobank bubble burst? Withstanding the challenges for sustainable biobanking in the digital era. BMC Med Ethics. 2016;17:39. https://doi.org/10.1186/s12910-016-0124-2.
53. Caulfield T, Borry P, Gottweis H. Industry involvement in publicly funded biobanks. Nat Rev Genet. 2014;15:220. https://doi.org/10.1038/nrg3704.
54. Watson PH, Mossback SY, Carter C, O'Donoghue S, Cheah S, Matzke LA, et al. A framework for biobank sustainability. Biopreserv Biobank. 2014;12:60–8. https://doi.org/10.1089/bio.2013.0064.
55. Hofman P, Bréchot C, Zatloukal K, Dagher G, Clément B. Public-private relationships in biobanking: a still underestimated key component of open innovation. Virchows Arch. 2014;464:3–9. https://doi.org/10.1007/s00428-013-1524-z.
56. Zawati MH, Borry P, Howard HC. Closure of population biobanks and direct-to-consumer genetic testing companies. Hum Genet. 2011;130:425–32. https://doi.org/10.1007/s00439-011-1019-4.
57. Dorsey ER, de Roulet J, Thompson JP, Reminick JI, Thai A, White-Stellato Z, et al. Funding of US biomedical research, 2003-2008. JAMA. 2010;303:137–43. https://doi.org/10.1001/jama.2009.1987.
58. Wellcome Trust. Public attitudes to commercial access to health data. 2016. https://wellcome.ac.uk/sites/default/files/public-attitudes-to-commercial-access-to-health-data-summary-wellcome-mar16.pdf
59. Hawkes N. NHS data sharing deal with Google prompts concern. BMJ. 2016;353:i2573. https://doi.org/10.1136/bmj.i2573.
60. Hunter P. The big health data sale: as the trade of personal health and medical data expands, it becomes necessary to improve legal frameworks for protecting patient anonymity, handling consent and ensuring the quality of data. EMBO Rep. 2016;17:1103–5. https://doi.org/10.15252/embr.201642917.
61. Regeneron Press Release. Regeneron and Geisinger Health System announce major human genetics research collaboration. 2014. Available at: http://investor.regeneron.com/releasedetail.cfm?releaseid=818844 (Accessed 12 Aug 2017).
62. Thorogood A, Bobe J, Prainsack B, Middleton A, Scott E, Nelson S, et al. APPLaUD: access for patients and participants to individual level uninterpreted genomic data. Hum Genomics. 2018;12:7. https://doi.org/10.1186/s40246-018-0139-5.
63. Sterkx S, Cockbain J. The UK National Health Service's 'innovation agenda': lessons on commercialization and trust. Med Law Rev. 2014;22:221–37.
64. Siu LL, Lawler M, Haussler D, Knoppers BM, Lewin J, Vis DJ, et al. Facilitating a culture of responsible and effective sharing of cancer genome data. Nat Med. 2016;22:464–71. https://doi.org/10.1038/nm.4089.
65. Stein LD, Knoppers BM, Campbell P, Getz G, Korbel JO. Data analysis: create a cloud commons. Nature. 2015;523:149–51. https://doi.org/10.1038/523149a.

20

Abundance of clinical variants in exons included in multiple transcripts

Sankar Subramanian

Abstract

Previous studies showed that the magnitude of selection pressure in constitutive exons is higher than that in alternatively spliced exons. The intensity of selection was also shown to be depended on the inclusion level of exons: the number of transcripts that include an exon. Here, we examined how the difference in selection pressure influences the patterns of clinical variants in human exons. Our analysis revealed a positive relationship between exon inclusion level and the abundance of pathogenic variants. The proportion of pathogenic variants in the exons that are included in > 10 transcripts was 6.8 times higher than those in the exons included in only one transcript. This suggests that the mutations occurring in the exons included in multiple transcripts are more deleterious than those present in the exons included in one transcript. The findings of this study highlight that the exon inclusion level could be used to predict the mutations associated with diseases.

Keywords: Constitutive exons, Alternatively spliced exons, Rate of protein evolution, Pathogenic variants

Background

One of the major tasks in clinical genomics is the identification of mutations associated with human genetic diseases. Typically, genome-wide genetic studies identify a large number of variants that have potential association with a disease [1]. However, to narrow this search and to pinpoint the variants that most likely cause a disease, a number of methods have been developed [2–7]. These methods use the evolutionary conservation of nucleotide positions and/or the functional consequences of mutations to distinguish disease-associated variants from neutral and benign variants. Some of these methods integrate a large number of functional annotations to identify deleterious mutations [2, 5], and hence, any new annotation will enhance the predictability of disease-associated mutations.

Previous studies showed that the rate of protein evolution in alternatively spliced exons was much higher than that observed in constitutive exons [8, 9]. Furthermore, the inclusion level of exons (the number or proportion of transcripts that include an exon) was found to be modulating the rate of evolution of proteins in mammals [8, 9]. These findings suggest that the magnitude of selection constraints is higher in exons included in multiple transcripts than that in exons included in a single transcript. Furthermore, a previous study showed that brain-expressed exons under purifying selection have more de novo mutations [10]. However, how the variation in selection intensity between different exons influence the distribution of deleterious and diseases-associated mutations is unclear. Hence, to investigate this, we obtained the alignment of the protein-coding genes for the human-macaque pair, population polymorphisms, and clinical pathogenic variations in human exomes. Using this large-scale data, we examined the relationship between exon inclusion levels and the fraction of deleterious and pathogenic variants.

Methods

Whole genome pairwise alignment of the human-macaque pair (hg38.rheMac3.net.axt - Dec. 2013) was downloaded from the UCSC genome data repository (https://genome.ucsc.edu/). Using the reference gene annotations, pairwise exonic alignments were extracted and the number of nonsynonymous and synonymous substitutions as well as sites were estimated for each exon. Nonsynonymous and synonymous substitutions observed for individual exons were summed separately for each class of exons, and Kimura two parameter correction [11] was applied to

Correspondence: ssankara@usc.edu.au
GeneCology Research Centre, The University of the Sunshine Coast, 90 Sippy Downs Drive, Sippy Downs, Qld 4556, Australia

estimate evolutionary distance at nonsynonymous and synonymous sites. We used the analytical variance to calculate the standard error [11].

The number of exons in each transcript, intron-exon boundaries and the number of transcript in each protein coding gene (Ensembl genes 92 – GRCh38.p12) were obtained from the *Ensembl* genome resource (www.ensembl.org). Exons were then grouped into 10 classes based on the number of transcripts that included them (1–10 transcripts), and the 11th class consists of the exons included in > 10 transcripts (exon inclusion level). We have also grouped exons into 10 categories based on the proportion of alternative transcripts that included them (exon inclusion ratio). Since our analysis is based on deleterious nonsynonymous SNVs, only the coding exons were included for the analysis.

Human variation data along with the annotations of functional consequences (Ensembl release 92 – GRCh38) was also downloaded from the *Ensembl* genome resource (https://www.ensembl.org/), and synonymous and nonsynonymous variations were extracted. Deleterious variations were determined based on the method, *PolyPhen2*, and only the variants designated as "probably deleterious" were included in the analysis [12]. Based on the annotations of the *ClinVar* database, variants that were denoted as "pathogenic" were used for further analysis [13]. Our final dataset included 5.1 million nonsynonymous variations of which 1.7 million were predicted to be deleterious by *PolyPhen2* and 25,883 were determined to be pathogenic by the *ClinVar* database. The proportion of deleterious nonsynonymous variants was calculated as the number of "probably deleterious" variations divided by the total number of nonsynonymous variations. Similar calculation was followed to obtain the proportion of pathogenic nonsynonymous variations, and the binomial variance was used to estimate the standard error. To examine the strength of correlations, the nonparametric Spearman's rank correlation was used.

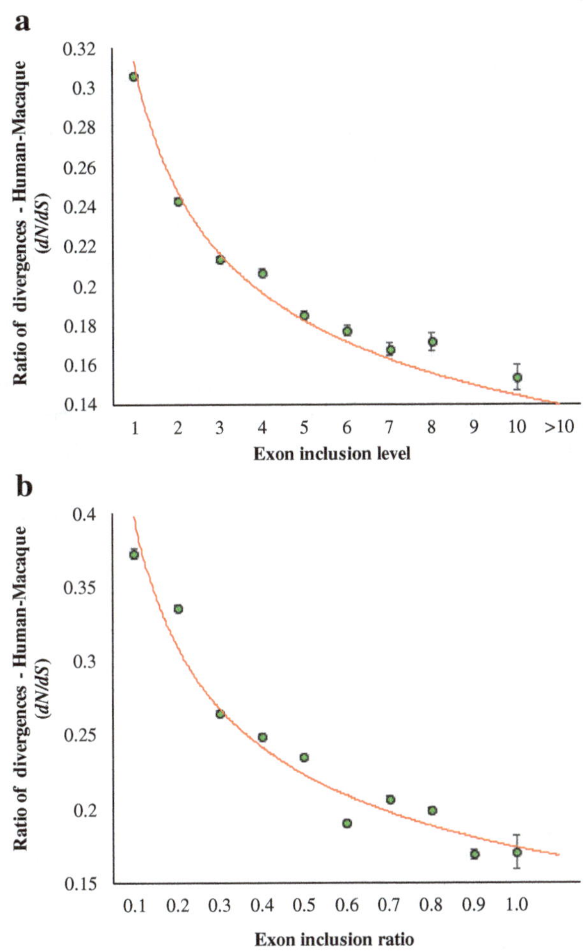

Fig. 1 Relationship between the exon inclusion measures and the ratio of nonsynonymous-to-synonymous divergences (*dN/dS*). **a** Exon inclusion level. **b** Exon inclusion ratio. Synonymous and nonsynonymous divergences were estimated using the Kimura two parameter model [11]. Error bars show the standard error of the mean, which were calculated using the analytical variance of the Kimura two parameter method [11]. The relationships were highly significant ($\rho = -0.98$ and $\rho = -0.95$ respectively; $P < 0.001$) using the Spearman's rank correlation. Note that in **a**, the last value (> 10 exons) on the *X*-axis was taken as 11 exons to calculate the correlation coefficient and significance

Results and discussion

To examine the effects of selection intensity on human exons, we estimated the divergence at nonsynonymous (*dN*) and synonymous (*dS*) positions of the protein-coding genes of the human-macaque comparison. We then plotted the ratio of divergences ($\omega = dN/dS$) against the number of transcripts that included the exon (exon inclusion level) (Fig. 1). This revealed a highly significant negative correlation between the exon inclusion level and dN/dS ratio ($P < 0.001$) (Fig. 1a). The *dN/dS* estimated for exons included in > 10 transcripts was 2.4 times smaller than that estimated for exons included in only one transcript. We also used another measure—exon inclusion ratio, which is the proportion of alternative transcripts that included an exon. Figure 1b shows that exon inclusion ratio also has a significant negative relationship with *dN/dS*. The *dN/dS* observed for exons included in > 90% of the transcripts was 2.2 times smaller than that estimated for exons included in 10% of the transcripts. The above results suggest that protein evolution was under high selection pressure for the exons included in many transcripts.

The higher selection pressure on exons included in many transcripts suggests the relative importance of these exons compared to those included in one or a few transcripts. Hence, any mutation in the former will be more deleterious than that in the latter. This was tested by examining the proportion of deleterious nonsynonymous variants: variants that were predicted by the method *PolyPhen2* based on sequence conservation levels and a number of functional annotations. Our results clearly showed a high significant positive correlation ($P < 0.001$) between the exon inclusion levels and the proportion of deleterious nonsynonymous variations (Fig. 2a). About 23% of the nonsynonymous variations observed in the exons included in one transcript were found to be deleterious in nature. However, this fraction was 57% for the exons included in > 10 transcripts, which is 2.5 times higher that observed for the exons included in only one transcript. A similar relationship ($P < 0.001$) was observed when exon inclusion ratio was used (Fig. 2b), and the magnitude of difference in the proportion of deleterious SNVs between the two extreme classes was 2.6 times (19% vs 50%). These population polymorphism-based results further confirm those obtained based on inter-species comparison.

We then examined the above relationship for pathogenic variations: variants in the *ClinVar* database that were well-known to be causing or associated with a genetic disease. Our results showed a similar positive correlation ($P < 0.001$) between the exon inclusion level and the fraction of pathogenic variations (Fig. 3a). However, the magnitude of this relationship was much larger than that observed for the predicted deleterious variants. The proportion of pathogenic nonsynonymous variations in exons included in > 10 transcripts was 1.96%, which is 6.8 times higher than that observed for the exons included in one transcript (0.29%). We performed similar analysis using exon inclusion ratio, which also produced a highly significant positive relationship ($P < 0.001$). We observed a fourfold difference

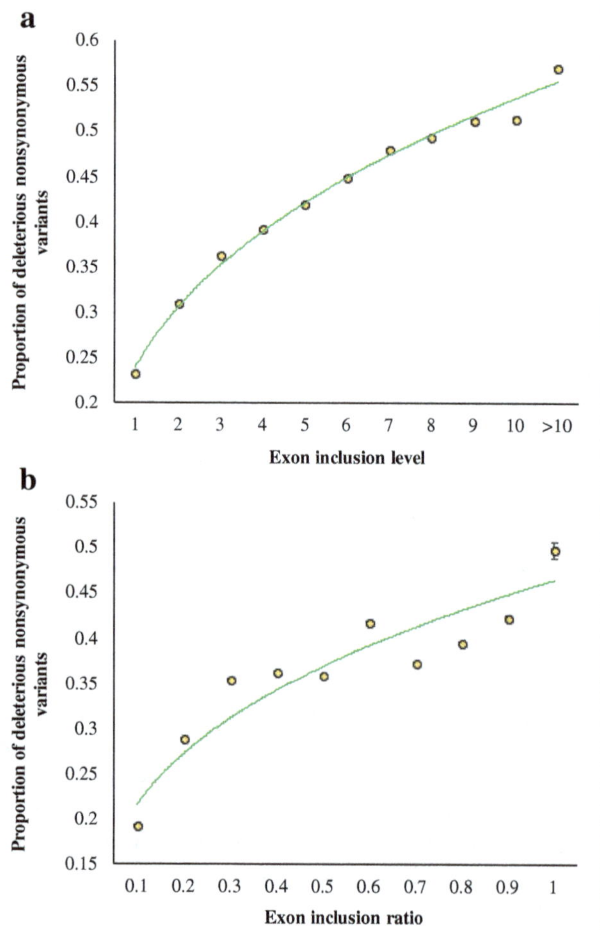

Fig. 2 Correlation between exon inclusion measures and the proportions of deleterious variants. **a** Exon inclusion level. **b** Exon inclusion ratio. Deleterious variants predicted by *PolyPhen2*. Error bars are the standard error of the mean, which were calculated using the binomial variance. The relationships were highly significant ($\rho = 1$; $P < 0.001$)

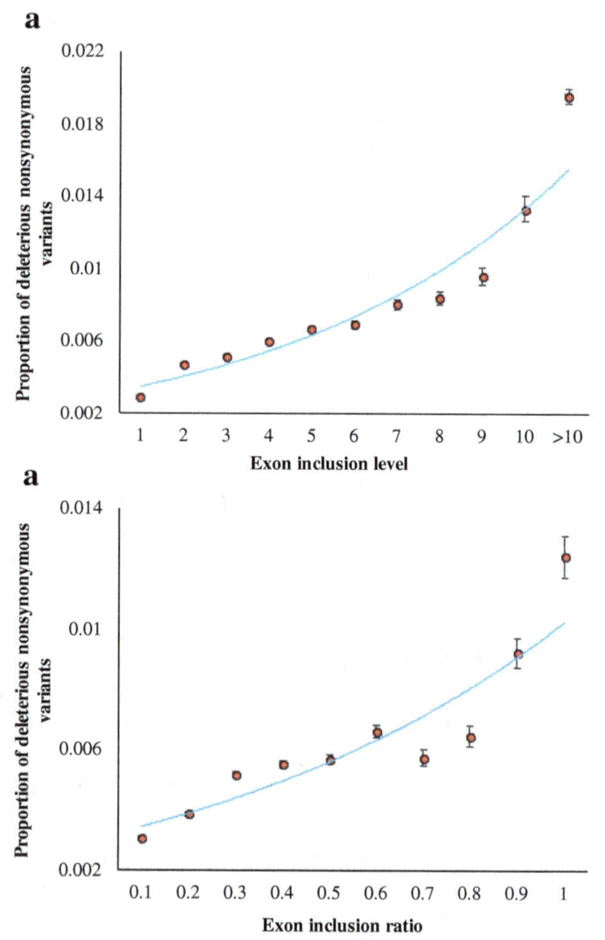

Fig. 3 Correlation between exon inclusion measures and the proportions of pathogenic variants. **a** Exon inclusion level. **b** Exon inclusion ratio. Clinical pathogenic variants were identified using the *ClinVar* database. Error bars are the standard error of the mean, which were calculated using the binomial variance. The relationships were highly significant ($\rho = 0.95$ and $\rho = 0.96$ respectively; $P < 0.001$)

Table 1 Proportion of deleterious SNVs and clinical variants in genes evolving under varying levels of selection intensity

Selection intensity dN/dS	Exon inclusion level (number of transcripts in which the exon is included)			Exon inclusion ratio (proportion of transcripts in which the exon is included)		
	1	2–5	> 5	0.1	0.2–0.5	> 0.5
Deleterious SNVs						
< 0.25	0.2466 (0.0006)	0.3748 (0.0004)	0.5155 (0.0010)	0.1598 (0.0028)	0.2785 (0.0010)	0.3417 (0.0019)
0.25–0.5	0.2243 (0.0008)	0.3391 (0.0006)	0.4538 (0.0015)	0.1956 (0.0015)	0.3248 (0.0006)	0.3728 (0.0012)
> 0.5	0.1972 (0.0012)	0.2994 (0.0010)	0.4301 (0.0026)	0.2027 (0.0010)	0.3666 (0.0004)	0.4257 (0.0008)
Clinical variants						
< 0.25	0.0034 (0.0001)	0.0062 (0.0001)	0.0116 (0.0002)	0.0015 (0.0003)	0.0027 (0.0001)	0.0036 (0.0002)
0.25–0.5	0.0025 (0.0001)	0.0041 (0.0001)	0.0065 (0.0002)	0.0018 (0.0002)	0.0041 (0.0001)	0.0044 (0.0002)
> 0.5	0.0016 (0.0001)	0.0028 (0.0001)	0.0056 (0.0004)	0.0034 (0.0001)	0.0059 (0.0001)	0.0079 (0.0002)

(1.24 vs 0.31%) in the fraction of pathogenic amino acid variations between the two extreme exon inclusion ratio categories (Fig. 3b).

We also investigated whether the patterns observed above hold true for genes evolving under different selection pressures. For this purpose, we separated genes based on the level of selection constraints measured by the *dN/dS* ratio and grouped them into three classes. We then compared the exon inclusion level and proportion of deleterious SNVs in the three gene classes (Table 1). In the case of highly constrained genes (*dN/dS* < 0.25), the proportion of deleterious SNVs in the exons included in > 5 transcripts was 2.1 times higher than that in the exons included in only one transcript (0.515 vs 0.247). A similar difference of 2.2 times (0.430 vs 0.197) was observed for the less constrained genes (*dN/dS* > 0.5) as well. Similar results were observed comparing the values based on the exon inclusion ratio (Table 1). The proportions of clinical variants in genes under varying selection pressure were also found to be comparable. For instance, the analysis of genes under high selection pressure (*dN/dS* < 0.25) showed that the fraction of pathogenic variants in the exons included in > 5 transcripts was 3.4 times higher than that estimated for the exons included in only one transcript (0.0116 vs 0.0034). In the case of less constrained genes (*dN/dS* > 0.5), this difference was 3.5 times (0.0056 vs 0.0016), which is very similar to the former. A very similar pattern was also observed for the results based on the exon inclusion ratio. These results clearly demonstrate that the patterns reported in this study are very similar across genes under varying levels of selection pressure.

Conclusions

The results of the present study highlight the abundance of clinical mutations associated with diseases in exons that are included in multiple transcripts. The excess of harmful mutations in these exons was attributed to the high magnitude of selective constraints on them [3, 14]. Because an exon required for many transcripts is more vital to an organism than that is needed for a single transcript. Hence, mutations in the former will have more severe deleterious effects than those in the latter. These findings could be useful in identifying pathogenic mutations, and exon inclusion level could be used as an indicator measure to detect deleterious variants.

Abbreviations

dN: Divergence at nonsynonymous sites; *dN/dS*: Ratio of divergences at nonsynonymous-to-synonymous sites; *dS*: Divergence at synonymous sites

Author's contribution

SS conceived the idea, designed the research, performed data analysis, and wrote the paper. The author read and approved the final manuscript.

Funding

This work was funded by the Australian Research Council (LP160100594) and the University of the Sunshine Coast.

Consent for publication

Not applicable.

Competing interests

The author declares that he has no competing interests.

References

1. Manolio TA. Genomewide association studies and assessment of the risk of disease. N Engl J Med. 2010;363:166–76.
2. Adzhubei IA, Schmidt S, Peshkin L, Ramensky VE, Gerasimova A, Bork P, et al. A method and server for predicting damaging missense mutations. Nat Methods. 2010;7:248–9.
3. Cooper GM, Goode DL, Ng SB, Sidow A, Bamshad MJ, Shendure J, et al. Single-nucleotide evolutionary constraint scores highlight disease-causing mutations. Nat Methods. 2010;7:250–1.
4. Cooper GM, Stone EA, Asimenos G, Program NCS, Green ED, Batzoglou S, et al. Distribution and intensity of constraint in mammalian genomic sequence. Genome Res. 2005;15:901–13.
5. Kircher M, Witten DM, Jain P, O'Roak BJ, Cooper GM, Shendure J. A general framework for estimating the relative pathogenicity of human genetic variants. Nat Genet. 2014;46:310–5.

6. Ng PC, Henikoff SSIFT. Predicting amino acid changes that affect protein function. Nucleic Acids Res. 2003;31:3812–4.
7. Schwarz JM, Cooper DN, Schuelke M, Seelow D. MutationTaster2: mutation prediction for the deep-sequencing age. Nat Methods. 2014;11:361–2.
8. Chen FC, Wang SS, Chen CJ, Li WH, Chuang TJ. Alternatively and constitutively spliced exons are subject to different evolutionary forces. Mol Biol Evol. 2006;23:675–82.
9. Xing Y, Lee C. Evidence of functional selection pressure for alternative splicing events that accelerate evolution of protein subsequences. Proc Natl Acad Sci U S A. 2005;102:13526–31.
10. Uddin M, Tammimies K, Pellecchia G, Alipanahi B, Hu P, Wang Z, et al. Brain-expressed exons under purifying selection are enriched for de novo mutations in autism spectrum disorder. Nat Genet. 2014;46:742–7.
11. Kimura M. A simple method for estimating evolutionary rates of base substitutions through comparative studies of nucleotide sequences. J Mol Evol. 1980;16:111–20.
12. Adzhubei I, Jordan DM, Sunyaev SR. Predicting functional effect of human missense mutations using PolyPhen-2. Curr Protoc Hum Genet. 2013;76:7.20.1–7.20.41.
13. Landrum MJ, Lee JM, Riley GR, Jang W, Rubinstein WS, Church DM, et al. ClinVar: public archive of relationships among sequence variation and human phenotype. Nucleic Acids Res. 2014;42:D980–5.
14. Subramanian S. The abundance of deleterious polymorphisms in humans. Genetics. 2012;190:1579–83.

A new bioinformatics tool to help assess the significance of *BRCA1* variants

Isabelle Cusin[1], Daniel Teixeira[1], Monique Zahn-Zabal[1], Valentine Rech de Laval[1,2], Anne Gleizes[1], Valeria Viassolo[3], Pierre O. Chappuis[3,4], Pierre Hutter[5], Amos Bairoch[1,2] and Pascale Gaudet[1,2*]

Abstract

Background: Germline pathogenic variants in the breast cancer type 1 susceptibility gene *BRCA1* are associated with a 60% lifetime risk for breast and ovarian cancer. This overall risk estimate is for all *BRCA1* variants; obviously, not all variants confer the same risk of developing a disease. In cancer patients, loss of BRCA1 function in tumor tissue has been associated with an increased sensitivity to platinum agents and to poly-(ADP-ribose) polymerase (PARP) inhibitors. For clinical management of both at-risk individuals and cancer patients, it would be important that each identified genetic variant be associated with clinical significance. Unfortunately for the vast majority of variants, the clinical impact is unknown. The availability of results from studies assessing the impact of variants on protein function may provide insight of crucial importance.

Results and conclusion: We have collected, curated, and structured the molecular and cellular phenotypic impact of 3654 distinct *BRCA1* variants. The data was modeled in triple format, using the variant as a subject, the studied function as the object, and a predicate describing the relation between the two. Each annotation is supported by a fully traceable evidence. The data was captured using standard ontologies to ensure consistency, and enhance searchability and interoperability. We have assessed the extent to which functional defects at the molecular and cellular levels correlate with the clinical interpretation of variants by ClinVar submitters. Approximately 30% of the ClinVar *BRCA1* missense variants have some molecular or cellular assay available in the literature. Pathogenic variants (as assigned by ClinVar) have at least some significant functional defect in 94% of testable cases. For benign variants, 77% of ClinVar benign variants, for which neXtProt Cancer variant portal has data, shows either no or mild experimental functional defects. While this does not provide evidence for clinical interpretation of variants, it may provide some guidance for variants of unknown significance, in the absence of more reliable data.
The neXtProt Cancer variant portal (https://www.nextprot.org/portals/breast-cancer) contains over 6300 observations at the molecular and/or cellular level for BRCA1 variants.

Keywords: *BRCA1*, Genetic variants, Molecular phenotypes, Functional defect assessment, Biological database, Cancer

Background

The breast cancer type 1 susceptibility gene *BRCA1* encodes a large protein of 1863 amino acids that acts as a tumor suppressor. Among other cellular functions, the BRCA1 protein is essential for maintaining the genome integrity by promoting DNA double-strand break repair via homologous recombination in response to DNA damage, critical for its tumor suppressor activity [1–3]. Pathogenic variants in *BRCA1* confer susceptibility to breast and ovarian cancer. By the age of 70, women carrying germline mutations in *BRCA1* have a 60% average cumulative risk for breast cancer and a 59% risk for ovarian cancer [4]. About 3–5% of all breast cancers and 10–15% of all ovarian cancers are associated with *BRCA1* germline pathogenic variants [5–8]. Since the identification of *BRCA1* pathogenic variants allows for specific preventive and surveillance measures, the establishment of the pathogenicity of *BRCA1* variants is crucial for clinical

* Correspondence: pascale.gaudet@sib.swiss
[1]CALIPHO group, SIB Swiss Institute of Bioinformatics, 1211 Geneva 4, Switzerland
[2]Department of Human Protein Sciences, Faculty of Medicine, University of Geneva, Geneva, Switzerland
Full list of author information is available at the end of the article

management of cancer patients and family members at risk of breast and ovarian malignancy. Indeed, prophylactic bilateral salpingo-oophorectomy from 35 years of age and prophylactic bilateral mastectomy in *BRCA1* carriers reduce the risk of developing breast cancer by 50% and by more than 90%, respectively [9, 10], although this has been recently challenged [11, 12]. In cancer patients, inactivation of BRCA1 in tumor tissue, either due to *BRCA1* germline or somatic pathogenic variants, epigenetic changes, or loss of wild-type alleles, is predictive for response to crosslinking chemotherapeutic agents, such as platinum-based drugs, and to PARP-inhibitors, leading to synthetic lethality in the presence of BRCA1/BRCA2 deficiency [13, 14]. Thus, two PARP inhibitors have been approved in the European Union and in the USA for the treatment of patients affected by advanced ovarian cancer with pathogenic or likely pathogenic *BRCA1* or *BRCA2* germline or somatic variants.

The American College of Medical Genetics and Genomics and the Association for Molecular Pathology (ACMG-AMP) have published guidelines for the interpretation of sequence variants [15]. Genetic variants are classified based on clinical assessment as pathogenic, likely pathogenic, variant of uncertain significance (VUS), likely benign, or benign. This interpretation often takes into account co-segregation, the variant frequency in unaffected individuals, and the variant impact analyzed with prediction tools such as SIFT [16] and PolyPhen-2 [17]. Of particular concern are the VUS, whose association with disease risk is unclear. For these, evidence from in vitro studies can provide insight of crucial importance for patient management.

Several public databases report clinical data for *BRCA1* variants: ClinVar,[1] NHGRI Breast Cancer Information Core (BIC),[2] Breast Cancer IARC database,[3] the ARUP database,[4] and the BRCA Share database (UMD)[5] [18]. The COSMIC database[6] (Catalog Of Somatic Mutations In Cancer) collects somatic variants that have been identified in cancer specimens. The Cancer Gene Census project within COSMIC is an effort to identify cancer-causing genes [19]. More recently, the BRCA Exchange site[7] has been providing information on cataloged *BRCA1* and *BRCA2* genetic variants. BRCA Exchange is a product of the BRCA Challenge[8] of the Global Alliance for Genomics and Health.[9] These resources are focused on the clinical impact of variants.

Some information on molecular and cellular impacts of variants is available at the *BRCA1* implementation of Leiden Open Variation Database (LOVD),[10] which, in addition to clinical relevance of variants, reports data from in vitro studies. BRCA Circos[11] [20] is a visualization resource that compiles and displays functional data on all documented *BRCA1* missense variants available at the time (679 variants).

While a large amount of information is available on *BRCA1* variants, their pathogenic classification may vary depending on how the assessment was done. In a recent study [21], classification of variants was entrusted to nine molecular diagnostic laboratories on 99 variants, using both the laboratory's own method and the ACMG-AMP criteria [15]. This study reports that there was only 34% concordance for either classification system across laboratories, and that the agreement was improved to 71% after discussions and detailed review of the ACMG-AMP criteria. Another study by [18] tested pairwise comparisons between BRCA Share™, ClinVar, and ARUP and found that BRCA Share™ and ClinVar agree on 72% of classifications, BRCA Share™ and ARUP on 81%, and ARUP and ClinVar on 60% of shared variants. Approximately 24% variants classified as VUS by BRCA Share™ were classified in another category by ClinVar, whereas 19% of variants classified as VUS by ClinVar were classified otherwise by BRCA Share™.

Hence, there is a need for an integrated and comprehensive resource that reports the current state of knowledge of the impact of variants at the molecular and/or cellular levels, in a format readily compatible with computational analysis [22]. This requires describing variants, functional data, and experimental details according to standard nomenclature and implementing ontologies. The data provenance should also be explicitly described, ensuring citing studies that only present original data.

In this paper, we describe the generation of a data corpus of *BRCA1* variants consisting of nearly 6300 observations at the molecular and/or cellular level on 3654 variants. We included two types of mutations: mutations found in patients, which we refer to as "variants," and mutations generated by site-directed mutagenesis to study specific aspects of protein function, since these may be found in patients as sequencing of individual genomes becomes more widespread for diagnostic and prognostic purposes. All variants are on the protein-coding region of BRCA1; most variants are missense (3455), as well as a small number of truncations, frameshifts, deletions, and indels.

BRCA1 structure and function

The molecular phenotypes reported in the literature relate to the normal function of the protein, which we briefly summarized here.

BRCA1 is composed of three parts: the amino-terminus, containing a RING-type zinc finger; a large central part that contains a nuclear location signal and a coiled coil region; and a carboxyl-terminus bearing two BRCT (BRCA1 C-terminus) domains (Fig. 1).

The helix (amino acids 65–90) immediately next to the RING domain (amino acids 24 to 65) at the *N-terminus* of the protein forms a heterodimer with

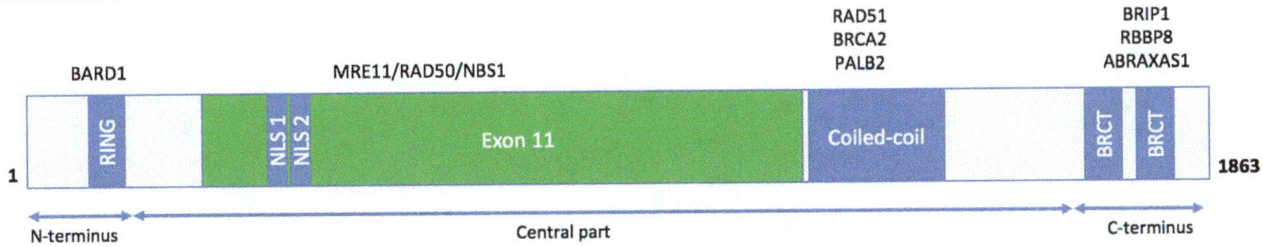

Fig. 1 Schematic representation of the BRCA1 primary structure. Major domains are highlighted, and the position of the binding of important interaction partners in shown on top

BARD1 [23], another RING zinc finger-containing protein [24–26]. The RING domain of BRCA1 possesses E3 ubiquitin ligase activity and interacts with E2 enzymes, allowing the transfer of ubiquitin from the E2 enzyme to the substrate [27]. The BRCA1/BARD1 heterodimer is a core component of all BRCA1 complexes [28]. BRCA1/BARD1 mediates the polyubiquitination via Lys6 of ubiquitin, which acts as a post-translational modification [29–31]. Ubiquitinated BRCA1/BARD1 substrates, including RBBP8 and NMP1, have been implicated in the assembly of protein complexes important for homologous recombination [32, 33]. BRCA1/BARD1 itself is a substrate for its own ubiquitin ligase E3 activity, which increases the stability and activity of the complex [30, 34]. Substrates of BRCA1/BARD1 include RBBP8, an end resection factor that generates 3′ single-stranded DNA tails essential for homologous recombination, and UIMC1 (RAP80), a component of the BRCA1-A complex (see section on the BRCT domains), which targets BRCA1 to DNA double strand breaks [35–37].

The *central part* of BRCA1 contains binding domains for several proteins including RAD50, RAD51, MYC, and PALB2. These interactions are important for homologous recombination. The central region also contains important regulatory phosphorylation sites: the CHEK2-dependent phosphorylation site Ser988 [38–40], required for the BRCA1/PALB2/BRCA2 complex function in RAD51-mediated homologous recombination [41]. The Serine Cluster Domain (SCD), spanning amino acids 1280 to 1524, is a Ser-Gln/Thr-Gln-rich cluster that contains approximately 10 ATM phosphorylation sites [42–44]. SCD phosphorylation by ATM is important for BRCA1-mediated G2/M and the G1/S-checkpoint activation.

The carboxyl terminus bears two *BRCT domains* (amino acids 1642 to 1736 and 1756 to 1855) that are phosphoprotein-binding modules [45]. Interaction partners BRIP1 [46], RBBP8 [47–50], and ABRAXAS1 [51, 52] contain a consensus BRCT-interacting motif (Ser*XX*Phe), which is phosphorylated at Ser to mediate the interaction [53–55]. BRCA1 is part of three distinct complexes, called BRCA1-A, BRCA1-B, and BRCA1-C [56] involved in multiple cellular functions, such as transcriptional regulation, cell-cycle checkpoint activation, and DNA repair. BRCA1 binds double-strand breaks through its association with ABRAXAS1, which recruits UIMC1, both components of the BRCA1-A complex that participates to the G_2-M phase checkpoint regulation [52]. The BRCA1-B complex contains, among other members, BRIP1 and TOPBP1, and binds to DNA damage sites [57]. The BRCA1-B complex is required for S-phase checkpoint activation when replication forks are stalled or collapsed [46, 58, 59], and thus involved in repair during DNA replication. BRCA1 binds RBBP8 within the BRCA1-C complex which facilitates DNA double-strand breaks resection, promotes ATR activation and homologous recombination [60–62].

Implementation

Data model

Annotation statements (Table 1A) are triplets composed of (1) a subject, which corresponds to the protein variation being annotated; (2) a predicate (or *relation*) describing how the property is affected (Table 1B); and (3) an object that describes the function, localization, or protein property being tested.

For functional phenotypes, the annotation *subjects* are variants, which can be of three different origins: germline, somatic, or artificial. All variants affecting the protein sequence are captured: non-synonymous codon, stop gained, frameshift, and in-frame codon loss variants. The *object* can correspond to the protein's molecular function or its localization, effect at the level of the organism, or interactions with proteins or small molecules. The relations linking subjects and objects are listed in Table 1 (also available from our ftp site).

We make extensive use of standard nomenclature, ontologies, and controlled vocabularies to capture data, to ensure consistency and unambiguity of the molecular entities and concepts captured. We capture three types of molecular entities: (i) *proteins*, which are captured using the entry accession number from neXtProt; for example BARD1 corresponds to NX_Q99728, which can be found on the neXtProt website at https://www.nextprot.org/

Table 1 Bioeditor data model: (A) Basic triplet statement; (B) Relations; (C) Evidence

Element	CV/ontology	Example
A. Annotation		
Subject	HGVS nomenclature	BRCA1-p.Cys61Gly
Relation	cv_modification_effect.obo	decreases
Object	Protein	BARD1 [neXtProt:NX_Q99728]
	ChEBI	Zn^{2+} [CHEBI:29105]
	GO	ubiquitin-protein transferase activity [GO:0004842]
	Protein property	protein abundance [PP:0001]
	Mammalian phenotype	premature death [MP:0002083]
B. Relations		
No impact	No significant effect observed compared to wild-type	
• Does not cause phenotype	No observable morphological, physiological and behavioral characteristics in the mutant compared to the wild-type	
Impacts	Some significant effect observed compared to wild-type	
• Causes phenotype	Some observable morphological, physiological and behavioral characteristics in the mutant compared to the wild-type	
• Increases	Some significant increase observed in a quantifiable measure compared to wild-type	
• Decreases	Some significant decrease observed in a quantifiable measure compared to wild-type	
• Gains function	Mutant protein acquires a property absent from the wild-type (new substrate, new cellular localization, etc.)	
C. Evidence		
Evidence code(s)	ECO	Immunoprecipitation evidence used in manual assertion [ECO:0005644]
Protein origin	NCBI taxonomy	*Homo sapiens* [NCBITaxID:9606]
Biological model species, cell type, anatomy, cell line	NCBI taxonomy	HEK293T [CVCL_0063]
	CALOHA anatomy ontology	
	Cellosaurus	
Phenotype intensity	Mild/moderate/severe	Severe
Evidence quality	Gold/Silver	Gold
Reference	Cross-reference to PubMed	PUBMED:20103620

CV Controlled vocabulary, *HGVS* Human Genome Variation Society, *ChEBI* Chemical Entities of Biological Interest, *GO* Gene Ontology, *ECO* Evidence and Conclusion Ontology

entry/NX_Q99728; (ii) *variants*, described using the HGVS nomenclature, a standard for unambiguously describing mutations at the DNA, RNA, and protein level developed by the Human Genome Variation Society [63], and (iii) *small molecules*, captured using the ChEBI dictionary of molecular entities, an ontology of molecular entities focused on "small" chemical compounds [64]).

Concepts are captured using either Gene Ontology [65] that provides a logical structure of biological functions ("terms") and their relationships to one another; phenotypic observations are captured with the mammalian phenotype ontology [66], while changes in protein stability or abundance are captured with in-house vocabulary available on our FTP site (ftp://ftp.nextprot.org/pub/current_release/controlled_vocabularies/). Example uses of these different vocabularies are shown in Table 1B.

For each annotation, detailed information about the experimental support of each statement is captured as evidence statements (Table 1C). The annotation evidence is composed of (1) one or more terms from ECO, Evidence and Conclusion Ontology [67], describing the experiment performed, (2) the Protein origin, which represents the species from which the protein was obtained for the experiment described using the NCBI taxonomy (http://www.ncbi.nlm.nih.gov/taxonomy); (3) the biological system in which the experiment was done that may contain one or more of these elements: the organism from the NCBI taxonomy; the tissue or cell type, from the CALOHA human anatomy vocabulary (ftp://ftp.nextprot.org/pub/current_release/controlled_vocabularies/caloha.obo) or the cell line, from the Cellosaurus database (http://web.expasy.org/cellosaurus/); (4) a qualitative assessment of the severity of the phenotype, either "mild," "moderate," or "severe"; and (5) a quality flag: each evidence is labeled as either Gold (high quality) or Silver (good quality). For experiments that involved statistical analyses (such as proteomics studies), Gold quality is assigned for $p \leq 0.01$, and Silver for $0.01 < p < 0.05$. Data is not integrated for p values greater than 0.05. In most cases, however, the decision to assign a Gold or Silver tag is based on the curator's judgment. Decision factors include parameters such as the lack of qualitative and/or statistical evaluation when that would be expected, very large errors in replicates, low confidence assay (for example, low replicate number, and poorly defined experimental systems), or experiments are carried out using non-human proteins that is evolutionarily distant from the human protein; and (6) a reference, captured as a cross-link to PubMed.

Selection of data for curation

The effects of *BRCA1* variants found in breast and ovarian cancer patients, as well as the effect of experimental amino acid mutations, were manually annotated based on in vitro data from the primary literature. Variants include non-synonymous and nonsense substitutions, in-frame deletions, and frameshifts. Papers describing the functional impact of variants and mutants were obtained from PubMed.

Quality control

Both automated and manual checks are performed on the annotations to ensure data integrity. For example, for variants, our software checks that the original amino acid at the position annotated is found in the sequence being annotated. For the annotations, automated checks ensure that the annotation is complete, i.e., that it contains a subject, a relation, an object, a reference, at least one evidence code, and the species in which the experiment was done. Additional sanity checks are performed, for example to ensure that the evidence codes are consistent with the annotation made, e.g., protein levels cannot be detected by Northern blots.

Results

Using the information derived from 100 publications, the functional impact of 3654 unique *BRCA1* variants was captured: 431 natural variants (both somatic and germline) and 3223 mutants generated by site-directed mutagenesis. The mutants generated by site-directed mutagenesis were annotated as such if they had never been identified as natural variants at the time of annotation. Of these, 3453 variants are missense mutations. A total of 6317 observations, including 6020 distinct triplet statements, were captured.

The most assayed phenotypes for *BRCA1* variants (Fig. 2) are its ubiquitin-protein transferase activity and its binding to BARD1. Most of this data is the work of Starita et al. [68], who have performed extensive mutational analysis of the first 300 amino acids of BRCA1. As shown in Fig. 3, there is a clear overlap in BARD1/UBE2D1 binding defects and defects in ubiquitin transferase activity. Also, the mutations in the RING domain most often cause severe defects in BRCA1 function (Fig. 3). Apart from the ubiquitin transferase activity, the most frequently tested phenotypes are defects in transcriptional regulation, defects in DNA damage response (survival, checkpoints, DNA repair, etc.), changes in protein stability, changes in the nuclear localization, and impact on the regulation of cell proliferation.

Correlation between molecular phenotypes and clinical severity of variants

The number of possible variants over a large gene such as *BRCA1* is in the tens of thousands. However, only about 50 *BRCA1* missense variants are clearly documented in the literature as pathogenic. There is a strong

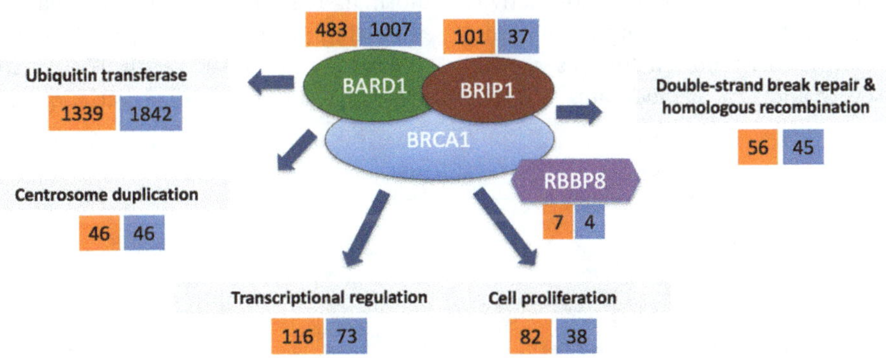

Fig. 2 Overview of the BRCA1 phenotypes captured at the molecular and biological process levels in the neXtProt Cancer variant portal. The number of unique variants with the most representative phenotypic observations is shown. Numbers in orange background represent variants with some deleterious effect, and numbers in blue background represent variants with no impact for the assayed function

correlation between defects in protein function and clinical pathogenicity [69]. While this correlation is not absolute, it provides useful insight for estimating the potential pathogenicity of a variant of unknown significance.

To determine the correlation between the clinical significance of variants and their functional defects, we have compared the ClinVar pathogenicity assessments with the severity of the defect on the protein function. The vast majority of variants in a high confidence classes "pathogenic" and "benign" have evidence from clinical tests, thus avoiding potential issues of circular reasoning in the assessment of our work. Unfortunately, in many cases the evidence is not provided, as much of the data comes from testing done by genetic screening companies. Nevertheless, this clinical information does provide an independent benchmark to evaluate the predictive value of the functional impact of variants.

As of June 2017, ClinVar listed 1546 missense variants for *BRCA1*, broken down into 50 pathogenic/likely pathogenic, 105 benign, 188 with conflicting evidence, 1126 VUS, and 77 variants for which no pathogenicity assessment was provided. In the neXtProt Cancer variant portal, we have captured data for 466, i.e., 30% of the *BRCA1* missense variants available in ClinVar (Table 2). Out of the 50 ClinVar pathogenic or likely pathogenic missense variants, 11 variants are adjacent to splice junctions (Arg71Gly/Lys/Met/Thr, Arg1495Met/Thr, Glu1559Gln/Lys, Asp1692Asn/His/Tyr) and 4 on the first methionine of the protein (Met1Arg/Ile/Thr/Val). These 15 variants are thus expected to be pathogenic for reasons unrelated to a missense substitution in the encoded protein, but are likely to result in a nonfunctional truncated product. These were excluded from our analysis because they are almost never tested in vitro. Of the remaining 35, 31 have experimental data testing the BRCA1 function, 29 (94%) of which having at least one severe or moderate defect in functional assays. For example, Ala1708Glu affects BRCA1's binding to BRIP1, which impacts its transcription factor activity and its role in DNA recombination. Among the 33 function and phenotype evidences reported for this variant, 72% are tagged as severe and 12% as moderate.

We have found experimental data for 49 variants out of the 103 missense variants (48%) located in protein coding regions and annotated as benign or likely benign in ClinVar. There are 14 variants (23%) classified as benign in ClinVar that have at least some moderate or severe functional defect in the Cancer Variant Portal. When we looked more closely at the data, we noticed that these variants affected phenotypes of a relatively minor function, or in a "Silver" grade assay. This highlights the fact that any pathogenicity predictor that could be developed from the data presented here should not be a binary classifier. None of these 14 variants looked reliably pathogenic based on the functional data we have captured.

Four of these variants have at one severe functional defect: Thr826Lys, Met1652Thr, Gly1706Ala, and Val1804Asp; while one has a severe defect in two assays, Gln356Arg. We took a closer look at these variants to understand how these apparently conflicting data could be reconciled with the ClinVar assessments. The classification as benign seems appropriate for three variants: Gln356Arg affects estrogen receptor-dependent transcriptional repressor function [70]; this function may not be important for the tumor-suppressor role of BRCA1. The other severe defect for this protein is a defect in binding to a transcription factor, ZNF350 [71]. This interaction is not very well studied and there is no evidence that it provides any predictive value for pathogenicity. Moreover, Gln356Arg has been identified as a polymorphism in several studies [72–74], indicating that it is very likely benign.

Met1652Thr impairs cell proliferation in a yeast assay. This assay is not very reliable since yeast lacks a *BRCA1* ortholog. The other assays examining transcription, BRIP1 binding, and protein stability are not majorly impaired.

Gly1706Ala gave contradictory results in two different transcriptional assays in one article; in one case, it has normal activity; and in another experiment, it is severely impaired [75]. Two other papers found no defect in this function [40, 76], indicating that this function is likely normal. This variant is also normal in seven other tests, including protein stability, nuclear localization [76], and double-strand break repair [77], further supporting its classification as a benign variation. However, according

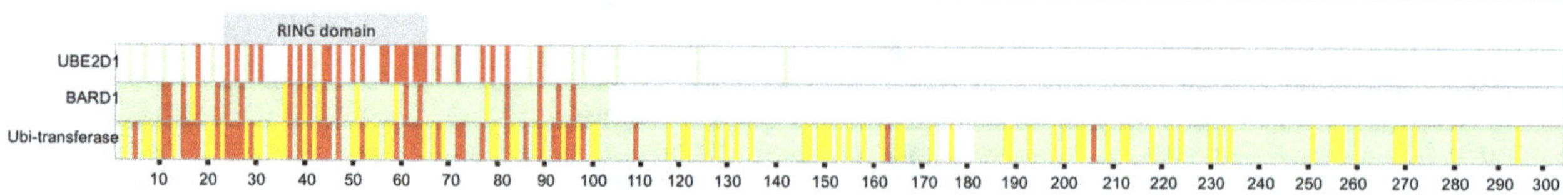

Fig. 3 Position of the variants with defects in ubiquitin transferase activity, BARD1 binding, and UBE2D1 binding for the first 300 BRCA1 residues. Positions where variations have no or mild impact are shown in green, those with moderate effects in yellow, and those with severe defects in red. The positions with no data are in white. The RING domain is indicated (positions 24 to 65)

Table 2 Correlation between ClinVar pathogenicity assessment and functional defects of *BRCA1* variants annotated in neXtProt Cancer variant portal. Only missense variants are compared (that is, variants causing potential aberrantly spliced products were excluded). The percentage of variants having severe/moderate or normal/mild functional phenotypes for each ClinVar pathogenicity class is shown

ClinVar missense variants		ClinVar missense variants with functional data in neXtProt		
ClinVar classification	Total	Total	Severe/ moderate	Normal/ mild
Pathogenic	50	31	29 (93%)	2 (7%)
Benign	105	60	14 (24%)	46 (77%)
Conflicting data	188	99	49 (50%)	50 (50%)
Uncertain significance	1126	244	74 (30%)	170 (70%)
Unassigned	77	32	12 (38%)	20 (62%)
Total	1546	466	178	288

to the AGCM guidelines, when two criteria for pathogenicity assessment are contradictory, the variant is classified as a VUS.

Classification of Thr826Lys and Val1804Asp as benign has less support. Thr826Lys has little evidence for pathogenicity assessment, either functional or clinical, but has been found in patients and not in control populations [78, 79], so it should be further investigated before being assigned as benign. Val1804Asp shows embryonic lethality in mouse embryonic stem cells [80] and was described as potentially deleterious.

VUS and variants with conflicting interpretations

For 53% of the ClinVar variants with conflicting interpretations, the neXtProt Cancer variant portal has identified functional data. Approximately half of these variants have severe to moderate functional defects. The neXtProt Cancer variant portal has data for 42% of the ClinVar variants of unassigned pathogenicity, 37% of which have severe to moderate functional defects. Out of the 1126 ClinVar VUS, we have functional data for 244 variants, of which 30% have at least severe to moderate functional defects.

Data access and visualization

The functional impact of *BRCA1* variants is available on our neXtProt Cancer variant portal (Fig. 4), accessible at https://www.nextprot.org/portals/breast-cancer. The data is presented in table form, with the following information:

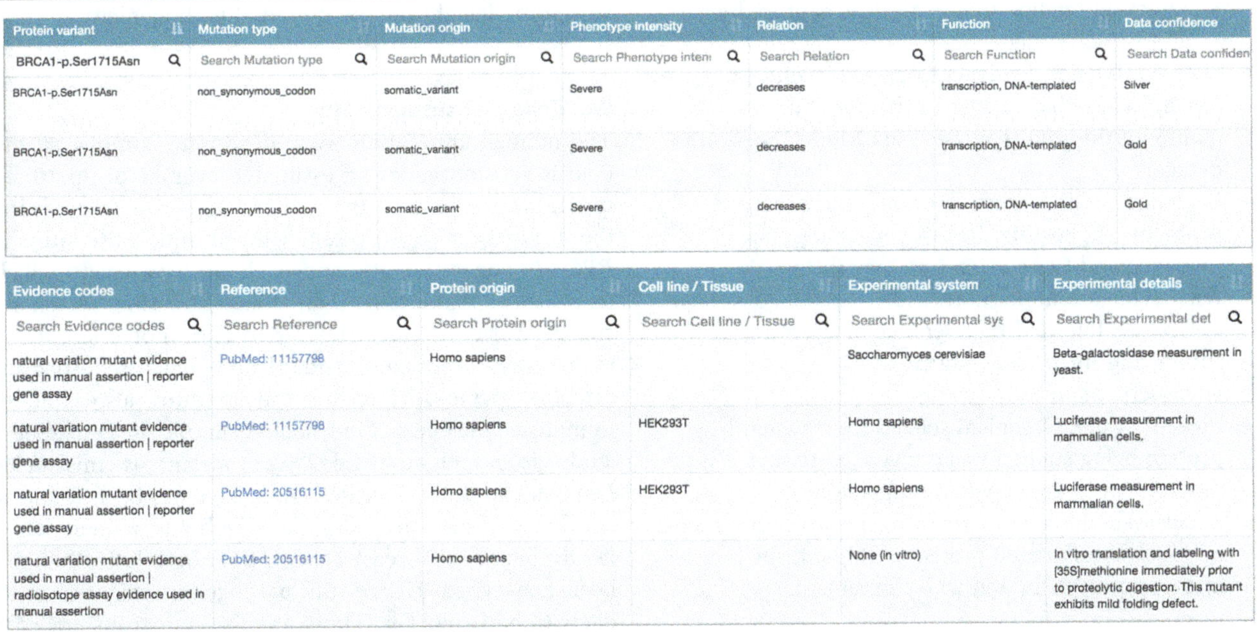

Fig. 4 Screenshot of the neXtProt Cancer variant portal. Evidence for the triplet "Ser1715Asn decreases transcription, DNA-templated". There are three evidences supporting this statement based on two papers, annotated as "Severe" because of the amplitude of the activity reduction in each study. One of the evidences is tagged as "Silver" because the human *BRCA1* variant was analyzed in a yeast system, which the curator judged less reliable since yeast does not have a *BRCA1* ortholog

- Position: Position of the mutation on the canonical protein sequence
- Protein variation: Protein mutation name according to HGVS nomenclature (http://varnomen.hgvs.org/recommendations/protein/)
- Mutation type: The mutation type describes the impact of the mutation on the protein, according to Sequence Ontology (http://www.sequenceontology.org) [81]
- Mutation origin: The mutation origin describes either inherited mutation (germline_variant), acquired mutation (somatic_variant) or mutations generated by site-directed mutagenesis (mutated_-variant_site) according to Sequence Ontology
- Phenotype intensity: Amplitude of the functional defect/phenotype observed: severe, moderate or mild. Not applicable for observation where the mutant has no significant impact: N/A
- Relation: In-house vocabulary of relations describing whether there is a functional defect/phenotype (Impact), or the absence of functional defect/phenotype (No impact) for a variant relative to a Function.
- Function:
  - Effect on protein function/biological process/cellular localization is captured with Gene Ontology terms
  - Effect on binding to proteins and protein complexes is captured with neXtProt entry accessions
  - Effect on binding to chemicals is captured with ChEBI entry accessions
- Data confidence: Evidence is tagged "Gold" or "Silver" according to curator judgment on the quality of the data (see the "Data Model" section for details)
- Evidence codes: Terms describing the experimental protocols supporting the evidence using the Evidence and Conclusion ontology (http://www.evidenceontology.org/) [67]
- Reference: PubMed ID reference of the study supporting the evidence http://www.ncbi.nlm.nih.gov/pubmed
- Protein origin: Organism species from which the protein being studied was derived. Note that it is different from the experimental system.
- Experimental system: Organism species of the model in which the mutated protein is studied, such as cell lines, primary cells, and whole organism.

Each column of the table can be filtered for specific information and sorted alphabetically or numerically, according to the data type. The entire dataset can be downloaded in cvs format.

Discussion

Correlation between functional defects and variant pathogenicity

Our data shows that there is a very good correlation between defects in protein function and the clinical classification of variants (Table 2). For ClinVar pathogenic variants for which neXtProt Cancer variant portal has data, 94% of variants are reported with severe to moderate functional defects. About 77% of ClinVar benign variants, for which neXtProt Cancer variant portal has data, shows either no or mild experimental functional defects.

We detailed the discrepancies of the functional studies and the ClinVar variants for the five benign variants having at least one functional defect in the results section. This analysis leads to a number of observations: first, not all phenotypes are of equal value in determining the potential pathogenicity of a variant. Also, the additional information that we are integrating (phenotype severity and quality) can be very valuable in evaluating the potential pathogenicity. Clearly, a binary classifier that would put any variant with an aberrant phenotype as potentially pathogenic would not perform very well; a much finer decision mechanism must be developed. We are developing a pathogenicity prediction tool that gives different weights to different phenotypes for different targets, with promising results.

The neXtProt Cancer variant portal data, although not conclusive for clinical decisions, may provide guidance for variant classification. Hence, for the 375 variants classified as VUS, unassigned, and having conflicting interpretations having functional data, that data may provide some insight for the potential pathogenicity.

Workload and sustainability

The manual annotation work needed to compile all this data is substantial: at an estimated average of up 10 annotations per hour, it takes about 15 weeks to complete the annotation of a protein with as much literature as *BRCA1*. The systematic approach we have used is likely to be more exhaustive than doing literature search for specific variants, since the variants are not easily found in the literature using standard nomenclature, especially for older papers. Moreover, the literature also contains numerous mistakes. One such example is Leu22Ser a study in which the Leu22Ter variant is mislabeled Leu22Ser in Table 2 in [82]. Leu22Ser has been found in another clinical study [83] in which the patient has a family history of breast cancer, but the relative has not been genotyped. Hence, the pathogenic variant is more likely to be Leu22Ter. There are also numerous errors in converting the one-letter amino acids code to the three-letter code, errors in the reference sequence provided, lack of a reference sequence, etc. We have tried to resolve these inconsistencies whenever possible.

This important effort is amply justified by the benefits gained by researchers and clinicians in having the variants annotated in a standardized, computable manner. While the current study does not aim to provide pathogenicity assessments for those variants, we believe that the functional phenotype data can provide a most useful additional source of information to help experts refine their final decision based on the corpus of criteria that need to be aggregated for variant prioritization. The neXtProt Cancer variant portal provides an easily accessible overview of experimental variant's phenotypic impact, which provides useful information to assess a VUS' potential pathogenicity. Clinicians might consider a closer monitoring of patients bearing variants with some evidence of a functional defect.

Limitations

As mentioned earlier, the best evidence for the pathogenicity of a genetic variation is its strong co-occurrence with the associated disease phenotype(s). In most patients, clinical decisions must nevertheless be made based on available evidence. While evidence that a genetic variation may be pathogenic based on functional assays should provide incentive for a close monitoring of the patient's condition, researchers and clinicians should be highly aware that the functional assays captured in the present work may not relate to the in situ effect of the variants. To avoid misinterpretation of the effect of a variant based on functional or predictive methods alone, the BRCA1 portal should be used as supporting data to validate clinical observations, as appropriate, but not to guide clinical decisions.

Conclusion

The neXtProt Cancer variant portal we have developed provides an exhaustive list of *BRCA1* variants for which molecular phenotypes are available, curated in a highly structured model, without redundancy in the data and with complete traceability to the original experimental results. Researchers, as well as clinical geneticists will be able to consult this database to have a comprehensive overview of the available data. We are capturing the functional defects in variants of other cancer genes, including *BRCA2* and the Lynch syndrome genes (*MSH2*, *MSH6*, and *MLH1*), among others. These annotations are available in the neXtProt Cancer variant portal.

Abbreviations

ACGM: American College of Medical Genetics and Genomics;
AMP: Association for Molecular Pathology; BRCT: BRCA1 carboxyl terminus domain; DNA: Doexyribonucleic acid; ECO: Evidence and Conclusion Ontology; HGVS: Human Genome Variation Society; NCBI: National Center for Biotechnology Information; VUS: Variant of uncertain (or unknown) significance

Acknowledgements

We thank the members of our teams for useful discussions and the reviewers for constructive suggestions.

Funding

The work was funded by the Recherche Suisse Contre le Cancer (Grant #KFS-3297-08-2013 to AB and PH).

Authors' contributions

IC collected the data and contributed to the redaction of the manuscript. DT, VRdL, and AG designed the database and the annotation tools. MZZ performed quality control on the annotations and the exported data. VV and POC contributed to the redaction of the manuscript. PH and AB contributed to the study design and to the redaction of the manuscript. PG supervised the work and contributed to the study design and to the redaction of the manuscript. All authors read and approved the final manuscript.

Consent for publication

Not applicable.

Competing interests

The authors declare that they have no competing interests.

Author details

[1]CALIPHO group, SIB Swiss Institute of Bioinformatics, 1211 Geneva 4, Switzerland. [2]Department of Human Protein Sciences, Faculty of Medicine, University of Geneva, Geneva, Switzerland. [3]Oncogenetics and Cancer Prevention Unit, Division of Oncology, University Hospitals of Geneva, 1205 Geneva, Switzerland. [4]Division of Genetic Medicine, University Hospitals of Geneva, 1205 Geneva, Switzerland. [5]Sophia Genetics, Rue du Centre 172, 1025 Saint Sulpice, Switzerland.

References

1. Moynahan ME, Chiu JW, Koller BH, Jasin M. Brca1 controls homology-directed DNA repair. Mol Cell. 1999;4(4):511–8.
2. Li ML, Greenberg RA. Links between genome integrity and BRCA1 tumor suppression. Trends Biochem Sci. 2012;37(10):418–24.
3. Roy R, Chun J, Powell SN. BRCA1 and BRCA2: different roles in a common pathway of genome protection. Nat Rev Cancer. 2012;12(1):68–78.
4. Mavaddat N, Peock S, Frost D, Ellis S, Platte R, Fineberg E, Evans DG, Izatt L, Eeles RA, Adlard J, et al. Cancer risks for BRCA1 and BRCA2 mutation carriers: results from prospective analysis of EMBRACE. J Natl Cancer Inst. 2013;105(11):812–22.
5. Walsh T, Casadei S, Lee MK, Pennil CC, Nord AS, Thornton AM, Roeb W, Agnew KJ, Stray SM, Wickramanayake A, et al. Mutations in 12 genes for inherited ovarian, fallopian tube, and peritoneal carcinoma identified by massively parallel sequencing. Proc Natl Acad Sci U S A. 2011;108(44):18032–7.
6. ACOG Committee on Practice Bulletins. Hereditary breast and ovarian cancer syndrome. Gynecol Oncol. 2009;113(1):6–11.
7. Kuchenbaecker KB, Neuhausen SL, Robson M, Barrowdale D, McGuffog L, Mulligan AM, Andrulis IL, Spurdle AB, Schmidt MK, Schmutzler RK, et al. Associations of common breast cancer susceptibility alleles with risk of breast cancer subtypes in BRCA1 and BRCA2 mutation carriers. Breast Cancer Res. 2014;16(6):3416.

8. Cancer Genome Atlas Research Network. Integrated genomic analyses of ovarian carcinoma. Nature. 2011;474(7353):609–15.
9. Stuckey AR, Onstad MA. Hereditary breast cancer: an update on risk assessment and genetic testing in 2015. Am J Obstet Gynecol. 2015; 213(2):161–5.
10. Hartmann LC, Lindor NM. The role of risk-reducing surgery in hereditary breast and ovarian cancer. N Engl J Med. 2016;374(5):454–68.
11. Heemskerk-Gerritsen BA, Seynaeve C, van Asperen CJ, Ausems MG, Collee JM, van Doorn HC, Gomez Garcia EB, Kets CM, van Leeuwen FE, Meijers-Heijboer HE, et al. Breast cancer risk after salpingo-oophorectomy in healthy BRCA1/2 mutation carriers: revisiting the evidence for risk reduction. J Natl Cancer Inst. 2015;107(5).
12. Kotsopoulos J, Huzarski T, Gronwald J, Singer CF, Moller P, Lynch HT, Armel S, Karlan B, Foulkes WD, Neuhausen SL, et al. Bilateral oophorectomy and breast cancer risk in BRCA1 and BRCA2 mutation carriers. J Natl Cancer Inst. 2017;109(1).
13. Fong PC, Boss DS, Yap TA, Tutt A, Wu P, Mergui-Roelvink M, Mortimer P, Swaisland H, Lau A, O'Connor MJ, et al. Inhibition of poly(ADP-ribose) polymerase in tumors from BRCA mutation carriers. N Engl J Med. 2009; 361(2):123–34.
14. Byrski T, Gronwald J, Huzarski T, Grzybowska E, Budryk M, Stawicka M, Mierzwa T, Szwiec M, Wisniowski R, Siolek M, et al. Pathologic complete response rates in young women with BRCA1-positive breast cancers after neoadjuvant chemotherapy. J Clin Oncol. 2010;28(3):375–9.
15. Richards S, Aziz N, Bale S, Bick D, Das S, Gastier-Foster J, Grody WW, Hegde M, Lyon E, Spector E, et al. Standards and guidelines for the interpretation of sequence variants: a joint consensus recommendation of the American College of Medical Genetics and Genomics and the Association for Molecular Pathology. Genet Med. 2015;17(5):405–24.
16. Choi Y, Sims GE, Murphy S, Miller JR, Chan AP. Predicting the functional effect of amino acid substitutions and indels. PLoS One. 2012;7(10):e46688.
17. Adzhubei IA, Schmidt S, Peshkin L, Ramensky VE, Gerasimova A, Bork P, Kondrashov AS, Sunyaev SR. A method and server for predicting damaging missense mutations. Nat Methods. 2010;7(4):248–9.
18. Beroud C, Letovsky SI, Braastad CD, Caputo SM, Beaudoux O, Bignon YJ, Bressac-De Paillerets B, Bronner M, Buell CM, Collod-Beroud G, et al. BRCA share: a collection of clinical BRCA gene variants. Hum Mutat. 2016;37(12):1318–28.
19. Futreal PA, Coin L, Marshall M, Down T, Hubbard T, Wooster R, Rahman N, Stratton MR. A census of human cancer genes. Nat Rev Cancer. 2004;4(3):177–83.
20. Jhuraney A, Velkova A, Johnson RC, Kessing B, Carvalho RS, Whiley P, Spurdle AB, Vreeswijk MP, Caputo SM, Millot GA, et al. BRCA1 Circos: a visualisation resource for functional analysis of missense variants. J Med Genet. 2015;52(4):224–30.
21. Amendola LM, Jarvik GP, Leo MC, McLaughlin HM, Akkari Y, Amaral MD, Berg JS, Biswas S, Bowling KM, Conlin LK, et al. Performance of ACMG-AMP variant-interpretation guidelines among nine laboratories in the Clinical Sequencing Exploratory Research Consortium. Am J Hum Genet. 2016;98(6):1067–76.
22. Toland AE, Andreassen PR. DNA repair-related functional assays for the classification of BRCA1 and BRCA2 variants: a critical review and needs assessment. J Med Genet. 2017;54(11):721–31.
23. Atipairin A, Canyuk B, Ratanaphan A. The RING heterodimer BRCA1-BARD1 is a ubiquitin ligase inactivated by the platinum-based anticancer drugs. Breast Cancer Res Treat. 2011;126(1):203–9.
24. Ayi TC, Tsan JT, Hwang LY, Bowcock AM, Baer R. Conservation of function and primary structure in the BRCA1-associated RING domain (BARD1) protein. Oncogene. 1998;17(16):2143–8.
25. Meza JE, Brzovic PS, King MC, Klevit RE. Mapping the functional domains of BRCA1. Interaction of the ring finger domains of BRCA1 and BARD1. J Biol Chem. 1999;274(9):5659–65.
26. Wu LC, Wang ZW, Tsan JT, Spillman MA, Phung A, Xu XL, Yang MC, Hwang LY, Bowcock AM, Baer R. Identification of a RING protein that can interact in vivo with the BRCA1 gene product. Nat Genet. 1996;14(4):430–40.
27. Lorick KL, Jensen JP, Fang S, Ong AM, Hatakeyama S, Weissman AM. RING fingers mediate ubiquitin-conjugating enzyme (E2)-dependent ubiquitination. Proc Natl Acad Sci U S A. 1999;96(20):11364–9.
28. Prakash R, Zhang Y, Feng W, Jasin M. Homologous recombination and human health: the roles of BRCA1, BRCA2, and associated proteins. Cold Spring Harb Perspect Biol. 2015;7(4):a016600.
29. Nishikawa H, Ooka S, Sato K, Arima K, Okamoto J, Klevit RE, Fukuda M, Ohta T. Mass spectrometric and mutational analyses reveal Lys-6-linked polyubiquitin chains catalyzed by BRCA1-BARD1 ubiquitin ligase. J Biol Chem. 2004;279(6):3916–24.
30. Chen A, Kleiman FE, Manley JL, Ouchi T, Pan ZQ. Autoubiquitination of the BRCA1*BARD1 RING ubiquitin ligase. J Biol Chem. 2002;277(24):22085–92.
31. Wu-Baer F, Ludwig T, Baer R. The UBXN1 protein associates with autoubiquitinated forms of the BRCA1 tumor suppressor and inhibits its enzymatic function. Mol Cell Biol. 2010;30(11):2787–98.
32. Ohta T, Sato K, Wu W. The BRCA1 ubiquitin ligase and homologous recombination repair. FEBS Lett. 2011;585(18):2836–44.
33. Sharma B, Preet Kaur R, Raut S, Munshi A. BRCA1 mutation spectrum, functions, and therapeutic strategies: the story so far. Curr Probl Cancer. 2018;42(2):189–207.
34. Mallery DL, Vandenberg CJ, Hiom K. Activation of the E3 ligase function of the BRCA1/BARD1 complex by polyubiquitin chains. EMBO J. 2002;21(24):6755–62.
35. Huen MS, Grant R, Manke I, Minn K, Yu X, Yaffe MB, Chen J. RNF8 transduces the DNA-damage signal via histone ubiquitylation and checkpoint protein assembly. Cell. 2007;131(5):901–14.
36. Yan J, Jetten AM. RAP80 and RNF8, key players in the recruitment of repair proteins to DNA damage sites. Cancer Lett. 2008;271(2):179–90.
37. Yan J, Kim YS, Yang XP, Li LP, Liao G, Xia F, Jetten AM. The ubiquitin-interacting motif containing protein RAP80 interacts with BRCA1 and functions in DNA damage repair response. Cancer Res. 2007;67(14):6647–56.
38. Lee JS, Collins KM, Brown AL, Lee CH, Chung JH. hCds1-mediated phosphorylation of BRCA1 regulates the DNA damage response. Nature. 2000;404(6774):201–4.
39. Stolz A, Ertych N, Kienitz A, Vogel C, Schneider V, Fritz B, Jacob R, Dittmar G, Weichert W, Petersen I, et al. The CHK2-BRCA1 tumour suppressor pathway ensures chromosomal stability in human somatic cells. Nat Cell Biol. 2010; 12(5):492–9.
40. Zhang J, Willers H, Feng Z, Ghosh JC, Kim S, Weaver DT, Chung JH, Powell SN, Xia F. Chk2 phosphorylation of BRCA1 regulates DNA double-strand break repair. Mol Cell Biol. 2004;24(2):708–18.
41. Sy SM, Huen MS, Chen J. PALB2 is an integral component of the BRCA complex required for homologous recombination repair. Proc Natl Acad Sci U S A. 2009;106(17):7155–60.
42. Cortez D, Wang Y, Qin J, Elledge SJ. Requirement of ATM-dependent phosphorylation of brca1 in the DNA damage response to double-strand breaks. Science. 1999;286(5442):1162–6.
43. Xu B, O'Donnell AH, Kim ST, Kastan MB. Phosphorylation of serine 1387 in Brca1 is specifically required for the Atm-mediated S-phase checkpoint after ionizing irradiation. Cancer Res. 2002;62(16):4588–91.
44. Kang Y, Cheong HM, Lee JH, Song PI, Lee KH, Kim SY, Jun JY, You HJ. Protein phosphatase 5 is necessary for ATR-mediated DNA repair. Biochem Biophys Res Commun. 2011;404(1):476–81.
45. Wu Q, Jubb H, Blundell TL. Phosphopeptide interactions with BRCA1 BRCT domains: more than just a motif. Prog Biophys Mol Biol. 2015; 117(2–3):143–8.
46. Cantor SB, Bell DW, Ganesan S, Kass EM, Drapkin R, Grossman S, Wahrer DC, Sgroi DC, Lane WS, Haber DA, et al. BACH1, a novel helicase-like protein, interacts directly with BRCA1 and contributes to its DNA repair function. Cell. 2001;105(1):149–60.
47. Wong AK, Ormonde PA, Pero R, Chen Y, Lian L, Salada G, Berry S, Lawrence Q, Dayananth P, Ha P, et al. Characterization of a carboxy-terminal BRCA1 interacting protein. Oncogene. 1998;17(18):2279–85.
48. Drikos I, Nounesis G, Vorgias CE. Characterization of cancer-linked BRCA1-BRCT missense variants and their interaction with phosphoprotein targets. Proteins. 2009;77(2):464–76.
49. Yu X, Wu LC, Bowcock AM, Aronheim A, Baer R. The C-terminal (BRCT) domains of BRCA1 interact in vivo with CtIP, a protein implicated in the CtBP pathway of transcriptional repression. J Biol Chem. 1998;273(39): 25388–92.

50. Yu X, Chen J. DNA damage-induced cell cycle checkpoint control requires CtIP, a phosphorylation-dependent binding partner of BRCA1 C-terminal domains. Mol Cell Biol. 2004;24(21):9478–86.
51. Kim H, Huang J, Chen J. CCDC98 is a BRCA1-BRCT domain-binding protein involved in the DNA damage response. Nat Struct Mol Biol. 2007;14(8):710–5.
52. Liu Z, Wu J, Yu X. CCDC98 targets BRCA1 to DNA damage sites. Nat Struct Mol Biol. 2007;14(8):716–20.
53. Rodriguez M, Yu X, Chen J, Songyang Z. Phosphopeptide binding specificities of BRCA1 COOH-terminal (BRCT) domains. J Biol Chem. 2003; 278(52):52914–8.
54. Mohammad DH, Yaffe MB. 14-3-3 proteins, FHA domains and BRCT domains in the DNA damage response. DNA Repair (Amst). 2009;8(9):1009–17.
55. Lee MS, Green R, Marsillac SM, Coquelle N, Williams RS, Yeung T, Foo D, Hau DD, Hui B, Monteiro AN, et al. Comprehensive analysis of missense variations in the BRCT domain of BRCA1 by structural and functional assays. Cancer Res. 2010;70(12):4880–90.
56. Wang B, Matsuoka S, Ballif BA, Zhang D, Smogorzewska A, Gygi SP, Elledge SJ. Abraxas and RAP80 form a BRCA1 protein complex required for the DNA damage response. Science. 2007;316(5828):1194–8.
57. Cantor SB, Andreassen PR. Assessing the link between BACH1 and BRCA1 in the FA pathway. Cell Cycle. 2006;5(2):164–7.
58. Litman R, Peng M, Jin Z, Zhang F, Zhang J, Powell S, Andreassen PR, Cantor SB. BACH1 is critical for homologous recombination and appears to be the Fanconi anemia gene product FANCJ. Cancer Cell. 2005;8(3):255–65.
59. Greenberg RA, Sobhian B, Pathania S, Cantor SB, Nakatani Y, Livingston DM. Multifactorial contributions to an acute DNA damage response by BRCA1/ BARD1-containing complexes. Genes Dev. 2006;20(1):34–46.
60. Williams RS, Dodson GE, Limbo O, Yamada Y, Williams JS, Guenther G, Classen S, Glover JN, Iwasaki H, Russell P, et al. Nbs1 flexibly tethers Ctp1 and Mre11-Rad50 to coordinate DNA double-strand break processing and repair. Cell. 2009;139(1):87–99.
61. Limbo O, Chahwan C, Yamada Y, de Bruin RA, Wittenberg C, Russell P. Ctp1 is a cell-cycle-regulated protein that functions with Mre11 complex to control double-strand break repair by homologous recombination. Mol Cell. 2007;28(1):134–46.
62. Sartori AA, Lukas C, Coates J, Mistrik M, Fu S, Bartek J, Baer R, Lukas J, Jackson SP. Human CtIP promotes DNA end resection. Nature. 2007; 450(7169):509–14.
63. den Dunnen JT, Dalgleish R, Maglott DR, Hart RK, Greenblatt MS, McGowan-Jordan J, Roux AF, Smith T, Antonarakis SE, Taschner PE. HGVS recommendations for the description of sequence variants: 2016 update. Hum Mutat. 2016;37(6):564–9.
64. Hastings J, Owen G, Dekker A, Ennis M, Kale N, Muthukrishnan V, Turner S, Swainston N, Mendes P, Steinbeck C. ChEBI in 2016: improved services and an expanding collection of metabolites. Nucleic Acids Res. 2016;44(D1):D1214–9.
65. Gene Ontology Consortium. Gene Ontology Consortium: going forward. Nucleic Acids Res. 2015;43(Database issue):D1049–56.
66. Smith CL, Eppig JT. The mammalian phenotype ontology as a unifying standard for experimental and high-throughput phenotyping data. Mamm Genome. 2012;23(9–10):653–68.
67. Chibucos MC, Mungall CJ, Balakrishnan R, Christie KR, Huntley RP, White O, Blake JA, Lewis SE, Giglio M. Standardized description of scientific evidence using the Evidence Ontology (ECO). Database (Oxford). 2014;2014.
68. Starita LM, Young DL, Islam M, Kitzman JO, Gullingsrud J, Hause RJ, Fowler DM, Parvin JD, Shendure J, Fields S. Massively parallel functional analysis of BRCA1 RING domain variants. Genetics. 2015;200(2):413–22.
69. Woods NT, Baskin R, Golubeva V, Jhuraney A, De-Gregoriis G, Vaclova T, Goldgar DE, Couch FJ, Carvalho MA, Iversen ES, et al. Functional assays provide a robust tool for the clinical annotation of genetic variants of uncertain significance. NPJ Genom Med. 2016;1.
70. Schoumacher F, Glaus A, Mueller H, Eppenberger U, Bolliger B, Senn HJ. BRCA1/2 mutations in Swiss patients with familial or early-onset breast and ovarian cancer. Swiss Med Wkly. 2001;131(15–16):223–6.
71. Zheng L, Pan H, Li S, Flesken-Nikitin A, Chen PL, Boyer TG, Lee WH. Sequence-specific transcriptional corepressor function for BRCA1 through a novel zinc finger protein, ZBRK1. Mol Cell. 2000;6(4):757–68.
72. Tavtigian SV, Deffenbaugh AM, Yin L, Judkins T, Scholl T, Samollow PB, de Silva D, Zharkikh A, Thomas A. Comprehensive statistical study of 452 BRCA1 missense substitutions with classification of eight recurrent substitutions as neutral. J Med Genet. 2006;43(4):295–305.
73. Johnston JJ, Rubinstein WS, Facio FM, Ng D, Singh LN, Teer JK, Mullikin JC, Biesecker LG. Secondary variants in individuals undergoing exome sequencing: screening of 572 individuals identifies high-penetrance mutations in cancer-susceptibility genes. Am J Hum Genet. 2012;91(1):97–108.
74. Dombernowsky SL, Weischer M, Freiberg JJ, Bojesen SE, Tybjaerg-Hansen A, Nordestgaard BG. Missense polymorphisms in BRCA1 and BRCA2 and risk of breast and ovarian cancer. Cancer Epidemiol Biomark Prev. 2009;18(8):2339–42.
75. Phelan CM, Dapic V, Tice B, Favis R, Kwan E, Barany F, Manoukian S, Radice P, van der Luijt RB, van Nesselrooij BP, et al. Classification of BRCA1 missense variants of unknown clinical significance. J Med Genet. 2005;42(2):138–46.
76. Lovelock PK, Healey S, Au W, Sum EY, Tesoriero A, Wong EM, Hinson S, Brinkworth R, Bekessy A, Diez O, et al. Genetic, functional, and histopathological evaluation of two C-terminal BRCA1 missense variants. J Med Genet. 2006;43(1):74–83.
77. Bouwman P, van der Gulden H, van der Heijden I, Drost R, Klijn CN, Prasetyanti P, Pieterse M, Wientjens E, Seibler J, Hogervorst FB, et al. A high-throughput functional complementation assay for classification of BRCA1 missense variants. Cancer Discov. 2013;3(10):1142–55.
78. Tonin PN, Mes-Masson AM, Futreal PA, Morgan K, Mahon M, Foulkes WD, Cole DE, Provencher D, Ghadirian P, Narod SA. Founder BRCA1 and BRCA2 mutations in French Canadian breast and ovarian cancer families. Am J Hum Genet. 1998;63(5):1341–51.
79. Meindl A. Comprehensive analysis of 989 patients with breast or ovarian cancer provides BRCA1 and BRCA2 mutation profiles and frequencies for the German population. Int J Cancer. 2002;97(4):472–80.
80. Chang S, Biswas K, Martin BK, Stauffer S, Sharan SK. Expression of human BRCA1 variants in mouse ES cells allows functional analysis of BRCA1 mutations. J Clin Invest. 2009;119(10):3160–71.
81. Cunningham F, Moore B, Ruiz-Schultz N, Ritchie GR, Eilbeck K. Improving the Sequence Ontology terminology for genomic variant annotation. J Biomed Semantics. 2015;6:32.
82. Katagiri T, Kasumi F, Yoshimoto M, Nomizu T, Asaishi K, Abe R, Tsuchiya A, Sugano M, Takai S, Yoneda M, et al. High proportion of missense mutations of the BRCA1 and BRCA2 genes in Japanese breast cancer families. J Hum Genet. 1998;43(1):42–8.
83. Sweet K, Senter L, Pilarski R, Wei L, Toland AE. Characterization of BRCA1 ring finger variants of uncertain significance. Breast Cancer Res Treat. 2010; 119(3):737–43.

22

How to create innovation by building the translation bridge from basic research into medicinal drugs: an industrial perspective

Paul G Germann[1*], Alexander Schuhmacher[2], Juan Harrison[3], Ronald Law[4], Kevin Haug[4] and Gordon Wong[5]

Abstract

The global healthcare industry is undergoing substantial changes and adaptations to the constant decline of approved new medical entities. This decrease in internal research productivity is resulting in a major decline of patent-protected sales (patent cliff) of most of the pharmaceutical companies. Three major global adaptive trends as driving forces to cope with these challenges are evident: cut backs of internal research and development jobs in the western hemisphere (Europe and USA), following the market growth potential of Asia by building up internal or external research and development capabilities there and finally, 'early innovation hunting' with an increased focus on identifying and investing in very early innovation sources within academia and small start-up companies. Early innovation hunting can be done by different approaches: increased corporate funding, establishment of translational institutions to bridge innovation, increasing sponsored collaborations and formation of technology hunting groups for capturing very early scientific ideas and concepts. This emerging trend towards early innovation hunting demands special adaptations from both the pharmaceutical industry and basic researchers in academia to bridge the translation into new medicines which deliver innovative medicines that matters to the patient. This opinion article describes the different modalities of cross-fertilisation between basic university or publicly funded institutional research and the applied research and development activities within the pharmaceutical industry. Two key factors in this important translational bridge can be identified: preparation of both partnering organisations to open up for new and sometime disruptive ideas and creation of truly trust-based relationships between the different groups allowing long-term scientific collaborations while acknowledging that value-creating differences are an essential factor for successful collaboration building.

Keywords: Healthcare industry, Corporate venture capital, Open innovation, New frontier science, Translational development, Technology platforms

Introduction

The human population is facing substantial challenges in the next coming decades with respect to their healthcare: We see an increasing size of the ageing populations, especially in the industrial countries like North America, Europe and Japan. On the other side, there is a clear 'globalisation' of healthcare accompanied by an increasing need for improved medication in developing countries. In addition, the constantly increasing costs for the healthcare system leads to a focus towards 'precise' medicines. These medicines must have a better therapeutic window, should be personalised to patients needs and accompanied by a validated biomarker concept and might even be combined with other medicines. Therefore, the scope of new research activities in the healthcare system is even broadened by the need to address potentially unfamiliar and complex diseases, new modes of action and challenges like smaller but more distinct multiple patient populations. New therapies will combine pharmaceuticals, diagnostics and devices, with an increase reporting and monitoring of effects via an enhanced IT environment. An increase in innovation is one answer to the upcoming challenges just mentioned. Here, it is important to note that the majority of innovation occurs outside of the pharmaceutical industry. With these upcoming challenges in mind, the global

* Correspondence: Paul-Georg.Germann@takeda.com
[1]New Frontier Science, Takeda GmbH, Constance, 78462, Germany
Full list of author information is available at the end of the article

healthcare industry is undergoing substantial changes and adaptations to the constant decline of approved new medical entities (see Figure 1) [1-3].

This decrease in the internal research productivity within most of the larger pharmaceutical companies will prospectively result in a major decline of patent-protected sales (so called 'patent cliff') of most of the pharmaceutical companies.

Three major global adaptive trends as driving forces are evident:

1. Cut backs of internal research and development jobs in the western hemisphere (Europe and USA, see Table 1),
2. Following the market growth potential of Asia by building up internal or external research and development capabilities there and
3. 'Early innovation hunting' with an opening of the pharmaceutical companies towards very early innovation sources within academia and small start-up companies. This can be done by different means: increased corporate funding, translational institutions to bridge innovation, increasing sponsored collaborations and technology hunting groups for front leading very early scientific ideas and concepts.

Especially, this trend of early innovation hunting demands special adaptations not only from pharmaceutical industry, but also from basic research in academia to bridge the translation into new medicines which matters to the patient.

On the other side of this innovation bridge, the universities and research institutions will see a static or even a decline in governmental funding, while corporate venture funding takes an increasing stake of importance in the financial system of these research institutions. Corporations are increasingly investing into healthcare as shown in Figure 2.

Main text

This opinion article describes the different modalities of cross-fertilisation between basic university or publicly funded research institutions and the applied research and development activities within the pharmaceutical industry. Some key phases in this important translational bridge can be identified:

1. *Prepare* the organisations on both sides for opening up for new ideas
2. *Find* the opportunities and *open the doors* to innovation
3. *Create trust* within the scientific collaboration
4. *Develop and select* the winning project as a team
5. *Translate the innovation* into the value chain of a big pharmaceutical company

Prepare the organisations

The need for a substantial increase of innovative ideas in the health care sector has led to a higher awareness and a

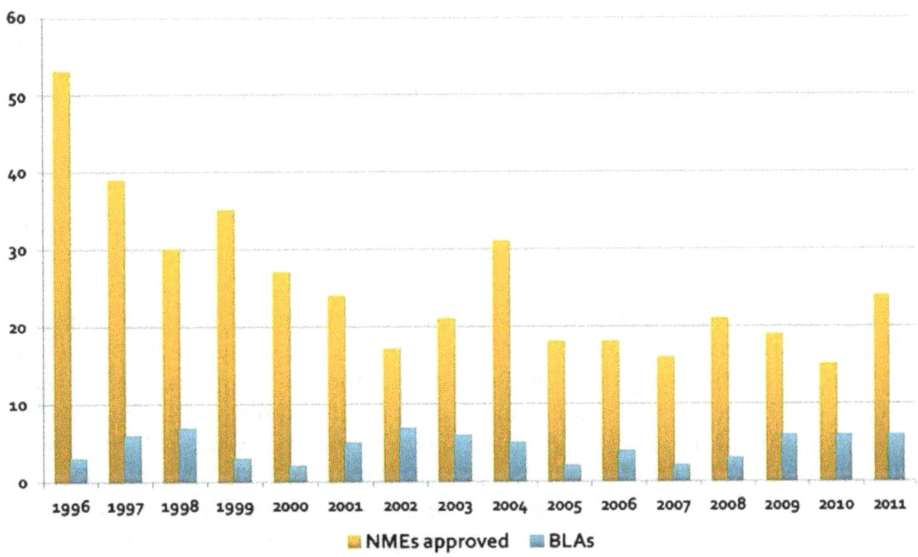

NME (New Molecular Entity), BLA (Biologic License Application)

Source: Hughes B. (2009) Nature Reviews Drug Discovery 8: 93-96; Mullard A. (2012) Nature Reviews Drug Discovery 11:91-94; www. fda.org

Figure 1 FDA drug approvals.

Table 1 Cut backs of internal research and development jobs in the western hemisphere (Europe and USA), September 2012

Recent layoffs in big pharmaceutical companies			
Ranking by 2011 sales	**Company**	**Date**	**Notes**
1	Novartis	January 2012	2,000 US sales jobs
2	Sanofi	Imminent	Reportedly up to 2,000 French jobs
3	Pfizer	2005	Still another 12,100 of planned 60,000 jobs to be cut
4	Roche	June 2012	Nutley site to close, 1,000 R and D jobs
5	GlaxoSmithKline	NA	Ongoing restructuring, no specific job target announced
6	Merck & Co	July 2011	12% to13% workforce reduction, in addition to earlier cuts following Schering-Plough takeover
7	Johnson & Johnson	November 2009	7,000 to 8,200 jobs
8	Abbott Laboratories	January 2012	700 manufacturing jobs
9	Bristol-Myers Squibb	NA	Ongoing, 295 jobs cut so far in 2012
10	AstraZeneca	Feb 2012	7,300 jobs, including 2,200 in R and D

NA not applicable, *R and D* research and development. Source: Takeda Media Monitoring 19 September 2012.

closer collaboration between academic institutions and the pharmaceutical industry. The universities/institutions with their technology transfer offices (TTO) are working here as change agents in two directions: by exposing the academics towards external interested partners via 'open research days' and business development conferences and by using their manifold networks outside the universities; a mindset change towards a customer orientation is the ultimate goal. In the external direction, fostering of their relationships to newly interested partners is an attempt to seek attention of potential new collaborations and ultimately, funding and partners for the research assets. A challenging point here is the current focus of many TTO and pharmaceutical companies on developed projects with the aim to generate on a fast track mode intellectual property (IP) and a licence option to be granted. Very embryonic assets are normally not in the focus of these kinds of TTO activities.

The hunting and scouting groups of pharmaceutical companies have the critical task to prepare the internal organisation for additional projects to supplement a much-focused high project load of the internal discovery, development and project management organisation. An environment in which external ideas are viewed as threatening competitors to internal project resources needs to be changed by constant communication flow into an open-minded welcoming spirit, which sees the new ideas coming from external as a critical success factor for the whole company. The term 'landing path' pictures well this attempt to prepare the internal pharmaceutical company organisation as an open, embracing and welcoming path towards external innovation.

Find the opportunities and open the doors

Innovation is available in all academic institutions all over the world. Comparing the total sizes of organisations and the total budget spent, academic institutions are outpacing the capacities of the pharmaceutical industry by far. Finding the 'right' innovation opportunities, which suits the company's needs, should use strategic competitive intelligence approaches in a smart and efficient way. The term 'right opportunity' will be addressed later. A good general overview of the academic landscape with respect to grant, publication and technology and therapeutic field ranking is the basis. A broad personal network of the company scientists within the selected scientific community is the second important factor to access scientific partners. Thirdly, the building of personal relationships between company and key academic scientists of the selected hot spots of interests are an important factor, which might help to open the right door to the right innovation.

To create trust within the scientific collaboration is the key factor of creating a joined success story between academic and pharmaceutical scientists. First of all, in the first introductory meetings, the innovative idea needs to be fully understood by both sides. This means that the colleagues from the pharmaceutical industry have to generate a deep insight into the basic biology or technology to get accepted by the academic collaborator. On the other side, their project and development knowledge and the strategic health benefit perspective, which they bring to the table, might be very beneficial for the academic side as an eye-opener. This kind of relationship building might take several meetings where ongoing discussions might shape more and more the possible joint project. In addition, the pharmaceutical company as a partner can support the academic innovator by giving him/her access to the company compound libraries and connect them to specialised experts and additional technologies. Especially in the case of very early innovative ideas, this phase is a very important process of relationship building as the 'way forward towards a medicine that matters' is often not evident and straightforward.

Develop and select the winning project as a team

During the idea-shaping discussions, the development and translational project knowledge of the pharmaceutical

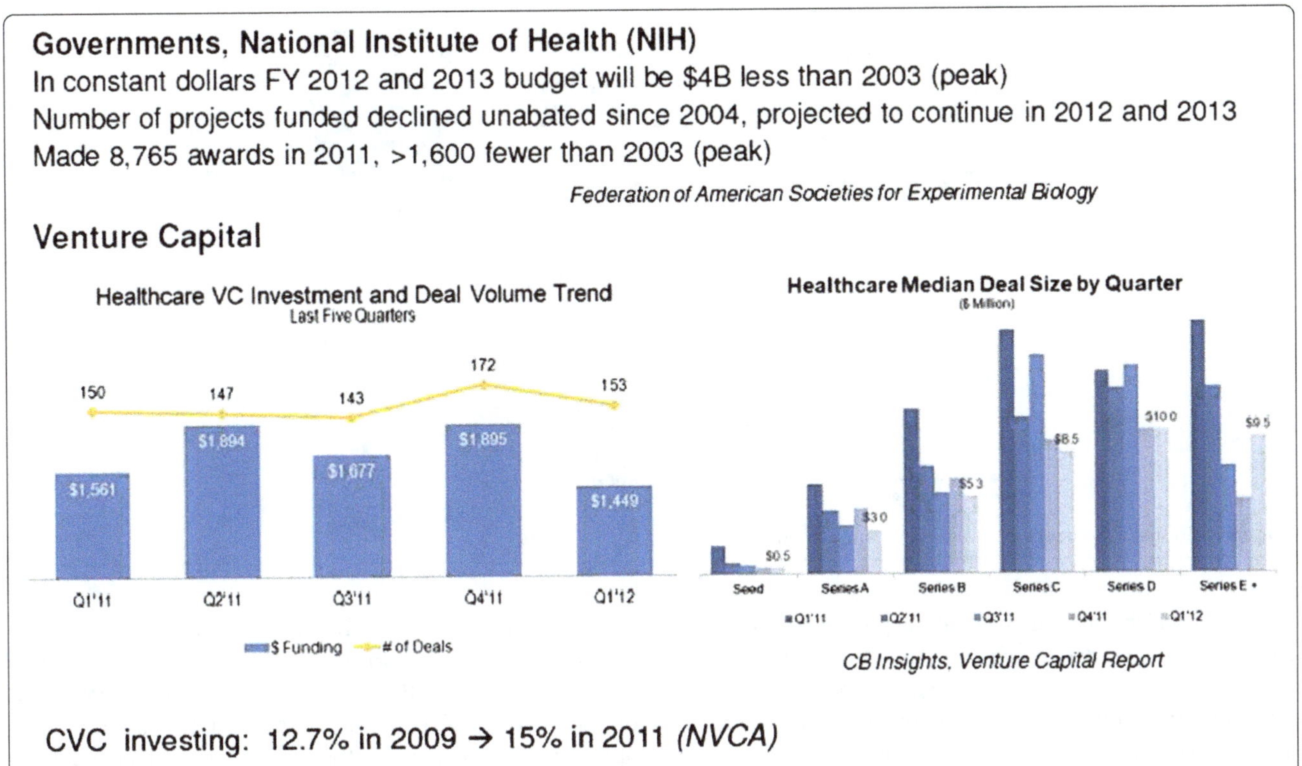

Figure 2 Trends in innovation funding: a US perspective.

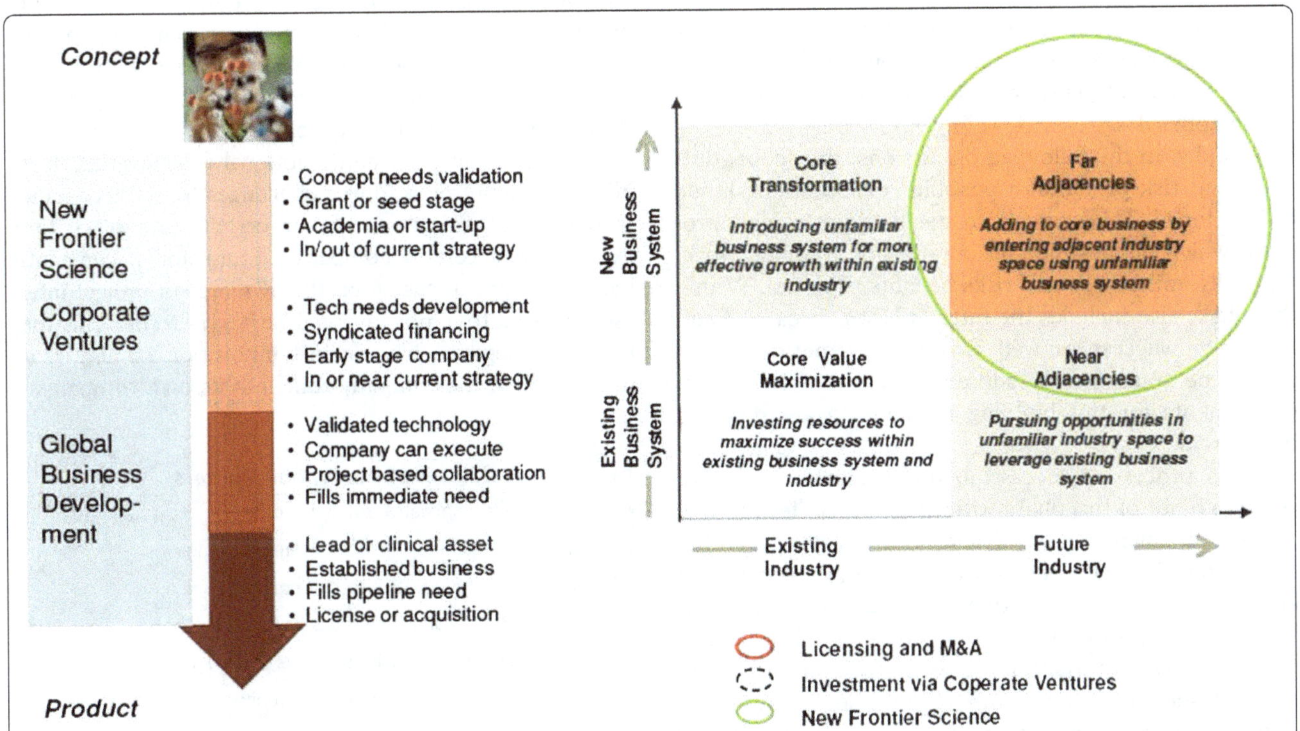

Figure 3 Important deliverables and dependencies in innovation management.

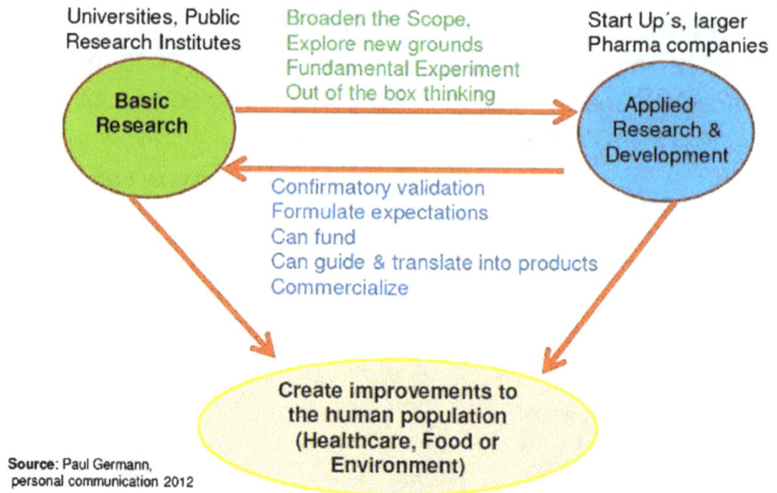

Figure 4 Strategic elements in innovation management.

colleagues will be used to generate a project proposal together with the academic inventor. Here three components are essential: in an open and transparent atmosphere, the pharmaceutical company offers support to the academic institution to generate, if not already done, their (academic side!) IP. This should be a unidirectional support from the pharmaceutical company to the academic inventor as a trust-building exercise. This approach of 'the helping hand' is not the normal current practice, which might be the reason why a trust building within this early part of a relationship is currently not the easiest way forward. On the other hand, if the project is successful and positive for both sides, then a later licence option already mentioned as the first right of refusal will generate a joined vision for success sharing on both sides.

Secondly, in the following discussions, the scope, duration and risk profile of a possible collaboration should be developed. This exercise creates the joint project proposal which defines the collaboration by framing, working tasks, milestones and risks benefits proposal. Within this phase also includes the future phases, in case of collaboration success as well as failure scenarios, which should be transparently addressed. The basic different components for this building relationship are depicted in Figure 3.

If this process is successful, the academic innovator should go out of this phase with the spirit of 'feeling well supported', 'having a partner' and 'seeing further than before'. The pharmaceutical partner see the spirit as 'we are a partner in this project', 'let us work on this innovation opportunity'.

Thereby, an important aspect is the 'buy-in' process of internal stakeholders in both organisations. Buy-in by both partnering organisations is also a supportive factor for a strong relationship building process.

Translate innovation into the value chain

To find the right opportunity is an easy sentence with a difficult translation. From the pharmaceutical perspective of pharmaceutical companies, the aim to find the right opportunity and to open the right door is dependent on the corporate strategy. A strong focus on the existing strategic (small molecular entities, also called smols, biologics, therapeutics and diagnostics) and/or therapeutic areas will automatically lead to narrowing the window of innovation hunting. The opportunities found in these more narrow windows are easier to find, select, develop and translate into the own organisation of the pharmaceutical company because of the closeness of the idea towards the receiving organisation and the scientific expertise. Compared to this, innovation outside the 'comfort zone' bears a higher risk for scientific error and emotional (not invented here, NIH syndrome) or resource challenges to get acceptance within the organisation. After a certain amount of time exposed to a certain company culture and a constantly high work load, focusing on the own area of project interests can lead to a 'not invented here' syndrome. This may lead to a negative bias against innovation coming from the outside of the company zone into its own company.

Table 2 Soft skill set of innovation hunters

- Active search for innovative solutions to disease
- Articulate the disease or therapeutic area challenge
- Radars a range of innovative technologies and solutions
- Bridges a range risk and time spans to proof of concept
- Looking for engagement with scientists and inventors
- Seek engagement with drug discovery units and therapeutic areas
- Be critical

Source: Gordon Wong, personal communication 2012.

In addition, early innovative ideas which might need 5 to 15 years to come into product reality need a long breath and a constant internal 'branding and advertising' before they might get accepted within the receiving organisation. For example, innovation hunters within the Takeda organisation should work on innovation, which are 'far adjacencies' (see Figure 4; PG, personal communication, 2012) to fulfil the strategic focus of the New Frontier Science approach. These innovation hunters should have a special social and communication skills set as depicted in Table 2. To build this critical bridge, social skills like networking building capability are essentially important.

Conclusions

The healthcare industry needs a boost of innovative ideas coming from the academic institutions to overcome the current challenges. New ways of collaborations and closer connectivity between the basic research in academic and the applied research within the pharmaceutical industry are essential for a joint success. To build in this broader context, a respectful and trustful relationship between the partners is the key for a win-win situation between academic institutions and pharmaceutical companies.

Competing interests

PG, JH, RL, KH and GW are employees of Takeda Pharmaceuticals. Therefore these authors, co-authors, would like to declare a conflict of interest in the description of the structural elements of the New Frontier Science concept and strategic elements. AS, employed by the government of the German federal state Baden-Württemberg, Germany, declares no conflict of interest.

Authors' contributions

PG drafted the first version of this commentary; the other authors provided editing feedback and main additional data sources. All authors read and approved the final manuscript.

Authors' information

PG is an exempt professor at the University for Veterinary Science, Hannover Foundation and currently working as the vice president for New Frontiers Science Europe for Takeda GmbH, Germany.

Acknowledgements

The authors wish to thank Mrs. Delli-Bovi for formatting this publication.

Author details

[1]New Frontier Science, Takeda GmbH, Constance, 78462, Germany. [2]University of Reutlingen, Reutlingen, 72760, Germany. [3]New Frontier Science, Takeda Pharmaceuticals, Palo Alto, CA94301, USA. [4]New Frontier Science, Takeda Pharmaceuticals, Chicago, IL 60601, USA. [5]New Frontier Science, Takeda Pharmaceuticals, Boston, MA 02467, USA.

References

1. Hughes B: **FDA drug approvals.** *Nature Rev Drug Discov* 2009, **8:**93–96.
2. Mullard A: **2011 FDA drug approvals.** *Nature Rev Drug Discov* 2012, **11:**91–94.
3. FDA: *FDA.org. The center for health and wellness.* http://fda.org/.

23

Transcriptomics to study the effect of a Mediterranean-inspired diet on inflammation in Crohn's disease patients

Gareth Marlow[1,2], Stephanie Ellett[1,2], Isobel R Ferguson[1], Shuotun Zhu[3], Nishi Karunasinghe[3], Amalini C Jesuthasan[1,2], Dug Yeo Han[1,2], Alan G Fraser[2,4] and Lynnette R Ferguson[1,2*]

Abstract

Background: Inflammation is an essential immune response; however, chronic inflammation results in disease including Crohn's disease. Therefore, reducing the inflammation can yield a significant health benefit, and one way to achieve this is through diet. We developed a Mediterranean-inspired anti-inflammatory diet and used this diet in a 6-week intervention in a Crohn's disease population. We examined changes in inflammation and also in the gut microbiota. We compared the results of established biomarkers, C-reactive protein and the micronuclei assay, of inflammation with results from a transcriptomic approach.

Results: Data showed that being on our diet for 6 weeks was able to reduce the established biomarkers of inflammation. However, using transcriptomics, we observed significant changes in gene expression. Although no single gene stood out, the cumulative effect of small changes in many genes combined to have a beneficial effect. Data also showed that our diet resulted in a trend of normalising the microbiota.

Conclusions: This study showed that our Mediterranean-inspired diet appeared to benefit the health of people with Crohn's disease. Our participants showed a trend for reduced markers of inflammation and normalising of the microbiota. The significant changes in gene expression after 6 weeks highlighted the increased sensitivity of using transcriptomics when compared to the established biomarkers and open up a new era of dietary intervention studies.

Keywords: Inflammation, Crohn's disease, Transcriptomics, Dietary intervention

Background

Nutrigenomics studies the effect of a specific food or diet on gene and expression using the omic technologies. This will lead to a better understanding of the mechanism of how specific dietary components affect specific gene and proteins resulting in an understanding of how metabolism is influenced [1].

Determining the effects of intervention studies can be difficult, as the change in gene expression for an individual gene may be low but the number of genes affected could be large, resulting in a cumulative beneficial effect as a result of the intervention. Such trials are costly and time consuming and have required a prior hypothesis and ideally pilot data before commencement, to ensure that the correct genes were measured. The technology of transcriptomics has allowed non-hypothesis-based studies to be undertaken. This technique allows the study of thousands of genes simultaneously, and the sensitivity allows the detection of a small change in the expression of a gene. The other advantage of such a sensitive technique is that the results allow intervention trials to be conducted over a much shorter time frame and with fewer participants. The non-hypothesis-based approach and the reduced cost of a shorter smaller trial would allow smaller food companies to prove efficacy of functional foods or novel diets and thus make a substantiated health claim.

* Correspondence: l.ferguson@auckland.ac.nz
[1]Discipline of Nutrition, Faculty of Medical and Health Sciences, The University of Auckland Private Bag 92019, Auckland 1142, New Zealand
[2]Nutrigenomics New Zealand, University of Auckland, Private Bag 92019, Auckland 1142, New Zealand
Full list of author information is available at the end of the article

Inflammation is a necessary immune response; however, chronic inflammation can lead to chronic diseases including cardiovascular disease, rheumatoid arthritis, Alzheimer's, Crohn's disease and even some cancers [2-4]. Therefore, reducing the inflammation can yield a significant health benefit [2,5,6]. Crohn's disease is a chronic intestinal disorder, typified by chronic inflammation of the gastrointestinal tract. While it has a clear genetic susceptibility, lifestyle factors including diet are important factors in disease development [7-9]. If diet is a cause of symptoms, then it stands to reason that diet can also relieve symptoms, and therefore, Crohn's disease would be a good target for nutrigenomics [1,10].

As Crohn's disease is localised to the gastrointestinal tract, one would expect to find dysbiosis of the intestinal microbiome [11-13]. The interplay between diet, intestinal microbiota, genetics and health is complex [14]. In recent years, the role of the microbiota has become of greater importance in understanding human health and disease. Six bacterial phyla, comprising over 1,000 species, have been identified as the predominant inhabitants of the human gut [15,16]. While previously considered a static entity, it is now emerging that the ratio of the bacterial phyla and species in the gut is constantly changing in response to external influences like diet. Different diseases also have a deviation from what is being considered a 'normal' ratio of bacterial phyla [17]. Whether change to the microbiota is a cause or effect of disease is currently unknown.

A healthy intestinal mirobiome consists of six bacterial phyla—Firmicutes, Bacteroidetes, Actinobacteria, Proteobacteria, Fusobacteria and Verrucomicrobia, with species of Firmicutes and Bacteriodetes being the most abundant at approximately 65% and 25%, respectively. Variations are observed in healthy individuals by the abundance of the different species within each phylum; however, disease association is observed by variations in the abundance of the six phyla [18]. Manichanh [19] and Sokol [20] both reported a reduction in faecal microbial diversity of patients with Crohn's disease, particularly a reduction in the number of species of the phyla Firmicutes (specifically *Clostridium* clusters IV and XIVa) and Bacteroidetes, with a corresponding increase in Proteobacteria and *Bacillus* [21] (Table 1). We developed an anti-inflammatory diet based upon a Mediterranean-inspired diet, which is well-known for its protective ability towards chronic disease [2,5,22-26]. To this base diet, we added foods that previous research has shown to be beneficial in reducing inflammation and removed foods that are known to be detrimental to Crohn's disease patients [27,28]. We conducted a pilot study in early 2012 [29], using both the established validated biomarkers, C-reactive protein (CRP) [30,31] and micronucleus assay (MN) [32], and transcriptomics to test the ability of this Mediterranean-inspired diet to reduce inflammation in healthy people [29]. Based on the success of this trial as determined by a statistically significant reduction in CRP in this healthy group, a similar trial was undertaken in participants with Crohn's disease. In this second study, we hoped to prove that the diet reduced inflammation and was beneficial to patients with Crohn's disease. We also hoped to show that the transcriptomic technique was more sensitive and thus required fewer subjects over a shorter time frame than the established biomarkers [5,33,34].

Table 1 The relative abundance of bacteria in a healthy and Crohn's disease microbiome

Bacterial phyla	'Healthy' microbiome (%)	'Crohn's disease' microbiome
Bacteroidetes	Approximately 25	Decreased expression
Firmicutes	Approximately 65	Decreased expression in *Clostridium* clusters IV and XIVa and increased expression in *Bacillus*
Actinobacteria	Approximately 5	
Proteobacteria	Approximately 8	Increased expression
Fusobacteria	Approximately 1	
Verrucomicrobia	Approximately 2	

Results

Adherence to the diet

All eight participants completed the 6-week diet and in a self-reported questionnaire felt they adhered to the diet well. Based on participant responses to the food diaries, we were able to show that the average total energy consumption reduced from 8,189 to 6,716 kJ, and cholesterol levels were reduced by 20%. There was also a reduction in average intake of saturated fat (43.9% to 32.1%) and a corresponding increase in mono- (38.9% to 46.6%) and poly-unsaturated fats (17% to 21.1%).

Biomarkers

The established biomarkers, CRP and micronuclei numbers, showed a trend of reduction after the 6-week diet; however, this was not significant. The change in CRP level as a result of dietary intervention is shown in Figure 1. Overall, there was a reduction after the 6-week diet, but this was not statistically significant ($p = 0.39$). Cytokinesis-blocked micronuclei numbers before and after dietary intervention are shown in Figure 2. Although numbers decreased after intervention, this reduction did not reach statistical significance ($p = 0.15$).

Gene expression

Using the Affymetrix PrimeView™ microarray (Santa Clara, CA, USA), we found that gene expression was significantly affected (Figure 3). In total, we found that 3,551 genes had significantly ($p < 0.05$) altered expression as a result of the

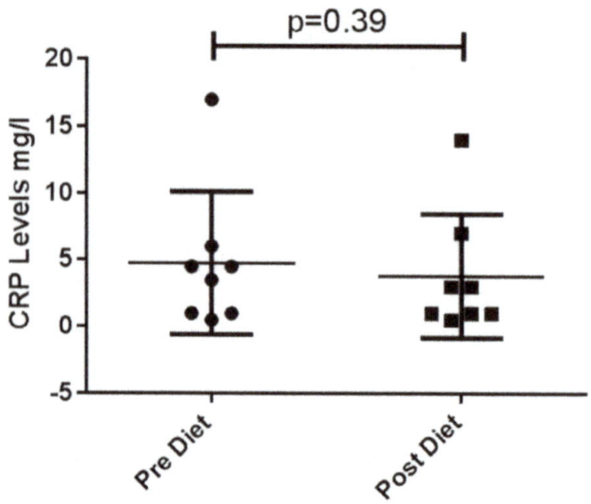

Figure 1 **Mean (±SE) levels of C-reactive protein pre- and post-dietary intervention for each participant.**

dietary intervention, with 1,902 genes being up-regulated and 1,649 down-regulated. These results highlight the increased sensitivity in this methodology.

Just changing gene expression is of no benefit; we expect our diet to change inflammation-relevant genes. We used pathway analysis software (Ingenuity Pathway Analysis (IPA)) to examine these differentially expressed genes in more detail. Table 2 shows the top functions and the number of differentially expressed genes for each. The functions were grouped into three categories by IPA: (1) diseases and disorders, (2) molecular and cellular function and (3) physiological system development and function.

Table 3 summarises the significantly affected canonical pathways for the dietary intervention, calculated by IPA.

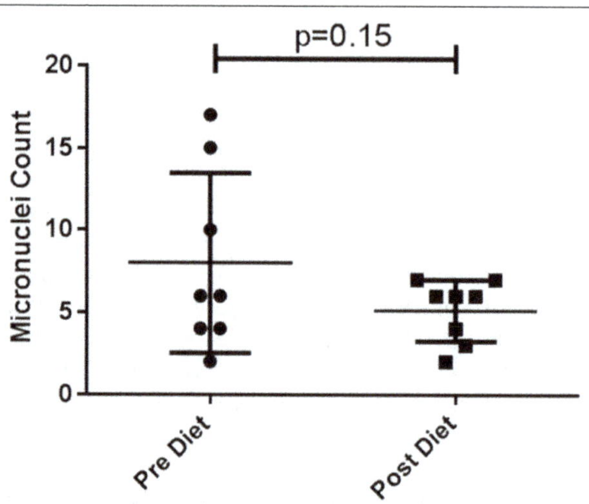

Figure 2 **Mean (±SE) micronuclei scored in 1,100 cytokinesis-blocked cells for each participant pre- and post-dietary intervention.**

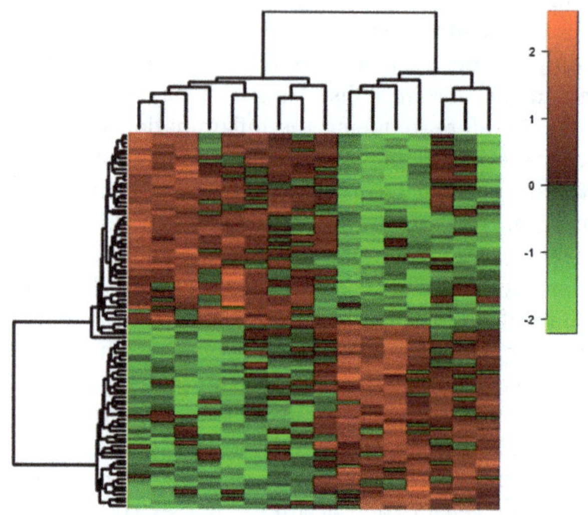

Figure 3 **Differential expression of top 100 genes ($p < 0.002$) pre- and post-dietary intervention.** Based on analysis of the top differentially expressed transcripts, it is clear that transcription expression is changed over time, with expression being both increased (*red*) and decreased (*green*) significantly in just 6 weeks.

The results are ranked according to significance (Fischer's exact test). The ratio for each pathway is also given. The ratio is the number of genes in the dataset that are in the canonical pathway divided by the total number of genes in that pathway.

In order to better understand the connections between the differentially regulated genes, we mapped the genes into a network diagram based on interactions as determined by the IPA Knowledge Base, using the upstream regulator interferon regulatory factor 2 (IRF2) (Figure 4). IRF2 has been shown to regulate NF-κB activity, which is essential in control of immune response and inflammation [35] and within the network to indirectly interact with signal transducer and activator of transcription 3 (STAT3). STAT3 is an important transcription factor in the JAK/STAT pathway and has been shown to be affected in inflammatory bowel disease (IBD) [36,37].

Microbiota abundance

The expression of the six bacterial phyla of the study participants was not too dissimilar from the healthy specimens (Figure 5) or from the theoretical diversity of a normal microbiome. However, before the diet, there was a tendency towards a reduction in bacterial diversity, indicative of Crohn's disease. This is noted by a combined relative abundance of Bacteroidetes at 17.89% in the study participants compared to 22.64% in the healthy individuals, Bacillaceae at 4.65% compared to 3.44% in the healthy individuals and a 5.93% relative abundance of Proteobacteria in the study participants compared to 1.67% in the healthy individuals. The

Table 2 Key functions associated with dietary intervention

Top function	Number of genes	*p* value
Diseases and disorders		
Neurological disease	122	8.67E – 09 to 9.70E – 03
Skeletal and muscular disorders	138	8.67E – 09 to 7.60E – 03
Infectious disease	126	8.67E – 08 to 1.41E – 02
Psychological disorders	91	1.27E – 05 to 9.70E – 03
Cancer	358	1.37E – 05 to 1.37E – 02
Molecular and cellular function		
Cellular growth and proliferation	218	1.23E – 07 to 1.47E – 02
Cellular development	177	1.81E – 07 to 1.40E – 02
Cell cycle	84	9.24E – 07 to 1.24E – 02
Cell-to-cell signalling and interaction	108	1.76E – 06 to 1.46E – 02
Cellular movement	120	1.76E – 06 to 1.37E – 02
Physiological system development and function		
Hematological system development and function	136	1.76E – 06 to 1.40E – 02
Immune cell trafficking	66	1.76E – 06 to 1.24E – 02
Tissue development	124	1.76E – 06 to 1.46E – 02
Organismal survival	154	3.81E – 06 to 3.81E – 06
Cardiovascular system development and function	110	3.90E – 06 to 1.32E – 02

relative abundance of Firmicutes was unchanged between the study group (72.8%) and the healthy individuals (73%).

When combining all data from Crohn's disease participants ($n = 8$) and making pre- and post-diet comparisons of each bacterial cluster, there is a forward trend, yet no significant improvement in the expression of the bacteria that were known to have an altered relative abundance in Crohn's disease (Figure 5). There was an increase in the expression of Bacteroidetes (17.89% to 18.74%), *Clostridium* cluster IV (19.2% to 21.86%) and *Clostridium* cluster XIVa (26.78% to 28.79%) and a decrease in the abundance of Proteobacteria (5.93% to 5.48%) and Bacillaceae (4.65% to 4.21%).

Discussion

As previously stated, inflammation can cause chronic disease; therefore, it is important to identify and reduce inflammation, one such way is through diet. We found that in this pilot study, there was a small reduction in the established biomarkers of inflammation after consuming our diet for 6 weeks. Using the transcriptomic approach, we did see significant changes in gene expression. In total, we found 3,551 genes that were differentially expressed in our study as a result of a 6-week dietary intervention. The most common candidates were not the genes that were affected, and although results for individual genes were not spectacular, it is the combination of affected genes that is interesting. The data highlighted the difference in sensitivity between the established biomarkers and the transcriptomic approach and confirmed that conducting a short-term trial with a small number of participants is feasible.

Table 3 Key canonical pathways affected by intervention

Name	*p* value	Ratio
EIF2 signalling	4.24E – 04	17/200 (0.085)
B cell development	9.31E – 04	6/33 (0.182)
T helper cell differentiation	3.55E – 03	8/72 (0.111)
Uracil degradation II (reductive)	7.6E – 03	2/11 (0.182)
Thymine degradation	7.6E – 03	2/11 (0.182)

The patients who volunteered for this study were selected based on strict criteria. Several of them already used diet as a way of controlling symptoms and so for transcriptomics to still show an effect highlights how sensitive this technique is. This increased sensitivity allows for short-term studies with fewer study numbers than traditional trials to be performed, which has significant implications for future human clinical trials.

The ratio of the six bacterial phyla or families from the faecal microbiome of healthy individuals has been determined. It is well documented that deviation from this 'norm' occurs in individuals who have Crohn's disease. Normalising the intestinal microbiota through diet is a step towards potentially reducing inflammation and thus restoring health and improving the quality of life for people with Crohn's disease.

After 6 weeks on our Mediterranean-inspired diet, there was some 'normalising' of the intestinal microbiota. As previously stated, the participants were already managing

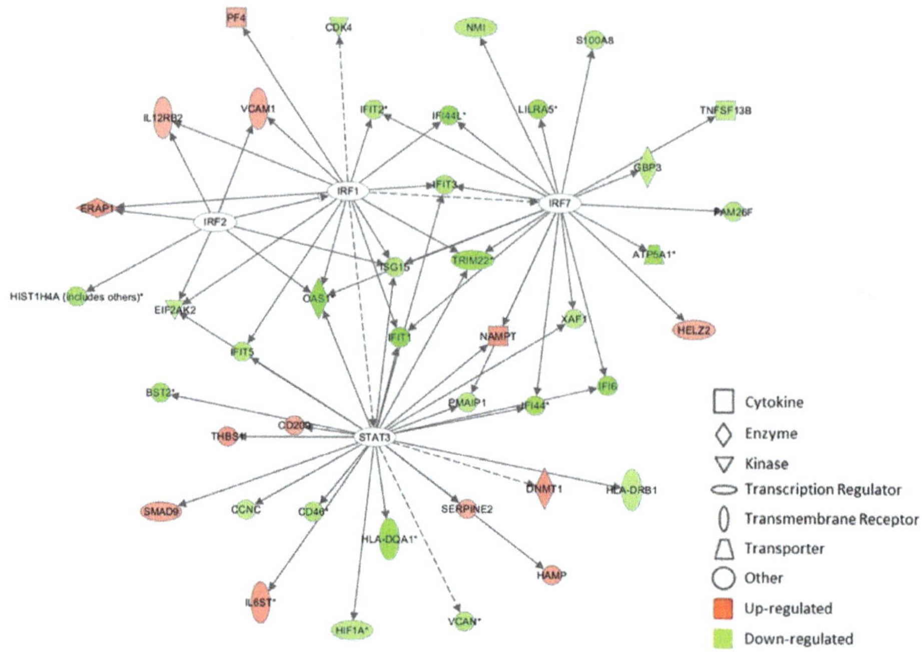

Figure 4 Generation of a biological network of genes related to the upstream regulator IRF2. Network was generated by IPA. Connections were applied based on known interactions within the Ingenuity Pathway Knowledge Base. *Solid lines* between genes represent direct interactions and the *dashed lines* indirect. Genes are represented by *nodes*, with the *red* and *green colours* indicating up- or down-regulated expression; the greater the colour intensity, the higher the level of differential expression.

their disease through diet, so the expression of the microbiota was not too dissimilar from that documented in a healthy group. However, as a group, the microbiota before the diet was tending towards that expected for people with Crohn's disease, notably a reduction in the presence of Bacteroidetes and an increase in the presence of Proteobacteria and Bacillaceae.

Consuming the Mediterranean-inspired anti-inflammatory diet for 6 weeks was able to influence the intestinal microbiota of our study population, although this improvement should be noted as a forward trend rather than any statistically significant change. There was an observed increase in Bacteroidetes and the *Clostridium* clusters and a decrease in Protebacteria and Bacillaceae.

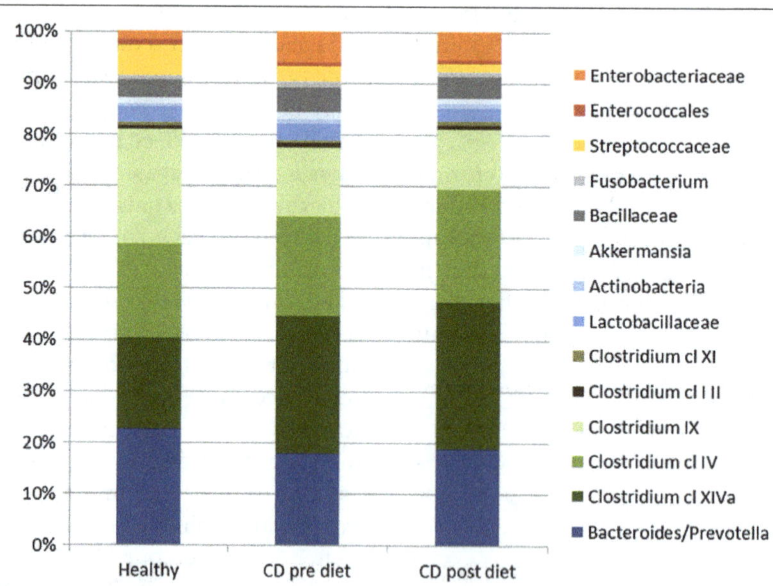

Figure 5 Relative abundance of microbiota pre- and post-dietary intervention. Healthy samples ($n = 2$), CD pre-diet ($n = 8$) and CD post-diet ($n = 8$).

Conclusions

One of the aims of this pilot study was to compare the data obtained from traditional biomarkers of inflammation with that of transcriptomics. The Affymetrix GeneChip® PrimeView™ arrays were selected as they provide complete coverage of the human genome. We were impressed by the increased sensitivity provided by the arrays over the biomarkers.

Peripheral blood mononuclear cells (PBMCs) can be easily obtained from a venepuncture, which allows for easy and repeated collection unlike biopsies of other tissues [38]. PBMCs have been used to examine gene expression in numerous diseases including inflammation [39-45] and have also been shown to act as a biomarker of nutritional interventions [22,46,47] and used to predict inflammatory response to functional foods [48]. The increased sensitivity of transcriptomics and the fact that PBMCs can be used as a model to study the expression of inflammatory genes [40] make this methodology attractive for non-hypothesis-based studies.

One of the drawbacks of this study was the small study population, which resulted in observing a trend in effect of the diet rather than significant results. However, one of the benefits of using transcriptomics is the ability to conduct dietary interventions over a shorter time frame and requiring fewer subject numbers. This subsequently reduce costs which will open up the area of health-based food claims to a wider market, meaning that more companies and more products could be tested. This could lead to a better understanding of the mechanism of action and thus substantiated health claims benefiting both the companies and the population.

The data from this pilot study, although not significant, does highlight that by choosing an anti-inflammatory diet, even for a short time, can have an effect on reducing inflammatory markers, changing gene expression and normalising the microbiota.

Methods

Study design

This study was granted ethical approval by the Northern Regional Ethics Committee of New Zealand (reference NTY/11/11/109). Requirements for inclusion in the study were very strict and were intentionally so given the aetiology of Crohn's disease and the potential bias from medication and surgical interventions. Selection criteria included the following: had no bowel surgery, was not taking prednisone or similar anti-inflammatory medication, had no changes to their medication over the last 3 months, indicating a stable condition, were willing to provide samples at the beginning and end of the study and were willing to change their diet. This was self-reported by the participants.

All participants consumed the Mediterranean-inspired anti-inflammatory diet for 6 weeks. They were provided with food items including salmon, organic avocados, kumara, a variety of vegetables, gluten-free bread, New Zealand extra virgin olive oil, green tea, honey and fish oil capsules. The majority of these foods were grown and produced in New Zealand and were used to supplement the participant's diet. A reduction in the consumption of red meat, white flour, high-fat foods and sugar was also expected. All participants provided a blood and faecal sample at the beginning and end of the study and completed food diaries.

Subject selection/eligibility

Eight participants, from Auckland, New Zealand, who had active yet stable Crohn's disease symptoms and passed the selection criteria (see above) were selected to participate following an initial invitation to all Crohn's disease participants in the Diet and Gene Database administered by Nutrigenomics New Zealand.

Our participants were six females and two males, aged between 31 and 60 years (mean age 45.4 years), and the length of time since diagnosis with Crohn's disease ranged from 7 to 36 years.

Study outcomes

Levels of C-reactive protein, a systemic measure of inflammation [31] and changes in DNA damage in peripheral blood lymphocyte cells by the micronucleus assay (in accordance with OECD guidelines 487) were scored before and after the diet, along with comparisons of RNA gene expression profiles.

C-reactive protein

A blood sample collected in serum-separating tubes was analysed for C-reactive protein. C-reactive protein is found in the blood in response to inflammation and is a biomarker for potential disease development. Specimens were analysed by a medical testing laboratory, Labtests Auckland, according to their protocols for the latex-enhanced immunoturbidimetric assay.

DNA damage—micronucleus assay

The cytokinesis-block micronucleus assay [32], a validated method for determining DNA damage in peripheral blood lymphocytes cells, was used to observe any changes in DNA damage before and after the diet intervention. DNA damage was determined by the presence of micronuclei (MN) in the cytoplasm of bi-nucleated lymphocyte cells. Whole blood treated with anticoagulant (heparin) was collected, stored at room temperature and cultured within 24 h. Duplicate cultures containing 0.6 ml whole blood and 9.25 ml alpha MEM and 15% foetal calf serum (Gibco New Zealand Ltd., Auckland, New Zealand) were prepared, to which 150 μl phytohaemaglutinin (PHA, Gibco New Zealand Ltd.) was added to stimulate lymphocyte replication. The cells were incubated in a humidified incubator containing 5% carbon dioxide for 44 h. Cytochalasin B (Sigma Chemical Co., St. Louis, MO, USA) was added to give a final concentration of 4.5 μg/ml, and the culture was incubated for an additional 26 h. The cytochalasin B would halt any further cell growth. Cells were harvested using standard protocols as outlined [49], including centrifugation, swelling of the cells using hypotonic KCl and fixing in a solution of methanol and acetic acid before dropping onto slides. Once dried, the slides were stained with Diff-Quik (Dade Behring Inc., Sacramento, CA, USA) according to staining protocols. Two thousand bi-nucleated cells were scored for micronuclei using the criteria outlined by Heddle et al. [50] and Fenech [51].

Transcriptomics

RNA isolation and storage

Whole blood was collected in a PAXgene Blood RNA Tube (PBRT) (PreAnalytiX) following the manufacturer's recommended protocol. The blood was incubated at room temperature for 2 h, after collection to improve RNA yield, before being stored at −70°C.

RNA extraction was performed according to the recommended protocol PAXgene Blood RNA System Kit (Qiagen). The quantity of RNA was determined using the NanoDrop ND-1000 Spectrophotometer (NanoDrop Technologies, Wilmington, DE, USA) and the quality of RNA by the Experion RNA StdSens Analysis Kit (Biorad, Hercules, CA, USA). For successful gene expression microarray hybridization, a concentration of >100 ng/μl of RNA and a RNA quality indicator (RQI) of >8 are required.

Gene expression arrays

Microarray hybridization was performed on GeneChip® PrimeView™ Human Gene Expression arrays (Affymetrix) following the manufacturer's protocol by The Ramaciotti Centre, University of New South Wales, Sydney, Australia, using the Affymetrix GeneChip® Instrument System.

Gene expression data analysis

Affymetrix Primeview array data was read using the 'affy' package in the statistical language R and normalised using the RMA method. QA of the data showed that it was of good quality and free of obvious artifacts or outliers. The 'limma' package was used to compare gene expression pre- and post-diet, paired by participant code.

Further analyses of the differentially expressed genes, including network, pathway and functional analysis, were carried out using IPA (Ingenuity Systems Inc., USA; http://www.ingenuity.com).

Microbiota analysis

A faecal sample was provided by each study participant before and after the diet. The samples were frozen at −80°C until required for analysis. Total DNA from the faecal matter was extracted according to the protocol published by Candela et al. [18] in combination with the DNAeasy Blood and Tissue Kit 50 (Qiagen). The final DNA concentration and purity were determined using the NanoDrop ND-1000 Spectrophotometer (NanoDrop Technologies). The extracted DNA was standardised to 50 ng/μl and stored at −20°C. These samples were then sent to the Department of Pharmaceutical Science, University of Bologna, Italy for analysis. The amplification and purification of DNA and the subsequent HTF-Microbi.Array were conducted according to protocols defined by Candela et al. [18]. Briefly, amplification of the DNA by PCR was achieved using 16 s rDNA sequencing, facilitated by Taq polymerase (Promega, Madison, WI, USA) and the universal forward primer f27 (5′-AGAGTTTGATCMTGGCTCAG-3′) and reverse primer 1492r (5′-TACGGYTACCTTGTTACGACTT-3′). The resultant PCR product was purified using the PCR Clean-up System Kit (Promega) and concentration of the purified DNA determined by nanodrop.

Specific detection and quantification of 32 phylogenetically related groups of the human intestinal microbiome were achieved by the HTF-Microbi.Array, an adaption to the Ligase Detection Reaction [18]. DNA probes specific for each of the currently identified bacteria of the intestinal microbiome are embedded on the array slide. Successful hybridisation of the DNA product to the probe results in fluorescence. The fluorescence intensities (IF) were normalised to the ligation control signal and background IF values, removing outlier signals that were 2.5-fold above or below the average of the repeated signals (four repeats of each probe on every array). The results were compared to two healthy control samples which were obtained at the start of the study.

Abbreviations

CRP: C-reactive protein; IBD: Inflammatory bowel disease; IPA: Ingenuity pathway analysis; IRF2: Interferon regulatory factor 2; JAK: Janus kinase; KCl: Potassium chloride; MEM: Minimum essential media; MN: Micronuclei; NF-κB: Nuclear factor kappa-light-chain-enhancer of activated B cells; PBMCs: Peripheral blood mononuclear cells; PBRT: PAXgene Blood RNA Tube; RMA: Reliabilty, maintainability and availability; RQI: RNA quality indicator; STAT3: Signal transducer and activator of transcription 3.

Competing interests

The authors declare that they have no competing interests.

Authors' contributions

GM and ACJ carried out the gene expression studies. SE carried out the microbiota analysis. SZ, NK and IRF carried out the biomarker work. DYH participated in the design of the study and performed the statistical analysis. GM and SE participated in study design and drafted the manuscript. LRF and AGF conceived of the study and participated in its design and coordination and helped draft the manuscript. All authors read and approved the final manuscript.

Acknowledgements

We would like to thank all the volunteers who took part in this study and the companies who generously supplied food for the study, New Zealand King Salmon, Venerdi, Red Seal Natural Health, Plant & Food Research, Cereal Partners Worldwide: Nestle & General Mills, Fonterra, New Zealand Avocado, Matiatia Grove, Vegetables.co.nz and The New Zealand Merino Company. Nutrigenomics New Zealand is a collaboration between The University of Auckland and AgResearch Limited and Plant & Food Research and is funded by the Ministry of Business, Innovation and Employment. The microbota work was supported by REINFORCE and was conducted in Professor Patrizia Brigidi's laboratory at the University of Bologna, Italy.

Author details

[1]Discipline of Nutrition, Faculty of Medical and Health Sciences, The University of Auckland Private Bag 92019, Auckland 1142, New Zealand. [2]Nutrigenomics New Zealand, University of Auckland, Private Bag 92019, Auckland 1142, New Zealand. [3]Faculty of Medical and Health Sciences, The University of Auckland, 85 Park Road, Grafton, Auckland 1023, New Zealand. [4]Department of Medicine, University of Auckland, Private Bag 92019, Auckland 1142, New Zealand.

References

1. Ferguson LR: **Potential value of nutrigenomics in Crohn's disease.** *Nat Rev Gastroenterol Hepatol* 2012, **9**(5):260–270.
2. Calder PC: **Fatty acids and inflammation: the cutting edge between food and pharma.** *Eur J Pharmacol* 2011, **668**(Suppl 1):S50–58.
3. Corfield AP, Wallace HM, Probert CS: **The molecular biology of inflammatory bowel diseases.** *Biochem Soc Trans* 2011, **39**(4):1057–1060.
4. Serhan CN: **The resolution of inflammation: the devil in the flask and in the details.** *FASEB J* 2011, **25**(5):1441–1448.
5. Bakker GC, van Erk MJ, Pellis L, Wopereis S, Rubingh CM, Cnubben NH, Kooistra T, van Ommen B, Hendriks HF: **An antiinflammatory dietary mix modulates inflammation and oxidative and metabolic stress in overweight men: a nutrigenomics approach.** *Am J Clin Nutr* 2010, **91**(4):1044–1059.
6. Bannenberg G, Serhan CN: **Specialized pro-resolving lipid mediators in the inflammatory response: an update.** *Biochim Biophys Acta* 2010, **1801**(12):1260 1273.
7. Gentschew L, Ferguson LR: **Role of nutrition and microbiota in susceptibility to inflammatory bowel diseases.** *Mol Nutr Food Res* 2012, **56**(4):524–535.
8. Amre DK, D'Souza S, Morgan K, Seidman G, Lambrette P, Grimard G, Israel D, Mack D, Ghadirian P, Deslandres C, Chotard V, Budai B, Law L, Levy E, Seidman EG: **Imbalances in dietary consumption of fatty acids, vegetables, and fruits are associated with risk for Crohn's disease in children.** *Am J Gastroenterol* 2007, **102**(9):2016–2025.
9. D'Souza S, Levy E, Mack D, Israel D, Lambrette P, Ghadirian P, Deslandres C, Morgan K, Seidman EG, Amre DK: **Dietary patterns and risk for Crohn's disease in children.** *Inflamm Bowel Dis* 2008, **14**(3):367–373.
10. Issa M, Saeian K: **Diet in inflammatory bowel disease.** *Nutr Clin Pract* 2011, **26**(2):151–154.
11. Brown K, DeCoffe D, Molcan E, Gibson DL: **Diet-induced dysbiosis of the intestinal microbiota and the effects on immunity and disease.** *Nutrients* 2012, **4**(8):1095–1119.
12. Frank DN, St Amand AL, Feldman RA, Boedeker EC, Harpaz N, Pace NR: **Molecular-phylogenetic characterization of microbial community imbalances in human inflammatory bowel diseases.** *Proc Natl Acad Sci U S A* 2007, **104**(34):13780–13785.
13. Greenblum S, Turnbaugh PJ, Borenstein E: **Metagenomic systems biology of the human gut microbiome reveals topological shifts associated with obesity and inflammatory bowel disease.** *Proc Natl Acad Sci U S A* 2012, **109**(2):594–599.
14. Albenberg LG, Lewis JD, Wu GD: **Food and the gut microbiota in inflammatory bowel diseases: a critical connection.** *Curr Opin Gastroenterol* 2012, **28**(4):314–320.
15. Candela M, Rampelli S, Turroni S, Severgnini M, Consolandi C, De Bellis G, Masetti R, Ricci G, Pession A, Brigidi P: **Unbalance of intestinal microbiota in atopic children.** *BMC Microbiol* 2012, **12:**95.
16. Hattori M, Taylor TD: **The human intestinal microbiome: a new frontier of human biology.** *DNA Res* 2009, **16**(1):1–12.
17. Candela M, Biagi E, Maccaferri S, Turroni S, Brigidi P: **Intestinal microbiota is a plastic factor responding to environmental changes.** *Trends Microbiol* 2012, **20**(8):385–391.
18. Candela M, Consolandi C, Severgnini M, Biagi E, Castiglioni B, Vitali B, De Bellis G, Brigidi P: **High taxonomic level fingerprint of the human intestinal microbiota by Ligase Detection Reaction - Universal Array approach.** *BMC Microbiol* 2010, **10:**116.
19. Manichanh C, Rigottier-Gois L, Bonnaud E, Gloux K, Pelletier E, Frangeul L, Nalin R, Jarrin C, Chardon P, Marteau P, Roca J, Dore J: **Reduced diversity of faecal microbiota in Crohn's disease revealed by a metagenomic approach.** *Gut* 2006, **55**(2):205–211.
20. Sokol H, Lay C, Seksik P, Tannock GW: **Analysis of bacterial bowel communities of IBD patients: what has it revealed?** *Inflamm Bowel Dis* 2008, **14**(6):858–867.
21. Rajilic-Stojanovic M, Heilig HG, Molenaar D, Kajander K, Surakka A, Smidt H, de Vos WM: **Development and application of the human intestinal tract chip, a phylogenetic microarray: analysis of universally conserved phylotypes in the abundant microbiota of young and elderly adults.** *Environ Microbiol* 2009, **11**(7):1736–1751.
22. Bouwens M, van de Rest O, Dellschaft N, Bromhaar MG, de Groot LC, Geleijnse JM, Muller M, Afman LA: **Fish-oil supplementation induces antiinflammatory gene expression profiles in human blood mononuclear cells.** *Am J Clin Nutr* 2009, **90**(2):415–424.
23. Esposito K, Di Palo C, Maiorino MI, Petrizzo M, Bellastella G, Siniscalchi I, Giugliano D: **Long-term effect of mediterranean-style diet and calorie restriction on biomarkers of longevity and oxidative stress in overweight men.** *Cardiol Res Pract* 2011, **2011:**293916.
24. Esposito K, Kastorini CM, Panagiotakos DB, Giugliano D: **Mediterranean diet and weight loss: meta-analysis of randomized controlled trials.** *Metab Syndr Relat Disord* 2011, **9**(1):1–12.
25. Kastorini CM, Milionis HJ, Esposito K, Giugliano D, Goudevenos JA, Panagiotakos DB: **The effect of Mediterranean diet on metabolic syndrome and its components: a meta-analysis of 50 studies and 534,906 individuals.** *J Am Coll Cardiol* 2011, **57**(11):1299–1313.
26. Sola R, Fito M, Estruch R, Salas-Salvado J, Corella D, de La Torre R, Munoz MA, Lopez-Sabater Mdel C, Martinez-Gonzalez MA, Aros F, Ruiz-Gutierrez V, Fiol M, Casals E, Wärnberg J, Buil-Cosiales P, Ros E, Konstantinidou V, Lapetra J, Serra-Majem L, Covas MI: **Effect of a traditional Mediterranean diet on apolipoproteins B, A-I, and their ratio: a randomized, controlled trial.** *Atherosclerosis* 2011, **218**(1):174–180.
27. Nanau R, Neuman M: **Nutritional and probiotic supplementation in colitis models.** *Dig Dis Sci* 2012, **57**(11):2786–2810.
28. Triggs CM, Munday K, Hu R, Fraser AG, Gearry RB, Barclay ML, Ferguson LR: **Dietary factors in chronic inflammation: food tolerances and intolerances of a New Zealand Caucasian Crohn's disease population.** *Mutat Res* 2010, **690**(1–2):123–138.
29. Ellett S, Ferguson IR, Zhu S, Karunasinghe N, Marlow G, Hurley D, Lam WJ, Han DY, Ferguson LR: *Foodomics to study efficacy of human dietary interventions: proof of principle study. In Nutrigenomics and Nutrigenetics in Functional Foods and Personalized Nutrition. Edited by Ferguson LR.* Boca Raton, FL: CRC Press; 2013.
30. Bisoendial RJ, Boekholdt SM, Vergeer M, Stroes ES, Kastelein JJ: **C-reactive protein is a mediator of cardiovascular disease.** *Eur Heart J* 2010, **31**(17):2087–2091.
31. Karadag F, Kirdar S, Karul AB, Ceylan E: **The value of C-reactive protein as a marker of systemic inflammation in stable chronic obstructive pulmonary disease.** *Eur J Intern Med* 2008, **19**(2):104–108.
32. Thomas P, Fenech M: **Cytokinesis-block micronucleus cytome assay in lymphocytes.** *Methods Mol Biol* 2011, **682:**217–234.
33. de Graaf AA, Freidig AP, De Roos B, Jamshidi N, Heinemann M, Rullmann JA, Hall KD, Adiels M, van Ommen B: **Nutritional systems biology modeling: from molecular mechanisms to physiology.** *PLoS Comput Biol* 2009, **5**(11):e1000554.
34. Puiggros F, Sola R, Blade C, Salvado MJ, Arola L: **Nutritional biomarkers and foodomic methodologies for qualitative and quantitative analysis of bioactive ingredients in dietary intervention studies.** *J Chromatogr A* 2011, **1218**(42):7399–7414.

35. Chae M, Kim K, Park S-M, Jang I-S, Seo T, Kim D-M, Kim I-C, Lee J-H, Park J: **IRF-2 regulates NF-κB activity by modulating the subcellular localization of NF-κB.** *Biochem Biophys Res Commun* 2008, **370**(3):519–524.
36. Sugimoto K: **Role of STAT3 in inflammatory bowel disease.** *World J Gastroenterol* 2008, **14**(33):5110–5114.
37. Li Y, de Haar C, Peppelenbosch MP, van der Woude CJ: **New insights into the role of STAT3 in IBD.** *Inflamm Bowel Dis* 2012, **18**(6):1177–1183.
38. de Mello VD, Kolehmanien M, Schwab U, Pulkkinen L, Uusitupa M: **Gene expression of peripheral blood mononuclear cells as a tool in dietary intervention studies: what do we know so far?** *Mol Nutr Food Res* 2012, **56**(7):1160–1172.
39. Rudkowska I, Ponton A, Jacques H, Lavigne C, Holub BJ, Marette A, Vohl MC: **Effects of a supplementation of n-3 polyunsaturated fatty acids with or without fish gelatin on gene expression in peripheral blood mononuclear cells in obese, insulin-resistant subjects.** *J Nutrigenet Nutrigenomics* 2011, **4**(4):192–202.
40. Rudkowska I, Raymond C, Ponton A, Jacques H, Lavigne C, Holub BJ, Marette A, Vohl MC: **Validation of the use of peripheral blood mononuclear cells as surrogate model for skeletal muscle tissue in nutrigenomic studies.** *OMICS* 2011, **15**(1–2):1–7.
41. Bomprezzi R, Ringner M, Kim S, Bittner ML, Khan J, Chen Y, Elkahloun A, Yu A, Bielekova B, Meltzer PS, Martin R, McFarland HF, Trent JM: **Gene expression profile in multiple sclerosis patients and healthy controls: identifying pathways relevant to disease.** *Hum Mol Genet* 2003, **12**(17):2191–2199.
42. Connolly PH, Caiozzo VJ, Zaldivar F, Nemet D, Larson J, Hung SP, Heck JD, Hatfield GW, Cooper DM: **Effects of exercise on gene expression in human peripheral blood mononuclear cells.** *J Appl Physiol* 2004, **97**(4):1461–1469.
43. Dabek J, Kulach A, Wilczok T, Mazurek U, Jakubowski D, Gasior Z: **Transcriptional activity of genes encoding interferon gamma (IFNgamma) and its receptor assessed in peripheral blood mononuclear cells in patients with cardiac syndrome X.** *Inflammation* 2007, **30**(3–4):125–129.
44. Rokutan K, Morita K, Masuda K, Tominaga K, Shikishima M, Teshima-Kondo S, Omori T, Sekiyama A: **Gene expression profiling in peripheral blood leukocytes as a new approach for assessment of human stress response.** *J Med Invest* 2005, **52**(3–4):137–144.
45. van de Vijver MJ, He YD, van't Veer LJ, Dai H, Hart AA, Voskuil DW, Schreiber GJ, Peterse JL, Roberts C, Marton MJ, Parrish M, Atsma D, Witteveen A, Glas A, Delahaye L, van der Velde T, Bartelink H, Rodenhuis S, Rutgers ET, Friend SH, Bernards R: **A gene-expression signature as a predictor of survival in breast cancer.** *N Engl J Med* 2002, **347**(25):1999–2009.
46. Di Paolo S, Schena A, Stallone G, Grandaliano G, Soccio M, Cerullo G, Gesualdo L, Paolo Schena F: **Captopril enhances transforming growth factor (TGF)-beta1 expression in peripheral blood mononuclear cells: a mechanism independent from angiotensin converting enzyme inhibition? A study in cyclosporine-treated kidney-transplanted patients.** *Transplantation* 2002, **74**(12):1710–1715.
47. Fuchs D, Piller R, Linseisen J, Daniel H, Wenzel U: **The human peripheral blood mononuclear cell proteome responds to a dietary flaxseed-intervention and proteins identified suggest a protective effect in atherosclerosis.** *Proteomics* 2007, **7**(18):3278–3288.
48. Theuwissen E, Plat J, Mensink RP: **Consumption of oat beta-glucan with or without plant stanols did not influence inflammatory markers in hypercholesterolemic subjects.** *Mol Nutr Food Res* 2009, **53**(3):370–376.
49. Shelby MD: **A report on guidelines for mutagenicity testing. "Report of the UKEMS Sub-Committee on Guidelines for Mutagenicity Testing. Part 1: Basic Test Battery; Minimal Criteria; Professional Standards; Interpretation; Selection of Supplementary Assays," Brian J. Dean (ed). London: UKEMS, 1983.** *Environ Mutagen* 1983, **5**(6):941–943.
50. Heddle JA, Lue CB, Saunders EF, Benz RD: **Sensitivity to five mutagens in Fanconi's anemia as measured by the micronucleus method.** *Cancer Res* 1978, **38**(9):2983–2988.
51. Fenech M: **The cytokinesis-block micronucleus technique: a detailed description of the method and its application to genotoxicity studies in human populations.** *Mutat Res* 1993, **285**(1):35–44.

24

Improved drug therapy: triangulating phenomics with genomics and metabolomics

Andrew A Monte[1,2,3*], Chad Brocker[4], Daniel W Nebert[5,6], Frank J Gonzalez[4], David C Thompson[2] and Vasilis Vasiliou[2]

Abstract

Embracing the complexity of biological systems has a greater likelihood to improve prediction of clinical drug response. Here we discuss limitations of a singular focus on genomics, epigenomics, proteomics, transcriptomics, metabolomics, or phenomics—highlighting the strengths and weaknesses of each individual technique. In contrast, 'systems biology' is proposed to allow clinicians and scientists to extract benefits from each technique, while limiting associated weaknesses by supplementing with other techniques when appropriate. Perfect predictive modeling is not possible, whereas modeling of intertwined phenomic responses using genomic stratification with metabolomic modifications may greatly improve predictive values for drug therapy. We thus propose a novel-integrated approach to personalized medicine that begins with phenomic data, is stratified by genomics, and ultimately refined by metabolomic pathway data. Whereas perfect prediction of efficacy and safety of drug therapy is not possible, improvements can be achieved by embracing the complexity of the biological system. Starting with phenomics, the combination of linking metabolomics to identify common biologic pathways and then stratifying by genomic architecture, might increase predictive values. This systems biology approach has the potential, in specific subsets of patients, to avoid drug therapy that will be either ineffective or unsafe.

Keywords: Individualized medicine, Genomics, Metabolomics, Omics, Personalized medicine, Phenomics, Systems biology, Transcriptomics

Introduction

Recent advances in genomics, epigenomics, transcriptomics, proteomics, metabolomics, and phenomics have allowed identification of certain factors associated with variable drug responses. However, with few exceptions, high-fidelity prediction of drug efficacy and safety on a larger scale has proven elusive. We have experienced many failures with pharmacogenetic attempts to predict success of drug therapy; this is due to insufficient knowledge and oversimplification of experimental approaches, as well as failure to accept that even the simplest traits almost always reflect an intersection of multiple genetic, epigenetic, and environmental factors. Therefore, we make an argument for embracing complexity. Starting with a clinically relevant trait—the individual patient drug response, which we refer to as 'phenotype'—and then working backward to integrate biological data, is more likely to identify common pathways and inter-individual variability between patient responses. We propose that this integrated-systems biology approach, focused on drug response and adverse drug reactions (ADRs), might be the best way to improve drug efficacy and safety.

* Correspondence: andrew.monte@ucdenver.edu
[1]University of Colorado Department of Emergency Medicine, Leprino Building, 7th Floor Campus Box B-215, 12401 E. 17th Avenue, Aurora, CO 80045, USA
[2]Skaggs School of Pharmacy and Pharmaceutical Sciences, Aurora, CO 80045, USA
Full list of author information is available at the end of the article

Limitations of single biological associations

'Personalized medicine' has endured many failures. Clinical phenotype of complex diseases (defined as any biological, physiological, morphological, or behavioral trait) is difficult to predict because most common diseases represent multifactorial traits.

Use of pharmacogenomics in predicting drug efficacy or toxicity is more advanced in oncology than perhaps in any other area of medicine. A high degree of efficacy and toxicity can be predicted for chemotherapeutic agents in cancer, based partially upon patient and tumor genotyping. For example, 5-fluorouracil toxicity is associated with dihydropyrimidine dehydrogenase polymorphisms [1,2], erlotinib [3] or cetuximab [4] responsiveness is linked to epidermal growth factor receptor polymorphisms, and there are other examples [5]. However, because tumor cells mutate or the patient develops associated co-morbidities (e.g. renal failure, pulmonary hypertension), then efficacy and toxicity remain difficult to predict. Focusing on a single biological association can sometimes efficiently predict drug response within a subset of a large cohort of patients, but rarely, if ever, can we expect to predict drug response in the individual patient [6].

Genotype-phenotype associations

Virtually, all clinical traits are polygenic, raising the number of potential phenotypes factorially; even the simplest genetic predictors lead to a range of phenotypes. This was demonstrated in 1960 when the earliest pharmacogenomic association of polyneuropathy with slow acetylation of isoniazid by *N*-acetyltransferase-2 (NAT2) was reported [7]. Not all individuals with the slow-acetylator trait develop neuropathy, and there remains a range of serum drug concentrations within each group of *NAT2* genotypes. Currently, at least 190 different *NAT2* alleles have been identified, and these polymorphisms result in a large range from "no effect", to slow, to very efficient acetylation [8]. In addition, *NAT2* performs AcCoA-dependent *O*-acetylation of *N*-hydroxyarylamines and AcCoA-independent *N,O*-acetylation of *N*-hydroxy-*N*-acetylarylamines, which suggests a pleiotropic effect of this polymorphism, likely contributing to variable penetrance of the phenotype [9]. Prediction of the expressed phenotype is more complex than initially appreciated, due to the wide range of downstream modifications and environmental factors that can function to alter expression of the underlying genetic code—leading to the ultimate biological response.

If prediction of success is defined as 'high positive and high negative predictive value of the test,' then all single biological associations have failed miserably. Strong biological associations can be made in small homogenous cohorts; in larger, more diverse populations, however, these associations are inevitably poor predictors of phenotype.

The literature is replete with examples of small cohort or observational studies, later shown in larger prospective trials to be poorly predictive; *CYP2C9* and vitamin K oxidoreductase complex subunit-1 (*VKORC1*) polymorphism-guided warfarin anticoagulation is foremost among such examples. Several early studies demonstrated benefit to *CYPC9* and *VKORC1* genotyping for prediction of 'time in the therapeutic window' and 'dose' of warfarin [9–12]. These correlations did not hold up in larger randomized controlled trials [13–15].

Genome-wide association studies

Genome-wide association (GWA) studies have demonstrated a strong association between *HLA-B*1502* and carbamazepine-associated Stevens-Johnson Syndrome and toxic epidermal necrolysis in Asian [16], but not in European populations [17]. The epigenomic drug vorinostat, a histone deacetylatase inhibitor, was initially found to profoundly decrease lymphoid proliferation in human cell lines [18], but demonstrated only a 30% response rate in a small cohort, prior to US FDA approval for cutaneous T-cell lymphoma [19]. Initial studies had suggested that transcriptomic screening for rejection following cardiac transplantation might be more sensitive than endomyocardial biopsy [20]. In a larger prospective trial, fewer biopsies were necessary in transcriptome-tested patients, although this did not eliminate the need for biopsy and only 6 of 34 rejection episodes were identified by the gene profiling test [21].

Testing for such single biological associations is therefore clinically impractical, due to such poor predictive values. Single biological associations should not be viewed as predictive; failure should be expected because of the extraordinarily large number of steps required to yield a phenotype after drug ingestion [5,6,22,23]. Specifically, the amount of drug absorbed may vary due to intestinal metabolism or disease, unpredictable hepatic blood flow can change the rate that enzymes metabolize the drug, polymorphisms in transporters and metabolic enzymes can lead to variable amounts of drug delivered to the systemic circulation, the drug must be transported to the site-of-action, and the site-of-action itself may be altered by polymorphisms en route to the observed clinical response, and the rate of elimination may be variable due to altered renal clearance [5]. This is further complicated in multifactorial traits, which increase potential phenotypic variability.

Starting with phenomics

Phenomics, defined as the unbiased study of a large number of expressed traits across a population, is the logical starting point for biological association studies. Traditional biological experiments, such as GWA studies, begin with the investigator selecting a phenotype and then attempting to associate biological differences within a population. Significant resources have been devoted to characterize the individual patient's whole genome, epigenome, transcriptome, proteome, metabolome, as well as gut microbiome. This approach has been robust; GWA studies have identified more than 4,000 polymorphisms linked to more than 500 clinical traits [24]. Unfortunately, it remains possible that identified single-nucleotide variants (SNVs) are not the causative factor but rather are associated with some additional metabolic factor that is polygenic. This effect-modification phenomenon has been recognized for decades in epidemiologic studies [25].

Ultimately, the unequivocal phenotype is what patients and clinicians wish to predict. Therefore, studies should shift focus away from these single biological associations that are only statistically associated with a phenotype when studying a large cohort, to an approach that characterizes the biologic system starting with phenotypic variables. Initiating analysis from a wide number of characterized traits [termed phenome-wide association (PheWA) studies] allows the investigator to see the intertwined biological processes leading all the way back to genetic associations.

Phenomics captures pleiotropic associations (genes associated with several traits) that are often overlooked [26]. Examples include *HLA8.1* association with both myasthenia gravis and thymus hyperplasia [27] (and likely other autoimmune diseases), as well as lipid-gene associations with plasma glucose and insulin resistance [28]. Whereas two traits may both be associated with the same SNV, this association does not provide unequivocal information about the relationship between the traits.

Some traits may be the direct result of SNVs while others are secondarily associated, thereby confounding the relationship. The aldehyde dehydrogenase-2 (ALDH2) Glu504Lys polymorphism is a classic example of this phenomenon; this amino-acid change is associated with a disulfiram-like reaction in Asians [29], one of the strongest genotype-phenotype associations. This polymorphism can also be associated with alcohol intolerance, but this is not the causal phenotype of the *ALDH2* polymorphism. Instead, a decrease in ALDH2-dependent metabolism is the associated phenotype, and decreased tolerance is likely due to the unpleasant disulfiram-like reaction rather than an inability to develop alcohol tolerance [30]. The clinically-relevant phenotype of alcohol intolerance may be modified by co-linearity with other metabolism enzyme gene polymorphisms such as *CYP2E1* [31,32], with genotypic factors dictating body mass index [33], and/or with addictive behaviors [34].

Examination of a wide range of phenotypes can identify which pathways are causal, and which are secondary effects. Specialized analysis techniques for PheWA studies must be utilized because phenomic data structure varies significantly, comprising binary as well as continuous variables when compared with other large datasets such as GWA studies [35,36]. At present, we are not aware of any phenomics studies that have been applied to drug therapy, although we predict this will happen soon. Detailed electronic medical record (EMR) data will allow for large-scale phenomic studies, when paired with GWA studies or other biological databases [37].

Phenomics demands a systems biology approach. Phenotypes must be associated with biological pathways, which in turn reflect genomic architecture. For example, a systems biology approach, starting with the trait 'sepsis survival', has identified new metabolic pathways characterizing survival [38]. This breakthrough gives us a more comprehensive understanding of the metabolite markers of survival as well as numerous genetic contributors, thereby permitting identification of biomarkers and potential therapeutic targets. Lack of a full understanding of all involved biological pathways can lead to false prioritization of phenotypes. For example, for years, the 'cataplexy' phenotype in rodents was targeted for the development of neuropsychiatric drugs. Unfortunately, this narrow focus appears to have led to the development of more drugs that produce extrapyramidal symptoms than provide antipsychotic efficacy [39].

Adding metabolomics to your arsenal

Metabolomics is the study of small molecules in biologic fluids or tissues. This methodology has been used to discover metabolites that act as diagnostic tools for a growing number of medical conditions. For example, metabolite profiles from human tissue, urine and plasma accurately predicted differentiated benign prostate hypertrophy from clinically-localized prostate cancer and metastatic disease [40]. In this case, complex and overlapping clinical phenotypes are tightly correlated with specific changes in metabolite homeostasis, which could then be further segregated into precise, distinguishable disease states. A similar scenario has been seen for metabolomic studies of ovarian cancer progression [41]. Moreover, urinary and serum biomarkers may also serve as a non-invasive and rapid means of identifying and monitoring phenotype-metabotype relationships during the onset and progression of disease [42,43]. Performed in an unbiased manner, addition of metabolomics to systems biology has provided insight into gene networks, resultant metabolic changes, and genotype-phenotype relationships [44]. These studies highlight the need for unbiased metabolomics to link phenomic data with genomic data.

Metabolomics: linking genomics with phenomics

Small molecules identified by metabolomics represent the substrates, intermediates, and products of all biochemical pathways. Consequently, this technique represents an integrated snapshot-in-time of all upstream biologic processes, ultimately leading to a clinical phenotype. Therefore, the metabolome may be the closest biological representation of a clinical trait. Indeed, metabolomics has identified possible biomarkers for cardiac [45], kidney [46], liver [47], and gastrointestinal [48] diseases, as well as many other pathophysiological conditions.

Metabolomics profiling is incredibly sensitive and can detect femtomolar to attomolar changes in metabolite concentrations [49]. Anything from small dietary changes, increased physical activity, elevated stress, or even seasonal variables can significantly alter the composition of metabolomic profiles. This profound sensitivity has obvious advantages: small metabolomic changes can account for complex physiological changes. However, because of increased sensitivity, specificity may be sacrificed, thus decreasing the predictive value of the test.

In some cases, large metabolic changes are able to maintain stability of a clinical trait; these findings can identify potential areas of metabolic decompensation. For instance, elevated lactate is a marker of impaired gluconeogenesis, as are increased concentrations of other gluconeogenic substrates, such as pyruvate and alanine, which are preferentially metabolized to lactate [50,51]. Mildly elevated levels of these metabolites are not clinically significant, but instead represent compensated buffer activity. If further stress is placed on the system, lactic acid itself can overwhelm the buffered system and lead to decompensated metabolic acidosis with high mortality [52]. Metabolic changes, such as lactic acidosis, can be the result of numerous upstream responses; post-exposure monitoring may predict severe disease processes and ADRs prior to phenotypic manifestation.

Therefore, the metabolome may be viewed as an overly sensitive tool with insight into adaptive physiology [53]. This sensitivity can serve to identify a wider range of genomic polymorphisms that contribute to expressed phenotypes, even if only under specific circumstances. Unbiased metabolomics has identified novel pathways in hypertension that include microbiome associations and sex steroid mediators previously not appreciated to contribute to the hypertensive phenotype [54]. Metabolomics identified the mechanism of anti-retroviral drug interaction mediated by the CYP3A4 enzyme through newly recognized enzymatic functions [55]. These mechanisms have implications for choosing drug therapy in HIV patients. The presence of five amino acids was correlated with the development of diabetes as well as an insulin-resistant phenotype in a cohort of initially normoglycemic patients followed for 12 years [56]. Similar findings identified new pathways in insulin resistance identified by the oral glucose tolerance test [57]. Metabolomics was able to predict poor response to insulin; thus, metabolomics has potential to predicting development of disease and therapeutic success [58]. Metabolomics can be a powerful tool to elucidate complex mechanisms of drug-modified clinical traits [59].

Genomic architecture

Despite the claim that pharmacogenetics has 'at best, a marginal benefit' [60], genetics represents a constant in any biological system on which we can build models and stratify expected phenotypes. As noted above, limitations of GWA studies must be recognized, but stratification of clinical traits can be accomplished with a systems biology approach. Pharmacogenetics may allow stratification of starting doses for drugs and identification of patients who are unlikely to respond at the recommended prescribed dose or who are at risk for serious ADRs.

Elucidation of such 'extreme discordant phenotypes' (EDPs) [61] is useful to physicians because EDP methodology can lead to decreased healthcare expense and lower patient morbidity. Seventy-four percent of all physician office visits involve drug therapy. In 2008, prescriptions accounted for $234.1 billion in patient costs [62]. Forty-eight percent of people in the USA take at least one prescription; more than 76% of people 60 years and older take two or more [62–64]. Despite the remarkable number of prescribed drugs, many of these medications are ineffective. For instance, hypertension is the most common chronic disease in the USA, yet 64% of patients receiving antihypertensive therapy fail to achieve blood pressure control [65]. Another factor beyond the scope of this review is the issue of 'non-compliance': the patient failing to adhere to his prescribed drug regimen. Non-compliance can easily be misinterpreted by the investigator as drug failure, thereby leading to increased 'noise' in any study of genotype-phenotype associations [6]. This confounder can be addressed by metabolomic screening to confirm drug ingestion [66].

If patients can be stratified with an EDP approach and clinical phenotypes modeled using sensitive metabolomics, it may be possible to reduce the number of office visits for ineffective therapy or ADRs. However, virtually, all clinical traits are multifactorial, with each haplotype contributing only a small fraction (0.1%–0.0001%) to the ultimate phenotype. For example, in a GWA study of almost 184,000 subjects, 180 loci associated with 'height' as the trait were identified; however, these loci together contributed only approximately 10% to variation in the phenotype [67]. This underscores the need to account for downstream modifying factors, and to assess the individual as a sum of his phenotypic parts.

Another major problem in all genotype-phenotype association studies is that our present-day methods can capture only additive genetic variance, which probably accounts for 70%–80% of heritability for any multifactorial trait. The remaining 20%–30% represents non-additive genetic variance. At this time, we have no methodology for finding this 'missing heritability' [*cf.* [68,69] for further details].

Triangulating phenomics with genomics and metabolomics

Combining metabolomic and GWA databases has resulted in identification of new biological pathways in cardiovascular, kidney disorders, type-2 diabetes, cancer, gout, venous thromboembolism, and Crohn's disease [70]. Phenomics has not yet been overlaid upon these analyses. Thus, important pleiotropic clinical traits with common biological pathways remain to be discovered.

By viewing each phenotype as a node within a systems biology model, linked by metabolic pathways and dictated by genetic architecture, we can more fully understand the relationship between biological processes that result in variable clinical traits. Proof of this concept has been demonstrated in the KORA F4 cohort that identified several SNVs associated with type-2 diabetes by way of metabolomics association studies [71]. Preliminary metabolomic studies have also proved useful in helping to differentiate phenotypically heterogeneous disorders, such as Parkinson's disease (PD). PD can present as either slowly or rapidly progressive forms, which can be distinguished early by comparing metabolite profiles. Identified metabolites might subsequently be used to shed light on the underlying metabolic abnormalities and pathway perturbations driving phenotypic variation [72]. Only by embracing the complexity of the biological system can we improve predictive accuracy.

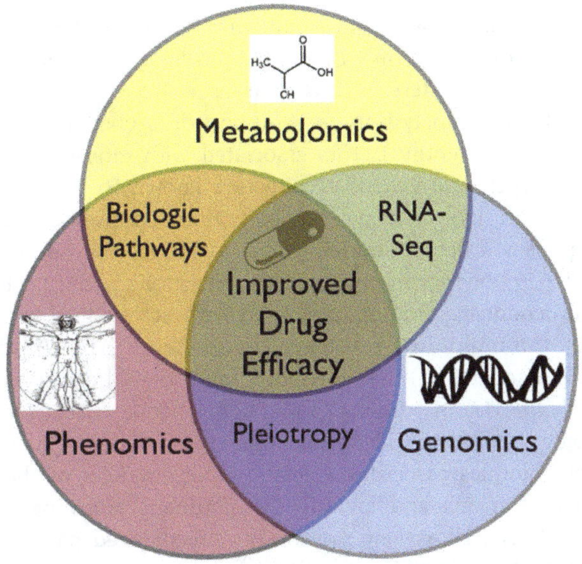

Figure 1 Illustration of an integrated systems biology approach to improve drug therapy. Using phenomics to fully characterize clinical traits associated with drug therapy. When combined with metabolomics, common biological pathways can be identified, providing insight into mechanisms of efficacy and safety. When phenomic data associated with genomics data are also combined, pleiotropic associations can be further identified and contribute to our understanding of underlying biological pathways. Other techniques, such as RNA-seq, can be integrated to add depth to the pathway data and supplement our understanding of genomic expression.

Combining transcriptomics and metabolomics

Other methodologies will undoubtedly need to be integrated. For instance, transcriptome analysis using RNA sequencing (RNA-seq) can be used to quantitatively identify global changes in gene expression in tissues and serum. Integration of transcriptomics and metabolomics data allows accurate identification of genes and enzymatic pathways driving downstream alterations in metabolite distribution, production, and degradation. These data can provide profound insight into a given phenotype by positioning biochemical compounds within metabolic pathways as substrates, intermediates or products. In addition, compensatory mechanisms can be identified during pathway analysis and help explain the absence of an expected phenotype. Integration of transcriptomics-metabolomics data provides a means to track how metabolic pathways change, in response to disease and/or therapy, and then directly tie those alterations with phenotypic outcomes.

Multilayer systems biology is still an emerging field, but initial studies using combined transcriptomics and metabolomics data look promising with regard to identifying phenotype-genotype-metabotype relationships (Figure 1), including those observed during pancreatic cancer progression, melanoma response to chemotherapy, as well as others [73–77].

Technically, the biggest bottleneck confronting the utilization of extremely large combined datasets is the difficulty in analysis and processing bioinformatics. In other words, there can be drawbacks to adding too much data. We will likely experience an 'hourglass effect' as we integrate more variables into predictive models. Initially, more data may improve such a model. As too many factors become integrated into the model, overfitting becomes problematic and the model becomes inherently unstable, sacrificing predictive accuracy. This phenomenon has been well documented in climate modeling. This argues for simplification of the model variables at points distant from the phenotypic outcome, as well as elimination of factors that contribute only marginally. New software systems, such as GenAMAP have been developed specifically for this purpose. GenAMAP allows for integration of genomics, transcriptomics, and phenomics data accounting for differences in dataset structure when one uses multivariate structured association-mapping algorithms [78].

A clinical example

Ideally, the approach starts with phenomics, then is stratified by genetic associations, and finally, further refined with metabolomic associations. This will require following thousands of patients with full characterization of biological samples and clinical outcomes for every commonly prescribed drug. For example, if we consider hydrocodone efficacy and safety phenotypes, we can build a model based on genetics/genomics and metabolomics factors. Consider patients given 10 mg of hydrocodone with careful characterization of phenotypic clinical responses and ADRs (Figure 2). Adding RNA-seq transcriptomic data from serum may allow determination of human opioid *mu*-1 receptor expression (*OPRM1*), which would differentiate chronic users from naïve users. Metabolomic analysis in pre- and post-drug-challenged patients may identify factors associated with efficacy, ADR phenotypes, and genetic architecture known to be associated with hydrocodone variability in response. Clinical responses can be stratified by genetic factors such as *CYP2D6* polymorphisms, principle metabolic pathways for hydrocodone activation associated with active drug levels [79], the multi-drug resistance transporter-1 (*MDR1*; official name *ABCB1*) that transports many opioid drugs [80], and *OPRM1*, in which 118A/A homozygous patients exhibit a correlation with hydrocodone pain relief [81]. Again, metabolomics associations may provide markers of these polymorphisms and identify the pertinent pathways involved, as well as new previously unrecognized pathways that might serve to identify additional associations.

Ultimately, this stratification of data can be distilled into an integrated model using programs that raise the receiver operator characteristic (ROC) curve for determining rate of efficacy and risk of ADRs. Some clinical factors may contribute to the ultimate drug-response phenotype, to varying degrees between patients. For instance, stomach acidity may affect drug dissolution; this complex trait (among other factors) can be influenced by inter-individual gene expression, concomitant drug therapy, and even the time of the day. Consequently, it should be obvious that specific factors may contribute significantly to the ultimate phenotype in some patients, provide only a minor contribution in others, and only contribute under certain circumstances (e.g. suppression of stomach acid with a proton pump inhibitor), in a third group. Because many of these complex relationships are present in each drug-patient interaction, a perfect predictive model will never be possible.

Conclusions

Whereas perfect prediction of efficacy and safety of drug therapy is not possible, improvements can be achieved by embracing the complexity of the biological system. Starting with phenomics, linking metabolomics to identify common biologic pathways, and stratifying by genomic architecture—this combination can increase predictive values. We believe that this systems biology approach has the potential to eliminate drug therapy that will either be ineffective or unsafe, in specific subsets of patients.

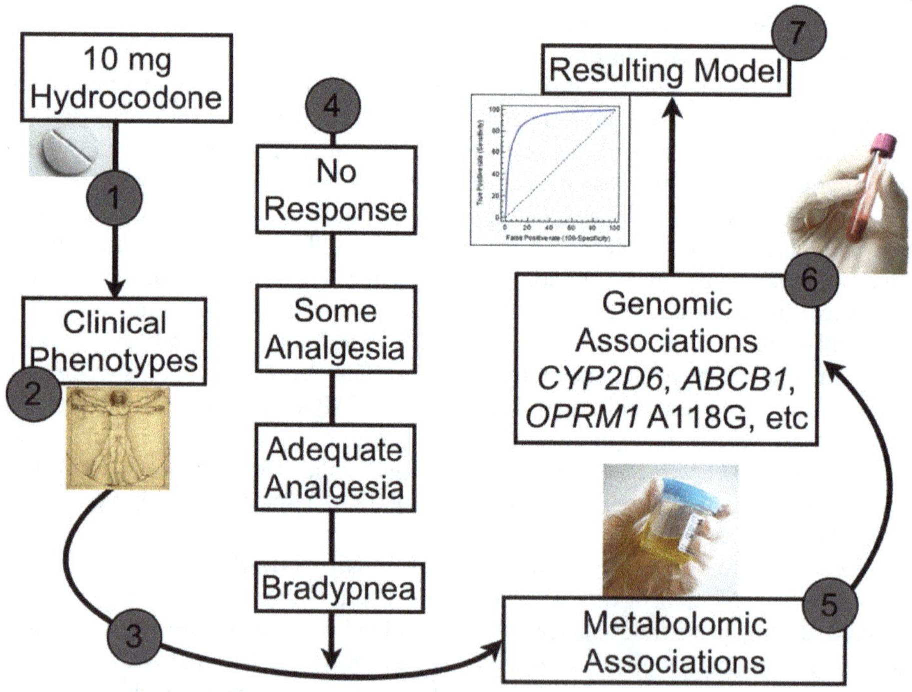

Figure 2 A clinical example of the proposed integrated method for predicting drug response. (1) Patients are given 10 mg of hydrocodone. (2) Clinical phenotypes are captured fully and completely. These may include (among others) development of ADRs, chronicity of treatment, ethnic differences, and demographic factors. (3) Association studies may contribute to characterization of the clinical phenotypes (e.g. RNA-sequencing may help distinguish chronicity of treatment). (4) The drug response is categorized into phenotypically pertinent groups. (5) Relevant biological pathways are identified and linked by individual metabolomic markers. (6) Stratification of drug response is refined by accounting for biological pathway polymorphisms and controlled for phenotypic variables captured in #2 above. (7) The final stepwise model is built, allowing for a high, although not perfect, receiver operating characteristic (ROC).

Competing interests

The authors declare that they have no competing interests.

Authors' contributions

All authors contributed knowledge and expertise in the writing of this review. All authors read and approved the final manuscript.

Acknowledgements

This work was supported in part by the National Institutes of Health Grants K23 GM110516 (A.A.M), P30 ES06096 (D.W.N.), R24 AA022057 and R01 EY14390 (V.V). Dr. Monte is supported by the Emergency Medicine Foundation Research Training Grant.

Author details

[1]University of Colorado Department of Emergency Medicine, Leprino Building, 7th Floor Campus Box B-215, 12401 E. 17th Avenue, Aurora, CO 80045, USA. [2]Skaggs School of Pharmacy and Pharmaceutical Sciences, Aurora, CO 80045, USA. [3]Rocky Mountain Poison & Drug Center, Denver, CO 80204, USA. [4]Laboratory of Metabolism, Center for Cancer Research, National Institute of Cancer, Bethesda, MD 20892, USA. [5]Division of Human Genetics, Department of Pediatrics and Molecular Developmental Biology, University of Cincinnati Medical Center, Cincinnati, OH 45220, USA. [6]Department of Environmental Health and Center for Environmental Genetics, University of Cincinnati Medical Center, Cincinnati, OH 45220, USA.

References

1. Ciaparrone M, Quirino M, Schinzari G, Zannoni G, Corsi DC, Vecchio FM, Cassano A, La Torre G, Barone C: **Predictive role of thymidylate synthase, dihydropyrimidine dehydrogenase and thymidine phosphorylase expression in colorectal cancer patients receiving adjuvant 5-fluorouracil.** *Oncology* 2006, **70:**366–377.
2. Lee A, Ezzeldin H, Fourie J, Diasio R: **Dihydropyrimidine dehydrogenase deficiency: impact of pharmacogenetics on 5-fluorouracil therapy.** *Clin Adv Hematol Oncol* 2004, **2:**527–532.
3. Gaughan EM, Costa DB: **Genotype-driven therapies for non-small cell lung cancer: focus on EGFR, KRAS and ALK gene abnormalities.** *Ther Adv Med Oncol* 2011, **3:**113–125.
4. Cappuzzo F, Finocchiaro G, Rossi E, Janne PA, Carnaghi C, Calandri C, Bencardino K, Ligorio C, Ciardiello F, Pressiani T, Destro A, Roncalli M, Crino L, Franklin WA, Santoro A, Varella-Garcia M: **EGFR FISH assay predicts for response to cetuximab in chemotherapy refractory colorectal cancer patients.** *Ann Oncol* 2008, **19:**717–723.
5. Monte AA, Heard KJ, Vasiliou V: **Prediction of drug response and safety in clinical practice.** *J Med Toxicol* 2012, **8:**43–51.
6. Nebert DW, Zhang G, Vesell ES: **From human genetics and genomics to pharmacogenetics and pharmacogenomics: past lessons, future directions.** *Drug Metab Rev* 2008, **40:**187–224.
7. Evans DA, Manley KA, Mc KV: **Genetic control of isoniazid metabolism in man.** *Br Med J* 1960, **2:**485–491.
8. McDonagh EM, Boukouvala S, Aklillu E, Hein DW, Altman RB, Klein TE: **PharmGKB summary: very important pharmacogene information for N-acetyltransferase 2.** *Pharmacogenet Genomics* 2014, **24:**409–425.
9. Anderson JL, Horne BD, Stevens SM, Grove AS, Barton S, Nicholas ZP, Kahn SF, May HT, Samuelson KM, Muhlestein JB, Carlquist JF: **Randomized trial of genotype-guided versus standard warfarin dosing in patients initiating oral anticoagulation.** *Circulation* 2007, **116:**2563–2570.
10. Burmester JK, Berg RL, Yale SH, Rottscheit CM, Glurich IE, Schmelzer JR, Caldwell MD: **A randomized controlled trial of genotype-based Coumadin initiation.** *Genet Med* 2011, **13:**509–518.
11. Caraco Y, Blotnick S, Muszkat M: **CYP2C9 genotype-guided warfarin prescribing enhances the efficacy and safety of anticoagulation: a prospective randomized controlled study.** *Clin Pharmacol Ther* 2008, **83:**460–470.
12. Wang M, Lang X, Cui S, Fei K, Zou L, Cao J, Wang L, Zhang S, Wu X, Wang Y, Ji Q: **Clinical application of pharmacogenetic-based warfarin-dosing algorithm in patients of Han nationality after rheumatic valve replacement: a randomized and controlled trial.** *Int J Med Sci* 2012, **9:**472–479.
13. Kimmel SE, French B, Kasner SE, Johnson JA, Anderson JL, Gage BF, Rosenberg YD, Eby CS, Madigan RA, McBane RB, Abdel-Rahman SZ, Stevens SM, Yale S, Mohler ER 3rd, Fang MC, Shah V, Horenstein RB, Limdi NA, Muldowney JA 3rd, Gujral J, Delafontaine P, Desnick RJ, Ortel TL, Billett HH, Pendleton RC, Geller NL, Halperin JL, Goldhaber SZ, Caldwell MD, Califf RM, *et al*: **A pharmacogenetic versus a clinical algorithm for warfarin dosing.** *N Engl J Med* 2013, **369:**2283–2293.
14. Pirmohamed M, Burnside G, Eriksson N, Jorgensen AL, Toh CH, Nicholson T, Kesteven P, Christersson C, Wahlstrom B, Stafberg C, Zhang JE, Leathart JB, Kohnke H, Maitland-van der Zee AH, Williamson PR, Daly AK, Avery P, Kamali F, Wadelius M: **A randomized trial of genotype-guided dosing of warfarin.** *N Engl J Med* 2013, **369:**2294–2303.
15. Verhoef TI, Ragia G, de Boer A, Barallon R, Kolovou G, Kolovou V, Konstantinides S, Le Cessie S, Maltezos E, van der Meer FJ, Redekop WK, Remkes M, Rosendaal FR, van Schie RM, Tavridou A, Tziakas D, Wadelius M, Manolopoulos VG, Maitland-van der Zee AH: **A randomized trial of genotype-guided dosing of acenocoumarol and phenprocoumon.** *N Engl J Med* 2013, **369:**2304–2312.
16. Chung WH, Hung SI, Hong HS, Hsih MS, Yang LC, Ho HC, Wu JY, Chen YT: **Medical genetics: a marker for Stevens-Johnson syndrome.** *Nature* 2004, **428:**486.
17. McCormack M, Alfirevic A, Bourgeois S, Farrell JJ, Kasperaviciute D, Carrington M, Sills GJ, Marson T, Jia X, de Bakker PI, Chinthapalli K, Molokhia M, Johnson MR, O'Connor GD, Chaila E, Alhusaini S, Shianna KV, Radtke RA, Heinzen EL, Walley N, Pandolfo M, Pichler W, Park BK, Depondt C, Sisodiya SM, Goldstein DB, Deloukas P, Delanty N, Cavalleri GL, Pirmohamed M: **HLA-A*3101 and carbamazepine-induced hypersensitivity reactions in Europeans.** *N Engl J Med* 2011, **364:**1134–1143.
18. Sakajiri S, Kumagai T, Kawamata N, Saitoh T, Said JW, Koeffler HP: **Histone deacetylase inhibitors profoundly decrease proliferation of human lymphoid cancer cell lines.** *Exp Hematol* 2005, **33:**53–61.
19. Mann BS, Johnson JR, He K, Sridhara R, Abraham S, Booth BP, Verbois L, Morse DE, Jee JM, Pope S, Harapanhalli RS, Dagher R, Farrell A, Justice R, Pazdur R: **Vorinostat for treatment of cutaneous manifestations of advanced primary cutaneous T-cell lymphoma.** *Clin Cancer Res* 2007, **13:**2318–2322.
20. Horwitz PA, Tsai EJ, Putt ME, Gilmore JM, Lepore JJ, Parmacek MS, Kao AC, Desai SS, Goldberg LR, Brozena SC, Jessup ML, Epstein JA, Cappola TP: **Detection of cardiac allograft rejection and response to immunosuppressive therapy with peripheral blood gene expression.** *Circulation* 2004, **110:**3815–3821.
21. Pham MX, Teuteberg JJ, Kfoury AG, Starling RC, Deng MC, Cappola TP, Kao A, Anderson AS, Cotts WG, Ewald GA, Baran DA, Bogaev RC, Elashoff B, Baron H, Yee J, Valantine HA: **Gene-expression profiling for rejection surveillance after cardiac transplantation.** *N Engl J Med* 2010, **362:**1890–1900.
22. Monte AA, Vasiliou V, Heard KJ: **Omics screening for pharmaceutical efficacy and safety in clinical practice.** *J Pharmacogenomics Pharmacoproteomics* 2012, **S5.**
23. Nebert DW, Jorge-Nebert L, Vesell ES: **Pharmacogenomics and "individualized drug therapy": high expectations and disappointing achievements.** *Am J Pharmacogenomics* 2003, **3:**361–370.
24. **A catalog of published genome wide association studies.** [http://www.genome.gov/page.cfm?pageid=26525384&clearquery=1#result_table]
25. Davis CE: **The effect of regression to the mean in epidemiologic and clinical studies.** *Am J Epidemiol* 1976, **104:**493–498.
26. Wagner GP, Kenney-Hunt JP, Pavlicev M, Peck JR, Waxman D, Cheverud JM: **Pleiotropic scaling of gene effects and the 'cost of complexity'.** *Nature* 2008, **452:**470–472.
27. Vandiedonck C, Beaurain G, Giraud M, Hue-Beauvais C, Eymard B, Tranchant C, Gajdos P, Dausset J, Garchon HJ: **Pleiotropic effects of the 8.1 HLA haplotype in patients with autoimmune myasthenia gravis and thymus hyperplasia.** *Proc Natl Acad Sci U S A* 2004, **101:**15464–15469.
28. Li N, van der Sijde MR, Study LC, Bakker SJ, Dullaart RP, van der Harst P, Gansevoort RT, Elbers CC, Wijmenga C, Snieder H, Hofker MH, Fu J: **Pleiotropic effects of lipid genes on plasma glucose, HbA1c and HOMA-IR levels.** *Diabetes* 2014. Epub ahead of print.
29. >Jones GL, Teng YS: **A chemical and enzymological account of the multiple forms of human liver aldehyde dehydrogenase. Implications for ethnic differences in alcohol metabolism.** *Biochim Biophys Acta* 1983, **745:**162–174.
30. Newlin DB: **The skin-flushing response: autonomic, self-report, and conditioned responses to repeated administrations of alcohol in Asian men.** *J Abnorm Psychol* 1989, **98:**421–425.

31. Howard LA, Ahluwalia JS, Lin SK, Sellers EM, Tyndale RF: **CYP2E1*1D regulatory polymorphism: association with alcohol and nicotine dependence.** *Pharmacogenetics* 2003, **13**:321–328.
32. Tang K, Li X, Xing Q, Li W, Feng G, He L, Qin S: **Genetic polymorphism analysis of cytochrome P4502E1 (CYP2E1) in Chinese Han populations from four different geographic areas of Mainland China.** *Genomics* 2010, **95**:224–229.
33. Brondani LA, Assmann TS, de Souza BM, Boucas AP, Canani LH, Crispim D: **Meta-analysis reveals the association of common variants in the uncoupling protein (UCP) 1-3 genes with body mass index variability.** *PLoS One* 2014, **9**:e96411.
34. Ehlers CL, Gizer IR: **Evidence for a genetic component for substance dependence in Native Americans.** *Am J Psychiatry* 2013, **170**:154–164.
35. Carroll RJ, Bastarache L, Denny JC: **R PheWAS: data analysis and plotting tools for phenome-wide association studies in the R environment.** *Bioinformatics* 2014, **30**:2375–2376.
36. Neuraz A, Chouchana L, Malamut G, Le Beller C, Roche D, Beaune P, Degoulet P, Burgun A, Loriot MA, Avillach P: **Phenome-wide association studies on a quantitative trait: application to TPMT enzyme activity and thiopurine therapy in pharmacogenomics.** *PLoS Comput Biol* 2013, **9**:e1003405.
37. Denny JC, Bastarache L, Ritchie MD, Carroll RJ, Zink R, Mosley JD, Field JR, Pulley JM, Ramirez AH, Bowton E, Basford MA, Carrell DS, Peissig PL, Kho AN, Pacheco JA, Rasmussen LV, Crosslin DR, Crane PK, Pathak J, Bielinski SJ, Pendergrass SA, Xu H, Hindorff LA, Li R, Manolio TA, Chute CG, Chisholm RL, Larson EB, Jarvik GP, Brilliant MH, *et al*: **Systematic comparison of phenome-wide association study of electronic medical record data and genome-wide association study data.** *Nat Biotechnol* 2013, **31**:1102–1110.
38. Langley RJ, Tsalik EL, van Velkinburgh JC, Glickman SW, Rice BJ, Wang C, Chen B, Carin L, Suarez A, Mohney RP, Freeman DH, Wang M, You J, Wulff J, Thompson JW, Moseley MA, Reisinger S, Edmonds BT, Grinnell B, Nelson DR, Dinwiddie DL, Miller NA, Saunders CJ, Soden SS, Rogers AJ, Gazourian L, Fredenburgh LE, Massaro AF, Baron RM, Choi AM, *et al*: **An integrated clinico-metabolomic model improves prediction of death in sepsis.** *Sci Transl Med* 2013, **5**:95–113.
39. Bilder RM, Sabb FW, Cannon TD, London ED, Jentsch JD, Parker DS, Poldrack RA, Evans C, Freimer NB: **Phenomics: the systematic study of phenotypes on a genome-wide scale.** *Neuroscience* 2009, **164**:30–42.
40. Sreekumar A, Poisson LM, Rajendiran TM, Khan AP, Cao Q, Yu J, Laxman B, Mehra R, Lonigro RJ, Li Y, Nyati MK, Ahsan A, Kalyana-Sundaram S, Han B, Cao X, Byun J, Omenn GS, Ghosh D, Pennathur S, Alexander DC, Berger A, Shuster JR, Wei JT, Varambally S, Beecher C, Chinnaiyan AM: **Metabolomic profiles delineate potential role for sarcosine in prostate cancer progression.** *Nature* 2009, **457**:910–914.
41. Denkert C, Budczies J, Kind T, Weichert W, Tablack P, Sehouli J, Niesporek S, Konsgen D, Dietel M, Fiehn O: **Mass spectrometry-based metabolic profiling reveals different metabolite patterns in invasive ovarian carcinomas and ovarian borderline tumors.** *Cancer Res* 2006, **66**:10795–10804.
42. Manna SK, Tanaka N, Krausz KW, Haznadar M, Xue X, Matsubara T, Bowman ED, Fearon ER, Harris CC, Shah YM, Gonzalez FJ: **Biomarkers of coordinate metabolic reprogramming in colorectal tumors in mice and humans.** *Gastroenterology* 2014, **146**:1313–1324.
43. Mathe EA, Patterson AD, Haznadar M, Manna SK, Krausz KW, Bowman ED, Shields PG, Idle JR, Smith PB, Anami K, Kazandjian DG, Hatzakis E, Gonzalez FJ, Harris CC: **Noninvasive urinary metabolomic profiling identifies diagnostic and prognostic markers in lung cancer.** *Cancer Res* 2014, **74**:3259–3270.
44. Widmann P, Reverter A, Fortes MR, Weikard R, Suhre K, Hammon H, Albrecht E, Kuehn C: **A systems biology approach using metabolomic data reveals genes and pathways interacting to modulate divergent growth in cattle.** *BMC Genomics* 2013, **14**:798.
45. Rhee EP, Gerszten RE: **Metabolomics and cardiovascular biomarker discovery.** *Clin Chem* 2012, **58**:139–147.
46. Weiss RH, Kim K: **Metabolomics in the study of kidney diseases.** *Nat Rev Nephrol* 2012, **8**:22–33.
47. Chen S, Kong H, Lu X, Li Y, Yin P, Zeng Z, Xu G: **Pseudotargeted metabolomics method and its application in serum biomarker discovery for hepatocellular carcinoma based on ultra high-performance liquid chromatography/triple quadrupole mass spectrometry.** *Anal Chem* 2013, **85**:8326–8333.
48. Kim JH, Yamaori S, Tanabe T, Johnson CH, Krausz KW, Kato S, Gonzalez FJ: **Implication of intestinal VDR deficiency in inflammatory bowel disease.** *Biochim Biophys Acta* 1830, **2013**:2118–2128.
49. Veenstra TD: **Metabolomics: the final frontier?** *Genome Med* 2012, **4**:40.
50. Bailey CJ, Turner RC: **Metformin.** *N Engl J Med* 1996, **334**:574–579.
51. Sirtori CR, Pasik C: **Re-evaluation of a biguanide, metformin: mechanism of action and tolerability.** *Pharmacol Res* 1994, **30**:187–228.
52. Seidowsky A, Nseir S, Houdret N, Fourrier F: **Metformin-associated lactic acidosis: a prognostic and therapeutic study.** *Crit Care Med* 2009, **37**:2191–2196.
53. Johnson CH, Gonzalez FJ: **Challenges and opportunities of metabolomics.** *J Cell Physiol* 2012, **227**:2975–2981.
54. Zheng Y, Yu B, Alexander D, Mosley TH, Heiss G, Nettleton JA, Boerwinkle E: **Metabolomics and incident hypertension among blacks: the atherosclerosis risk in communities study.** *Hypertension* 2013, **62**:398–403.
55. Li F, Wang L, Guo GL, Ma X: **Metabolism-mediated drug interactions associated with ritonavir-boosted tipranavir in mice.** *Drug Metab Dispos* 2010, **38**:871–878.
56. Wang TJ, Larson MG, Vasan RS, Cheng S, Rhee EP, McCabe E, Lewis GD, Fox CS, Jacques PF, Fernandez C, O'Donnell CJ, Carr SA, Mootha VK, Florez JC, Souza A, Melander O, Clish CB, Gerszten RE: **Metabolite profiles and the risk of developing diabetes.** *Nat Med* 2011, **17**:448–453.
57. Ho JE, Larson MG, Vasan RS, Ghorbani A, Cheng S, Rhee EP, Florez JC, Clish CB, Gerszten RE, Wang TJ: **Metabolite profiles during oral glucose challenge.** *Diabetes* 2013, **62**:2689–2698.
58. Bain JR, Muehlbauer MJ: **Metabolomics reveals unexpected responses to oral glucose.** *Diabetes* 2013, **62**:2651–2653.
59. Johnson CH, Patterson AD, Idle JR, Gonzalez FJ: **Xenobiotic metabolomics: major impact on the metabolome.** *Annu Rev Pharmacol Toxicol* 2012, **52**:37–56.
60. Furie B: **Do pharmacogenetics have a role in the dosing of vitamin K antagonists?** *N Engl J Med* 2013, **369**:2345–2346.
61. Nebert DW: **Extreme discordant phenotype methodology: an intuitive approach to clinical pharmacogenetics.** *Eur J Pharmacol* 2000, **410**:107–120.
62. Gu Q, Dillon CF, Burt VL: **Prescription drug use continues to increase: U.S. prescription drug data for 2007-2008.** *NCHS Data Brief* 2010:1-8.
63. Kaufman DW, Kelly JP, Rosenberg L, Anderson TE, Mitchell AA: **Recent patterns of medication use in the ambulatory adult population of the United States: the Slone survey.** *JAMA* 2002, **287**:337–344.
64. Tinetti ME, Bogardus ST Jr, Agostini JV: **Potential pitfalls of disease-specific guidelines for patients with multiple conditions.** *N Engl J Med* 2004, **351**:2870–2874.
65. Cutler JA, Sorlie PD, Wolz M, Thom T, Fields LE, Roccella EJ: **Trends in hypertension prevalence, awareness, treatment, and control rates in United States adults between 1988-1994 and 1999-2004.** *Hypertension* 2008, **52**:818–827.
66. Monte AA, Heard KJ, Hoppe JA, Vasiliou V, Gonzalez FJ: **The accuracy of self-reported drug ingestion histories in emergency department patients.** *J Clin Pharmacol* 2014. Epub ahead of print.
67. Lango Allen H, Estrada K, Lettre G, Berndt SI, Weedon MN, Rivadeneira F, Willer CJ, Jackson AU, Vedantam S, Raychaudhuri S, Ferreira T, Wood AR, Weyant RJ, Segre AV, Speliotes EK, Wheeler E, Soranzo N, Park JH, Yang J, Gudbjartsson D, Heard-Costa NL, Randall JC, Qi L, Vernon Smith A, Magi R, Pastinen T, Liang L, Heid IM, Luan J, Thorleifsson G, *et al*: **Hundreds of variants clustered in genomic loci and biological pathways affect human height.** *Nature* 2010, **467**:832–838.
68. Lander ES: **Initial impact of the sequencing of the human genome.** *Nature* 2011, **470**:187–197.
69. Nebert DW, Zhang G, Vesell ES: **Genetic risk prediction: individualized variability in susceptibility to toxicants.** *Annu Rev Pharmacol Toxicol* 2013, **53**:355–375.
70. Suhre K, Shin SY, Petersen AK, Mohney RP, Meredith D, Wagele B, Altmaier E, Deloukas P, Erdmann J, Grundberg E, Hammond CJ, de Angelis MH, Kastenmuller G, Kottgen A, Kronenberg F, Mangino M, Meisinger C, Meitinger T, Mewes HW, Milburn MV, Prehn C, Raffler J, Ried JS, Romisch-Margl W, Samani NJ, Small KS, Wichmann HE, Zhai G, Illig T, Spector TD, *et al*: **Human metabolic individuality in biomedical and pharmaceutical research.** *Nature* 2011, **477**:54–60.
71. Illig T, Gieger C, Zhai G, Romisch-Margl W, Wang-Sattler R, Prehn C, Altmaier E, Kastenmuller G, Kato BS, Mewes HW, Meitinger T, de Angelis MH, Kronenberg F, Soranzo N, Wichmann HE, Spector TD, Adamski J, Suhre K:

A genome-wide perspective of genetic variation in human metabolism. *Nat Genet* 2010, **42:**137–141.

72. Roede JR, Uppal K, Park Y, Lee K, Tran V, Walker D, Strobel FH, Rhodes SL, Ritz B, Jones DP: **Serum metabolomics of slow vs. rapid motor progression Parkinson's disease: a pilot study.** *PLoS One* 2013, **8:**e77629.
73. Jun HJ, Lee JH, Kim J, Jia Y, Kim KH, Hwang KY, Yun EJ, Do KR, Lee SJ: **Linalool is a PPARalpha ligand that reduces plasma TG levels and rewires the hepatic transcriptome and plasma metabolome.** *J Lipid Res* 2014, **55:**1098–1110.
74. Morvan D, Demidem A: **Metabolomics and transcriptomics demonstrate severe oxidative stress in both localized chemotherapy-treated and bystander tumors.** *Biochim Biophys Acta* 1840, **2014:**1092–1104.
75. Mukherjee K, Edgett BA, Burrows HW, Castro C, Griffin JL, Schwertani AG, Gurd BJ, Funk CD: **Whole blood transcriptomics and urinary metabolomics to define adaptive biochemical pathways of high-intensity exercise in 50-60 year old masters athletes.** *PLoS One* 2014, **9:**e92031.
76. Zhang G, He P, Tan H, Budhu A, Gaedcke J, Ghadimi BM, Ried T, Yfantis HG, Lee DH, Maitra A, Hanna N, Alexander HR, Hussain SP: **Integration of metabolomics and transcriptomics revealed a fatty acid network exerting growth inhibitory effects in human pancreatic cancer.** *Clin Cancer Res* 2013, **19:**4983–4993.
77. Zhang Y, Deng Y, Zhao Y, Ren H: **Using combined bio-omics methods to evaluate the complicated toxic effects of mixed chemical wastewater and its treated effluent.** *J Hazard Mater* 2014, **272:**52–58.
78. Xing EP, Curtis RE, Schoenherr G, Lee S, Yin J, Puniyani K, Wu W, Kinnaird P: **GWAS in a box: statistical and visual analytics of structured associations via GenAMap.** *PLoS One* 2014, **9:**e97524.
79. Jannetto PJ, Bratanow NC: **Utilization of pharmacogenomics and therapeutic drug monitoring for opioid pain management.** *Pharmacogenomics* 2009, **10:**1157–1167.
80. Lotsch J, Skarke C, Liefhold J, Geisslinger G: **Genetic predictors of the clinical response to opioid analgesics: clinical utility and future perspectives.** *Clin Pharmacokinet* 2004, **43:**983–1013.
81. Boswell MV, Stauble ME, Loyd GE, Langman L, Ramey-Hartung B, Baumgartner RN, Tucker WW, Jortani SA: **The role of hydromorphone and OPRM1 in postoperative pain relief with hydrocodone.** *Pain Physician* 2013, **16:**E227–E235.

25

Strong interaction between T allele of endothelial nitric oxide synthase with B1 allele of cholesteryl ester transfer protein TaqIB highly elevates the risk of coronary artery disease and type 2 diabetes mellitus

Zohreh Rahimi[1,2*], Reza Nourozi-Rad[3], Ziba Rahimi[1] and Abbas Parsian[4]

Abstract

Background: The present study was conducted to investigate the possible outcome of interaction between endothelial nitric oxide (NOS3) G894T and cholesteryl ester transfer TaqIB variants on the risk of coronary artery disease (CAD) and type 2 diabetes mellitus (T2DM). The sample included a total of 207 CAD patients (102 CAD patients with T2DM and 105 CAD patients without T2DM). There were also 101 patients with T2DM and 92 age- and sex-matched healthy individuals as controls. All study participants were from Western Iran. The sample was genotyped by polymerase chain reaction-restriction fragment length polymorphism.

Results: The presence of NOS3 T allele was not associated with the risk of CAD or T2DM, and the CETP B1 allele was only significantly associated with the increased risk of CAD in total CAD patients (odds ratio (OR) = 5.1, $p = 0.019$). However, the concomitant presence of both CETP B1 and NOS3 T alleles significantly increased the risk of CAD in total CAD patients (OR = 18.1, $p < 0.001$), in CAD patients without T2DM (OR = 27.1, $p = 0.03$), and in CAD patients with T2DM (OR = 13.5, $p = 0.002$). Also, the presence of both alleles increased the risk of T2DM (OR = 12, $p = 0.004$).

Conclusions: Our findings, for the first time, indicate that NOS3 T allele strongly interacts with CETP B1 allele to augment the risk of CAD and T2DM in the population of Western Iran.

Keywords: NOS3 G894T, CETP TaqIB, CAD, T2DM, Western Iran

Introduction

Cholesteryl ester transfer protein (CETP) participates in reverse cholesterol transport by transfering cholesteryl esters from high-density lipoprotein-cholesterol (HDL-C) to apolipoprotein-B containing particles in exchange for triglycerides (TG), thereby reducing the concentration of HDL-C [1-3].

CETP gene located on chromosome 16q21 consists of 16 exons and 15 introns and has several genetic polymorphisms affecting CETP activity among which TaqIB polymorphism has been most widely studied. This polymorphism results from G to A base pair change at nucleotide 277 in intron 1 of the CETP gene which disrupts TaqI restriction site (single-nucleotide polymorphism (SNP) rs708272). The allele containing the TaqI endonuclease site is called B1, while the allele without the restriction site is called B2. The less common B2 allele has been associated with increased HDL-C levels and decreased CETP activity and levels [4,5]. The association of CETP variants with coronary artery disease (CAD) and type 2 diabetes mellitus (T2DM) has been

* Correspondence: zrahimi@kums.ac.ir
[1]Medical Biology Research Center, Medical School, Kermanshah University of Medical Sciences, Daneshgah Avenue, P.O. Box 67148-69914, Kermanshah, Iran
[2]Department of Biochemistry, Medical School, Kermanshah University of Medical Sciences, Daneshgah Avenue, P.O. Box 67148-69914, Kermanshah, Iran
Full list of author information is available at the end of the article

investigated in several studies without consistent results [1,6-9].

Nitric oxide synthase (NOS) synthesizes NO through the oxidation of L-arginine to L-citrulline which is an important regulator of vasodilator tone and blood pressure [10,11]. One of the most clinically important polymorphisms of NOS3, the G894T polymorphism, results from G to T conversion at nucleotide 894 of exon 7 of gene that changes Glu298Asp (SNP rs1799983). The presence of this polymorphism reduces the NO production. There are several studies reporting controversial results related to the role of NOS3 variants on the susceptibility to CAD and T2DM [12-17].

Recently, we reported that the B1 allele of CETP increased the risk of CAD and T2DM 1.65- and 1.7-fold, respectively [18]. Also, we indicated that the risk of CAD was increased by 2.15-fold in the presence of T allele of NOS3 in our population [19]. To our knowledge, there is no report related to the influence of concomitant presence of CETP variants and NOS3 G894T polymorphism on the risk of CAD and T2DM in the literature.

The aim of the present study was to examine the interaction between CETP TaqIB and NOS3 G894T variants and its effect on the risk of CAD and T2DM in the population of Western Iran.

Materials and methods

The sample consisted of 308 patients and 92 controls. There were 207 total CAD patients including 113 males and 94 females with the mean age of 56.9 ± 8.6 years from whom there were 102 CAD patients with T2DM (CAD/T2DM) and 105 CAD patients without T2DM. There were 101 patients with T2DM including 51 males and 50 females with the mean age of 56.5 ± 9.8 years. The controls were 92 non-diabetic individuals that consisted of 47 males and 45 females with the mean age of 54.3 ± 8.5 years who were evaluated by angiography for suspected CAD but had normal coronary arteries. All patients and controls were recruited from Imam Ali Hospital of Kermanshah University of Medical Sciences and were from Western Iran with Kurdish ethnic background.

Patients were referred to the Cardiology Division of the Imam Ali Hospital of the Kermanshah University of Medical Sciences to undergo their first coronary angiography to evaluate the presence and extent of CAD. Coronary artery involvement was defined as a ≥50% diameter obstruction of a major coronary vessel. The diagnosis of diabetes in patients was confirmed using WHO criteria [20]. Written informed consent was obtained from each individual before participation in the study. The study was approved by the Ethics Committee of Kermanshah University of Medical Sciences and was in accordance with the principles of the Declaration of Helsinki (2000).

Genotype analysis

DNA was extracted from the leukocytes of the whole blood by the phenol-chloroform method as previously described in [21]. The NOS3 G894T polymorphism was detected by amplification of a region in exon 7 of the gene using the forward primer of 5′-AAG GCA GGA GAC AGT GGA TGG A-3′ and the reverse primer of 5′-CCC AGT CAA TCC CTT TGG TGC TCA-3′ and subsequent digestion with MboI restriction enzyme as previously described in [22].

For the detection of the CETP TaqIB genotypes, the following primers were used: 5′-CACTAGCCCAGAGA GAGGAGTGCC-3′ and 5′ CTGAGCCCAGCCGCACA CTAAC-3′ to amplify the 535-bp fragment in intron 1 of the CETP gene which was amplified by PCR, and the products were digested with TaqIB restriction endonuclease as previously described in [18].

Chemical analysis

Plasma total cholesterol (TC) and TG were measured by the standard enzymatic method (Pars Azmoon kit, Pars Azmoon Inc., Tehran, Iran), using an automated Technicon RA-1000 (Technicon Instruments Corporation, NY, USA). The plasma low-density lipoprotein-cholesterol (LDL-C) and HDL-C levels were measured using commercially available enzyme assay kits (Pars Azmoon kit, Iran).

Statistical analysis

The allelic frequencies were calculated by the chromosome counting method. The genotype and allele frequencies of CETP and NOS3 in CAD and T2DM patients were compared to controls, and the significance of differences calculated using χ^2 test. Odds ratios (OR) were calculated as estimates of relative risk for disease and 95% confidence intervals (CI) obtained by SPSS logistic regression software. A two-tailed Student's t test was used to compare quantitative data. Statistical significance was assumed at the $p < 0.05$ level. The SPSS statistical software package version 16 was used for the statistical analysis.

Results

The biochemical characteristics of patients and controls are presented in Table 1. The plasma level of LDL-C and TG was significantly higher, and HDL-C level was significantly lower in both CAD and T2DM patients compared to controls. In Table 2, the lipid profile of CAD/T2DM patients has been compared to CAD, T2DM, and controls. Significantly higher level of TG and lower level of HDL-C were observed in CAD/T2DM patients

Table 1 Demographic and biochemical parameters of the controls and patients

Parameters	CAD patients with and without diabetes ($n = 207$)	T2DM ($n = 101$)	Control subjects ($n = 92$)
Age (years)	56.9 ± 8.6*NS	56.5 ± 9.8	54.3 ± 8.5
Sex (M/F)	113/94*NS	51/50	47/45
FBS (mg/dl)	136.2 ± 59.6, $p < 0.001$	162.9 ± 71.3, $p < 0.001$	97.0 ± 20.1
History of hypertension (%)	102 (49.6), $p < 0.001$	29 (28.7), $p = 0.68$	24 (26.1)
LDL-C (mg/dl)	96 ± 28, $p < 0.001$	98.5 ± 38.4, $p < 0.001$	83 ± 18
HDL-C(mg/dl)	47 ± 9.3, $p = 0.007$	45.2 ± 10.2, $p < 0.001$	49.8 ± 5.8
TC (mg/dl)	186 ± 42, $p = 0.046$	185.9 ± 45.8, $p = 0.09$	177 ± 26
TG (mg/dl)	177 ± 89, $p = 0.038$	200.8 ± 99.3, $p = 0.001$	156 ± 48
BMI (kg/m^2)	26 ± 2.7*NS	26.2 ± 2.7*NS	26.6 ± 3.7

Plasma fasting blood sugar (FBS), LDL-C, HDL-C, TC, and TG levels, as well as age and BMI were compared between patients and controls using two-tailed Student's *t* test. The sex was compared between two groups by the χ^2-test. NS, not significant; *$p > 0.05$.

compared to those in CAD patients and controls. Although the level of LDL-C was higher in CAD/T2DM patients compared to those in CAD and control groups, the differences reached statistically significant values only with controls. Plasma total cholesterol was insignificantly increased in CAD/T2DM group compared to those in all studied groups. The same results were obtained when the levels of TG, HDL-C, and LDL-C were compared between T2DM patients with CAD and controls. In CAD patients, the level of LDL-C was significantly increased when compared to that in controls (Table 2). The plasma lipid and lipoprotein profiles categorized based on gender in each group are shown in Table 2. Comparison of genders in each group for lipid and lipoprotein levels indicated that women with T2DM had significantly higher plasma total cholesterol than males with T2DM (Table 2). Table 3 indicates the synergistic effect of both CETP B1 and NOS3 T alleles on the risk of CAD and T2DM. The concomitant presence of both alleles increased the risk of CAD significantly by 27.1-, 18.1-, and 13.5-fold in CAD patients without T2DM, total CAD, and CAD patients with T2DM, respectively. Also, the presence of both alleles (B1 and T) increased the risk of T2DM by 12-fold ($p = 0.004$) (Table 3). However, as demonstrated in Table 3, the presence of NOS3 T allele alone did not increase the risk of CAD or T2DM. Further, the presence of CETP B1 allele was significantly ($p = 0.019$) associated with 5.1-fold increased risk of CAD in total CAD patients.

Discussion

Diabetes mellitus is a strong risk factor for the development of atherosclerosis [6] that is related to dyslipidemia linked to insulin resistance characterized by a high triglyceride level, a high LDL-C, and a low HDL-C level [23]. In fact, decreased concentrations of HDL-C have been reported to be significantly related to CAD in patients with type 2 diabetes mellitus [7]. The significant

Table 2 Comparison of plasma lipid and lipoprotein levels in patients and controls

Patients (*n*)	TG (mg/dl)	TC (mg/dl)	LDL-C (mg/dl)	HDL-C (mg/dl)
CAD with T2DM	202.2 ± 87.9*	207.6 ± 185.4	97.8 ± 30.8**	44.7 ± 10.5*
Males (52)	206.4 ± 85.9	225.8 ± 253.6	98.6 ± 25.9	43.8 ± 8.2
Females (50)	197.8 ± 90.6	188.6 ± 56.2	96.8 ± 35.3	45.6 ± 12.5
CAD without T2DM	151.8 ± 83.2***	182.8 ± 36.1	94.1 ± 25.9**	49.2 ± 7.5***
Males (61)	150.3 ± 93.3	184.2 ± 37.7	97.2 ± 27.6	48.2 ± 8.2
Females (44)	153.9 ± 67.5	180.8 ± 34.1	89.8 ± 23.1	50.4 ± 6.1
T2DM	200.8 ± 99.3*	185.9 ± 45.8	98.5 ± 38.4**	45.2 ± 10.2*
Males (51)	198.4 ± 110.6	175.9 ± 41.2****	90.9 ± 31.3*	42.5 ± 9.7*
Females (50)	203.2 ± 87.1	196.2 ± 48.3	106.2 ± 43.3	47.9 ± 10.1
Controls	161.5 ± 64.5	176.8 ± 25.8	82.8 ± 17.8	49.8 ± 5.8
Males (47)	161.1 ± 53.5	179.7 ± 27.2	85.3 ± 17.4	48.4 ± 5*
Females (45)	161.8 ± 74.8	173.7 ± 24.2	80 ± 17.9	51.3 ± 6.1

*$p < 0.05$ compared to CAD without T2DM and controls; **$p < 0.05$ compared to controls; ***$p < 0.05$ compared to CAD with T2DM and T2DM; ****$p < 0.05$ compared between males and females in each group.

Table 3 The carrier odds ratio interaction between CETP B1 and NOS3 894 T alleles

CETP B1	NOS3 T	Total CAD patients *n* (%) ORs (95% CI) *n* = 207	CAD with T2DM *n* (%) ORs (95% CI) *n* = 102	CAD without T2DM *n* (%) ORs (95% CI) *n* = 105	T2DM patients *n* (%) ORs (95% CI) *n* = 101	Controls *n* (%) *n* = 92
–	–	3 (1.4)	2 (2)	1 (1)	2 (2)	8 (8.7)
–	+	3 (1.4)	3 (2.9)	0	2 (2)	12 (13)
		0.67 (0.11–4.17, $p = 0.67$)	1 (0.14–7.4, $p = 1$)		0.67 (0.1–5.7, $p = 0.71$)	
+	–	113 (54.6)	53 (52)	60 (57.1)	58 (57.4)	59 (64.2)
		5.1 (1.3–20, $p = 0.019$)	3.6 (0.73–17.7, $p = 0.11$)	8.14 (1–67, $p = 0.05$)	3.9 (0.8–19.3, $p = 0.09$)	
+	+	88 (42.6)	44 (43.1)	44 (41.9)	39 (38.6)	13 (14.1)
		18.1 (4.2–76.8, $p < 0.001$)	13.5 (2.6–71.8, $p = 0.002$)	27.1 (3.1–237, $p = 0.003$)	12 (2.25–63.8, $p = 0.004$)	

Interaction with respect to B2 or G alleles in CAD and T2DM patients compared with controls. Overall distribution of interaction between CETP B1 and NOS3 T alleles in total CAD compared to controls ($\chi^2 = 42.4$, df = 3, $p < 0.001$) and between CAD with T2DM compared to controls ($\chi^2 = 25.7$, df = 3, $p < 0.001$), as well as comparison between CAD without T2DM and controls ($\chi^2 = 33.6$, df = 3, $p < 0.001$). Overall distribution of interaction between CETP B1 and NOS3 T alleles in T2DM patients compared to controls ($\chi^2 = 23.4$, df = 3, $p < 0.001$).

higher level of TG and lower level of HDL-C observed in CAD patients with T2DM compared to those in CAD patients without diabetes in the present study confirm the role of dyslipidemia for predicting the risk of CAD in T2DM patients.

Both genetics and environmental factors have important roles in the pathogenesis of CAD and T2DM [24]. The role of genetic factors appears to be considerably different between various populations [25].

The most commonly studied polymorphism of CETP is TaqIB with a frequency of 0.44 in Caucasian populations and is associated with decreased CETP mass, an increase in HDL-cholesterol, and modulating the risk for diabetic complications in patients with T2DM. The presence of homozygous B1 allele is associated with lowest while in B2B2 carriers there is highest HDL-cholesterol concentration [5,26]. The role of CETP TaqIB polymorphism on the risk of CAD and T2DM either through its influence on lipid metabolism or independent of its effect on lipid profile has been reported in various populations [1,6-9]. Previously, we reported an association between the B1 allele of CETP and the risk of CAD and T2DM independent of HDL-C level [18]. Endothelial NOS gene through coding endothelial NOS enzyme has a role in maintaining normal endothelial function. Endothelial NOS through synthesis of NO affects the relaxation of vascular smooth muscle, inhibition of adhesion of platelets and leukocytes to the endothelium, reduction of vascular smooth muscle cell migration and proliferation, and limitation of the oxidation of LDL-C [27,28]. There are several reports indicating an association between the NOS3 G894T polymorphism and the risk of CAD [13,14]. However, some studies demonstrated the lack of association between this polymorphism and the risk of CAD [15,17,29]. Our recent work indicated that the risk of CAD is elevated in the presence of NOS3 T allele [19]. In the present work, we examined the influence of concomitant presence of NOS3 T and CETP B1 alleles on the risk of CAD and T2DM. We noticed that the risk of CAD augments in the presence of both alleles in total CAD and in CAD patients with and without T2DM to the level of 18.1-, 13.5-, and 27.1-fold, respectively. Also, the combined presence of both alleles increased the risk of T2DM by 12-fold. Our study demonstrated that the presence of variations in more than one gene play an important role in the susceptibility to CAD and T2DM.

The presence of hypercholesterolemia and oxidized LDL-C downregulates NOS expression and rapid degradation of NO. The exact mechanism of influence of CETP variants and its interaction with NOS3 G894T polymorphism on the risk of CAD and T2DM is unclear. However, it has been suggested that contribution of CETP to the formation of small dense LDL-C particles and impairment of NO synthesis in the presence of NOS3 G894T variants that are enhanced in hypercholesterolemia might lead to endothelial dysfunction and atherosclerosis [30].

Briefly, our study indicated that the B1 allele of CETP TaqIB polymorphism in combination with NOS3 T allele augments the risk of CAD and T2DM in our population. The results of the present study emphasize the role of gene-gene interaction in the pathogenesis of complex disorders such as CAD and T2DM that need to be confirmed in further studies from other populations.

Competing interests

The authors declare that they have no competing interests.

Authors' contributions

ZoR designed and supervised the research, analyzed and interpreted the data, and drafted the manuscript. RNR and ZiR carried out the molecular genetic studies. AP revised the manuscript. All authors read and approved the final manuscript.

Acknowledgments

This work was performed in partial fulfillment of the Master of Science requirements of RNR in Kermanshah University of Medical Sciences and was financially supported by a grant from Kermanshah University of Medical Sciences office of Vice Chancellor for Research, Kermanshah, Iran. We would like to thank Dr. Mansour Rezaei for his statistical comments.

Author details
[1]Medical Biology Research Center, Medical School, Kermanshah University of Medical Sciences, Daneshgah Avenue, P.O. Box 67148-69914, Kermanshah, Iran. [2]Department of Biochemistry, Medical School, Kermanshah University of Medical Sciences, Daneshgah Avenue, P.O. Box 67148-69914, Kermanshah, Iran. [3]Department of Biochemistry, Medical School, Dezful University of Medical Sciences, Azadegan Avenue, P.O. Box 6461653476, Dezful, Iran. [4]Division of Neuroscience & Behavior, NIAAA, National Institutes of Health, Rockville, Maryland 20852, USA.

References

1. Boekholdt SM, Sacks FM, Jukema JW, Shepherd J, Freeman DJ, McMahon AD, Cambien F, Nicaud V, de Grooth GJ, Talmud PJ, Humphries SE, Miller GJ, Eiriksdottir G, Gudnason V, Kauma H, Kakko S, Savolainen MJ, Arca M, Montali A, Liu S, Lanz HJ, Zwinderman AH, Kuivenhoven JA, Kastelein JJ: **Cholesteryl ester transfer protein TaqIB variant, high-density lipoprotein cholesterol levels, cardiovascular risk, and efficacy of pravastatin treatment individual patient meta-analysis of 13677 subjects.** *Circulation* 2005, **111**:278–287.
2. de Grooth GJ, Klerkx AHEM, Stroes ESG, Stalenhoef AF, Kastelein JJ, Kuivenhoven JA: **A review of CETP and its relation to atherosclerosis.** *J lipid Res* 2004, **45**:1967–1974.
3. Padmaja N, Kumar RM, Balachander J, Adithan C: **Cholesteryl ester transfer protein TaqIB, −629C → A and I405V polymorphisms and risk of coronary heart disease in an Indian population.** *Clin Chim Acta* 2009, **402**:139–145.
4. Kashani Farid MA, Azizi F, Hedayati M, Daneshpour MS, Shamshiri AR, Siassi F: **Association between CETP Taq1B and LIPC -514C/T polymorphisms with the serum lipid levels in a group of Tehran's population: a cross sectional study.** *Lipids in Health and Disease* 2010, **9**:96.
5. Dixit M, Bhattacharya S, Mittal B: **Association of CETP TaqI and APOE polymorphisms with type II diabetes mellitus in North Indians: a case control study.** *BMC Endocrine Disorders* 2005, **5**:7.
6. Chaaba R, Hammami S, Attia N, Smaoui M, Masmoudi AS, Mahjoub S, Ben Hamda K, Hammami M: **Association of plasma cholesteryl ester transfer protein activity and polymorphism with coronary artery disease extent in Tunisian type II diabetic patients.** *Clin Biochem* 2005, **38**:373–378.
7. Hsieh MC, Tien KJ, Chang SJ, Lo CS, Hsin SC, Hsiao JY, Hsu SC, Liang HT, Chen HC, Shin SJ, Lin SR: **Cholesteryl ester transfer protein B1B1 genotype as a predictor of coronary artery disease in Taiwanese with type 2 diabetes mellitus.** *Metabolism* 2007, **56**:745–750.
8. Relvas WG, Izar MC, Helfenstein T, Fonseca MI, Colovati M, Oliveira A, Ihara SS, Han SW, Jr Las Casas AA, Fonseca FA: **Relationship between gene polymorphisms and prevalence of myocardial infarction among diabetic and non-diabetic subjects.** *Atherosclerosis* 2005, **178**:101–105.
9. Kawasaki I, Tahara H, Emoto M, Shoji T, Nishizawa Y: **Relationship between TaqIB cholesteryl ester transfer protein gene polymorphism and macrovascular complications in Japanese patients with type 2 diabetes.** *Diabetes* 2002, **51**:871–874.
10. Zintzaras E, Papathanasiou AA, Stefanidis I: **Endothelial nitric oxide synthase gene polymorphisms and diabetic nephropathy: A HuGE review and meta-analysis.** *Genet Med* 2009, **11**:695–706.
11. Miyamoto Y, Saito Y, Kajiyama N, Yoshimura M, Shimasaki Y, Nakayama M, Kamitani S, Harada M, Ishikawa M, Kuwahara K, Ogawa E, Hamanaka I, Takahashi N, Kaneshige T, Teraoka H, Akamizu T, Azuma N, Yoshimasa Y, Yoshimasa T, Itoh H, Masuda I, Yasue H, Nakao K: **Endothelial nitric oxide synthase gene is positively associated with essential hypertension.** *Hypertension* 1998, **32**:3–8.
12. Tamemoto H, Ishikawa S, Kawakami M: **Association of the Glu298Asp polymorphism of the eNOS gene with ischemic heart disease in Japanese diabetic subjects.** *Diabetes Res Clin Pract* 2008, **80**:275–279.
13. Kerkeni M, Addad F, Chauffert M, Myara A, Ben Farhat M, Miled A, Maaroufi K, Trivin F: **Hyperhomocysteinemia, endothelial nitric oxide synthase polymorphism, and risk of coronary artery disease.** *Clin Chem* 2006, **52**:53–58.
14. Motawi T, Shaker O, Taha M, Sedrak H, Nabil M: **Endothelial nitric oxide synthase and angiotensinogen gene polymorphism in coronary artery diseases in Egypt.** *Angiology* 2011, **62**:191–197.
15. Liyou N, Simons L, Friedlander Y, Simons J, McCallum J, O'Shaughnessy K, Davis D, Johnson A: **Coronary artery disease is not associated with the E298D variant of the constitutive, endothelial nitric oxide synthase gene.** *Clin Genet* 1998, **54**:528–529.
16. Jaramillo PC, Lanas C, Lanas F, Salazar LA: **Polymorphisms of the NOS3 gene in Southern Chilean subjects with coronary artery disease and controls.** *Clin Chim Acta* 2010, **411**:258–262.
17. Andrikopoulos GK, Grammatopoulos DK, Tzeis SE, Zervou SI, Richter DJ, Zairis MN, Gialafos EJ, Sakellariou DC, Foussas SG, Manolis AS, Stefanadis CI, Toutouzas PK, Hillhouse EW, GEMIG study investigators: **Association of the 894 G → T polymorphism in the endothelial nitric oxide synthase gene with risk of acute myocardial infarction.** *BMC Med Genet* 2008, **9**:43.
18. Rahimi Z, Nourozi-Rad R, Vaisi-Raygani A, Saidi MR, Rahimi Z, Ahmadi R, Yarani R, Hamzehee K, Parsian A: **Association between cholesteryl ester transfer protein TaqIB variants and risk of coronary artery disease and diabetes mellitus in the population of Western Iran.** *Genet Test Mol Biomarkers* 2012, **15**:813–819.
19. Rahimi Z, Nourozi-Rad A: **Association of endothelial nitric oxide synthase gene variant (G894T) with coronary artery disease in Western Iran.** *Angiology* 2012, **63**:131–137.
20. World Health Organization: **Part 1. Diagnosis and classification of diabetes mellitus.** In *Definition, Diagnosis and Classification of Diabetes Mellitus.* Geneva: WHO; 1999:1–59.
21. Rahimi Z, Ghaderi M, Nagel RL, Muniz A: **Prevalence of thrombotic risk factors among β-thalassemia patients from Western Iran.** *J Thromb Thrombolysis* 2008, **26**:229–233.
22. Jafari Y, Rahimi Z, Vaisi-Raygani A, Rezaei M: **Interaction of eNOS polymorphism with MTHFR variants increase the risk of diabetic nephropathy and its progression in type 2 diabetes mellitus patients.** *Mol Cell Biochem* 2011, **353**:23–34.
23. Meguro S, Takei I, Murata M, Hirose H, Takei N, Mitsuyoshi Y, Ishii K, Oguchi S, Shinohara J, Takeshita E, Watanabe K, Saruta T: **Cholesteryl ester transfer protein polymorphism associated with macroangiopathy in Japanese patients with type 2 diabetes.** *Atherosclerosis* 2001, **156**:151–156.
24. Felehgari V, Rahimi Z, Mozafari H, Vaisi-Raygani A: **ACE gene polymorphism and serum ACE activity in Iranians type II diabetic patients with macroalbuminuria.** *Mol Cell Biochem* 2011, **346**:23–30.
25. Liu SM, Zhou X, Zheng F, Li X, Liu F, Zhang HM, Xie Y: **Novel mutations found in mitochondrial diabetes in Chinese Han population.** *Diabetes Res & Clin Practice* 2007, **76**:425–435.
26. Heilbronn LK, Noakes M, Clifton PM: **Association between HDL-cholesterol and the Taq1B polymorphism in the cholesterol ester transfer protein gene in obese women.** *Atherosclerosis* 2002, **162**:419–424.
27. Bellini MH, Figueira MN, Piccoli MF, Marumo JT, Cendoroglo MS, Neto MC, Dalboni MA, Batista MC, Goes MA, Schor N: **Association of endothelial nitric oxide synthase gene intron 4 polymorphism with end-stage renal disease.** *Nephrology* 2007, **12**:289–293.
28. Möllsten A, Lajer M, Jorsal A, Tarnow L: **The endothelial nitric oxide synthase gene and risk of diabetic nephropathy and development of cardiovascular disease in type 1 diabetes.** *Molecular Genetics and Metabolism* 2009, **97**:80–84.
29. Ragia G, Nikkolaidis E, Tavridou A, Arvanitidis KI, Kanoni S, Dedoussis GV, Bougioukas G, Manolopoulos VG: **Endothelial nitric oxide synthase gene polymorphisms −786 T → C and 894 G → T in coronary artery bypass graft surgery patients.** *Hum Genomics* 2010, **4**:375–383.
30. Goff WL, Guerin M, Chapman MJ: **Pharmacological modulation of cholesteryl ester transfer protein, a new therapeutic target in atherogenic dyslipidemia.** *Pharmacology & Therapeutics* 2004, **101**:17–38.

Permissions

All chapters in this book were first published in JNI, by BioMed Central; hereby published with permission under the Creative Commons Attribution License or equivalent. Every chapter published in this book has been scrutinized by our experts. Their significance has been extensively debated. The topics covered herein carry significant findings which will fuel the growth of the discipline. They may even be implemented as practical applications or may be referred to as a beginning point for another development.

The contributors of this book come from diverse backgrounds, making this book a truly international effort. This book will bring forth new frontiers with its revolutionizing research information and detailed analysis of the nascent developments around the world.

We would like to thank all the contributing authors for lending their expertise to make the book truly unique. They have played a crucial role in the development of this book. Without their invaluable contributions this book wouldn't have been possible. They have made vital efforts to compile up to date information on the varied aspects of this subject to make this book a valuable addition to the collection of many professionals and students.

This book was conceptualized with the vision of imparting up-to-date information and advanced data in this field. To ensure the same, a matchless editorial board was set up. Every individual on the board went through rigorous rounds of assessment to prove their worth. After which they invested a large part of their time researching and compiling the most relevant data for our readers.

The editorial board has been involved in producing this book since its inception. They have spent rigorous hours researching and exploring the diverse topics which have resulted in the successful publishing of this book. They have passed on their knowledge of decades through this book. To expedite this challenging task, the publisher supported the team at every step. A small team of assistant editors was also appointed to further simplify the editing procedure and attain best results for the readers.

Apart from the editorial board, the designing team has also invested a significant amount of their time in understanding the subject and creating the most relevant covers. They scrutinized every image to scout for the most suitable representation of the subject and create an appropriate cover for the book.

The publishing team has been an ardent support to the editorial, designing and production team. Their endless efforts to recruit the best for this project, has resulted in the accomplishment of this book. They are a veteran in the field of academics and their pool of knowledge is as vast as their experience in printing. Their expertise and guidance has proved useful at every step. Their uncompromising quality standards have made this book an exceptional effort. Their encouragement from time to time has been an inspiration for everyone.

The publisher and the editorial board hope that this book will prove to be a valuable piece of knowledge for researchers, students, practitioners and scholars across the globe.

List of Contributors

Ryan L Parr and Luis H Martin
Mitomics Inc, Thunder Bay, Ontario P7A 7T1, Canada

Madhuchhanda Bhattacharjee
School of Mathematics and Statistics, University of Hyderabad, Hyderabad 500046, India

Mangalathu S. Rajeevan
Division of High-Consequence Pathogens & Pathology, Centers for Disease Control and Prevention, Atlanta 30333, USA

Mikko J. Sillanpää
Departments of Mathematical Sciences, Biocenter Oulu, University of Oulu, Oulu FIN-90014, Finland

Konstantinos Mitropoulos
The Golden Helix Foundation, London, UK

Angela Brand
University of Maastricht, Maastricht, The Netherlands

Bassam R. Ali
Department of Pathology, College of Medicine and Health Sciences, United Arab Emirates University, Al-Ain, United Arab Emirates

Hayat Al Jaibeji
University of Maastricht, Maastricht, The Netherlands
Department of Pathology, College of Medicine and Health Sciences, United Arab Emirates University, Al-Ain, United Arab Emirates

Diego A. Forero
Laboratory of NeuroPsychiatric Genetics, Biomedical Sciences Research Group, School of Medicine, Universidad Antonio Nariño, Bogotá, Colombia

Paul Laissue
Unidad de Genética, Grupo GENIUROS, Escuela de Medicina y Ciencias de la Salud, Universidad del Rosario, Bogotá, Colombia

Ambroise Wonkam
Division of Human Genetics, Faculty of Health Sciences, University of Cape Town, Cape Town, South Africa

Catalina Lopez-Correa
Genome Quebec, Montreal, Canada

Zahurin Mohamed
Department of Pharmacology, Faculty of Medicine, University of Malaya, Kuala Lumpur, Malaysia

Wasun Chantratita
Department of Pathology, Medical Genomic Center, Ramathibodi Hospital, Faculty of Medicine, Mahidol University, Bangkok, Thailand

Ming Ta Michael Lee
Laboratory for International Alliance on Genomic Research, RIKEN Center for Integrative Medical Sciences, Yokohama, Japan
Institute of Biomedical Sciences, Academia Sinica, Taipei, Taiwan

Adrian Llerena
CICAB Clinical Research Center, Extremadura University Hospital and Medical School, Badajoz, Spain

George P. Patrinos
Department of Pharmacy, University of Patras School of Health Sciences, Patras, Greece

Andrew Mallett
Kidney Health Service & Conjoint Kidney Research Laboratory, Royal Brisbane and Women's Hospital, Butterfield Street, Herston, Brisbane, Qld 4029, Australia
Centre for Kidney Disease Research, CKD.QLD and Centre for Chronic Disease, School of Medicine, The University of Queensland, Brisbane, Australia
Centre for Rare Diseases Research, Institute for Molecular Bioscience, The University of Queensland, Brisbane, Australia

Christopher Corney and Helen Healy
Kidney Health Service & Conjoint Kidney Research Laboratory, Royal Brisbane and Women's Hospital, Butterfield Street, Herston, Brisbane, Qld 4029, Australia
Centre for Kidney Disease Research, CKD.QLD and Centre for Chronic Disease, School of Medicine, The University of Queensland, Brisbane, Australia

Hugh McCarthy
Department of Paediatric Nephrology, Children's Hospital at Westmead, Sydney, Australia
Centre for Kidney Research, University of Sydney, Sydney, Australia

Stephen I. Alexander
Department of Paediatric Nephrology, Children's Hospital at Westmead, Sydney, Australia
Centre for Kidney Research, University of Sydney, Sydney, Australia
Discipline of Paediatrics and Child Health, University of Sydney, Sydney, Australia

Hongbin Dong and Vasilis Vasiliou
Department of Environmental Health Sciences, Yale School of Public Health, 60 College St, New Haven, CT 06250, USA

Daniel W. Nebert
Department of Environmental Health and Center for Environmental Genetics, University Cincinnati Medical Center, Cincinnati, OH 45267-0056, USA

Elspeth A. Bruford
HUGO Gene Nomenclature Committee (HGNC), European Bioinformatics Institute (EMBL-EBI), European Molecular Biology Laboratory, Hinxton CB10 1SD, UK

David C. Thompson
Department of Clinical Practice, University of Colorado Denver, Aurora, CO 80045, USA

Hans Joenje
Department of Clinical Genetics and the Cancer Center Amsterdam/VUmc Institute for Cancer and Immunology, VU University Medical Center, NL-1081 BT Amsterdam, The Netherlands

Xiaomin Chen
Cardiovascular Center of Ningbo First Hospital, Ningbo University, Ningbo, Zhejiang 315010, China

William Yang
Texas Advanced Computing Center, University of Texas at Austin, 10100 Burnet Road (R8700), Austin, TX 78758-4497, USA

Xiaoying Chen, Yan Xu, Nan Wu, Huadan Ye, Qingxiao Hong and Shiwei Duan
School of Medicine, Ningbo University, Ningbo, Zhejiang 315211, China

Yanfei Xin
Center of Safety Evaluation, Zhejiang Academy of Medical Sciences, Hangzhou, Zhejiang 310007, China

Mary Qu Yang and Jack Y. Yang
MidSouth Bioinformatics Center, Department of Information Science, George Washington Donaghey College of Engineering and Information Science, and Joint Bioinformatics Graduate Program, University of Arkansas at Little Rock and University of Arkansas for Medical Sciences, 2881 S. University Ave, Little Rock, AR 72204, USA

Youping Deng
Medical College, Wuhan University of Science and Technology, Wuhan 430064, China
Department of Internal Medicine and Biochemistry, Rush University Medical Center, Chicago, IL 60612, USA

Perciliz L. Tan and Nicholas Katsanis
Center for Human Disease Modeling, Duke University Medical Center, Durham, NC 27710, USA
Department of Cell Biology, Duke University Medical Center, Durham, NC 27710, USA

Catherine Bowes Rickman
Department of Cell Biology, Duke University Medical Center, Durham, NC 27710, USA
Department of Ophthalmology, Duke Eye Center, Duke University, Durham, NC 27710, USA

Binh Ho Duy
Hue University of Medicine and Pharmacy, Hue University, 06 Ngo Quyen, Hue city 530000, Vietnam
Department of Traumatology and Orthopaedics, University of Tartu, Puusepa 8, 51014 Tartu, Estonia
Clinic of Traumatology and Orthopaedics, Tartu University Hospital, Puusepa 8, 51014 Tartu, Estonia

Lidiia Zhytnik
Department of Traumatology and Orthopaedics, University of Tartu, Puusepa 8, 51014 Tartu, Estonia

Katre Maasalu and Aare Märtson
Department of Traumatology and Orthopaedics, University of Tartu, Puusepa 8, 51014 Tartu, Estonia
Clinic of Traumatology and Orthopaedics, Tartu University Hospital, Puusepa 8, 51014 Tartu, Estonia

Sulev Kõks
Centre of Translational Medicine, University of Tartu, Ravila 14a, Tartu 50411, Estonia
Department of Pathophysiology, University of Tartu, Ravila 19, Tartu 50411, Estonia

Ivo Kändla, Ele Prans and Ene Reimann
Department of Pathophysiology, University of Tartu, Ravila 19, Tartu 50411, Estonia

Ana R. Cardoso, Manuela Oliveira, Antonio Amorim and Luisa Azevedo
Instituto de Investigação e Inovação em Saúde, Universidade do Porto, Rua Alfredo Allen 208, 4200-135 Porto, Portugal
IPATIMUP-Institute of Molecular Pathology and Immunology, University of Porto, Rua Júlio Amaral de Carvalho 45, 4200-135 Porto, Portugal
Department of Biology, Faculty of Sciences, University of Porto, Rua do Campo Alegre S/N, 4169-007 Porto, Portugal

Angeliki Balasopoulou, Angeliki Panagiotara, Effrosyni Mendrinou, Apostolos Stratopoulos, Aigli Ioanna Legaki, Vasiliki Stathakopoulou, Aristoniki Tsolia, Nikolaos Govaris, Sofia Govari, Zoi Zagoriti, Konstantinos Poulas and Theodora Katsila
Department of Pharmacy, School of Health Sciences, University of Patras, University Campus, Rion, 265 04 Patras, Greece

Biljana Stanković, Gordana Nikčevic, Sonja Pavlovic and Branka Zukic
Institute of Molecular Genetics and Genetic Engineering, University of Belgrade, Belgrade, Serbia

Brock A. Peters and Radoje Drmanac
Complete Genomics Inc., Mountain View, CA, USA
BGI Shenzhen, Shenzhen 51803, People's Republic of China

George P. Patrinos
Department of Pharmacy, School of Health Sciences, University of Patras, University Campus, Rion, 265 04 Patras, Greece
Department of Pathology, College of Medicine and Health Sciences, United Arab Emirates University, Al Ain, United Arab Emirates

Anne John and Bassam R. Ali
Department of Pathology, College of Medicine and Health Sciences, United Arab Emirates University, Al Ain, United Arab Emirates

Maria Kanariou, Nikki Constantinidou and Kleopatra Spanou
Department of Immunology and Histocompatibility, "Aghia Sophia" Children's Hospital, Athens, Greece

Maro Krini, George Chrousos and Eleftheria Roma
First Department of Pediatrics, National and Kapodistrian University of Athens Medical School, Athens, Greece

Nedeljko Radlovic
Department of Gastroenterology and Nutrition, University Children's Hospital, Medical Faculty, University of Belgrade, Belgrade, Serbia

Joseph Borg
Department of Applied Biomedical Science, Faculty of Health Sciences, University of Malta, Msida, Malta

Ana Lígia Buzolin, Caroline Mônaco Moreira, Patricia Rossi Sacramento, Andre Yuji Oku, Alexandre Ricardo dos Santos Fornari, David Santos Marco Antonio, Caio Robledo D Angioli Costa Quaio, Wagner Rosa Baratela and Miguel Mitne-Neto
Research and Development, Fleury Group, Av. General Valdomiro de Lima, 508, São Paulo/SP 04344-070, Brazil

Simranjeet Kaur
CPH-DIRECT, Department of Pediatrics, Herlev University Hospital, Herlev Ringvej 75, DK-2730 Herlev, Denmark

Aashiq H. Mirza and Flemming Pociot
CPH-DIRECT, Department of Pediatrics, Herlev University Hospital, Herlev Ringvej 75, DK-2730 Herlev, Denmark
Faculty of Health and Medical Sciences, University of Copenhagen, Copenhagen, Denmark
Center for non-coding RNA in Technology and Health, University of Copenhagen, Copenhagen, Denmark

Maynard V. Olson
Department of Medicine, University of Washington, Seattle, Washington 98195, USA
Department of Genome Sciences, University of Washington, Seattle, Washington 98195, USA

Jyothi Thrivikraman
POLARIS, Genome Institute of Singapore, Agency for Science, Technology and Research, Singapore, Singapore

Yasmin Bylstra
POLARIS, Genome Institute of Singapore, Agency for Science, Technology and Research, Singapore, Singapore
SingHealth Duke-NUS Institute of Precision Medicine, Singapore, Singapore
Inherited Cardiac Clinic, National University Hospital, Singapore, Singapore

Patrick Tan
SingHealth Duke-NUS Institute of Precision Medicine, Singapore, Singapore
Cancer and Stem Biology, Duke-NUS Medical School, Singapore, Singapore
Biomedical Research Council, Agency for Science, Technology and Research, Singapore, Singapore

Tamra Lysaght and Sangeetha Watson
Centre for Biomedical Ethics, Yong Loo Lin School of Medicine, National University of Singapore, Singapore, Singapore

Caroline H. Johnson and Vasilis Vasiliou
Department of Environmental Health Sciences, Yale School of Public Health, New Haven, CT, USA

Toby J. Athersuch
Department of Surgery and Cancer, Faculty of Medicine, Imperial College London, London, UK
MRC-PHE Centre for Environment and Health, School of Public Health, Imperial College Norfolk Place, London, UK

Gwen W. Collman
Division of Extramural Research and Training, National Institute of Environmental Health Sciences, National Institutes of Health, Morrisville, NC, USA

Suraj Dhungana
Waters Corporation, Metabolomics and Translational Research, Milford, MA, USA

David F. Grant
Department of Pharmaceutical Sciences, University of Connecticut, Storrs, CT, USA

Dean P. Jones
Department of Medicine, Emory University School of Medicine, Atlanta, GA, USA

Chirag J. Patel
Department of Biomedical Informatics, Harvard Medical School, Boston, MA, USA

Jarrett D. Morrow, Weiliang Qiu, Xiaobo Zhou and Kimberly Glass
Channing Division of Network Medicine, Brigham and Women's Hospital, 181 Longwood Avenue, Boston, MA 02115, USA

Michael H. Cho, Dawn L. DeMeo, Edwin K. Silverman and Craig P. Hersh
Channing Division of Network Medicine, Brigham and Women's Hospital, 181 Longwood Avenue, Boston, MA 02115, USA
Division of Pulmonary and Critical Care Medicine, Brigham and Women's Hospital, Boston, MA 02115, USA

Bartholome Celli and George R. Washko
Division of Pulmonary and Critical Care Medicine, Brigham and Women's Hospital, Boston, MA 02115, USA

John Platig and John Quackenbush
Department of Biostatistics and Computational Biology, Dana-Farber Cancer Institute, Boston, MA 02115, USA

Nathaniel Marchetti and Gerard J. Criner
Division of Pulmonary and Critical Care Medicine, Temple University, Philadelphia, PA 19140, USA

Raphael Bueno
Division of Thoracic Surgery, Brigham and Women's Hospital, Boston, MA 02115, USA

U. Plöckinger, A. Ziagaki and N. Tiling
Kompetenzzentrum Seltene Stoffwechselkrankheiten, Interdisziplinäres Stoffwechsel-Centrum: Endokrinologie, Diabetes und Stoffwechsel, Charité Universitätsmedizin Berlin, Augustenburger Platz 1, Campus Virchow-Klinikum, 13352 Berlin, Germany

V. Prasad
Department of Nuclear Medicine, Charité Universitätsmedizin Berlin, Berlin, Germany
Department of Nuclear Medicine Universitätsklinik Ulm, Ulm, Germany

A. Poellinger
Department of Diagnostic, Interventional and Pediatric Radiology, Inselspital Bern University Hospital, University of Bern, Bern, Switzerland

Fida K. Dankar
College of IT, UAEU, Al Ain, UAE

Andrey Ptitsyn
Gloucester Marine Genomics Institute, Gloucester, MA, USA

Samar K. Dankar
Faculty of Sciences, University of Balamand, Souk El Ghareb, Lebanon

Jusaku Minari
Uehiro Research Division for iPS Cell Ethics, Center for iPS Cell Research and Application (CiRA), Kyoto University, Kyoto, Japan

Kyle B. Brothers
Kosair Charities Pediatric Clinical Research Unit, University of Louisville School of Medicine, Louisville, KY, USA

Michael Morrison
Centre for Health, Law and Emerging Technologies (HeLEX), Nuffield Department of Population Health, University of Oxford, Ewert House, Ewert Place, Banbury Road, Oxford OX2 7DD, UK

Sankar Subramanian
GeneCology Research Centre, The University of the Sunshine Coast, 90 Sippy Downs Drive, Sippy Downs, Qld 4556, Australia

Isabelle Cusin, Daniel Teixeira, Monique Zahn-Zabal and Anne Gleizes
CALIPHO group, SIB Swiss Institute of Bioinformatics, 1211 Geneva 4, Switzerland

Valentine Rech de Laval, Amos Bairoch and Pascale Gaudet
CALIPHO group, SIB Swiss Institute of Bioinformatics, 1211 Geneva 4, Switzerland
Department of Human Protein Sciences, Faculty of Medicine, University of Geneva, Geneva, Switzerland

Valeria Viassolo
Oncogenetics and Cancer Prevention Unit, Division of Oncology, University Hospitals of Geneva, 1205 Geneva, Switzerland

Pierre O. Chappuis
Oncogenetics and Cancer Prevention Unit, Division of Oncology, University Hospitals of Geneva, 1205 Geneva, Switzerland
Division of Genetic Medicine, University Hospitals of Geneva, 1205 Geneva, Switzerland

Pierre Hutter
Sophia Genetics, Rue du Centre 172, 1025 Saint Sulpice, Switzerland

Paul G Germann
New Frontier Science, Takeda GmbH, Constance, 78462, Germany

Alexander Schuhmacher
University of Reutlingen, Reutlingen, 72760, Germany

Juan Harrison
New Frontier Science, Takeda Pharmaceuticals, Palo Alto, CA94301, USA

Ronald Law and Kevin Haug
New Frontier Science, Takeda Pharmaceuticals, Chicago, IL 60601, USA

Gordon Wong
New Frontier Science, Takeda Pharmaceuticals, Boston, MA 02467, USA

Isobel R Ferguson
Discipline of Nutrition, Faculty of Medical and Health Sciences, The University of Auckland Private Bag 92019, Auckland 1142, New Zealand

Gareth Marlow, Stephanie Ellett, Amalini C Jesuthasan, Dug Yeo Han and Lynnette R Ferguson
Discipline of Nutrition, Faculty of Medical and Health Sciences, The University of Auckland Auckland 1142, New Zealand
Nutrigenomics New Zealand, University of Auckland Auckland 1142, New Zealand

Alan G Fraser
Nutrigenomics New Zealand, University of Auckland, Auckland 1142, New Zealand
Department of Medicine, University of Auckland, Auckland 1142, New Zealand

Shuotun Zhu and Nishi Karunasinghe
Faculty of Medical and Health Sciences, The University of Auckland, 85 Park Road, Grafton, Auckland 1023, New Zealand

Andrew A Monte
University of Colorado Department of Emergency Medicine, Leprino Building, 7th Floor Campus 12401 E. 17th Avenue, Aurora, CO 80045, USA
Skaggs School of Pharmacy and Pharmaceutical Sciences, Aurora, CO 80045, USA
Rocky Mountain Poison & Drug Center, Denver, CO 80204, USA

David C Thompson and Vasilis Vasiliou
Skaggs School of Pharmacy and Pharmaceutical Sciences, Aurora, CO 80045, USA

Chad Brocker and Frank J Gonzalez
Laboratory of Metabolism, Center for Cancer Research, National Institute of Cancer, Bethesda, MD 20892, USA

Daniel W Nebert
Division of Human Genetics, Department of Pediatrics and Molecular Developmental Biology, University of Cincinnati Medical Center, Cincinnati, OH 45220, USA
Department of Environmental Health and Center for Environmental Genetics, University of Cincinnati Medical Center, Cincinnati, OH 45220, USA

Ziba Rahimi
Medical Biology Research Center, Medical School, Kermanshah University of Medical Sciences, Daneshgah Avenue, Kermanshah, Iran

Zohreh Rahimi
Medical Biology Research Center, Medical School, Kermanshah University of Medical Sciences, Daneshgah Avenue, Kermanshah, Iran
Department of Biochemistry, Medical School, Kermanshah University of Medical Sciences, Daneshgah Avenue, Kermanshah, Iran

Reza Nourozi-Rad
Department of Biochemistry, Medical School, Dezful University of Medical Sciences, Azadegan Avenue, Dezful, Iran

Abbas Parsian
Division of Neuroscience & Behavior, NIAAA, National Institutes of Health, Rockville, Maryland 20852, USA

Index

www.ingramcontent.com/pod-product-compliance
Lightning Source LLC
LaVergne TN
LVHW080703210926
848485LV00003B/410